Asian Septorhinoplasty

Eun-Sang Dhong • Min-Wha Na

Asian Septorhinoplasty

Conundrums and Solutions

Springer

Eun-Sang Dhong
Department of Plastic and Reconstructive Surgery
Guro Hospital, College of Medicine
Korea University
Seoul
Korea (Republic of)

Min-Wha Na
Yerom Plastic Surgery Clinic
Seoul
Korea (Republic of)

ISBN 978-981-16-0544-4 ISBN 978-981-16-0542-0 (eBook)
https://doi.org/10.1007/978-981-16-0542-0

This Springer imprint is published by the registered company Springer Nature Singapore Pte Ltd.
The registered company address is: 152 Beach Road, #21-01/04 Gateway East, Singapore 189721, Singapore

Preface

The snow leopard in the Himalayas of India has leather that can withstand −29 °C and it hunts by starving for more than a week within a hunting range of 200 km. Still, hunting blue sheep on a high cliff at an altitude of 4800 m would fail dozens of times. It looks dangerous, as if falling down a cliff, but it challenges again and hunts for life. Winter is harder. When the temperature drops and the ibex descend from the snow-covered peak to the valley, the snow leopard runs through the thick snow and throws itself off the cliff to hunt. Ibex is quick and challenging to hunt. It needs food to get through the winter. It eventually throws itself in the rugged terrain by throwing all the remaining force, biting the neck of a Tibetan blue sheep and rolling down the cliff 60 m dozens of times, and descending. It seems to be lost for a moment but eventually wakes up, and the snow leopard fills the stomach. However, success comes at a tremendous cost. It is badly injured. However, the wild thing will never be sorry for itself. Still, it gets up again and goes on the way it was going. It is a scene of emotion. Indomitable determination is the life itself to live. I remember this video of "Bear Grylls' hostile planet-mountains" on the plane going back from one conference.

"Asian rhinoplasty is challenging." Which is more demanding, tissue reduction or tissue recruitment? No matter how low the dorsum and flat the tip, I think the unoperated nose is the most comfortable. Comforts and beauty are different in the rhinoplasty. The beauty is the emotional-social prejudice to be determined by the public, but the rhinoplasty surgeons should determine the beautiful nose.

After becoming a plastic surgeon, I studied through journals and attended academic conferences to learn. Rhinoplasty needs a long learning curve. I was fortunate. I learned the sincerity for the patients from my father, Dr. Young-song Dhong, a general surgeon, and septoplasty from my brother, Dr. Hun-jong Dhong, an ENT professor.

I don't think I am doing the rhinoplasty perfectly. Perhaps, by the day my practice ends, I would provide the fellow surgeons a more comfortable way to achieve agreeable results. Rhinoplasty requires a lot of time investment to get the best results. It is a surgery that involves a lot of thought before surgery and during the surgery. The nose is the prettiest just after the flap closure. Moreover, Asian rhinoplasty surgeon's hard work to overcome the alloplastic-implant-sequelae and autograft-resorption deserves praise from other plastic surgeons. If I don't look back, I probably do not have time to organize myself.

Now, as I clear it up, I want to share my knowledge and experience to move forward.

Nobody can attend the conference for a year now, but I hope that it will end soon.

I wish all those who read this book a meaningful accomplishment.

Seoul, Korea Eun-Sang Dhong

Contents

The Longevity of Alloplastic Implants

1

Pearls

- Bone resorption under the alloplastic implant is determined by (1) the implant's hardness, (2) the retention period, (3) implant location, and (4) the tension of the soft tissue envelope.
- Not only the tissue defects caused by the removal of the capsule, but the concavity induced by bone resorption should be considered when determining the dorsal on laying volume of the secondary surgery.
- The rhinion weakened by bone resorption makes the spreader graft very difficult and requires a long length.
- Unstable rhinion can induce saddle nose deformity after septorhinoplasty using autologous grafts.
- When correcting the mild hump nose, it is better to carve the implant than the bony dorsum by cutting the implants under part rather than resecting the bony dorsum.
- Putting an implant after medial and lateral osteotomies causes instability, which can cause long-term implant deviation.
- Dorsal implanting is not recommended after osteotomy. However, if necessary, the modification of leaving a broad platform in the rhinion area should be considered.
- Minor differences between the bony axis and the septal axis may be emphasized when the dorsum is projected, so care should be taken when implanting.
- In the secondary operation to solve complications caused by an implant, autografts should resolve the dorsum.

1.1 Bony Resorption Under Alloplastic Implants

Apart from the primary and secondary operation, there is no substitute as convenient and easy as the alloplastic implant in Asian rhinoplasty. As a way to increase the bony dorsum and cartilaginous dorsum at once, the surgeon only needs to pay attention to the tip plasty. Many Asian rhinoplasty surgeons' presentations at conferences focus exclusively on tip surgery and tend to overlook dorsum. The bony dorsum is rigid and immobile, but the cartilaginous dorsum provides a large amount of mobility. The mechanical effect of the rigid alloplastic implant on the underlying tissue is very different at each location. There are a myriad of alloplastic implants, but clinically, for dorsal projection, it is limited to three materials: boat-shaped Silicone, Gore-tex, and Alloderm. There are so many other hybrid products that are too diverse, so the author will not discuss them in this chapter. In general, it is widely used in this order, and among them, the use of Silicone solves the low nasion, which is the most used in Korea.

Bone resorption under the silicone implant applied to chin augmentation or malar augmenta-

E.-S. Dhong, M.-W. Na, *Asian Septorhinoplasty*, https://doi.org/10.1007/978-981-16-0542-0_1

tion has been reported. Methyl methacrylate and silicone are known to cause thinning of the skin on the top with bone resorption on the bottom. The bone under the polyfluoroethylene may also be resorbed [1]. It should be noted that both silicone and Gore-Tex, which are most commonly used in Asian rhinoplasty, may result in resorption of the underlying bone.

- The factors determining bone resorption degree are implant hardness, retention period, and implant location. Here, the pressure of the soft tissue envelope and the external physical force of the facial mimetic muscle play an essential role.
- Implantation through subperiosteal dissection of the nasal bone may decrease the implant's mobility but also a factor that promotes bone resorption.
- Concavity induced by removing capsules around the implant and bone resorption causes a vast amount of dorsal skin depression in secondary rhinoplasty. When preparing the autograft, surgeons should prepare a larger dorsal onlaying graft volume than the actual implant volume (Fig. 1.1).

The extensive bony resorption of the most critical rhinion can be observed in a long-lasting implant (Fig. 1.2).

1.2 Silicone Implant over Osteotomized Nasal Bone

Dorsal to tip projection is sometimes required after humpectomy and correcting a deviated nose. The method of using implants after the humpectomy is not recommended. Also, there is no evidence that it is safe to insert an alloplastic implant in the dorsum after the left or right lateral osteotomy [2]. The alloplastic implant tends to tilt to one side when inserted on the nasal bone in the patient who underwent medial and lateral osteotomy. This phenomenon is found in almost all patients who visited my clinic for the reoperation.

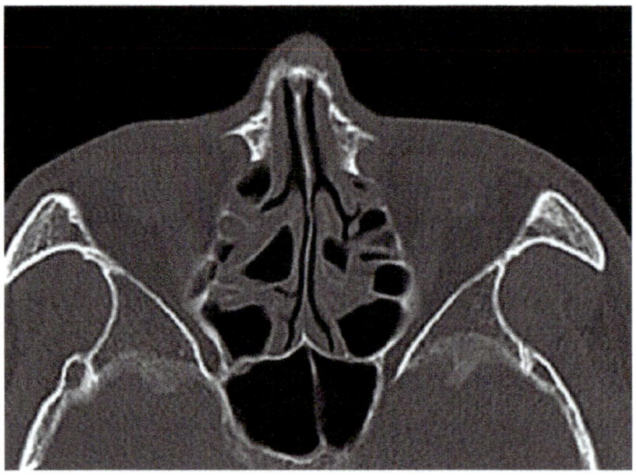

Fig. 1.2 Bone resorption under silicone implant: axial CT scan. Bone resorption with bone erosion

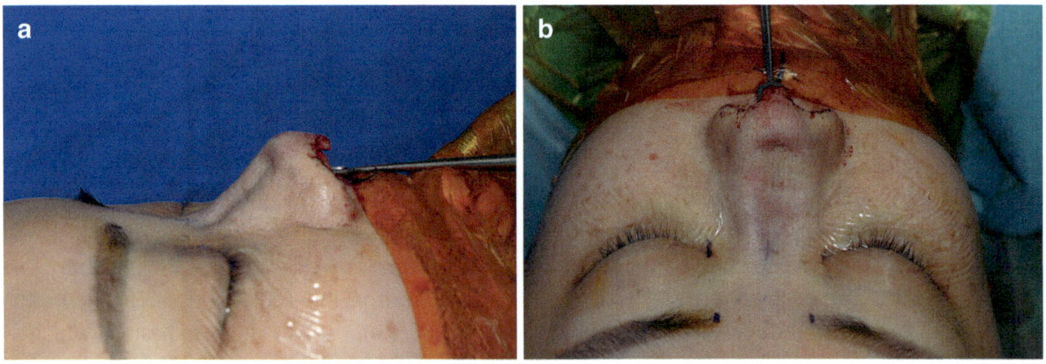

Fig. 1.1 Skin flap remaining after removing the silicone capsule. It created a massive concavity with bone resorption. (**a**) Lateral view, (**b**) frontal view

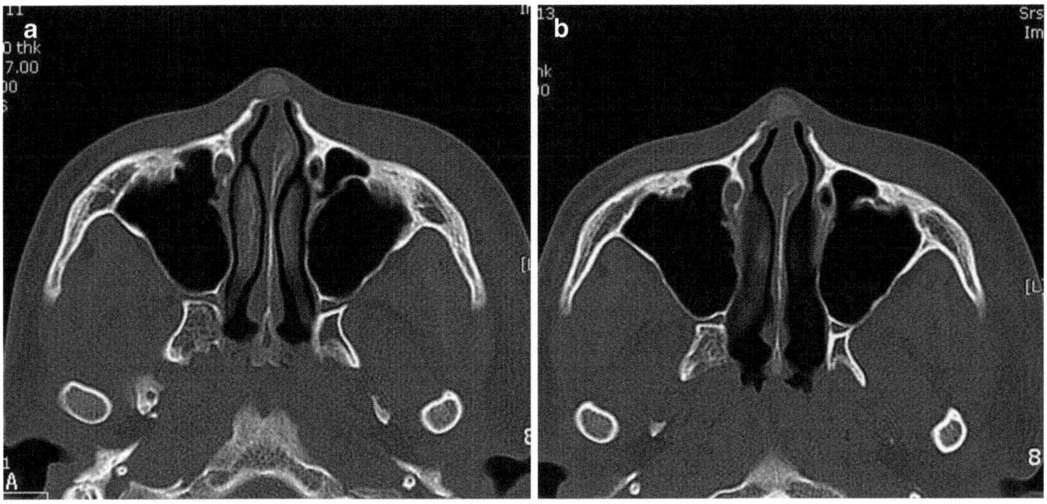

Fig. 1.3 Rhinion: destroyed by a silicone implant. (**a**) A rhinion destroyed by a 5 mm-thick silicone implant. (**b**) The base on the right side is pressing the nasal mucosa. This patient is presumed to be performed medial and lateral osteotomy

If you flatten the rhinion under the implant, as shown in the following picture, you can find that the rhinion is already weakened, and the bottom is severely destroyed. Also, the osteotomized lateral wall cannot be a safe platform for the dorsal implant (Fig. 1.3).

The weakened rhinion acts as an obstacle to reconstruction after implant removal.

However, in many Asian rhinoplasties, there is a tendency to correct the discrepancy by using an alloplastic implant after bony dorsum reduction. Even now, rather than excessive humpectomy, efforts should be made to fit the profile by carving the implant's undersurface.

The destruction of the rhinion makes the spreader graft very difficult. When applying the spreader graft, the length must be long enough; otherwise, anterior (high) septal instability may occur after surgery.

- When correcting the hump nose, the author focuses on the projection of the cartilaginous dorsum rather than reducing the hump excessively.
- Destruction of rhinion and nasal mucosa by the implant is believed to cause late-onset inflammation in the long term (Chap. 2).
- Unstable rhinion can induce saddle nose deformity after septorhinoplasty using autologous tissue. So the instability can later cause inverted V deformity.
- Do not use dorsal implants to cover any open roof deformity after humpectomy.

Medial oblique osteotomy is advantageous for implant support during corrective osteotomies. The Nasal bone can act as a platform on which an implant can be placed (Fig. 1.4). In the lateral osteotomy with medial osteotomy, a greenstick osteotomy is advantageous for the nasal pyramid's stability (Fig. 1.5).

The nasal platform above the rhinion can be preserved using the medial oblique osteotomy line for support.

- The lateral bone instability is often generated; the implant is sinking to the weak side. It can cause long-term implant deviation (Fig. 1.6).

It is difficult to find an implant that is located exactly in the midline on the nasal bone. Therefore, bone rasping may be more advantageous than osteotomy, but it cannot be applied in all cases. Ensuring a stable platform for implant placement is the most crucial key when projecting while reducing the wide nasal bone width. It is better to apply autograft to the dorsum when osteotome is accompanied.

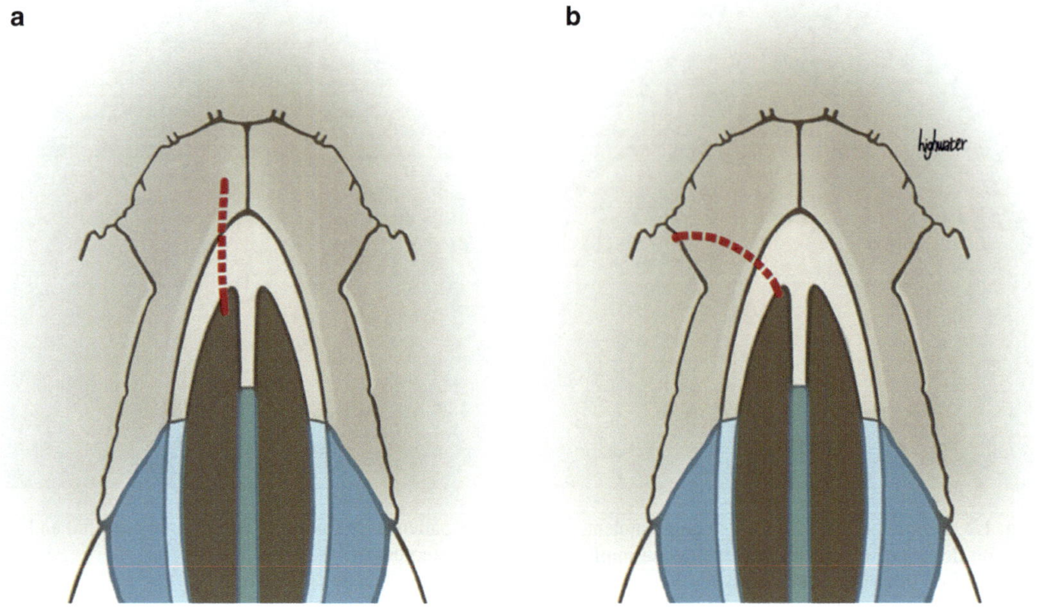

Fig. 1.4 Medial oblique osteotomy can preserve more bones for the stable implant platform. (**a**) Paramedian osteotomy. (**b**) Medial oblique osteotomy

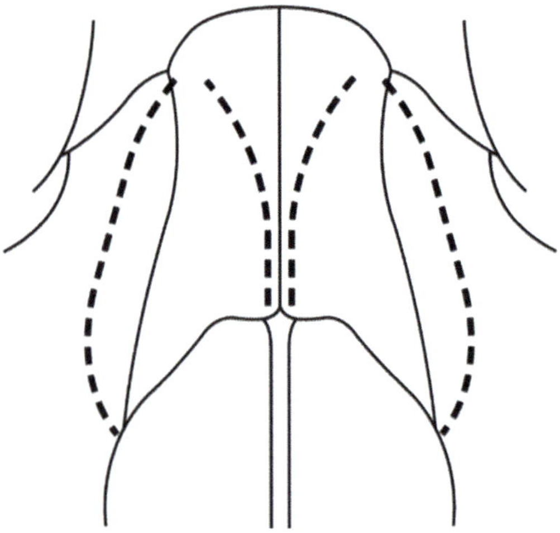

Fig. 1.5 Design of the greenstick fracture between medial oblique osteotomy and lateral low-high osteotomy

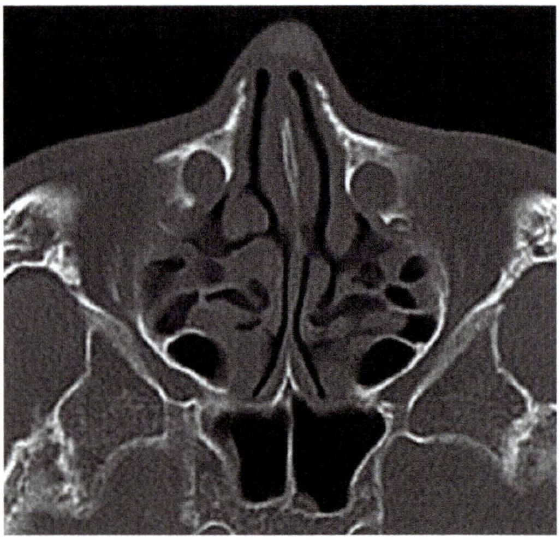

Fig. 1.6 Silicone implant dislocated to the left side with malunion of the lateral nasal bone

1.3 Implant Deviation

Longer Implant than the Pocket

The most significant cause of the deviation is the tension in the implant's longitudinal direction, generated by a longer implant than the pocket size. In this case, lateral capsulotomy is attempted as a closed technique, but this method is not very helpful unless the implant's length is shortened. Any means to reduce tension should be used. With the introduction of very soft silicone, implant deviation occurs even with less longitudinal pressure. Make sure to make enough soft tissue envelopes and use implants that are not too long. Note that implant mobility occurs when excessive dissection is performed.

Bony Axis Vs. Septal Axis

No matter how low the nose, the bony axis, and the axis of the cartilaginous dorsum are often different. If this is overlooked, the implant tilts according to the slope of the platform. Light axis discrepancy can be camouflaged with an appropriate implant-carving, but deviations are often seen again after swelling disappears.

Even patients with very low nasion can find that the cartilaginous dorsum is directed to one side from the rhinion. In this case, although silicone was inserted, there may be a discrepancy between the upper one-third and lower two-third postoperatively, resulting in cosmetic dissatisfaction (Fig. 1.7).

On the other hand, when the deviation of the septum is resolved with a spreader graft, a dorsal autograft yields a more stable result (Fig. 1.8).

However, applying the spreader graft under an implant to correct the deviation is a waste of cartilage. Although the spreader graft is functional and invisible, if covered by the dorsal implant, applying septal cartilage underneath the implant is ineffective. A dorsal implant may camouflage the deviation.

When the spreader graft is adopted, an autologous material is recommended at the dorsum. After the ULC and the septum are separated, an alloplastic implant is not recommended on it. Micromucosal damage after complete dissection between ULC from anterior septum can cause late-onset inflammation.

- There are many cases in augmenting very low nasion, in which alloplastic implants have to be used. In this situation, dissect the pocket more widely.
- Prepare a platform as flat as possible with a rasping. Bring the implant to the midline by sculpting the undersurface asymmetrically.
- It is advantageous not to perform septal dissection when implants must be used on the dorsum. In other words, without dissecting the ULC and anterior septum, the axis deviation of the lower two-third can be corrected by connecting the implant to the tip by appropriate suture rather than the spreader graft.
- Minor differences between the bony axis and the septal axis may be emphasized when the

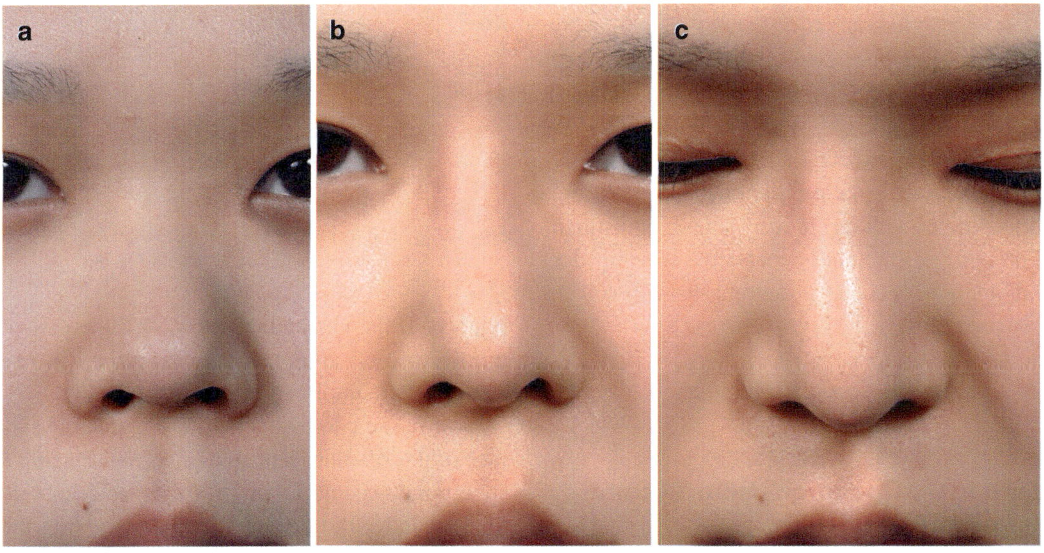

Fig. 1.7 Silicone deviation. (**a**) Very low nasion with axis discrepancy between the bony axis and the axis of the cartilaginous dorsum. (**b**) Frontal view. (**c**) Distinct deviation by the dorsal highlights

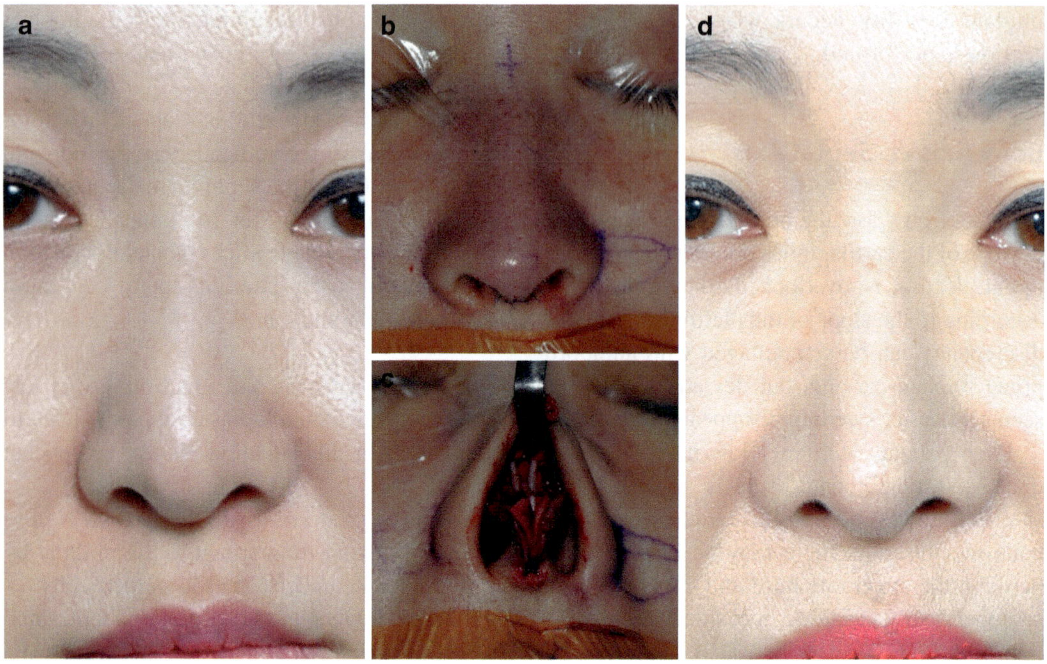

Fig. 1.8 Correction of deviation by autograft only. (**a**) Preoperative view. (**b**) After the spreader graft: correction of the high septum. (**c**) Dorsal highlight was focused on the Lt. side spreader graft. (**d**) Postoperative view

dorsum is projected, so care should be taken when applying a dorsal implant.

Implant-Dependent Dorsum

In Asian rhinoplasties, the techniques have been evolved on the premise that alloplastic materials augment the dorsum. The main methods have focused on tip projection and extension.

The severe deviation cannot achieve a straight dorsal line without proper septal adjustment. Furthermore, implant-dependent dorsum does not apply to secondary rhinoplasty with soft tissue problems.

– As the septum goes, the implant goes.

Secondary Operation Using Silicone Implant (Re-insertion)

In secondary operation, it is unavoidable to remove the silicone and re-insert the silicone implant. If the nasion is too low, or if the patient refuses to apply autograft, the last option is to use an alloplastic implant again.

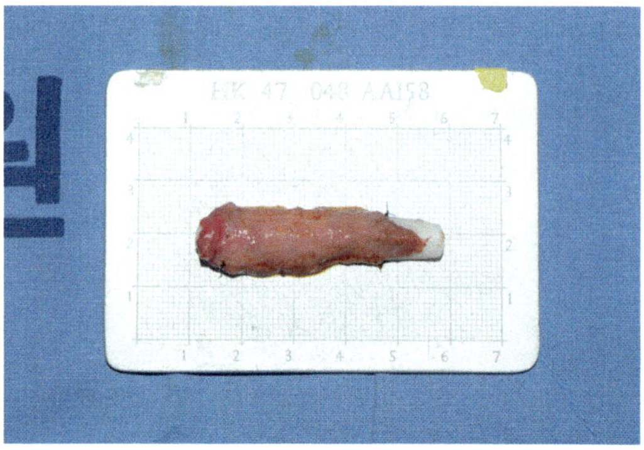

Fig. 1.9 The anterior surface of the silicone implant was covered with flattened superficial mastoid fascia

Soft tissue can be applied to the anterior surface of the silicone implant as a barrier. Placing a superficial mastoid fascia [3] on the anterior side implant fades the demarcation and supports the thin anterior skin (Fig. 1.9).

The indications of applying anterior soft tissue are:

1. After removing all capsules, if the anterior skin envelope remains very thin.
2. Surgery to correct implant demarcation.
3. In secondary operation, when the silicone must be re-inserted after removing the silicone.

1.4 Clinical Features of Complications

Silicone Implants

Capsule: Contracture

Silicone inevitably forms a capsule. If five silicone surgeries are performed, five different capsules are formed. If the capsules are not removed, those are not resorbed naturally (Fig. 1.10). The scar band of myofibroblast or fibroblast formed around the capsule is consistent with the inflammatory reaction. Some capsules are healthy and very thin; these can be used as soft tissues in secondary surgery. Nonhealthy capsules that are made up of very thick scars cause contractures that should be removed. In Chap. 2, the author will discuss the late-onset inflammation of nonhealthy capsules.

Calcification

Calcification is a characteristic feature on the surface of old silicone. It can be easily diagnosed on an X-ray, and in older cases, it may cause skin lesions.

It is essential to remove both the anterior and posterior capsules. When removing the anterior capsule, be careful of skin necrosis (Fig. 1.11).

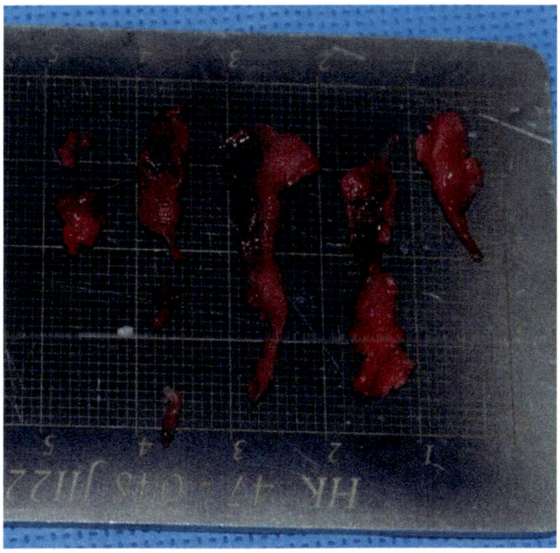

Fig. 1.10 Multilayers of silicone capsules were removed from a secondary surgery

Demarcation, Transparency

In patients with too low nasion, demarcation around the implant can be found. Also, in thin-skinned patients, the silicone is seen through the sunlight, making it appear transparent. The above method of applying the soft tissue to the anterior surface effectively controls demarcation and transparency (Fig. 1.12).

Gore-tex

Since Gore-tex has micropore, it has a high infection rate along with Medpor among alloplastic implants. In a proportion of 3% or more, implant removal is required due to infection. Surgeons might think that there is no contracture because it doesn't make a capsule, but the bigger problem is the use of silicone and Gore-tex alternately due to multiple surgeries.

- Contracture occurs even in Gore-tex inserted into a capsule made of silicone, and the late-onset inflammation that happens in this situation shows a very complex clinical feature.

Shrinkage and Demarcation

Shrinkage and demarcation of the implant is a phenomenon peculiar to Gore-tex that occurs when the micropore is reduced. It is characterized by a very hard leather-like degeneration when removed. Since it does not make a capsule, it is sometimes more difficult to remove. It should be noted that there is no such opportunity as the capsule can be used as some soft tissue in the case of a patient who has undergone multiple surgeries using a silicone implant. When removing Gore-tex, it also should be noted that the dorsal skin on the affected area is very thin. Such thin skin takes a very long time to regain its elasticity and return to its original shape (Fig. 1.13).

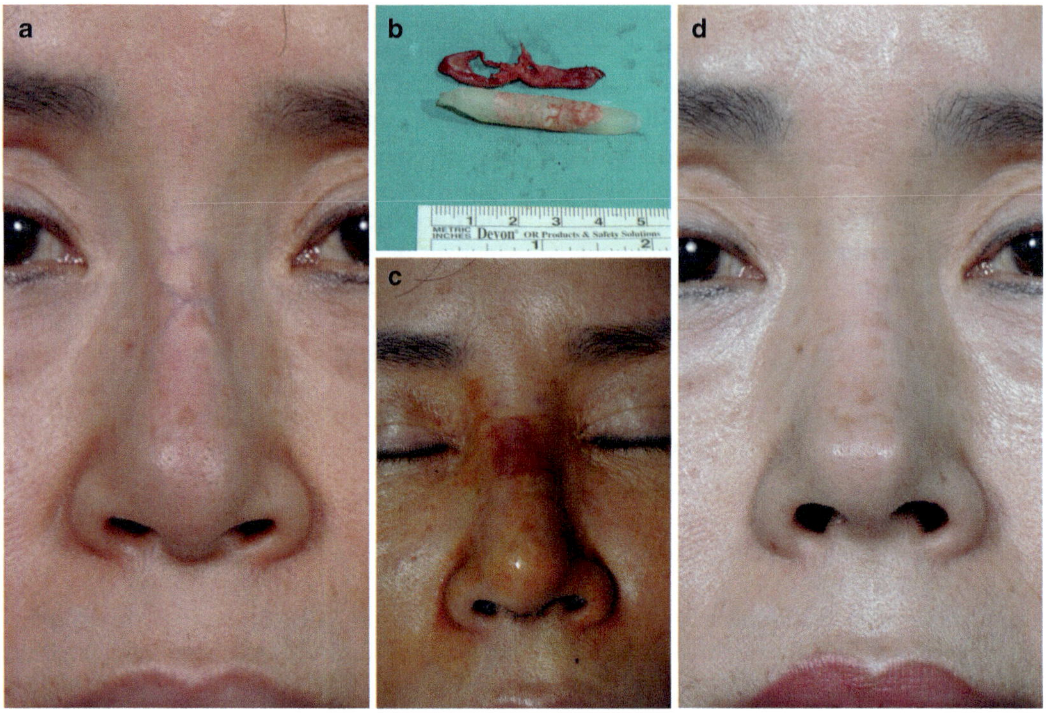

Fig. 1.11 Calcification of old silicone implant. (**a**) Preoperative view; skin thinning with venous engorgement. (**b**) Silicone and the capsule; the anterior surface of the silicone was covered with stone-like calcification. (**c**) Skin problem: the thin skin is in danger of necrosis, hyperbaric O^2 treatment is recommended. (**d**) Postoperative view

Along with demarcation, many patients complain of unknown pain due to this thin skin (Fig. 1.14).

Demarcation around the implant, accompanied by shrinkage, is also commonly found in silicone implants with healthy capsules (Fig. 1.15). In other words, demarcation around the implant may occur in both silicone and Gore-tex. Even too superficially inserted dermofat graft may be demarcated, so care should be taken to handle the thick dermis margin.

IHCC (Irradiated Homologous Cartilage)

Resorption: Fracture

The resorption was found to be the most problematic in the long-term follow-up of IHCC. The resorption rate of autologous costal cartilage is 3%, and that of IHCC is 30% [4]. There had been a problem with fracture-resorption, so the author no longer uses it [5]. Conclusively IHCC is not free from surgical site infection (SSI) and late-onset inflammation (LOI) other than resorption and fracture.

- When used for the nasal framework, many shape problems can occur due to resorption in the long term.
- It is not recommended to use as columellar struts, caudal septal extension grafts, lateral crural strut grafts, or alar rim grafts.
- It is relatively advantageous to use dorsal onlay graft, but there is also a problem of resorption.
- As it is a non-viable cartilage graft, it is not free from inflammation caused by long-term trauma [6]
- It has a complication rate of about 3%, and the frequency of resorption with or without infection is about 2% [7]

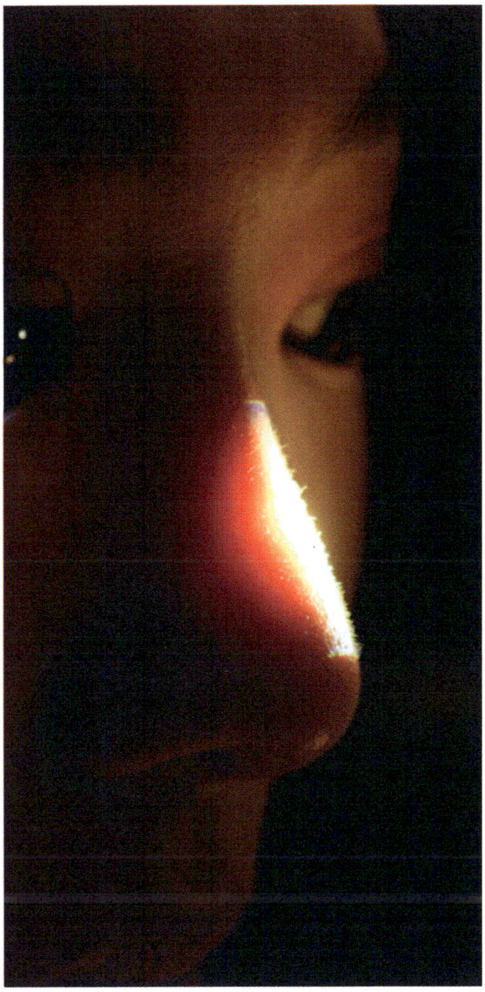

Fig. 1.12 Transparent silicone implant in thin skin

There are many situations in which IHCC has to be used because the amount of autologous cartilage that remains after multiple reoperations is insufficient. However, IHCC use in primary rhinoplasty is increasing enormously due to the convenience. Therefore, the complications of IHCC increase rapidly.

Alloderm

Alloderm is a suitable material that can be used conveniently without sacrificing the donor site, but it is not free from absorption [8]. It is reported that the relationship between multilayered application and absorption is trivial. Still, in Asian rhinoplasty, more than two layers are often used, and the hardness due to scar formation is more problematic than absorption clinically.

- Absorption of alloderm on the bony dorsum is more significant due to insufficient circulation during engraftment.
- Multiple layers of application create an intermediate avascular layer and remain as a stone-like scar.

Central Avascular Scar: Contracture Inside the Preexisting Capsule

An avascular layer or scar is formed in the center where several layers are applied, and a scar lump with a hardness that does not allow the scalpel to enter. An alloderm-contracture may occur when inserted in the capsule that has not been removed [9].

1.5 Surgical Site Infection Vs. Late-Onset Inflammation

The most significant complication of alloplastic implants is infection. According to the meta-analysis report, the infection rate of Gore-tex and Silicone was 4%, and the infection rate of Medpor was 6%, but it was not statistically significant. Relatively, the Mepor and Gore-tex were half as low [10].

Due to empirical antibiotics and the surgical environment's improvement, the infection rate will show very different patterns, so there will be errors in generalization. However, SSI (surgical site infection) and late-onset inflammation seen after wound healing should be distinguished (Chap. 2).

Above is the most crucial perspective of Asian rhinoplasty because most of the contractures come from inflammation.

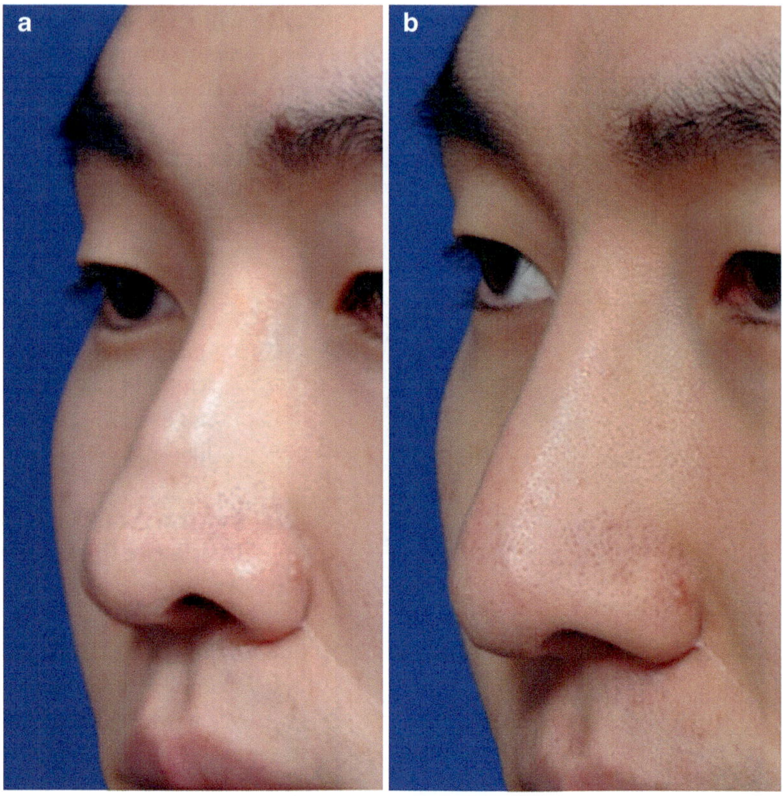

Fig. 1.13 Demarcated Gore-tex. (**a**) Preoperative quarter view, (**b**) postoperative view

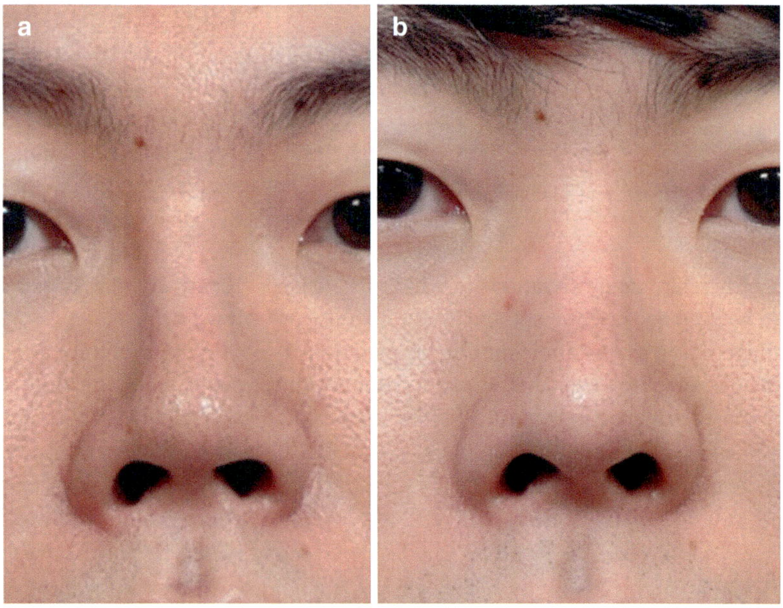

Fig. 1.14 A patient who suffered from unknown nasal pain. (**a**) Preoperative view, (**b**) Pain disappeared after removing dorsal Gore-tex and replaced with autologous dermis graft

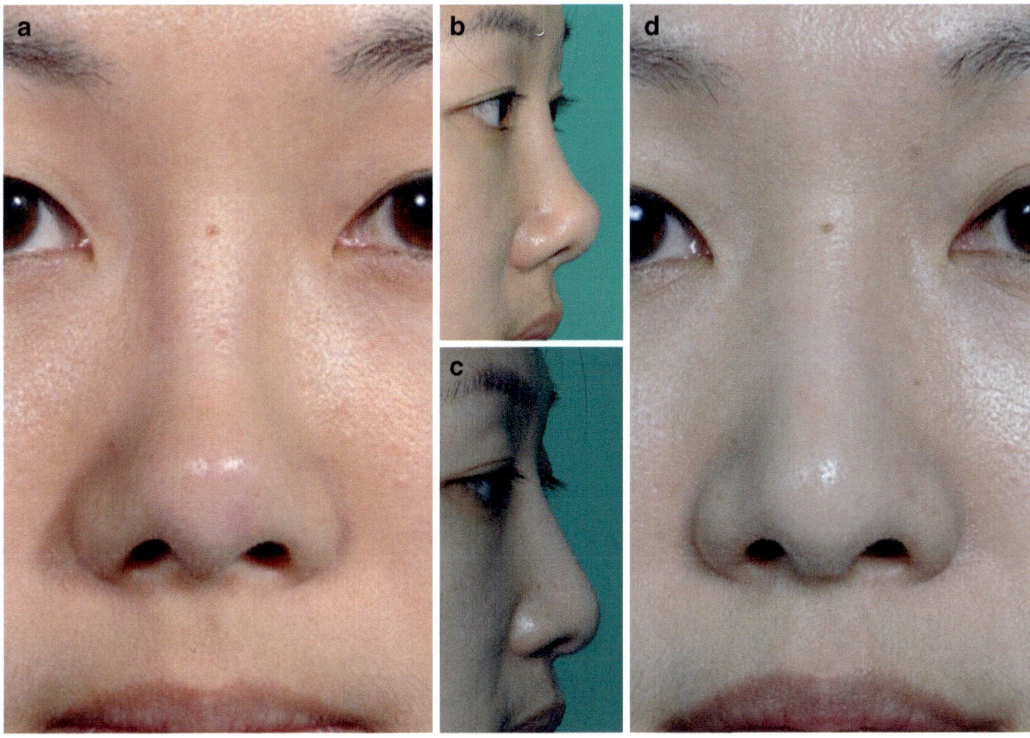

Fig. 1.15 Demarcated silicone implant with contracture (**a**, **b**) preoperative view, (**c**, **d**) postoperative view

References

1. Oliver JD, Eells AC, Saba ES, Boczar D, Restrepo DJ, Huayllani MT, et al. Alloplastic facial implants: a systematic review and meta-analysis on outcomes and uses in aesthetic and reconstructive plastic surgery. Aesthet Plast Surg. 2019;43(3):625–36.
2. Toriumi DM, Pero CD. Asian rhinoplasty. Clin Plast Surg. 2010;37(2):335–52.
3. Hong S-T, Kim D-W, Yoon E-S, Kim H-Y, Dhong E-S. Superficial mastoid fascia as an accessible donor for various augmentations in Asian rhinoplasty. J Plast Reconstr Aesthet Surg. 2012;65(8):1035–40.
4. Wee JH, Mun SJ, Na WS, Kim H, Park JH, Kim D-K, et al. Autologous vs irradiated homologous costal cartilage as graft material in rhinoplasty. JAMA Facial Plast Surg. 2017;19(3):183–8.
5. Suh M-K, Ahn E-S, Kim H-R, Dhong E-S. A 2-year follow-up of irradiated homologous costal cartilage used as a septal extension graft for the correction of contracted nose in Asians. Ann Plast Surg. 2013;71(1):45–9.
6. Toriumi DM. Choosing autologous vs irradiated homograft rib costal cartilage for grafting in rhinoplasty. JAMA Facial Plast Surg. 2017;19(3):188–9.
7. Kridel RWH, Ashoori F, Liu ES. Long-term use and follow-up of irradiated homologous costal cartilage grafts in the nose. Arch Facial Plast Surg [Internet]. 2009. https://jamanetwork.com/journals/jama/fullarticle/407629.
8. Gryskiewicz JM. Waste not, want not: the use of AlloDerm in secondary rhinoplasty. Plast Reconstr Surg [Internet]. 2005. https://journals.lww.com/plasreconsurg/Fulltext/2005/12000/Alloderm_Lip_Augmentation.24.aspx?casa_token=4n4K7vf5ObQAAAAA:PaVJJEk65rVrb351MEjlbHdUyg8slWclJhHq_hv9jxM94EK2oq4w11e167Ow_7F4CnZhxFa_149dXC2oxEpE5SOo.
9. Dhong E. 11 management of alloplast-related complications. Aesthetic Plastic Surgery of the East Asian Face [Internet]. 2016. https://pdfs.semanticscholar.org/fc9e/a8e751045e2e299c8649a38b57c80ded9b72.pdf#page=153.
10. Peled ZM, Warren AG, Johnston P, Yaremchuk MJ. The use of alloplastic materials in rhinoplasty surgery: a meta-analysis. Plast Reconstr Surg. 2008;121(3):85e–92e.

2 Surgical Site Infection (SSI) Vs. Late-Onset Inflammation (LOI)

Pearls

- A septorhinoplasty is a clean-contaminated surgery. In a sense, a septorhinoplasty using an alloplastic implant is contaminated surgery.
- Therefore, pre-, peri-, and postoperative antibiotics should be used.
- Asian septorhinoplasty is a complicated surgery combining submucosal resection (SMR), many cartilage grafts, and sometimes an alloplastic implant.
- Septal surgery is the most crucial factor in deciding the duration of antibiotic use.
- SSI that occurs in the acute postoperative phase and LOI that occurs after the long term should be treated separately.

SSI

- The treatment principle of SSI is rapid I&D and removal of implants and grafts.
- The SSI of open rhinoplasty begins with septum and the columella.
- Surgery can be salvaged with appropriate antibiotics, but all grafts and implants should be removed immediately when pus drains or the degree of cellulitis becomes severe.
- It is contraindicated to do the immediate secondary surgery during SSI.

LOI

- The first clinical manifestations are skin lesions such as cyst formations on the nasal dorsum, tip, and nasal cavity.
- Along with the above condition, a puncture is formed over time, or pus is drained.
- The criterion for deciding whether to perform only I&D or do the revision surgery is the degree of cellulitis of the skin envelope. The severity of cellulitis determines the timing of surgery.
- In the case of pus-draining patients, it is recommended to delay surgery after eradicating the pus with irrigation and antibiotics. However, if the severity of cellulitis is low, pus-drainage is not a contraindication of immediate reconstruction.
- The cyst is found in the operation field as a mucus-containing "mucocele" in a capsule.
- In the case of Gore-tex use, mucus-filled cyst patterns were also found.
- Damaged capsules and ingrowth of endothelium-like mucosa or de novo proliferation of granulation tissues and inflammatory cells play a crucial role in late-onset inflammation related to alloplastic implants.

2.1 The Differences by Definition

Surgical Site Infection (SSI)

Surgical site infection is an infection that occurs after any rhinoplasty. It is superficial infections involving a surgical pocket. It occurs during the wound-healing process and occurs within

E.-S. Dhong, M.-W. Na, *Asian Septorhinoplasty*, https://doi.org/10.1007/978-981-16-0542-0_2

2 weeks from 5 days postoperatively. In the acute phase, redness, swelling, and pain are accompanied, and eventually, pus drains. When septal surgery is performed simultaneously, the clinical picture may be completely different compared to the case without septal surgery.

SSI After a Septal Surgery

SSI from the septal surgical pocket can have serious consequences. The reason for this is the clinical risk of bacterial dissemination, rather than the vast extent of surgery.

The existing literature argues that antibiotics do not eradicate staphylococcus, which is the most problematic during septoplasty, disrupt intranasal physiology by changing the normal flora, concludes that septal surgery does not require any antibiotics [1, 2]. However, the author cannot fully agree with this. Asian septorhinoplasty (SRP) covered in this book is not a simple surgery mentioned in the papers, but a completely different surgical category. Although simple septoplasty shows a low infection rate, Asian SRP should be considered as a clean-contaminated surgery due to the surgery's nature [3]. Patients should receive prophylactic antibiotics appropriate for their specific procedures. In principle, antibiotics rather than the first generation of cephalosporin should be used prophylactically or perioperatively [4]. It is essential to keep in mind that the patient is in a temporary bacteremia state during surgery [5].

- Since the septum and external nose have two different surgical pockets, care must be taken to ensure that the two pus pockets communicate with each other or not.
- Septal mucosal flaps coapt sooner than the dorsal flap heals. However, the septal pocket lies in a dependent position, the pus often accumulates in the septum (Fig. 2.1).
- The pus pocket confined to the septum should be irrigated with external drainage.
- For septal abscess, systemic symptoms should be monitored. There have been reports of cases of severe sepsis, even death.

Septal mucosal flaps coapt sooner before the dorsal flap heals. When pus drains, if antibiotics had been treated just for one time, most cultures are found to be no bacteria, but susceptible antibiotics appropriate for the cultured strains should be prescribed.

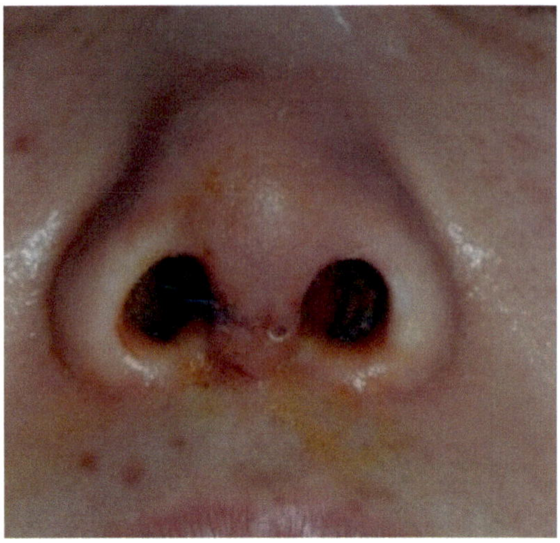

Fig. 2.1 SSI started from the septal abscess. The abscess pocket was connected from the septum to the dorsal pocket

- Monitoring the SSI begins with a flap color change of columella.
- Surgery can be salvaged with appropriate antibiotics, but all grafts and implants should be removed immediately when pus drains or the degree of cellulitis becomes severe.

SSI Without Septal Surgery

Since the surgical pocket is limited to the external nose, SSI is controlled by appropriate irrigation and systemic antibiotics. The essential principle is removing alloplastic implants and grafts quickly.

- As in the case of septal surgery above, immediate secondary surgery is avoided.
- The degree of dorsal cellulitis is the indicator of safe wound healing.

Late-Onset Inflammation (LOI)

Late-onset inflammation (LOI) is a rare complication that may occur several months to years

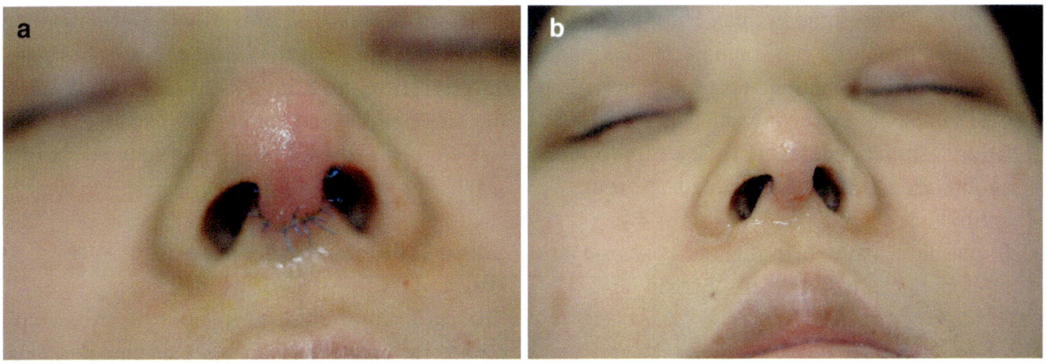

Fig. 2.2 Transient inflammation of the columella. (**a**) The redness was found 3 days postoperatively and changed the antibiotics from empirical cephalosporin to quinolone. (**b**) After 5 days, the redness improved without irrigation

after an uneventful rhinoplasty. It is an inflammatory stage utterly different from SSI, with or without pus-drainage seen in the acute stage of surgery. The inflammatory stage may progress to the last stage of infection that ends in pus-drainage. However, LOI is often accompanied by redness and mild repetitive swelling. Swelling subsides whenever empirical antibiotics are prescribed. LOI often occurs after pregnancy and when the patient's general condition is bad.

2.2 The Differences Between Clinical Features and Managements

Surgical Site Infection (SSI)

In case of simultaneous septal SMR, proper packing is critical. Nasal packing with appropriate antibiotics prevents hematoma, and at the same time it affects inhibiting colony [6]. The septal hematoma often results in a septal abscess. The causative agent of SSI, which occurs in the postoperative wound-healing process and occurs within 2 weeks from a few days after surgery, will be discussed in detail in Chap. 3.

In the early stages, redness usually begins from the columella. After removal of packing, endonasal inspection should be performed well. If the local fluctuation is found in the septum, actively do the puncture and drain. Besides, appropriate antibiotics should be started that match the culture. Whether columellar redness is temporary, cellulitis gets better, and the rhinoplasty will be salvaged in some cases (Fig. 2.2).

Adequate choice of antibiotics is the key, and the infected pocket usually improves within 1–2 days, so the wound should be observed daily. If an empirical antibiotic, first- to second-generation cephalosporin, was prescribed, it is necessary to switch to quinolones. If there is susceptibility, symptoms can improve after transient inflammation (Fig. 2.2b). However, when swelling gets worse or cellulitis progresses further, the breakage of the suture margin is observed. The pus starts to drain at an irreversible state, all graft materials and implants should be removed. Repeated irrigation is the only surgical maneuver.

Management of SSI

- Once the pus is drained, it is the principle to remove all implants and cartilages grafted from the nose.
- There are cases where an increase in CRP is found in the blood inflammation index (ESR

or CRP). These markers can help, especially CRP, but they are not a standard of treatment.
- As a general condition, fever, tiredness, and cold symptoms are accompanied by early onset.
- Efforts should be made to use appropriate antibiotics and willing to change unresponsive antibiotics.
- If antibiotics are being taken, bacteria are often not detected in the discharged pus.

Late-Onset Inflammation (LOI)

There has been debate on the status of "subclinical infection": A state in which swelling and improvement have fluctuated. A status of weak infection drains discharges but not the pus. However, this term should be redefined. Repeated swelling may be attributed to the biofilm formed around the implant. However, it can be observed that the clinical picture is more complicated than the inflammation caused by biofilm. It has been reported that coagulase-negative staphylococci found in the breast's capsular contracture are the leading cause of the biofilm [7]. The biofilm around the implant may be the cause of contracture, there are similarities, but the pathologic findings are slightly different. The LOI is characterized by intermittent nasal dorsal swelling and sometimes granuloma-like skin lesions. In severe cases, puncture with fluid drainage on the external or intranasal area may be present. There are many cases where pus is drained to the puncture site.

A "mucocele-like cyst"is a characteristic pathology that is not found in breast implants.

The stages of late-onset inflammation (LOI) can be divided into the following four stages:

1. The fluctuation of swelling, which is the mildest stage. The soft tissue starts to contract.
2. The granulation with skin lesions forms a thick scar around the pocket.
3. The stage of skin puncture, which is the opening of a "mucocele-like cyst."
4. Full infection with cellulitis.

If antibiotics are prescribed and sustained at the stage of one, the clinical pattern repeats deterioration and improvement, but finally, the stage of severity increases, so it is essential to perform surgical intervention before stage 3.

Stage 1: Fluctuation: Wax and Wane

The recurring pattern of swelling is frequently found in patients using alloplastic implants. Usually, empirical antibiotics are prescribed, and taking NSAIDs subsides swelling, and in some cases, this process lasts for years (Fig. 2.3). However, the swelling becomes more extensive in the end, and the capsule becomes irreversibly thick. Moreover, "the nose becomes shorter" (Fig. 2.4).

Regardless of the silicone or Gore-tex, the fluctuation is found, and no clear evidence of worsening and improving symptoms from the biofilm has not been found. Trauma history, drinking, pregnancy, and childbirth can be heard, but most of them are idiopathic. The appearance of gradually changing and thickening is the formation of scar tissue around the capsule, and when palpated, the fluid inside can be touched.

- It is recommended to perform a secondary operation before skin puncture, and the standard timing for this operation is when swelling is not severe and subsided.
- At this time, a CT scan can be helpful in planning the operation and in identifying the volume to be reconstructed.
- The soft tissue starts to contract.

It is advantageous to check the septal state to obtain full information about the type and method of alloplastic material used in the previous operation for the secondary operation.

It is essential to inspect the maximal swelling, and the height of the dorsum to be reconstructed can be predicted.

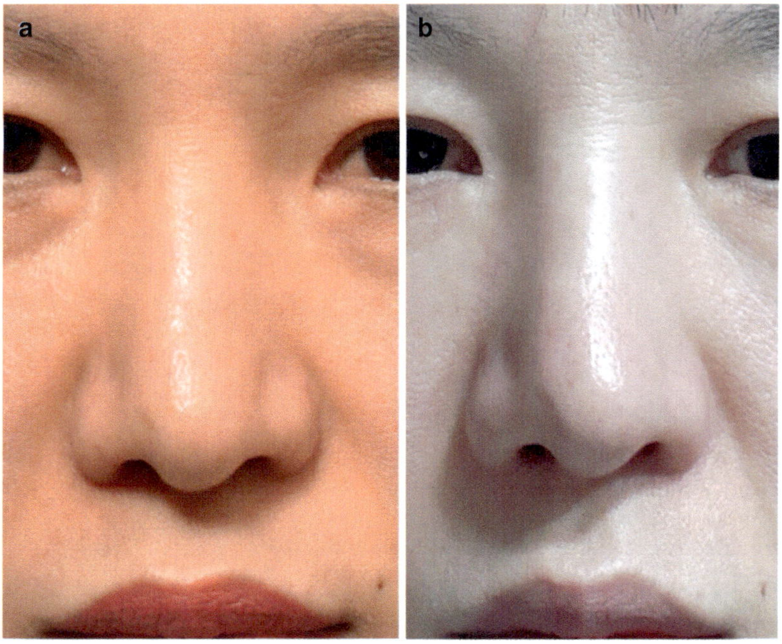

Fig. 2.3 The first stage of LOI: fluctuation. (**a**) Normal state after taking empirical oral antibiotics. (**b**) Swollen state

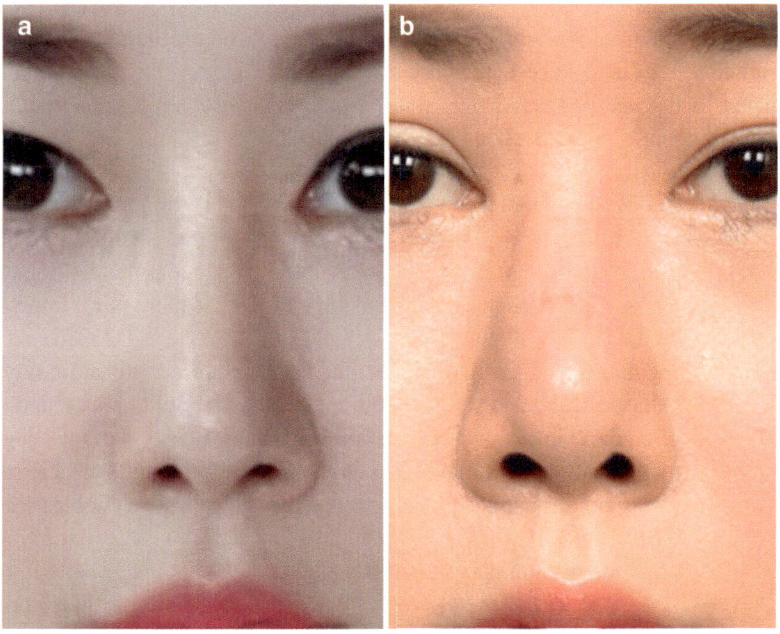

Fig. 2.4 The first stage of LOI: swelling does not subside. (**a**) The normal state, 1 year after the silicone implantation at another hospital. (**b**) Swollen state, which does not subside treated with quinolone. She was managed with secondary rhinoplasty using autologous materials

Stage 2: Skin Lesion: Out-Growth of the Granulation Tissue

The lesions found in the skin may show epidermal cyst patterns, but most are found as dark purple cysts with central thinning (Fig. 2.5a, b). It is found in various locations, even in the membranous septum (Fig. 2.5c).

Doctors who do not understand the LOI course perform skin biopsy or excision and encounter unpredicted sequels. This lesion's pathology is usu-

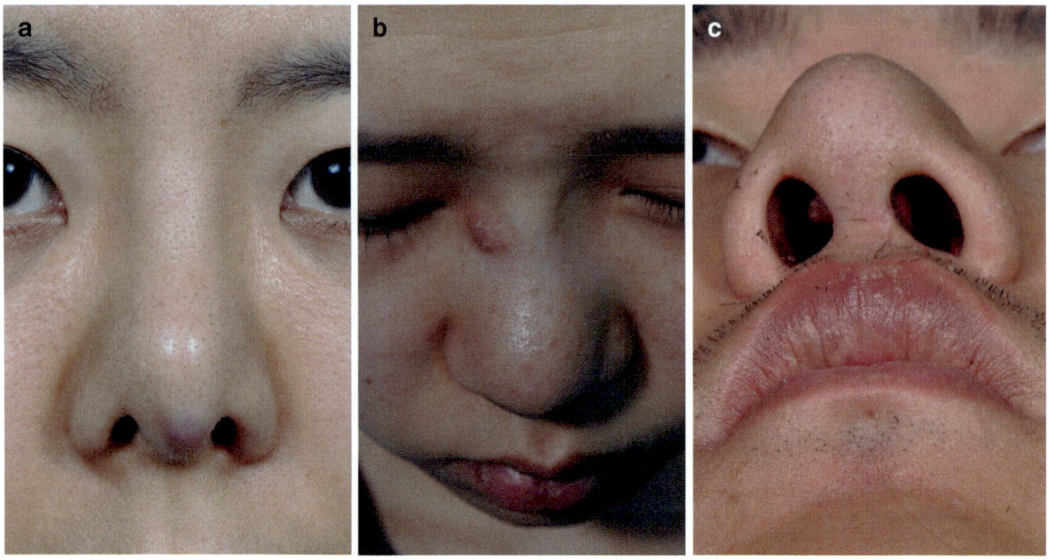

Fig. 2.5 The second stage of LOI: granuloma-like cysts. (**a**) Purple-colored thinning at the nasal tip. (**b**) Nasal root cyst misdiagnosed as an epidermal cyst by a dermatologist. (**c**) Granuloma-like cyst at the membranous septum

ally a granulomatous reaction with a mucous cyst, similar to the sinus mucoceles. Since this lesion is likely to become punctured over time, a definite septorhinoplasty should be considered at this stage.

- The mucous cyst should be eradicated from the whole lesion.
- Pockets made deep up to the anterior nasal spine or pockets connected to the nasion can be scraped with a small curette.
- The most challenging part is to dissect the thin dorsal skin surface. It is essential not to make a puncture on the skin as much as possible, but if it becomes punctured during surgery, it is necessary to apply appropriate soft tissue underneath. However, surprisingly it can be found that it heals well with the minimal scar left (Fig. 2.6).

Stage 3: Puncture with or Without Pus-Drainage

Discharge occurs at first and then develops into pus. The puncture heals by epithelization, but it requires a definitive excision. Only total resection is the solution (Fig. 2.7).

For pus, aggressive antibiotics should be treated, and for wounds with a puncture, the regimen should follow contaminated wounds. The first-generation cephalosporin cannot solve the problems overall. Ciprofloxacin (quinolone) meets the requirement of a single broad-spectrum antibiotic available in intravenous and oral form.

- If the primary choice of antibiotics should be made without the culture result, quinolone is recommended for stage 3 [8].
- If there is no improvement after using quinolone for 2–3 days, dual or triple antibiotics, including aminoglycoside or metronidazole, should be included.
- Besides many negative results in culture, selecting susceptible antibiotics as soon as possible enables secondary operation and prohibits soft tissue contracture.

This effort is for preparing secondary surgery and is not an end-point of treatment. If the underlying pathology containing mucocele is not resolved, improvement cannot be expected.

Level 4: Cellulitis with Pus-Drainage

Active irrigation and drainage are required. In principle, all grafts, along with alloplastic material in the nose, are removed. Check the cartilage condition, whether it is bleeding or not. It is essential to use appropriate antibiotics before

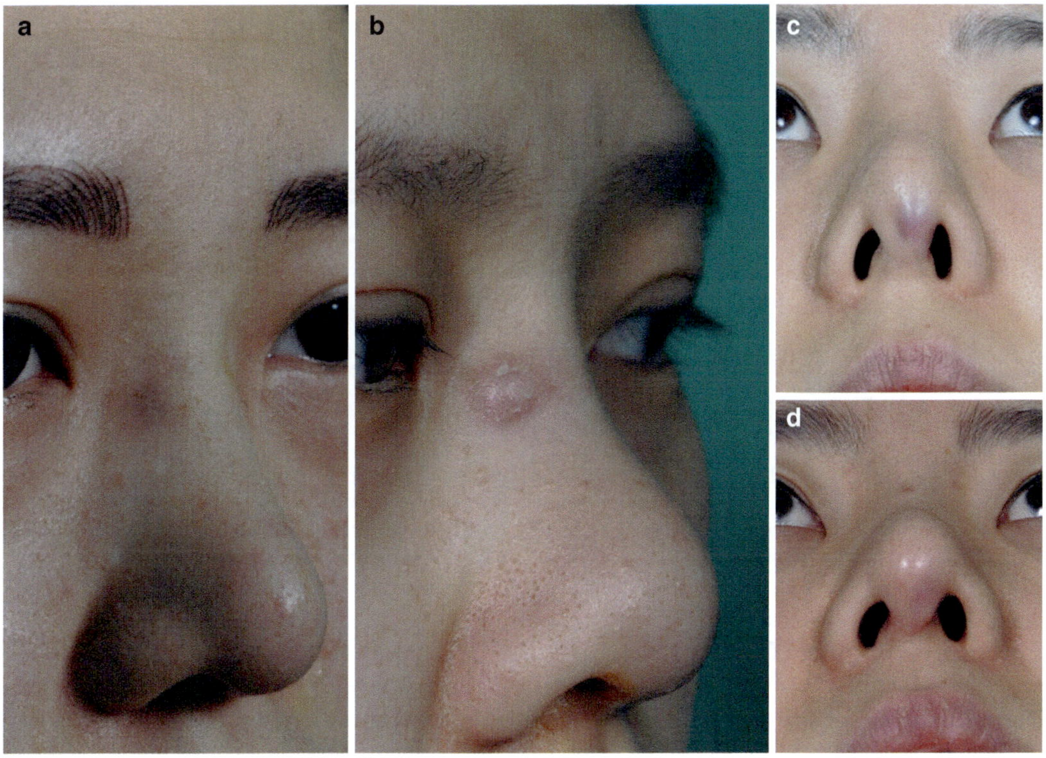

Fig. 2.6 Total excision of granuloma-like cysts that extends from root to tip inside the capsule. (**a**, **b**) Nasal root lesion, pre-, and postoperative state. (**c**, **d**) Columellar lesion, pre-, and postoperative state

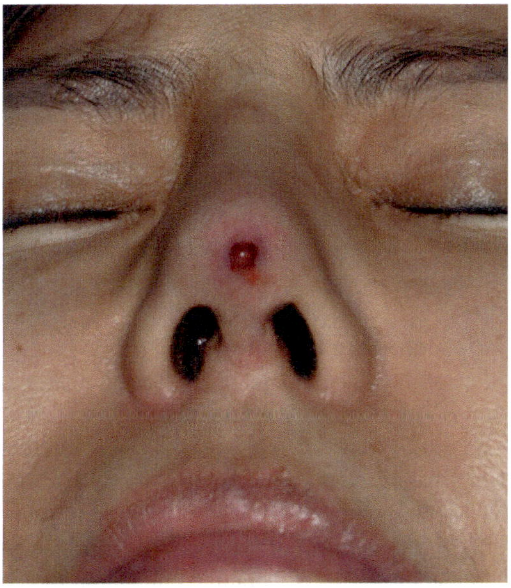

Fig. 2.7 The third stage of LOI: skin puncture, mucous cystic outbreak without pus-drainage

surgery, and it is crucial to reduce cellulitis as much as possible and undergo surgery.

- The degree of cellulitis is an index that determines whether a secondary operation is possible as in the SSI.
- Active reoperation is possible when cellulitis decreases, and the color of the skin flap returns to normal.
- However, if severe cellulitis is found, graft or septal surgery other than removing the pathogen is contraindicated (Fig. 2.8).
- It is good to plan step-by-step surgery, but note that if aggressive capsule removal is not performed, contracture occurs during the wound-healing period.
- The degree to which the nasal framework remains is a condition that determines the presence or absence of devastating deformation after surgery.

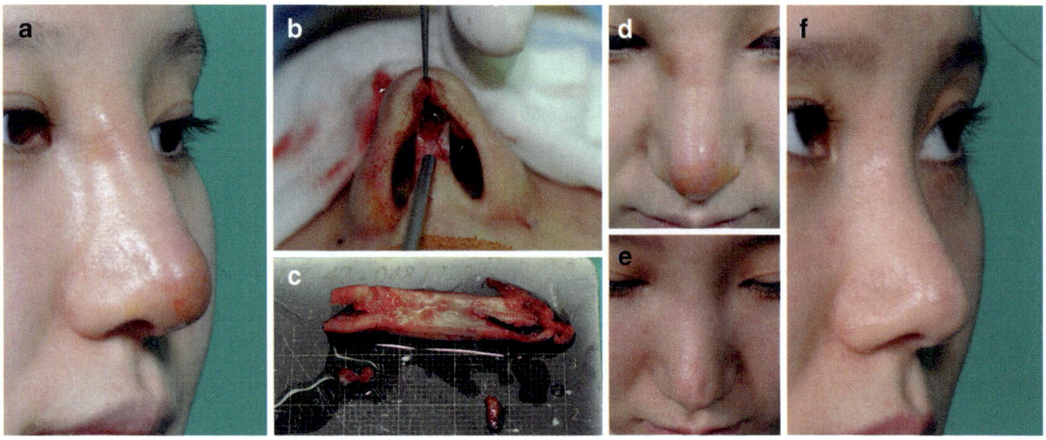

Fig. 2.8 The fourth stage of LOI: severe cellulitis with pus-drainage. (**a**, **d**) A 23-year-old female had been operated with a surgifoam. Her secondary operation was performed using dermofat graft replacing the surgifoam by the same doctor 1 year before visiting the author. Preoperative view. (**b**, **c**) Pus was drained after the incision. Old capsule with mucocele was excised above the scarred dermis. (**e**, **f**) Postoperative view

Pathophysiology of LOI

There have been no analytic reports of LOI in alloplastic implant patients. Most reports regarded the total infection rate. The complications that can occur due to silicone implants are reported to be 4–24% [9], but there is no detailed study on infection timing for all complications. One study reported a long-term infection of 1.3% in the primary operation in patients with Gore-tex and 4.3–5.4% in secondary operations [10].

Biofilm

Biofilm formation has been believed to be the most significant cause of subclinical infection. However, biofilm cannot be confirmed in the actual surgical field. A biofilm is defined as an assemblage of surface-associated microbial cells enclosed in a protective extracellular, primarily the polysaccharide matrix [11]. Abiotic surfaces surrounded by bacterially produced extracellular matrix established 3-D aggregates of polarized cells able to produce mucoglycoproteins and stimulate mucus production [12].

A large amount of mucus is formed in the biofilm, but it looks like a mucocele in the operation field.

- It is found as a cyst containing mucus in a silicone capsule.
- In the case of Gore-tex, mucus-filled cyst patterns were also found.
- In the case of patients who have undergone multiple operations, the clinical features are more complicated, so it is essential to listen to the detailed medical history and to estimate the cyst size and location of the mucocele by CT scan.
- By adjusting the CT contrast, the mucocele size and the soft tissue volume to be reconstructed can be estimated (Fig. 2.9).
- However, in multiple surgeries, more research is needed because there are many cases of putting Gore-tex back into the existing silicone capsule.

Mucocele-Like Pathology

Most of the mucus found in late-onset inflammation is formed in the capsule, so it shows an intricate pattern related to the biotic surface different from that of the mucus derived from the biofilm. Mucocele is mucus extravasation forming pseudocyst with epithelioid macrophages and a bunch of mucin actually without any epithelioid tissue. However, the mucocele-like cysts seen in LOI are different from typical ranula, and more similar to the pus containing mucocele of the nasal sinus.

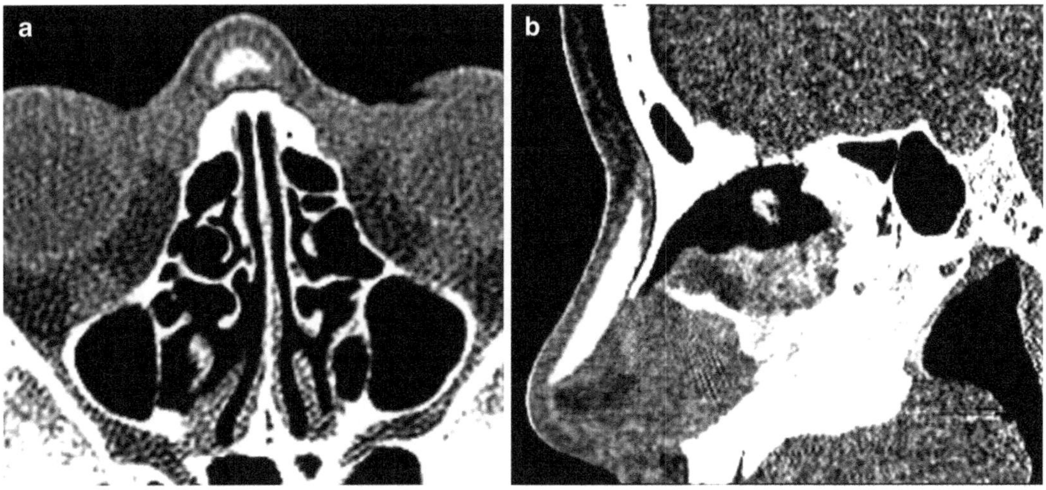

Fig. 2.9 Mucocele around the silicone implant, by adjusting the contrast, well-developed pericapsular space is identified. (**a**) Axial view. (**b**) Sagittal view

Histological Manifestations in Silicone Capsule

Healthy Capsule (HC)

The healthy capsule is in a stable state that does not show any aspect of LOI. Healthy silicone capsules with no inflammation signs are thin and can be separated as one layer during surgery. This capsule can be dissected well and used as a soft tissue graft. If necessary, the anterior capsule does not need to be removed when the anterior skin flap becomes too thin.

Thick capsules are not recommended to be used in situ because there is a risk of contracture. However, it is relatively safe to cut it out and use it on the tip or tissue depression.

Since the lateral capsulotomy alone can make a stable pocket, HC does not become a hurdle for secondary rhinoplasty.

Nonhealthy Capsule (NHC)

Nonhealthy capsules appear with LOI, and the capsules around the implants were thick and firmly adhered to the surrounding soft tissues of the nasal skin and cartilages. The thickness of the capsule depends on the patient's symptoms. Patients with contracture inflammation are found that the scar tissue around the capsule is thick (Fig. 2.10).

If this capsule and surrounding scar tissue are not removed, the nose will not be elongated comfortably. The capsule content has a fluctuation, and patients are divided into cases with or without surrounding cellulitis.

The Differences in the Histological Study [13]

Hematoxylin and Eosin Staining and Masson's Trichrome Staining

The HC group was organized into three tiers. The innermost layer adjacent to the implant is lined with a row of cells. Beyond this layer, synovial metaplasia was found. The outermost layer was a dense, regular layer of collagen (Masson's trichrome staining) with no signs of foreign body reaction or recruitment of inflammatory cells. All collagen layers were aligned relatively parallel to the implant compared to the NHC group (Fig. 2.11). In the NHC group, a synovial layer is found in the intermediate layer between the innermost silicone contacting layer, which is the contact surface with the implant, and the outermost granulation layer in a complex collagen arrangement. The outer layer looks similar to the granulation tissue. The content of inflammatory cells demon-

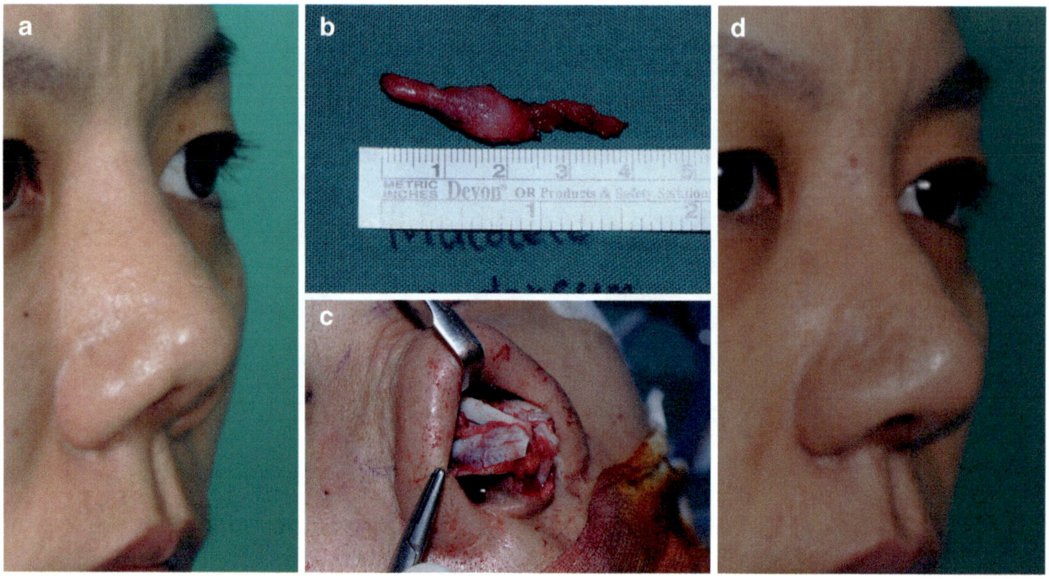

Fig. 2.10 Unhealthy capsule with contracture. (**a**) A 28-year-old female referred due to the severe contracture with dorsal fluctuation. (**b**) A thick pericapsular scar and a mucocele were removed. (**c**) Postoperative view. (**d**) Silicone was removed, and septal L-strut was extended using costal cartilage with anatomical crural batten graft

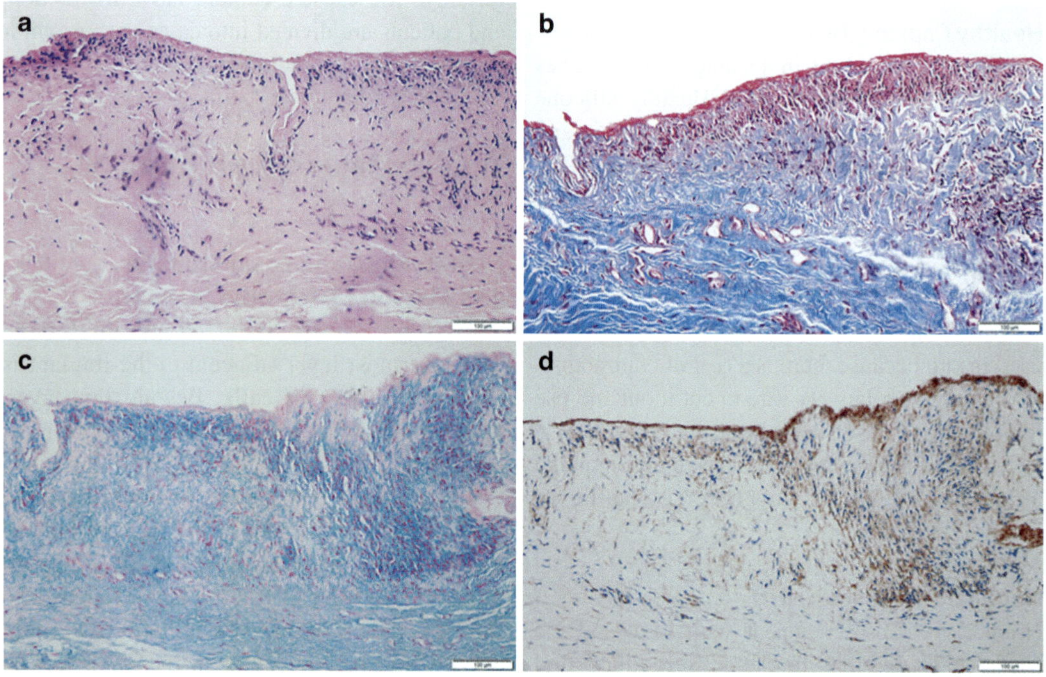

Fig. 2.11 Histology of a healthy capsule. (**a**) Hematoxylin and eosin staining, (**b**) Masson's trichrome staining, (**c**) Colloidal iron histochemical staining, (**d**) CD31 immunohistochemical staining of a healthy capsule at 200× magnification (Material from: Moon et al. Late-Onset Inflammation in Asian Rhinoplasty Using Alloplastic Implants, Aesthetic Plastic Surgery, 2020, Springer)

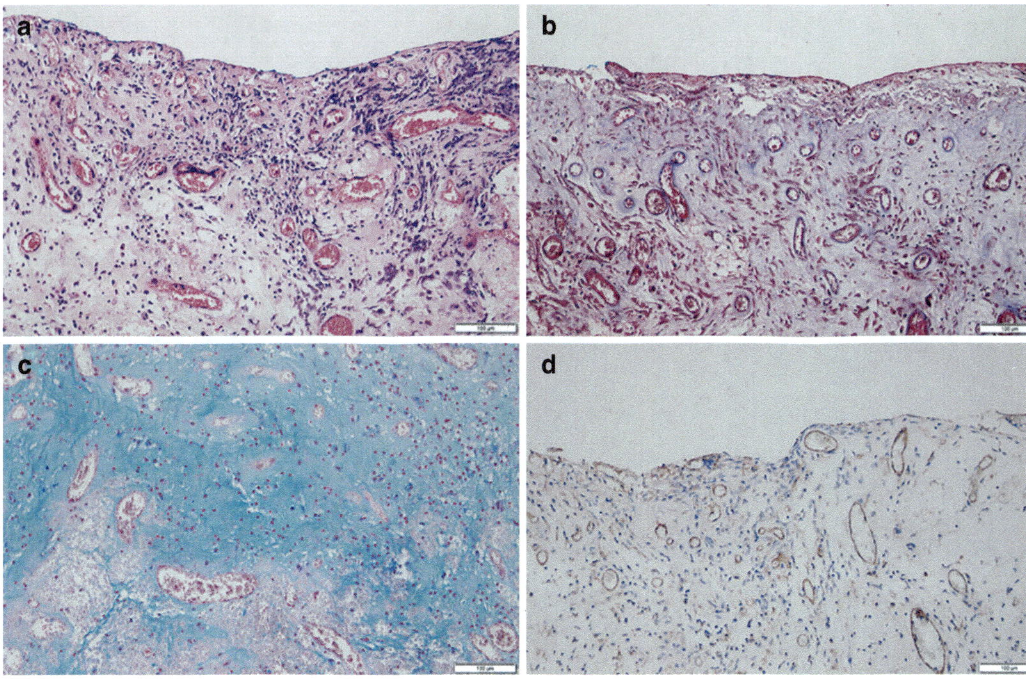

Fig. 2.12 Histology of a nonhealthy capsule. (**a**) Hematoxylin and eosin staining: irregular arrangement of collagen fibers. (**b**) Masson's trichrome staining: severe collagen degeneration. (**c**) Colloidal iron histochemical staining: intense blue staining shows mucin deposition. (**d**) CD31 immunohistochemical staining at 200× magnification. (Material from: Moon et al. Late-Onset Inflammation in Asian Rhinoplasty Using Alloplastic Implants, Aesthetic Plastic Surgery, 2020, Springer)

strated by the presence of macrophages and neutrophils also increased. However, no evidence of anaplastic large cell lymphoma or T cell proliferation was observed in the patients (Fig. 2.12).

Colloidal Iron Histochemical Staining

This staining determines the presence or absence of mucin. Mucin was found only in NHC; it was collected inside the capsule and lining. Although there was no evidence that the origin of mucin was from EPS of biofilm, the inner layer secreted it [14]. The endothelial component has grown in the capsule. Its vast amount and the multiple layers were found at the inner lining. The discovery of the endothelial layer found in the capsule's inner lining requires more research on whether it is endothelial metaplasia or mucosal metaplasia exposed during surgery (Fig. 2.12).

Immunohistochemical CD31 Staining

In the NHC group, the innermost layer, which was the surface in contact with the implant, consisted of the dense stratified lining of CD31-staining cells dispersed throughout the capsule. Breakage of endothelial or epithelial lining is also found, but it looks different depending on the site (Figs. 2.12 and 2.13).

The function of the inner layer and the synovial metaplasia around the implant can be seen as a good effect as a coating for sliding and lubrication between tissues and tissues to maintain synovial fluid around the implant. The late-onset inflammation response itself contributes to the development of tissue destruction through the continuous recruitment of pro-inflammatory cells such as macrophages and lymphocytes and the release of inflammatory mediators and proteases [15]. More research is needed to determine why complex inflammatory reaction

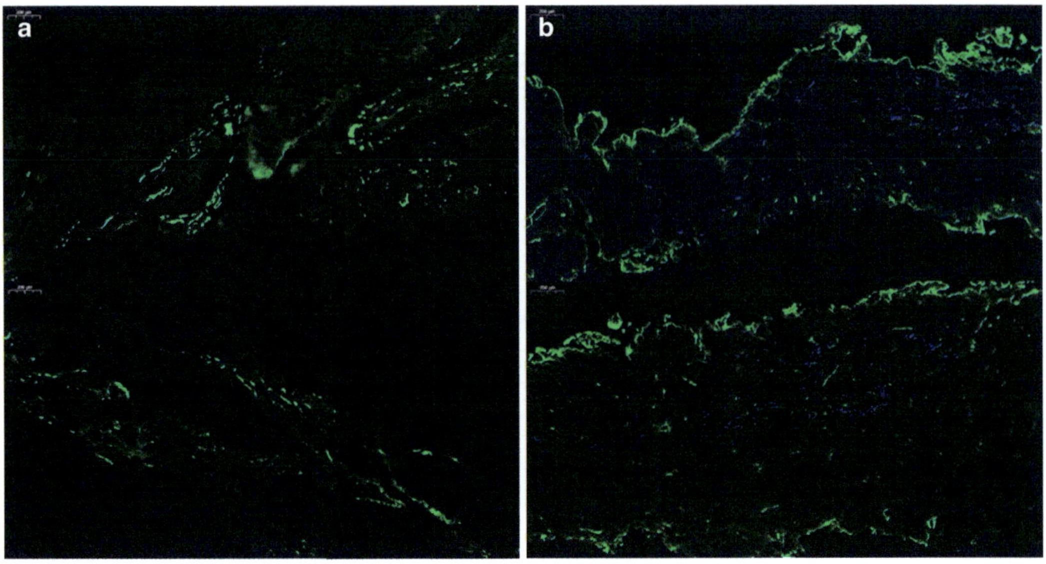

Fig. 2.13 Immunohistochemical staining of CD31 using a fluorescent dye at 200× magnification. (**a**) Healthy capsule: (**b**) Nonhealthy capsule: nonhealthy capsule shows continuous staining at the lumen with green color, which is endothelial hyperplasia of the inner layer

occurs in NHC, and mucus was accumulated inside while a thin single-layer capsule in HC does not. The author's conclusions to date are as follows.

- Damaged capsules and ingrowth of synovium-like mucosa or de novo proliferation of granulation tissues and inflammatory cells may play a crucial role in late-onset inflammation related to endothelial hyperplasia (or metaplasia).

Case Study 1: Granuloma-like Skin Lesion with Contracted Nose

A 28-year-old female underwent augmentation rhinoplasty using a silicone implant 8 years ago. During secondary septorhinoplasty, a silicone implant was found and removed. The lower lateral cartilages were mostly destroyed. The intracapsular space was filled with purulent fluids, and the capsule was totally excised. In the histological study, colloidal iron staining was markedly positive and Masson's trichrome staining showed collagen degeneration. She was managed with secondary septorhinoplasty using autogenous cartilage grafts after total release of contracted band (Fig. 2.14).

- A dense scar band forms the capsule in NHC. It attaches the upper lateral cartilage to the scroll area connecting the lower lateral cartilage.
- Resecting this contracture band is the surgical goal of the foreshortened nose correction.
- In some cases, until only the mucosal lining of the nasal cavity remains, LLC cannot be freely transferred to the caudal direction without tension. As more septal extension grafts are performed, the extent of release widens.

Case Study 2: LOI with the Loss of Mucosal Lining

A 22-year-old female patient was referred for intermittent swelling and a granuloma-like lesion on her right nasal mucosa that began 2 months ago. She underwent rhinoplasty using a silicone implant 2 years ago at another clinic. During secondary rhinoplasty, the capsule was filled with purulent fluid, and the capsule was totally

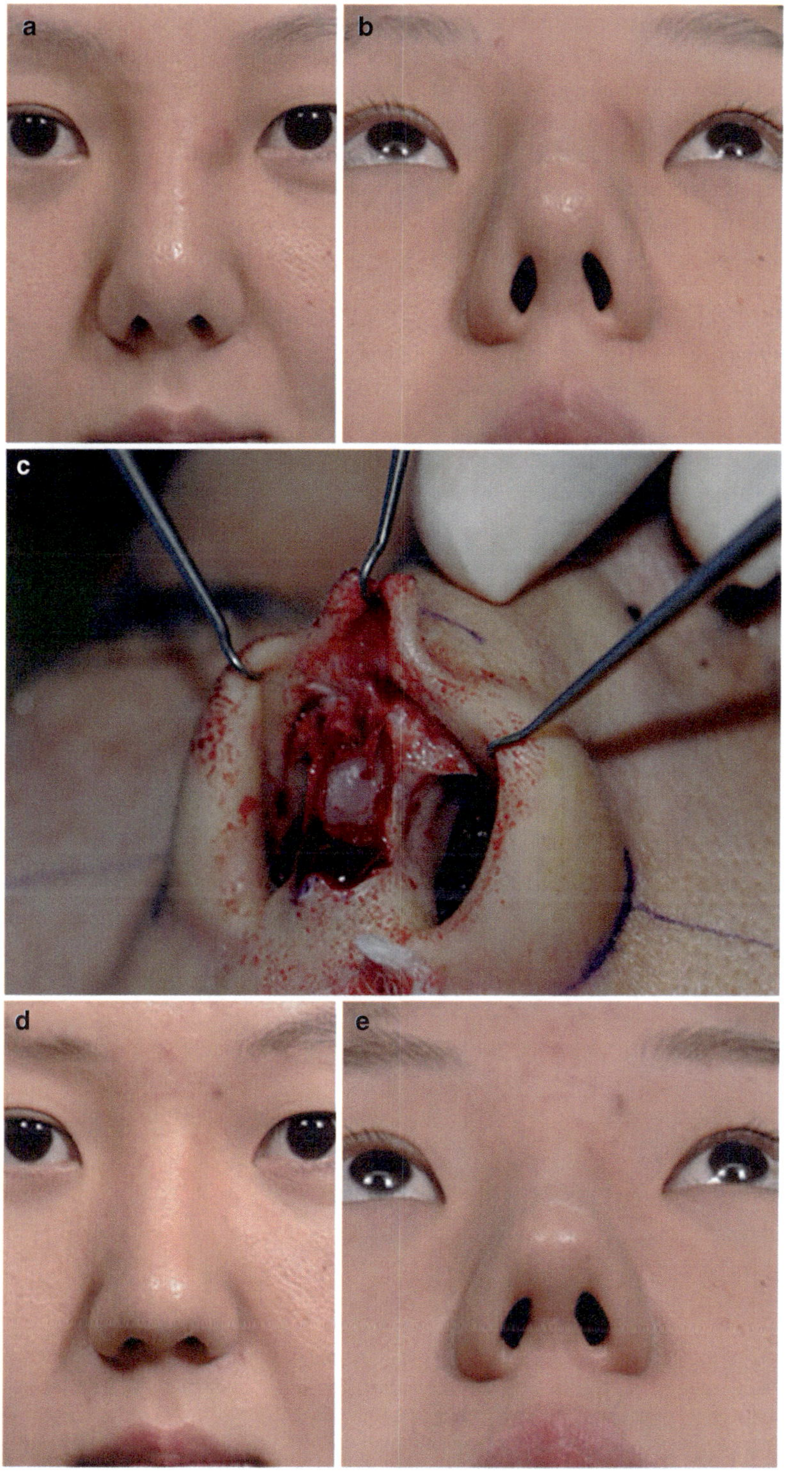

Fig. 2.14 Granuloma-like skin lesion with a contracted nose: A 28-year-old female underwent augmentation rhinoplasty using a silicone implant 8 years ago. (**a**, **b**) Preoperative views. (**c**) Intraoperative views. (**d**, Management of alloplast-related complications. Aesthetic Plastic Surgery of the East Asian Face) Six months after revisional septorhinoplasty. (Material from: Moon et al. Late-Onset Inflammation in Asian Rhinoplasty Using Alloplastic Implants, Aesthetic Plastic Surgery, 2020, Springer)

excised. For correction, two conchal cartilage were used. A sacral dermofat graft was grafted for nasal dorsal augmentation. The defect of the right membranous septum was sutured from inside and a small defect still remained after the repair. The wound was managed with wet dressing and prolonged antibiotics and healed after 5 days postoperatively.

- If the mucosal lining is damaged, the nasal cavity can be seen from the surgical pocket. It may not be possible to suture appropriately.
- Mucocele grows and ruptures into the nasal cavity, and the mucosal lining tends to be defective upon removal of a cyst.
- Care must be taken not to expose directly the graft cartilage and try to approximate the defect if the gap is located at the membranous septum.

Alloplastic materials should not be reused. Autograft should be adopted, and it is essential to use appropriate antibiotics for more days after the operation (Fig. 2.15).

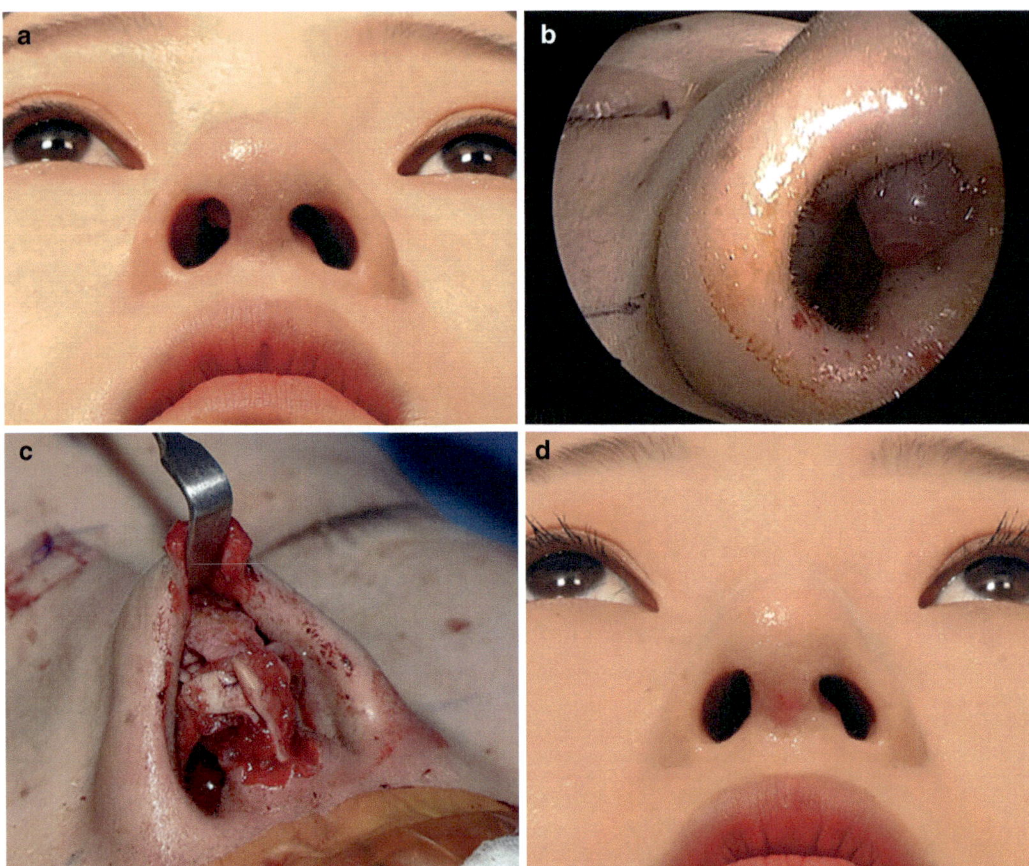

Fig. 2.15 LOI with the loss of mucosal lining: A 22-year-old female patient was referred for intermittent swelling and a granuloma-like lesion on her right nasal mucosa that began 2 months ago. Microbiological culture of the purulent fluid was identified as Staphylococcus aureus. She was successfully managed with purulent fluid drainage, silicone implant removal, capsulectomy, secondary septorhinoplasty using autogenous cartilage grafts, and intravenous antibiotics. (**a**) Preoperative views. (**b**, **c**) Intraoperative views. (**d**) Six months after revisional septorhinoplasty

References

1. Ottoline ACX, Tomita S, da Penha Costa Marques M, Felix F, Ferraiolo PN, Laurindo RSS. Antibiotic prophylaxis in otolaryngologic surgery. Int Arch Otorhinolaryngol. 2013;17(1):85–91.
2. Karaman E, Alimoglu Y, Aygun G, Kilic E, Yagiz C. Effect of septoplasty and preoperative antibiotic prophylaxis on nasal flora. B-ENT. 2012;8(1):13–9.
3. Mäkitie A. Postoperative infection following nasal septoplasty [Internet]. Acta Otolaryngolog. 2000;120:165–6. https://doi.org/10.1080/000164800454297.
4. Salkind AR, Rao KC. Antibiotic prophylaxis to prevent surgical site infections. Am Fam Phys. 2011;83(5):585–90.
5. Okur E, Yildirim I, Aral M, Ciragil P, Kiliç MA, Gul M. Bacteremia during open septorhinoplasty. Am J Rhinol. 2006;20(1):36–9.
6. Bandhauer F, Buhl D, Grossenbacher R. Antibiotic prophylaxis in rhinosurgery. Am J Rhinol. 2002;16(3):135–9.
7. Pajkos A, Deva AK, Vickery K, Cope C, Chang L, Cossart YE. Detection of subclinical infection in significant breast implant capsules. Plast Reconstr Surg. 2003;111(5):1605–11.
8. Patzakis MJ, Bains RS, Lee J, Shepherd L, Singer G, Ressler R, et al. Prospective, randomized, double-blind study comparing single-agent antibiotic therapy, ciprofloxacin, to combination antibiotic therapy in open fracture wounds. J Orthop Trauma. 2000;14(8):529–33.
9. Tham C, Lai Y-L, Weng C-J, Chen Y-R. Silicone augmentation rhinoplasty in an oriental population. Ann Plast Surg. 2005;54(1):1–5; discussion 6–7.
10. Jang YJ, Moon BJ. State of the art in augmentation rhinoplasty: implant or graft? Curr Opin Otolaryngol Head Neck Surg. 2012;20(4):280–6.
11. Donlan RM. Biofilms: microbial life on surfaces. Emerg Infect Dis. 2002;8(9):881–90.
12. Moreau-Marquis S, Stanton BA, O'Toole GA. Pseudomonas aeruginosa biofilm formation in the cystic fibrosis airway. Pulm Pharmacol Ther. 2008;21(4):595–9.
13. Moon K-C, Lee K-I, Lee J-S, Kim A-R, Dhong E-S, Kim D-W, et al. Late-onset inflammation in Asian rhinoplasty using alloplastic implants. Aesthetic Plast Surg [Internet]. 2020. https://doi.org/10.1007/s00266-020-01648-8.
14. Kasprzak A, Adamek A. Mucins: the old, the new and the promising factors in hepatobiliary carcinogenesis. Int J Mol Sci [Internet]. 2019;20(6). https://doi.org/10.3390/ijms20061288.
15. Galdiero M, Larocca F, Iovene MR, Martora F, Pieretti G, D'Oriano V, et al. Microbial evaluation in capsular contracture of breast implants. Plast Reconstr Surg. 2018;141(1):23–30.

3 Nasal Swab Culture: The Preparation for the Safe Surgery

Pearls

- Asian rhinoplasty can be categorized into two surgeries: septorhinoplasty and rhinoplasty that does not dissect the septum.
- Septorhinoplasty combining autografts is a clean-contaminated surgery that creates a complicated wound.
- Septorhinoplasty combining alloplastic implants is reasonably regarded as contaminated surgery.
- Reduction rhinoplasty is relatively safe from infection.
- A nasal swab is the simplest method and provides evidence of guidance for antibiotic therapy.
- SSI after the complicated septorhinoplasty results in a disastrous foreshortened nose.
- A nasal swab study showed that the prevalence rate of potentially infectious nasal flora (PINF) approximately 85%; MSSA and MSSE are most often identified.
- Using empirical antibiotics without a nasal swab study revealed the probability of resistance to these antibiotics up to 17%; In 3–17% of all patients, more than the first- and second-generation antibiotics are required for the undiagnosed PINF.
- According to the nasal swab results, applying mupirocin or quinolone ointment reduce PINF negative in 53% of positive patients.
- The nasal flora changes even after the surgery, so monitoring the bacterial change is necessary postoperatively, and if any inflammation is detected, efforts to change the primary antibiotics should be made.
- If the nasal swab is not available, quinolones will be appropriate for the complicated septorhinoplasty for the prevalent PINF.

Case Study 1

A 22-year-old female underwent primary septorhinoplasty with a dorsal silicone implant. SMR was performed for septal extension graft; since the nasion was low, a 3.5 mm-thick silicone implant was inserted into the dorsum. There were no other events during surgery, but the pocket bled more during septal surgery than others, but aPTT and BT were normal. Empirical first-generation cephalosporin was used from the day of surgery. The nasal packing was removed on the second day after surgery, and columellar stitches were removed on the fifth day. The septal hematoma was found at this time, and it was immediately drained, and the nose was repacked. However, she complained of generalized malaise and fever on the seventh postoperative day, and she was prescribed antipyretics. The packing was removed but swollen again. On the 11th postoperative day, pus was drained from the septum. Immediate revision underwent on that day, and all cartilages with the implant were removed. As a result of culture, pseudomonas aeruginosa was identified afterward. Antibiotics were changed to third-generation cephalosporin and aminoglycoside. After switching to susceptible antibiotics,

E.-S. Dhong, M.-W. Na, *Asian Septorhinoplasty*, https://doi.org/10.1007/978-981-16-0542-0_3

pus decreased, and cellulitis was also improved. However, cellulitis was improved entirely after switching to IV tobramycin and ceftazidime. For 3 months, pseudomonas was persistently cultured in the nasal swab (Fig. 3.1).

She later reconstructed using costal cartilage and is still awaiting more tip plasty (Fig. 3.2).

Case Study 2

A 46-year-old female visited the author with Lefort I and III fracture, and she underwent surgery. After 1 year, the L-shaped cantilever graft using costal cartilage was performed. An empirical second-generation cephalosporin was prescribed. On the fifth postoperative day, severe swelling and redness were noted. On the eighth day, cellulitis with the fluctuation deteriorated, so the pus was drained, and all rib cartilage was removed. As a result of culture, MRSA and MRSE were identified. After replacing the antibiotic with vancomycin, the amount of pus was reduced, and the cellulitis improved (Figs. 3.3 and 3.4). Subsequently, MRSA was intermittently identified in a nasal swab study until 1 year after the outpatient visit.

F/22 Primary: SRP: Septal extension + silicone
- Pseudomonas aeruginosa : for 3 months

Ticarc/K Clavulanate	S <= 16	**Gentamicin**	**I 8**
Amikacin	S 8	Imipenem	S <= 4
Aztreonam	S <= 8	Levofloxacin	R > 4
Ceftazidime	**S 4**	Meropenem	S <= 4
Ciprofloxacin	R > 2	**Tobramycin**	**S 2**
Ceftriaxone	I 32	Piperacillin/Tazobac	S <= 8
Cefotaxime	I 16		
Cefepime	S 4		

Fig. 3.1 Culture results of the pus drained; pseudomonas aeruginosa was positive by nasal swab study 3 months after the wound healed. (*R* resistant, *I* intermediate, *S* susceptible)

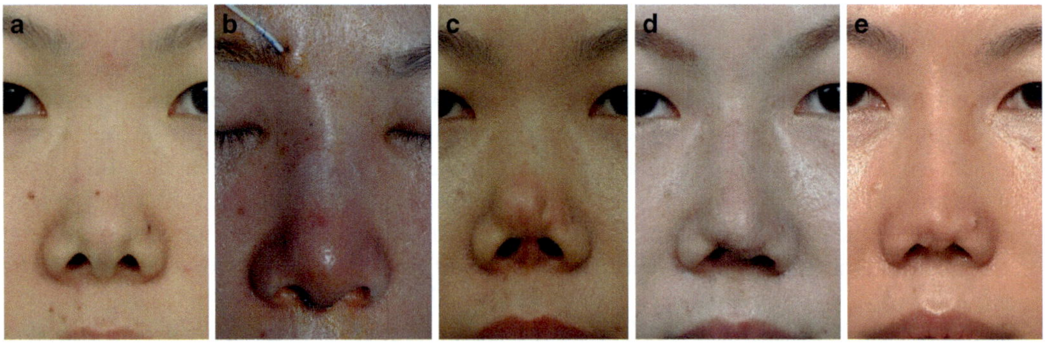

Fig. 3.2 Sequential AP photos. (**a**) Preoperative view. (**b**) After the pus was drained, all implants and grafts were removed, then a catheter was inserted for intermittent irrigation. (**c**) After the wound healed, severe foreshortening progressed. (**d**) After the nose was reconstructed using costal cartilages. (**e**) After the tip revision: The patient is awaiting a revision soon

Fig. 3.3 Culture results of the pus drained on the eighth postoperative day; MRSA was cultured by scheduled nasal swab study for one more year. (*R* resistant, *I* intermediate, *S* susceptible)

F/46 Revision: Costal Cartilage SRP.
- POD 8th day - For 1 year MRSA

Fusidic Acid	R > 16	Imipenem	R > 8
Teicoplanin	S < = 4	Meropenem	R > 8
Ticarc/K Clavulanate	R > 8	Ofloxacin	R > 4
Ampicillin	R > 8	**Oxacillin**	**R > 2**
Amox/K Clav(c)	R > 4/2	Penicillin	R > 8
Chloramphenicol	I 16	**Rifampin**	**S < = 1**
Clindamycin	R > 2	Trimethoprim/Sulfa	S < = 2/38
Cephalothin	R > 16	Synercid	S < = 1
Ciprofloxacin	R > 2	Tetracycline	R > 8
Cefotaxime	R > 32	**Vancomycin**	**S < = 2**
Cefuroxime	R > 16		
Cefazolin	R > 16		
Erythromycin	R > 4		
Cefepime	R > 16		
Gentamicin	R > 8		

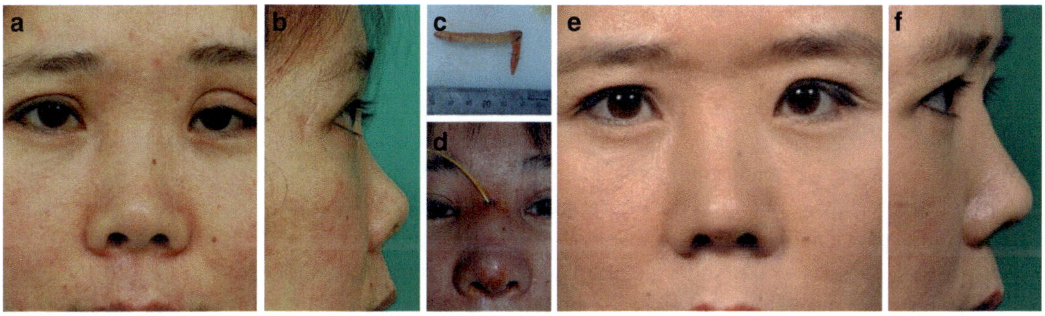

Fig. 3.4 Sequential photos. (**a**, **b**) Preoperative views: low nasion with foreshortening and Lt. eyelid ptosis. (**c**) Cantilever graft using costal cartilage before insertion. Ptosis correction was performed simultaneously. (**d**) After the pus was drained all grafts were removed, then a catheter was inserted for intermittent irrigation. (**e**, **f**) Three years later, she wanted a secondary rhinoplasty using silicone implants

3.1 What Did I Learn from these Patients?

The most painful moment in the author's Asian rhinoplasty-learning curve was the case of surgical site infection (SSI) involving septal pocket. These experiences are not well shared, but most doctors will have similar ones. Moreover, if a complex operation for several hours leads to bad results, the pain will be significant, and the patient's pain will be more profound.

- There are cases in which the surgical site infection cannot be prevented even with proper irrigation and antiseptic procedures.
- Empirical antibiotics are not enough.
- The complex wounds should be treated with susceptible antibiotics.
- A nasal swab study may be necessary for the procedure and preparation of the surgery.
- When pus-drainage occurs, it falls into an irreversible course, and there is no effect of continuous irrigation for cartilage salvage.

3.2 The Impact of SSI in Asian Septorhinoplasty

Framework Destruction

The technique of septal extension grafts in Asian rhinoplasty is increasing. Since submucosal resection (SMR) weakens the remaining septal strut, and even more frightening consequence is the septal framework's collapse after SSI (Fig. 3.1).

Once the framework collapses, continuous contraction or contracture occurs while waiting for a secondary operation, resulting in a foreshortened nose. The soft tissue results in irreversible contraction, which makes the secondary surgery difficult. Even when SSI is alleviated, inflammation of the soft tissues remains afterward.

Most secondary Asian rhinoplasty is an operation to lengthen the nose. Reconstruction of the framework is more difficult where the Medpor used.

- For patients who have undergone septal extension graft after SMR, the nasal dorsum is recommended to use autograft as possible.
- Conversely, patients who plan to use alloplastic materials for nasal dorsum are advised not to perform SMR concurrently.

3.3 The Potentially Infectious Normal Flora (PINF)

Among the potential bacterial pathogens (PBP), Staphylococcus aureus is the most problematic, and it has been reported that 33% and 41% were identified in the nasal vestibule and cavity, respectively. In other words, because Staphylococcus aureus was identified in the cavity where two-third of the total population was the vestibule, biofilms must also be taken into account in the nose. The inherent resistance to antimicrobial agents may be at the root of persistent and chronic bacterial infections [1].

However, many papers are claiming the uselessness of redundant antibiotic treatment in further studies. Assuming that the SSI rate after rhinoplasty is less than 1%, it is argued that antibiotic use is not supported [2, 3]. There is even a paper saying that topical antibiotics do not need to be used in rhinoplasty accompanied by septal surgery and do not need to be used pre- and postoperatively [4].

In a recent meta-analysis, similar conclusions have been drawn, and the use of antibiotics in nose surgery is discussed. Subsequently, the authors agree that there would have been no difference in SSI occurrence, whether used or not. Of course, when revision rhinoplasty and graft are required, there are cases where it is reported that the use of prophylactic antibiotics is meaningful [5]. However, as the author understands, the uselessness of antibiotic use has gained more sympathy until recently. There will be many refutations of the importance of the author's use of antibiotics in this chapter. The authors agree that redundant antibiotics lead to antibiotic resistance, while the patient's systemic condition deteriorates. However, reduction rhinoplasty should be distinguished from complex rhinoplasty. Reports are based on simple septoplasty-related surgeries, which quickly finish in a short time. If grafts and implants are not applied in Asian septorhinoplasty, the characteristics are entirely different. Asian septorhinoplasty is considered to be equivalent to or more complex than Western revision rhinoplasty.

PINF in Asian Septorhinoplasty

According to the author's study, Gram-positive microorganisms, such as Staphylococcus aureus (MSSA) and Staphylococcus epidermidis (MSSE), are frequently cultured. Among them, MRSA and MRSE strains cause problematic SSIs. Corynebacterium striatum is also cultured. Gram-negative microorganisms include Enterobacter aerogenes, Klebsiella pneumoniae, and Citrobacter spp. are frequently cultured [6] (Fig. 3.5). Among these, the problem would be the strain that resisted the first- and second-generation cephalosporin.

Fig. 3.5 Preoperative microbial profiles of nasal swab study; 72 patients in Cohort 2 and 326 patients in Cohort 3 were analyzed. (Material from: Moon et al. Preoperative Nasal Swab Culture: Is It Beneficial in Preventing Postoperative Infection in Complicated Septorhinoplasty?, Plastic and Reconstructive Surgery, 2020, Lippincott Williams & Wilkins)

Preoperative Microbiology Profiles

	Cohort 2 (%)	Cohort 3 (%)	*p*
No. of patients	72	326	
Negative	10 (13.9)	50 (15.3)	0.756*
Positive	62 (86.1)	276 (84.7)	0.756*
Gram-positive microorganisms	42 (58.3)	194 (59.5)	0.854*
Staphylococcus aureus (MSSA)	29 (40.3)	77 (23.6)	0.004*
Staphylococcus epidermidis (MSSE)	6 (8.3)	48 (14.7)	0.152*
Staphylococcus aureus (MRSA)	2 (2.8)	13 (4.0)	1.000†
Staphylococcus epidermidis (MRSE)	3 (4.2)	42 (12.9)	0.035*
Corynebacterium striatum	2 (2.8)	14 (4.3)	0.747†
Gram-negative microorganisms	20 (27.8)	82 (25.2)	0.978*
Enterobacter aerogenes	14 (19.4)	56 (17.2)	0.648*
Klebsiella pneumoniae	3 (4.2)	8 (2.5)	0.427†
Citrobacter spp.	1 (1.4)	8 (2.5)	1.000†
Others	2 (2.8)	10 (3.1)	1.000†

MSSA, methicillin-sensitive S. *aureus;* MSSE, methicillin-sensitive S. *epidermidis;* MRSA, methicillin-resistant S. *aureus;* MRSE, methicillin-resistant S. *epidermidis.*
*Pearson χ^2 test.
†Fisher's exact test.

Clean-Contaminated Wound

Septorhinoplasty should be considered a clean-contaminated surgery. Nose with late-onset inflammation (LOI) should be regarded as contaminated wounds if there is a puncture of the skin or drained discharge.

- For LOI with severe cellulitis, susceptible antibiotics should be used for at least 1 week before surgery. It is recommended to perform surgery after cellulitis decreases.

Complicated Septorhinoplasty for Asians

Among Asian septorhinoplasty, many surgeries correspond to septal surgery, cartilage graft, osteotomy, alloplastic material use, and secondary rhinoplasty. Most of them are considered complicated septorhinoplasty, and it is essential to take appropriate measures. The current description does not refer to a simple surgery that does not perform septal surgery with a simple rhinoplasty so that ULC and septum dissection are not performed.

Bacteremia During Operation

It is reasonable to assume that the patient is in a transient bacteremia during septal surgery. Of the septorhinoplasty, 13.5% of patients reported a bacteremia state, and the incidence was high in patients with severe postoperative bleeding. The bacteremia state worsened by nasal packing [7]. In most cases of head and neck surgery and maxillofacial surgery, it is essential to be aware that transient bacteremia may occur in patients from the moment of mucosal incision [8].

Nasal Packing: Intraoperative and Postoperative Management

Temporary nasal packing is essential during surgery. The author uses small-sized sponges soaked in a solution consisting of 50 CCs of 10% Povidone-iodine (Betadine), 1 g cefazolin, 80 mg gentamicin, and 500 CCs normal saline. Whenever transferring the instruments into the nasal vestibule, the instruments are cleansed with 70% alcohol. Cleansing is also applied when inserting and taking out an endoscope. While operating the external nose, the nasal cavity is packed with small sponges repeatedly. The author prefers much irrigation into the dissected pocket using the same solution 3–4 times (Fig. 3.6).

- While the external rhinoplasty is performed, the nasal cavity is packed with the soaked sponge. While the author performs septal surgery, packing is removed.
- All surgical instruments that have touched the nasal cavity should be cleaned with alcohol gauze during surgery.

For patients who underwent septal surgery, nasal packing is applied for 2–3 days postoperatively after surgery. The author uses a sufficient amount of susceptible ointment to the foam and pack. The authors prefer NasoPore® bioresorbable nasal dressing, which does not require packing out. On the second or third postoperative day, all packing is removed by suction.

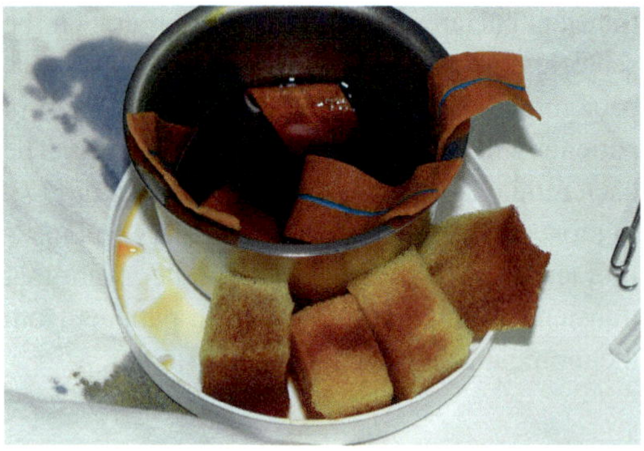

Fig. 3.6 Small sponges and nasal packing soaked in irrigation solution

3.4 Nasal Swab Study for PINF [6]

The efficacy of nasal swab study is high. One of the detection systems, VITEK2 (Biomérieux, Marcy-l'Étoile, France), reported excellent sensitivity/specificity of 99% and 96% for antibiotic susceptibility, according to MRSA, and the reporting time was quick within 6–18 h. Of course, there may be an error in the test method, and there is a possibility of a false-negative study. It is still the most convenient and rapid method of the nasal cavity in the existing and advantageous method for identifying vestibule strains. Although it costs, there is no reason not to do it for good results. Although extensive studies on septorhinoplasty have spoken about the ineffectiveness of antibiotics, the author cannot agree, at least in Asian septorhinoplasty [9].

Nasal Swab Negative

In our retrospective study, the number of patients with a culture-negative was 13.9–15.3% of the total when nasal swabs performed two weeks preoperatively. These patients do not experience SSI, even with empirical antibiotics. First- or second generation cephalosporin or amoxicillin-clavulanate may be prescribed.

Nasal Swab Positive

In the same study, the results of PINF were 84–86% of the total (Fig. 3.5). The prevalence of MSSA and MSSE was 23.6%–40.3% and 8.3%–14.7%, respectively. Then, MRSA and MRSE, which were not usually susceptible to empirical antibiotics, showed a frequency of 2.8%–4.0% and 4.2%–12.9%, respectively. Also, enterobacter aerogenes such as E-coli and Klebsiella pneumoniae showed 17.2%–19.4% and 2.5%–4.2% frequency, respectively. All these patients were identified to have resistant or intermediate sensitivity with empirical first or second-generation cephalosporin.

It is significant that MRSA, MRSE, and enterobacter, which are resistant to the empirical antibiotics of our hospital, were found at 4–17%. It was high, at least more than 4% of the total who undergo surgery, the empirical selection of antibiotics does not make any sense. At least it means that the antibiotic regimen of Quinolone or higher is correct.

Second Nasal Swab Positive

The results of the nasal swab performed immediately before surgery are shown in Fig. 3.7. MRSE was the most common at 9.8%, and the identification of MRSA was 1.8%, and the identification of Gram-negative microorganisms accounted for a large proportion of 8.9%. According to this result, antibiotics were changed and P.O. medication was also determined.

Changes in Microbiology

Positive to Negative Change

Two weeks before surgery, a susceptible ointment was applied to the found strain in the nasal cavity and swab again before the surgery to observe the change. As a result, the strain was no longer identified in 53.7% of the patients who showed positivity before surgery. There is no evidence that preoperative antibiotic ointment application to the nasal cavity prevents SIS. It is also risky that the application of lesional antibiotics with lesional irrigation may increase resistance to antibiotics. It has been reported that the effect of prophylactic antibiotic irrigation performed on intraoperative wounds is equivocal [10]. However, in terms of the effect of changing positive nasal swabs to negative, the authors judge that there is significant clinical significance (Fig. 3.8).

Negative to Positive Change

Instead, in the group of patients with negative cultures 2 weeks ago, 4.6% of patients showed positive nasal swab immediately before surgery. Here, there may be a new outbreak of PINF because ointment treatment was not performed before the surgery, or the first test may have been a false negative.

Positive to Positive

Even though the ointment was applied, 31% of patients showed identification of PINF. Most of them were identified with the same strain, and in a few, a change occurred as different strands. Because

Fig. 3.7 Microbiology profiles performed immediately before surgery; 326 patients in Cohort 3 were analyzed. (Material from: Moon et al. Preoperative Nasal Swab Culture: Is It Beneficial in Preventing Postoperative Infection in Complicated Septorhinoplasty?, Plastic and Reconstructive Surgery, 2020, Lippincott Williams & Wilkins)

Microbiology Profiles Performed Immediately before Surgery

	Cohort 3 (%)
No. of patients	326
Negative	210 (64.4)
Positive	116 (35.6)
Gram-positive microorganisms	88 (27.0)
Staphylococcus aureus (MSSA)	15 (4.6)
Staphylococcus epidermidis (MSSE)	23 (7.1)
Staphylococcus aureus (MRSA)	6 (1.8)
Staphylococcus epidermidis (MRSE)	32 (9.8)
Corynebacterium striatum	12 (3.7)
Gram-negative microorganisms	28 (8.9)
Enterobacter aerogenes	4 (1.2)
Klebsiella pneumoniae	5 (1.5)
Citrobacter spp.	0 (0.0)
Others	19 (5.8)

MSSA, methicillin-sensitive S. *aureus;* MSSE, methicillin-sensitive S. *epidermidis;* MRSA, methicillin-resistant S. *aureus;* MRSE, methicillin-resistant S. *epidermidis.*

Microbiology Profile changes in Cohort 3

	Cohort 3 (%)
No.	326
Negative → negative	35 (10.7)
Negative → positive	15 (4.6)
Positive → positive	101 (31.0)
Positive → negative	175 (53.7)

Fig. 3.8 Microbiology profile change in 326 patients of septorhinoplasty. (Material from: Moon et al. Preoperative Nasal Swab Culture: Is It Beneficial in Preventing Postoperative Infection in Complicated Septorhinoplasty?, Plastic and Reconstructive Surgery, 2020, Lippincott Williams & Wilkins)

the area where the ointment is applied is mainly the nostril, where the columella and marginal incision will be made, the bactericidal role may be insignificant. Applying ointment may not affect the nasal vestibule's bacteria, and there is a possibility that the bacteria will remain in the nasal cavity.

3.5 My Protocol for a *SAFE* Asian Septorhinoplasty

Nasal Swab Culture: Two Times

All patients underwent preoperative nasal swab cultures 2 weeks before surgery. After the internal nose was cleaned using a cotton swab wetted with saline solution, the nasal vestibule was swabbed using a culture swab. The nasal swab sample was immediately stored in an aseptic tube for subsequent culture. The nasal swab culture is repeated immediately before surgery in the operating room using the same method as the first preoperative nasal swab culture.

- The reason for doing two nasal swabs is that the strain of PINF may change in the timeline, or there may be false negatives in the initial nasal swab.
- If the second strain changes, an effort should be made to replace the primary antibiotics with a susceptible one.
- In our study, 4.6% of the total were negative in the first nasal swab and then changed to positive in the second, so empirical antibiotics may be of no use in some of this patient group.

Applying Antibiotic Ointment

Topical antibiotics were not applied in culture-negative patients. However, when microorganisms were isolated, the patients were taught to apply ointment at home for 5 days before the surgery at least three times a day. Two types of antibiotic ointments were used, mupirocin (Bactroban, GlaxoSmithKline, London, United Kingdom) and ofloxacin (Tarivid, Santen, Japan). In brief, mupirocin ointment was used for the decolonization of mupirocin-sensitive microorganisms. Ofloxacin ointment was used in sensitive microorganisms, including mostly such as MRSE, MRSA, and enterobacter.

- There are criticisms that the use of preoperative antibiotic ointment may lead to antibiotic resistance, but previous studies have reported that the identification of PINF decreased when antibiotic was applied to nasal packing during surgery.
- The author's study also confirmed that the strain found before surgery in 53.7% of patients disappeared, which is the basis [6].

The Choice of IV Antibiotics

The empirical antibiotics for the culture-negative patient and MSSA patients were the first-generation cephalosporin. In the case of patients whose strains were identified in the culture, susceptible antibiotics were administered pre- and postoperatively as a rule. Typically, many patients with MRSE and enterobacter were sensitive to ciprofloxacin. Simultaneously, MRSA mostly received vancomycin as the first-line prophylactic antibiotics. For patients with both methicillin- and ciprofloxacin-resistant S. aureus and S. epidermidis, intravenous teicoplanin, or vancomycin was administered.

However, when de novo bacteria were isolated in the second preoperative nasal swab cultures and were resistant to the previous prophylactic antibiotics, the intravenous prophylactic antibiotics were changed. The new antibiotic was administered intravenously for 3 days and then orally for the next 4 days (Fig. 3.9).

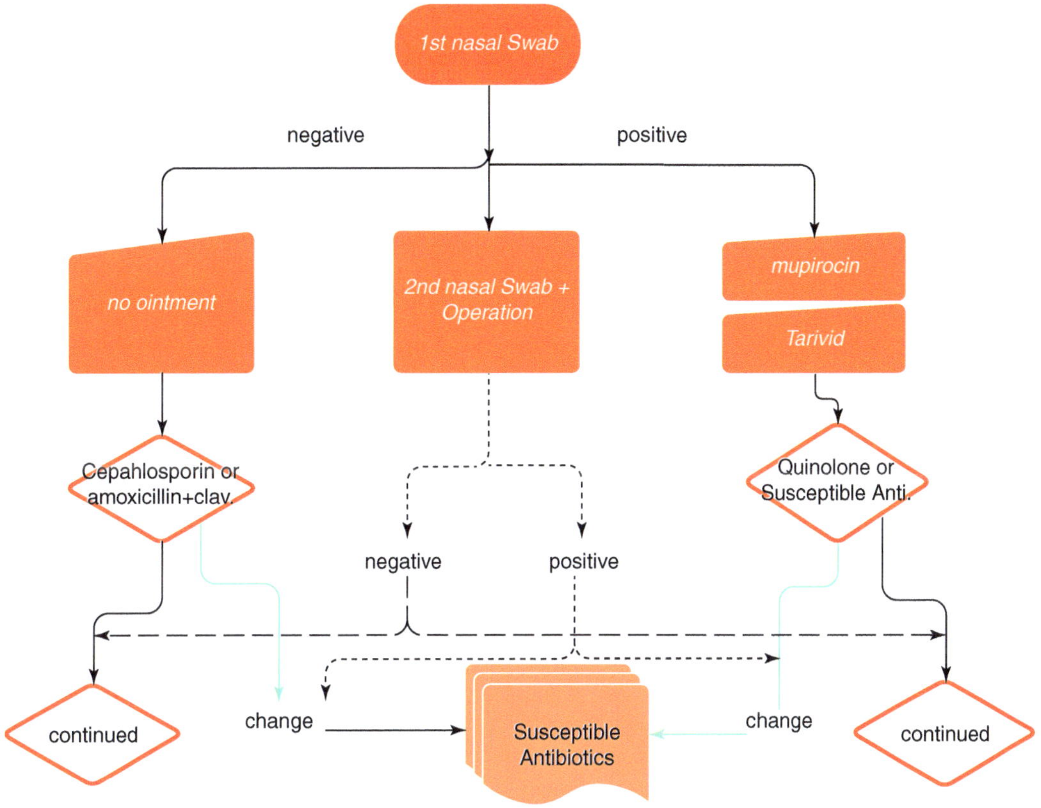

Fig. 3.9 Flow sheet of my protocol for a safe septorhinoplasty

References

1. Glück U, Gebbers JO. The nose as bacterial reservoir: important differences between the vestibule and cavity. Laryngoscope. 2000;110(3 Pt 1):426–8.
2. Nuyen B, Kandathil CK, Laimi K, Rudy SF, Most SP, Saltychev M. Evaluation of antibiotic prophylaxis in rhinoplasty: a systematic review and meta-analysis. JAMA Facial Plast Surg. 2019;21(1):12–7.
3. Georgiou I, Farber N, Mendes D, Winkler E. The role of antibiotics in rhinoplasty and septoplasty: a literature review. Rhinology. 2008;46(4):267–70.
4. Yoder MG, Weimert TA. Antibiotics and topical surgical preparation solution in septal surgery. Otolaryngol Head Neck Surg. 1992;106(3):243–4.
5. Schäfer J, Pirsig W. Preventive antibiotic administration in complicated rhinosurgical interventions—a double-blind study. Laryngol Rhinol Otol. 1988;67(4):150–5.
6. Moon K-C, Jung J-E, Dhong E-S, Jeong S-H, Han S-K. Preoperative nasal swab culture: is it beneficial in preventing postoperative infection in complicated septorhinoplasty? Plast Reconstr Surg. 2020;146(1):27e–34e.
7. Okur E, Yildirim I, Aral M, Ciragil P, Kiliç MA, Gul M. Bacteremia during open septorhinoplasty. Am J Rhinol. 2006;20(1):36–9.
8. Koc S, Uysal IO, Uysal EB, Yenişehirli G, Duygu F. The comparison of bacteremia and amount of bleeding during septoplasty. Eur Arch Otorhinolaryngol. 2012;269(4):1139–42.
9. Kullar R, Frisenda J, Nassif PS. The more the Merrier? Should antibiotics be used for rhinoplasty and septorhinoplasty?—a review. Plast Reconstr Surg Glob Open. 2018 Oct;6(10):e1972.
10. de Jonge SW, Boldingh QJJ, Solomkin JS, Allegranzi B, Egger M, Dellinger EP, et al. Systematic review and meta-analysis of randomized controlled trials evaluating prophylactic intra-operative wound irrigation for the prevention of surgical site infections. Surg Infect. 2017;18(4):508–19.

4 Medpor: The Hurdle of Secondary Rhinoplasty

Pearls

- Medpor has high tissue integration; the destruction of the surrounding tissue is devastating when the Medpor is removed.
- When Medpor was applied to the septum, the part that contacts the septal cartilage causes damage to the adjacent quadrangular cartilage, and the part that reaches the mucosa causes mucosal thinning and perforation.
- Extrusion or infection cannot be treated with antibiotics. Medpor should be removed.
- Micropore can be a breeding ground for bacterial growth, causing late-onset inflammation.
- Dorsal alloplastic implant and septal Medpor use are the worst combinations in late-onset inflammation communicating the septal pocket with dorsal implant capsule.

4.1 Physical Properties

The Medpor implant is made of a medical-grade, high-density polyethylene that is sintered to create a somewhat flexible framework of interconnecting pores [1]. The pore size ranges from 160 to 368 μm and more than half of these pores are larger than 150 μm in diameter. Since 1985, MEDPOR porous polyethylene implants have provided you with a range of off the shelf, biocompatible implant options for esthetic and reconstruction. Microthin, ultrathin, and sheet form is ready up to 0.25–3 mm. The vascular and fibrous ingrowth leads to excellent integration and stabilization of the implant and decreased rates of infection once the implant complex has formed [2]. Mainly, thin Medpor has been used for the nose in Asia. Thin Medpor is used for the septal application, and thick Medpor is used for nasal dorsum. Currently, it is mainly used for septal extension in Asian rhinoplasty.

4.2 Complication Reports

There are still many debates in the Asian rhinoplasty society. Medpor shortens surgery time, is easy to use for septal extension or extended septal extension, has an excellent functional outcome and reports that complication is not a problem in the long-term follow-up [3–6]. It is argued that only two of the 27 patients had a long-term extrusion, but due to their thin physical properties, the nasal cross-sectional area was wider than that of the septal cartilage after surgery. Here, two out of 27 are 7%. In one meta-analysis, the removal rate of silicone was 6.1%, and the removal rate of Medpor was 3.1%, and the safety of tissue integrating was reported [7]. However, the infection rate was reported as 4% for silicone and 6% for Medpor, and the extrusion of Medpor as 2%. The difference between these reports is that the

Supplementary Information The online version of this chapter (https://doi.org/10.1007/978-981-16-0542-0_4) contains supplementary material, which is available to authorized users.

E.-S. Dhong, M.-W. Na, *Asian Septorhinoplasty*, https://doi.org/10.1007/978-981-16-0542-0_4

Medpor use would be different. It remains unfortunate that this report comes only with complication rates. Each author might use Medpor at different sites such as the septum, membranous septum, columella, or dorsum.

The author has only bad memories of Medpor. Every single case was problematic due to the Medpor use. It is necessary to rethink the stability of this material based on science.

Due to the physical characteristics, Medpor provides stable support even with a thin thickness and maintains stability by the tissue's ingrowth. However, refutation on long-term stability without resorting to suture is below.

- The tissue ingrowth of Medpor, upon removal, destroys the surrounding tissue.
- When applied to the septum, the contact causes damage to the adjacent quadrangular cartilage and mucosal tear or perforation.
- Extrusion or infection cannot be treated with drugs. It must be removed.
- Silicone makes soft tissue called capsule or scar around, while Medpor is challenging to remove and cause soft tissue loss.
- The pore can be a breeding ground for bacterial growth.
- Secondary surgery is complicated due to adhesion.

The above reasons alone indicate that Medpor use is the leading cause of the most challenging complications in Asian septorhinoplasty. Any surgery cannot be convinced that it is the patient's last surgery.

Since the surgeon is not sure that he or she is the last surgeon, consideration should be given to reoperations that may occur next. Therefore, Medpor is not a good material for any septorhinoplasty.

As shown in Fig. 4.1, the vast high septal perforation is very difficult to reconstruct because of its location. Such complications would be a peculiar complication found only in Asia. Multiple septal perforations are also a typical complication due to Medpor. Septum reconstruction is impossible if these patients accompany framework collapse.

4.3 Why Is Medpor Such a Big Hurdle for Secondary Operation?

The physical characteristics of stiffness, micropores, and tissue integration are obstacles to the secondary operation.

The bilateral ingrowth of surrounding tissues should be removed and damaged while Medpor is removed.

- When Medpor is applied directly to the quadrangular cartilage, the septal cartilage and mucosa are simultaneously inflicted.
- If Medpor is applied to both sides of the quadrangular cartilage, the damage is more severe.

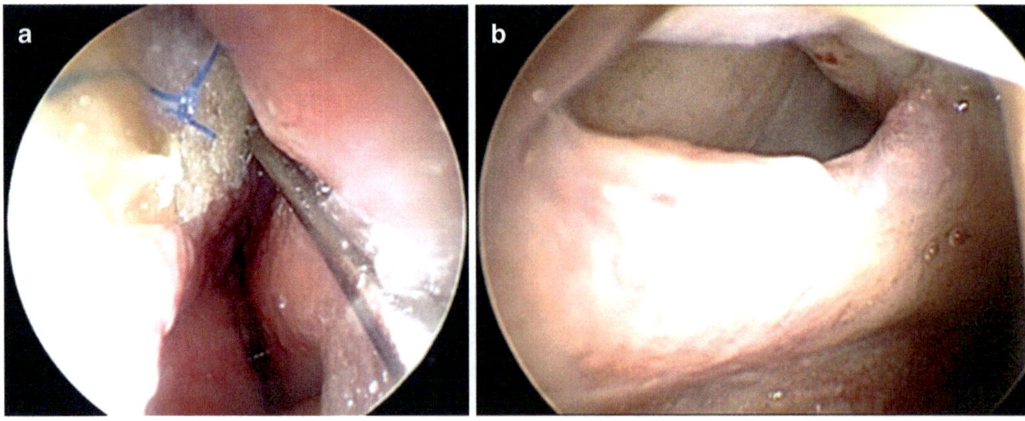

Fig. 4.1 Huge high septal perforation. (**a**) Before removing the Medpor and crust. (**b**) After removing the Medpor

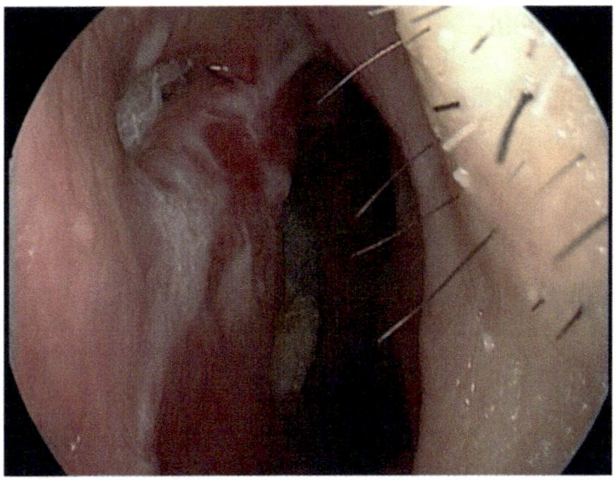

Fig. 4.2 Multiple perforations of the septum at the high septum and ethmoid-quadrangular cartilage junction

- In many cases, the reconstruction is impossible; multiple septal perforations would be the worst cases (Fig. 4.2).
- Microscopically, Medpor was covered with fibrous collagenous tissue, partially bridging through the pores. Inflammatory cells had infiltrated around the polyethylene [8].
- Micropores can cause late-onset inflammation.

In our study, 22% of the patients found Medpor in secondary septorhinoplasty. Of these patients, 28% had extrusion or puncture. In other words, in the author's experience, it is reasonable to say that Medpor can be found in one of five secondary surgeries in which the alloplastic materials are scheduled to be removed.

Patients are divided into cases with and without accurate previous operative information. 21% of them were draining pus or swollen with dorsal fluctuation. Most patients were inserted silicone or Gore-tex implants on the nasal dorsum and Medpor at their septum. Therefore, it is impossible to distinguish whether the cause of late-onset inflammation is Medpor or dorsal implant. However, based on the fact that the most pus pocket is connected to the Medpor, it is evident that the inflammation starts from Medpor.

- Since Medpor has high tissue integration, dorsal inflammation is not transferred to septal Medpor.
- Relatively, late-onset inflammation caused by Medpor is more likely to spread to the dorsal capsular pocket. This is why the LOI starts from septal Medpor.

The complication is characterized by intermittent nasal dorsal tenderness, swelling, and sometimes granuloma-like skin lesions. In severe cases, puncture with fluid drainage on the external or intranasal area may be present. Late-onset inflammation may result in significant esthetic and functional complications. In any case, the problem is fundamentally solved by removing the entire Medpor.

Dissectiblity

It is difficult to dissect the area where Medpor was applied. The greater the integration between tissues, the more difficult it is to dissect. If nasal framework damage occurs after excision, it may not be possible to remove the entire Medpor. It is advantageous for subsequent reconstruction leaving as much of the adjacent soft tissue as possible.

The preservation of mucosa is the most critical factor in the success or failure of the surgery.

4.4 What Do you Have to Prepare for the Reconstruction?

CT Scan: The Only Aid for Preoperative Diagnosis

It is impossible to obtain all surgical records or the history of accurate alloplastic use from patients with 3–6 previous surgeries. Of course, it is helpful for reoperation if there are detailed surgical records. However, if there is scanty information, computed tomography is the only diagnostic tool.

In the bone setting, there is no help other than checking the dorsum's alloplastic material. Changing the contrast to the abdomen (W 250 L50) or mediastinum (W450 L 45) and rotating the axial view would show "hypolucent Medpor shadow." Based on CT information, then the intranasal inspection should be accurately repeated by pressing the dorsum with a finger, and carefully observing the caudal septum through anterior rhinoscopy.

- A septal extension graft should be suspected if the caudal septal end cannot be observed with an anterior rhinoscope without the gap of the membranous septum.
- Pushing down with a finger touches the hardness or causes pain in the patients; suspects the Medpor use.

However, it is more important than anything else to control the contrast in CT scan and find a shadow with hypodensity (Video 4.1).

In the first case of each patient, the patient was not aware of Medpor use, and the actual operation for this image is shown (Fig. 4.3). Batten type septal extension graft can be seen in two layers under the silicone implant [9]. Since the pus pocket did not invade the septal Medpor, in this case, the pus was not drained from the septum, and the destruction was relatively small. Still, Medpor was in contact with the pus pocket, so the complete removal was necessary. In the second video, the operation was performed due to pain, and the anterior-caudal part of the septum was severely destroyed (Video 4.2, Fig. 4.4). In CT, Medpors with hypolucent density were found in a wide area.

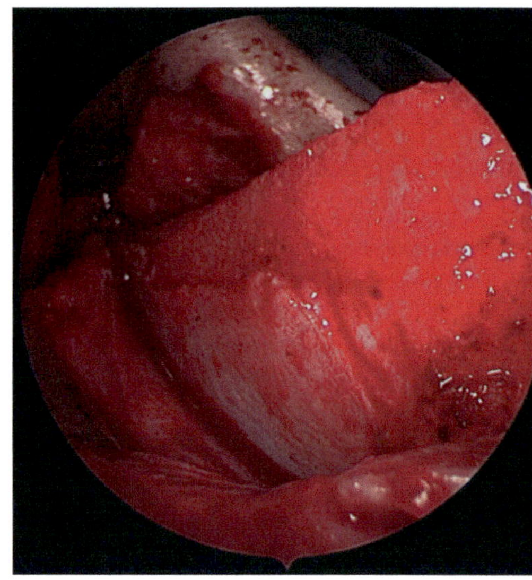

Fig. 4.4 A long and huge Medpor was found in one piece at the anterocaudal septum. The anterocaudal margin was destructed already before removing it

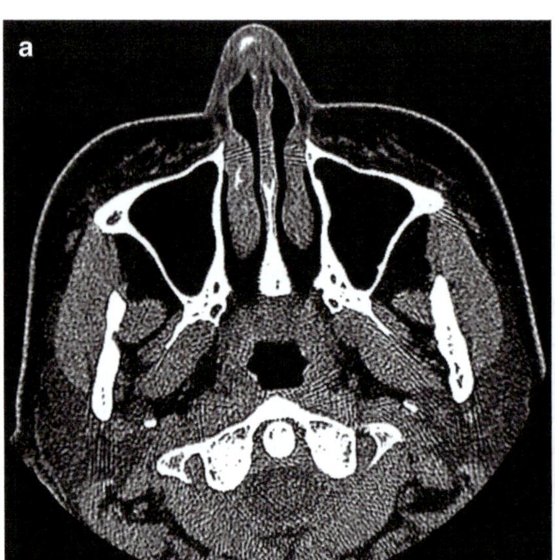

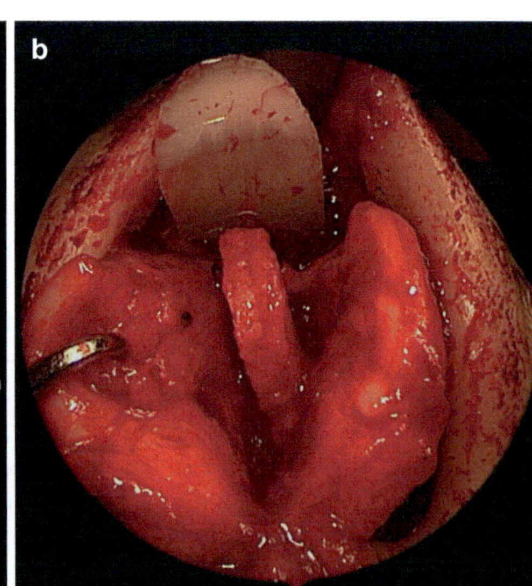

Fig. 4.3 Batten type septal extension by Medpor was found under the silicone implant. (**a**) Axial CT scan. (**b**) Intraoperative view

Autograft for the Septal Reinforcement

To rebulid the detroyed septum, the amount required should be larger than the actual size. Since the destruction of the rhinion weakens the fixation force, there is a high possibility of saddle nose deformity after surgery. Also, much effort is required to get the dorsal esthetic line smooth. There are many problems because the septal part is also fragile, and there is no supporting force. Significantly, the posterior septal angle is often required to obtain strong support. The extent to which the mucous membrane on the other side has been destroyed determines the operability.

4.5 Patterns of Medpor Application

Septal Application

Anterior Application

This is a method for applying Medpor in the same way as Dr. Byrd's spreader type septal extension. It leads to severe deficits, as shown in Fig. 4.1. Particularly crucial in part is that it involves the rhinion, which makes the reconstruction difficult. Ten years ago, this technique was popular in the form of a projection by emphasizing the boomerang type nasal tip. The high septal destruction is the most difficult of all complications.

Case Study 1: Deviation with Pain and Stiffness

A 24-year-old female underwent septorhinoplasty 2 years before the referral. The history described SMR, harvesting ear cartilage, and corrective osteotomies. One year later, 2 mm thick silicone was inserted for the esthetic dissatisfaction.

The patient complained of pain and stiffness in the nose and implant deviation in the nose.

The biggest problem was nasal congestion, and the NOSE score was 14/20 points. There were no records or information on Medpor use. A spreader type Medpor was found in the surgical pocket (Fig. 4.5).

The dorsal and tip projection did not change much, but all of the alloplastic materials were replaced with autografts. Pain has disappeared. That is a significant change (Figs. 4.6 and 4.7).

Caudal Application

Mainly Dr. Byrd's batten type, Medpor attaches to the caudal portion of the quadrangular cartilage, extends to the membranous septum, and projects the nasal tip. Injury to the cartilage in the caudal portion can be detected, and a severe reduction of the tip projection that loses support should be prepared after removal (Fig. 4.8).

Anterocaudal Application

Anterocaudal application yields the most severe case. The Medpor applied to the entire anterocaudal septum can be found along the patient's L-strut. Most patients complain of pain. The patient's nose is moving left to right but has restrictions in the anterocaudal direction. Therefore, even subtle nose movements can cause pain and discomfort. In particular, patients feel discomfort in mimetic movement, especially in making the "o" pronunciation. The tip of the nose is stiff. If Medpor is found in late-onset inflammation, salvaging the nose length would be difficult.

Case Study 2: Late-Onset Inflammation

A 31-year-old man, a patient with a nasal bone fracture 14 years ago was transferred to the author after four surgeries. Septoplasty was performed after a nasal bone fracture, but the exact history was not remembered. Two years ago, augmentation rhinoplasty underwent using silicone implants. One year later, the tip plasty and silicone were replaced twice. In history, the information of Medpor use was unclear, and for several months before the visit, the swelling and subside was repeated after taking empirical antibiotics. Just before the visit, the scar band and hard foreign body descending to the columella were palpable, and the skin thinning was found to the extent that impending puncture was suspicious

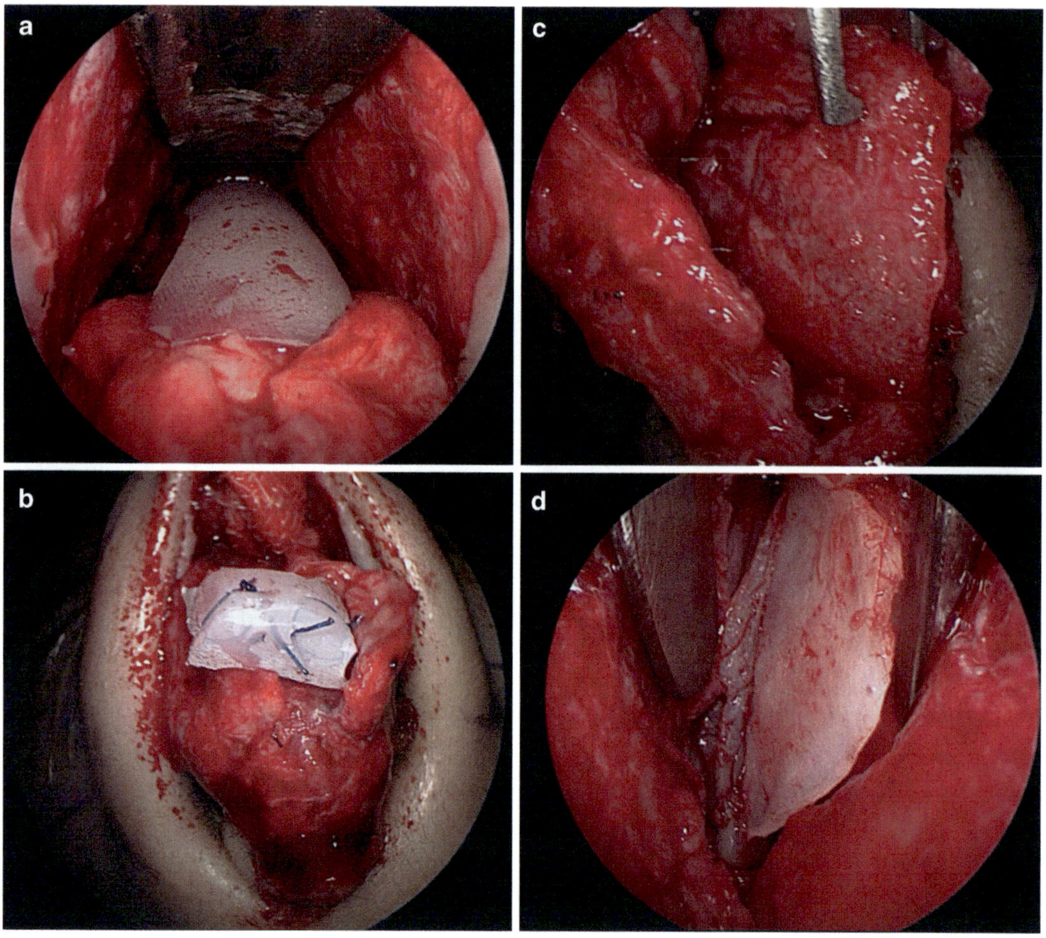

Fig. 4.5 Dorsal silicone implant with septal Medpor use. (**a**) Dorsal silicone. (**b**) Tip silicone was found first before approaching the dorsum. (**c**) Batten type one-piece Medpor at the right caudal margin. (**d**) After removing the Medpor, the caudal septal margin was attenuated and fractured

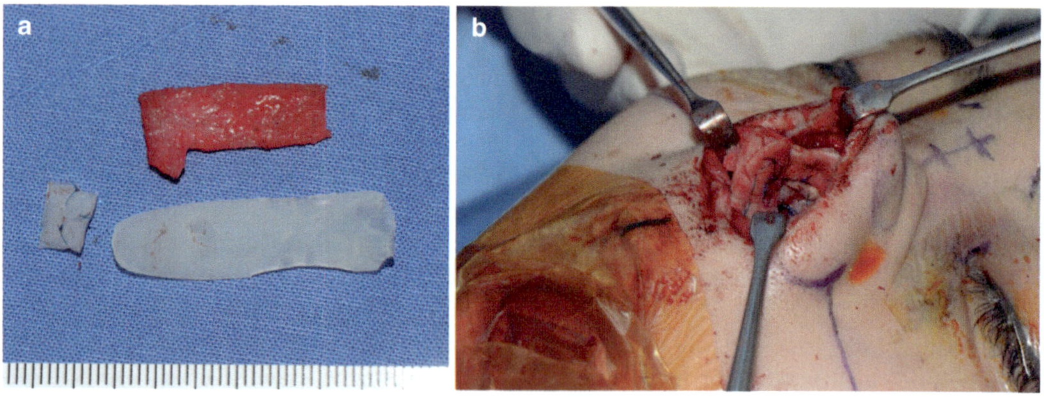

Fig. 4.6 Substitutes of the surgery. (**a**) Removing the alloplastic materials: dorsal silicone, tip silicone, and septal Medpor. (**b**) Reconstructing the L-strut using two conchas

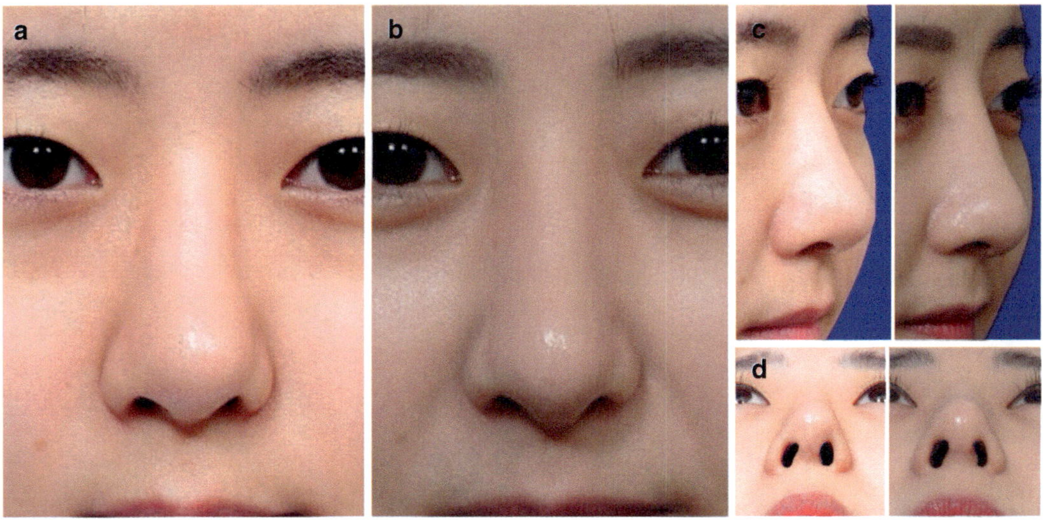

Fig. 4.7 Pre- and postoperative views. (**a**) Preoperative view: dorsal implant deviation to Lt. side. (**b**) Postoperative 1 year view. (**c**) Quarter view: Lt. preoperative, Rt. postoperative view. (**d**) Basal view: Lt. preoperative, Rt. postoperative view

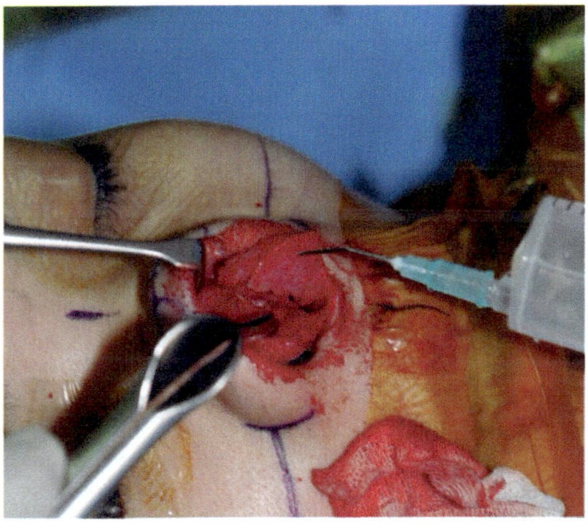

Fig. 4.8 Caudal unilateral batten type application of Medpor

(Fig. 4.9). Several silicone pieces were found in the surgical field, and Medpors applied in two layers to the anterior septum, and two layers to the caudal septum were found, and the capsule existing in the surrounding scar had to be removed (Fig. 4.10). Also, as shown in the following method, the septal L-strut was rebuilt using two ear cartilage. The superficial mastoid fascia was grafted to minimize dorsal irregularity (Fig. 4.11).

Case Study 3: Pain with Saddle Nose Deformity

A 21-year-old female patient came to the hospital with persistent discomfort after surgery. Recently, she felt a pulling down sensation and pain when speaking and laughing. A saddle nose and drooping nose deformity were found. In the surgical field, four pieces of Medpor were found at the anterocaudal portions of the L-strut. She underwent L-strut reconstruction using two conchal cartilage using the same technique (Figs. 4.12 and 4.13).

Columella Application

A relatively small amount of Medpor can be found in the columella, and if the LLC surrounds, it is relatively less in the case of extrusion. Even the smallest amount of Medpor cannot be said to be without problems.

Nasal Pain

A characteristic symptom of patients who are applied Medpor is unknown pain; pain is believed

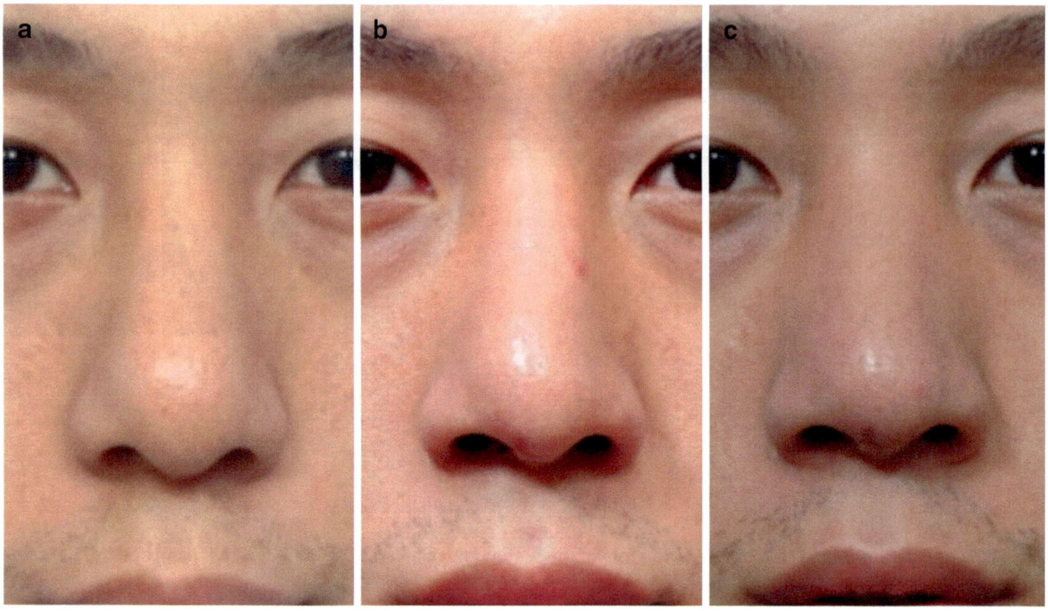

Fig. 4.9 Repetition of swelling and skin puncture due to Medpor. (**a**) He visited the author with a swollen nose. (**b**) He visited 2 months later for the secondary surgery. The swelling has subsided after the columellar discharge and antibiotics. (**c**) Postoperative view

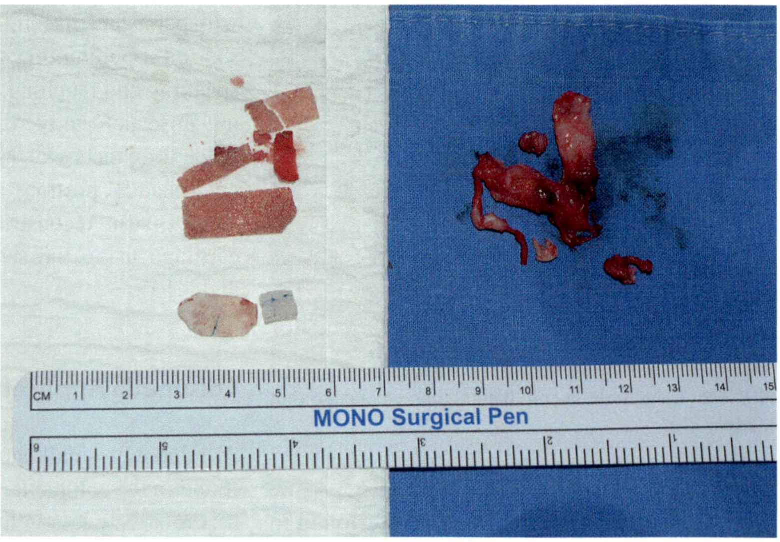

Fig. 4.10 Excised alloplastic materials: Medpors, two silicone pieces at the dorsum, and old nonhealthy capsules

to be due to the physical properties. The plate is more rigid than the autogenous tissue, so constant physical pressure is applied to the surrounding tissue. The good thing about tissue incorporation is that it is closely attached after the suture loses integrity. There must be constant movement in the normal scroll area or hinge area. However, the central component with Medpor is not as movable as the lateral component. Mucoperichondrium, Pitanguy ligaments, and mucosa trilogy connect the ULC and LLC to the septum enabling the micromovement central component of Medpor to make this impossible. Pain is proportional to the degree of stiffness at

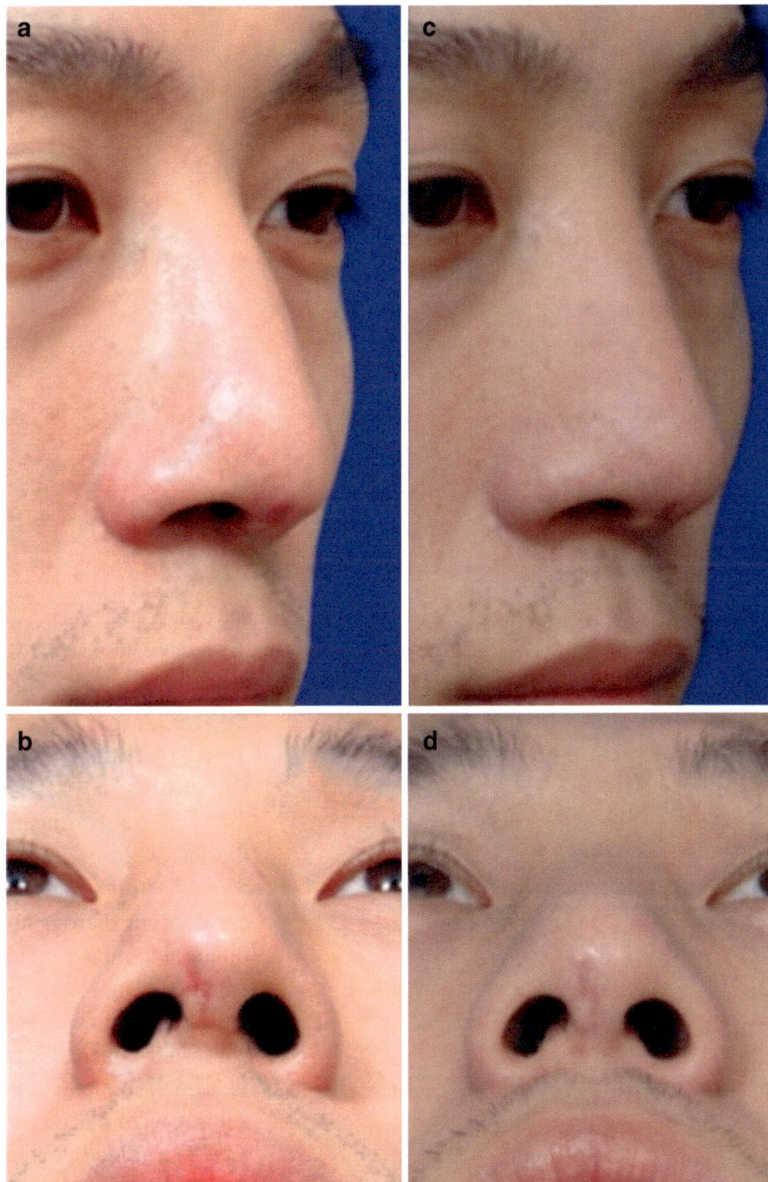

Fig. 4.11 Pre- and postoperative 1 year. (**a**, **b**) Preoperative views. (**c**, **d**) Postoperaive views

the tip and dorsum. The pain when breathing should be compared with the pain from its stiffness. Breading pain is related to nasal dryness and obstruction.

4.6 Operative Technique of Reconstruct the Collapsed Septum

There are two ways to restore nasal length: septal L-strut reconstruction and cantilever graft. It is impossible to reconstruct without cartilage transplantation at the site of destruction. Since Medpors is attached in various forms, it varies depending on the situation. However, when a thin Medpor is applied, the destruction of the tissue is relatively vast.

Septum Reconstruction

The cartilage that can be replaced is ear cartilage and costal cartilage.

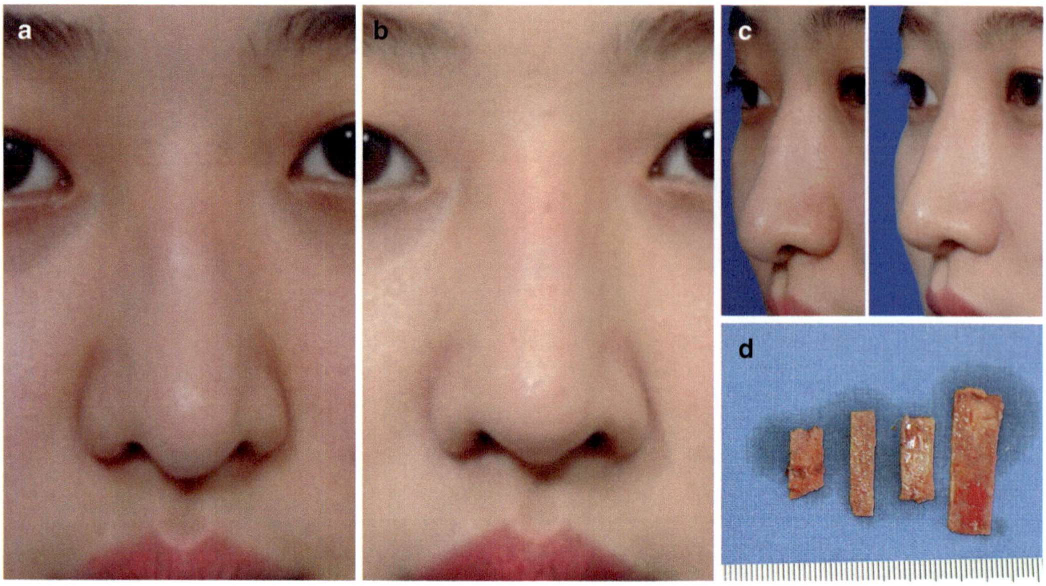

Fig. 4.12 Saddle nose with tip drooping: anterocaudal septal extension by Medpor. (**a**) Preoperative AP view, (**b**) Postoperative 1 year, (**c**) Quarter view, Lt. preoperative view, Rt. postoperative view. (**d**) Four pieces of Medpor

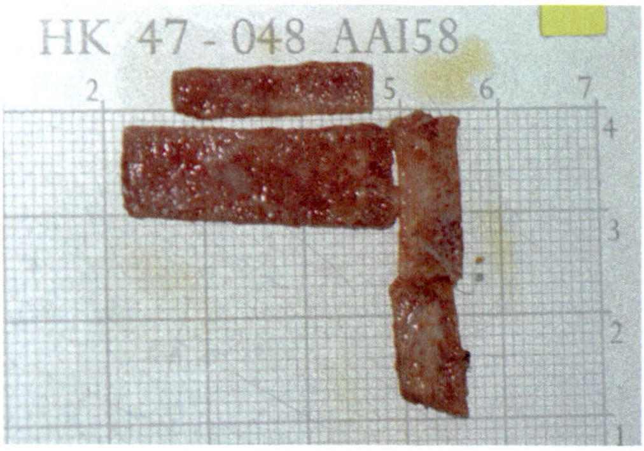

Fig. 4.13 Four pieces of Medpor: bilateral application anteriorly, and caudally

In the author's case, since most patients have a stiff nose, they want to change to a softer nose. Therefore, the first choice is ear cartilage, and the costal cartilage is chosen as the last choice. In many cases, since the ear cartilage has been used on one side, all cartilages are collected from the ear. Cymba concha is used where long cartilage is needed, and cavum concha is used where the relatively short cartilage is needed. Moreover, tragal cartilage can also be harvested.

Septal L-strut Reconstruction Using Two Conchal Cartilages [10]

Two conchal cartilage (cymba and cavum) from the ear were used as the primary selection for septal L-strut reconstruction. If the patient's ears are small or there is no cavum conchal cartilage, bilateral cymba conchal cartilage is used. If the patient did not have bilateral conchal cartilage, costal cartilage was used for reconstruction. This harvested conchal cartilage was folded face to face on the concave side. Two horizontal mattress sutures were placed using 5-0 or 6-0 polypropylene. The folded conchal cartilage was placed in the ANS (septal extension graft type) in a tongue-in-groove manner.

The folded cartilage was attached to the ANS's periosteum and surrounding soft tissue using 4-0 polydioxanone (PDS) without drill holes. Other conchal cartilage was also folded in the same manner and used in a tongue-in-groove method for the anterior septum (spreader type). The graft was sutured to the remaining anterior square cartilage using multiple fixation sutures with 4-0

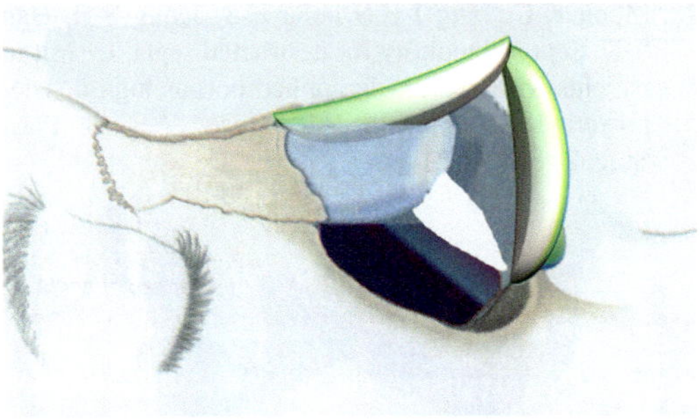

Fig. 4.14 Septal L-strut extension graft using two conchal cartilages

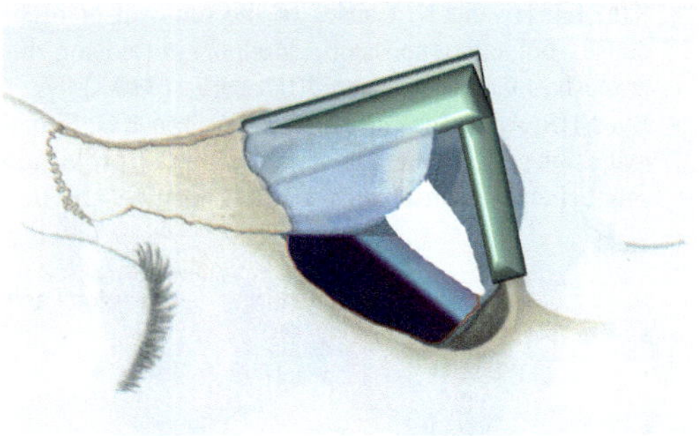

Fig. 4.15 Septal L-strut extension graft using sliced costal cartilages

Vicryl and 5-0 PDS. When severe destruction of the keystone was observed, cartilage was attached to the nasal bone through both drilled holes. After that, the two-folded conchal cartilage was sutured together to create a de novo anterior septal angle and suture to the middle crura using 4-0 PDS (Video 4.3). Small cartilage pieces, sculpted from previously harvested conchal cartilage, can be applied as reinforcing rafters between two folded conchal cartilage. After the reconstruction of the septal L-strut, tip plasty and dorsal autograft was performed (Fig. 4.14).

Septal L-strut Reconstruction Using Sliced Costal Cartilages

For reconstructing the septal L-strut, the seventh costal cartilage was usually used with an incised costal cartilage. Harvested rib cartilage was carved lengthwise. Divide into several pieces approximately 1–2 mm thick. The sculpted cartilage was immersed in a saline-filled container for at least an hour to reveal a tendency to warp. Two costal cartilages were applied facing the concave side of the anterior septum. The caudal septum was created and sutured to the anterior septum using the other two rib cartilage slices. The rectus abdominis fascia was taken and wrapped with a cut rib cartilage. They were applied onlay graft to project and smooth the nose dorsal profile (Fig. 4.15).

Cantilever Graft

If no septal reconstruction is possible, only the reconstruction of the external nose should be focused. This method without septal dissection may be more difficult as it is difficult to loosen enough constricted soft tissue. Considering that most Medpor is applied to the nasal septum, this is not a fundamental solution. The author does not use this method because the septal dissection has to be done to remove Medpor.

References

1. Frodel JL, Lee S. The use of high-density polyethylene implants in facial deformities. Arch Otolaryngol Head Neck Surg. 1998;124(11):1219–23.
2. Sclafani AP, Thomas JR, Cox AJ, Cooper MH. Clinical and histologic response of subcutaneous expanded polytetrafluoroethylene (Gore-Tex) and porous high-density polyethylene (Medpor) implants to acute and early infection. Arch Otolaryngol Head Neck Surg. 1997;123(3):328–36.
3. Kim YH, Kim BJ, Jang TY. Use of porous high-density polyethylene (Medpor) for spreader or extended septal graft in rhinoplasty: aesthetics, functional outcomes, and long-term complications. Ann Plast Surg. 2011;67(5):464–8.
4. Skouras A, Skouras G, Karypidis D, Asimakopoulou F-A. The use of Medpor© alloplastic material in rhinoplasty: experience and outcomes. J Plast Reconstr Aesthet Surg. 2012;65(1):35–42.
5. Sykes JM, Patel KG. Use of Medpor implants in rhinoplasty surgery. Oper Tech Otolaryngol Head Neck Surg. 2008;19(4):273–7.
6. Niechajev I. Facial reconstruction using porous high-density polyethylene (Medpor): long-term results. Aesthet Plast Surg. 2012;36(4):917–27.
7. Peled ZM, Warren AG, Johnston P, Yaremchuk MJ. The use of alloplastic materials in rhinoplasty surgery: a meta-analysis. Plast Reconstr Surg. 2008;121(3):85e–92e.

8. Kim JH, Hwang K. Causes of the removal of high-density polyethylene sheets (Medpor) in revision rhinoplasty. J Craniofac Surg. 2018;29(7):1730–2.
9. Byrd HS, Andochick S, Copit S, Walton KG. Septal extension grafts: a method of controlling tip projection shape. Plast Reconstr Surg. 1997;100(4):999–1010.
10. Moon K-C, Jung J-E, Dhong E-S, Jeong S-H, Han S-K. Septorhinoplasty for destructed septal L-strut in patients with previously applied porous high-density polyethylene implants (Medpor®). Aesthet Plast Surg. 2019;43(5):1286–94.

5 Nasal Obstruction in Asian Rhinoplasty

Pearls

- Patients with sudden worsening of symptoms or the presence of new symptoms with purulence on physical examination imply an acute exacerbation of CRS (chronic rhinosinusitis), and the operation should be postponed at least 4 weeks.
- Symptoms of nasal obstruction do not always coincide with those examined with nasal or nasal endoscopy and CT scans.
- The most important defense is to take a history of nasal congestion before surgery.
- Patients in the post-SMR state have weak L-strut. At this time, the pressure applied to the lower part of the implant in the tight soft tissue pocket worsens the septum's deviation.
- Atypical causes of nasal obstruction that can be seen after the Asian septorhinoplasty are mainly related to the exaggerated tip projection with dorsal augmentation.
- The most significant cause of functional deterioration is found at the minimal cross-sectional area (MCA) of the internal nasal valve (INV).
- "Exaggerated tip extension anchoring (sutures)" pushes down the INV.
- If the nasal framework is weak, dorsal alloplastic implants or thick dermis graft may destroy the healthy angle of the INV.
- Excessive tip projection causes a step ladder deformity from internal nares to MCA of INV area.
- To improve the function of INV, projection of the caudal portion of the ULC corresponding to the tip projection is necessary.

5.1 Diagnosis

History and Inspection

In nasal obstruction, the most important thing is taking the patient's history. The symptoms of nasal obstruction are not related as it looks. From the past, nasal obstruction is said to be located in the anterior part, visible by a nasoscope. However, the patient's subjective symptoms do not necessarily coincide with these findings. In other words, it is not what the patient feels as seen on the nasoscope or as seen on the CT scan. Always the patient's subjective symptom is more critical to the diagnosis. No objective measurement perfectly represents the subjective symptom [1, 2].

However, the use of minimal objective measurements to obtain surgical help or compare patients' surgical outcomes is necessary to protect the doctor's practice.

Supplementary Information The online version of this chapter (https://doi.org/10.1007/978-981-16-0542-0_5) contains supplementary material, which is available to authorized users.

E.-S. Dhong, M.-W. Na, *Asian Septorhinoplasty*, https://doi.org/10.1007/978-981-16-0542-0_5

Relying 100% on the subjective symptoms of the patient is because objectivity is poor.

Comparing the nasal airflow entirely to the intranasal cross-sectional area is not 100% physiologically correct, but too much worry is often detrimental to the surgery's decision. Based on the patient's symptoms, it is necessary to obtain appropriate auxiliary means for surgery. Even nasal inspiratory peak flow is not related to subjective symptoms, so it is challenging to implement accurate flow objectively [3]. Also, the limitations of acoustic rhinometry have been reported. It has been reported that there is a limit to the association of rhinomanometry with clinical symptoms [4].

There are various measurements for the patient's subjective symptoms, but the author mainly uses the NOSE scale (Nasal Obstruction Symptom Evaluation Scale© AAO-HNS Foundation 2002) and is used as the basis for clinical follow-up [5] (Fig. 5.1).

It is the simplest and most effective instrument for observing the patient's condition before and after surgery. It should be borne in mind that this single sheet can be a great resource to protect doctors from patients complaining of unexpected nasal obstruction after surgery.

Nasal Cycle

Naturally, everyone has a nasal cycle. It is an autonomous cycle and is affected by the patient's posture and emotion and shows a complex and subtle relationship such that the resting state and exercise, night and day, and left and right dominance exist [6]. It is necessary to listen to the patient's nasal cycle closely. Decongest to change the turbinate and closely observe the patient's nasal obstruction. It is recommended to visit the doctor when the patient's symptoms are the most severe and examine and compare even when there are no symptoms. It is also essential to accurately record the antihistamine formulation and nasal spray the patients are taking.

In the end, keep in mind that nasal obstruction, which can be improved with drugs, is contraindicated in surgery because the part that the doctor can help with is limited to the visible part.

Nasal Obstruction and Septoplasty Effectiveness Scale

Physician AAO-HNS#: __________ **Patient ID:** ________________ **Today's date:** __/__/_____

➔ **To the Patient:** Please help us to better understand the impact of nasal obstruction on your quality of life by **completing following survey.** Thank You!

Over the past *ONE* month, how much of a problem were the following conditions for you?

Please circle the most correct response

	Not a Problem	*Very Mild Problem*	*Moderate problem*	*Fairly Bad Problem*	*Severe problem*
1. Nasal congestion or stuffiness	0	1	2	3	4
2. Nasal blockage or obstruction	0	1	2	3	4
3. Trouble breathing through my nose	0	1	2	3	4
4. Trouble sleeping	0	1	2	3	4
5. TUnable to get enough air through my nose during exercise or exertion	0	1	2	3	4

Fig. 5.1 Nasal Obstruction Symptom Evaluation Scale © AAO-HNS Foundation 2002

Rhinitis and Sinusitis

The worse the atmospheric environment gets, the more patients' nasal function deteriorates. It is necessary to remove the vibrissae to observe the intranasal structure from external nares to deep turbinate at the first outpatient clinic.

Based on the patient's medical history, rhinitis and sinusitis should be treated separately. Depending on the type of rhinitis, the surgery needs to be postponed. For mucosal whitish discoloration and secretions, which are signs of typical allergic rhinitis, medical treatment prioritizes first. Symptoms should be released first, then structural problems are considered for the surgery.

Also, acute and chronic sinusitis should be diagnosed differentially. CT scans at this time are helpful. It is possible to diagnose space-occupying lesions of the sinus or polyps of the meatus. Of course, it is necessary to observe the nasal septal deviation that causes obstruction.

Bacterial and viral rhinosinusitis are difficult to distinguish on a clinical basis. The clinical diagnosis of acute bacterial rhinosinusitis should be reserved for patients with nasal sinusitis symptoms lasting more than 7 days with maxillary pain or tenderness in the face or teeth and purulent nasal secretion. Patients with body temperature less than 38.3 °C and mild pain can be prescribed by amoxicillin or trimethoprim/sulfamethoxazole.

However, if these symptoms come and go for more than 8–12 weeks, it is better to postpone the operation and perform the operation after sufficient antibiotic treatment for at least 3 weeks. In addition to chronic rhinosinusitis, it is recommended to use irrigation and topical therapy along with priority to regular treatment by an ENT doctor. If there is a schedule for surgery, one of the antibiotics such as amoxicillin-clavulanate, clindamycin, sulfamethoxazole/trimethoprim, and levofloxacin or ciprofloxacin should be selected and treated. If the symptoms do not improve during treatment, you should try changing it [7]. There are many thesis and disagreements regarding antibiotics, but the patients awaiting septorhinoplasty should be rhinosinus-symptoms-free. The problem is that sudden worsening of symptoms or the presence of new symptoms with purulence on physical examination implies an acute exacerbation of CRS, which should be treated. These patients are managed by microbiological culture, determination of antibiotic sensitivities, and appropriate antibiotic therapy [8].

CT Scan

In nasal obstruction, the most important thing is taking the patient's history. However, the doctor has no choice but to operate as seen by the intranasal inspection. It should be remembered again that nasal obstruction is not correlated 100% as it looks. CT is beneficial to see the relationship between the shape of the nasal septum and the surrounding inferior turbinate. It is also essential to observe the shape of the internal nasal valve (INV) and judge the possibility of reconstructing it. According to one report, the INV of Asians is broader than that of Caucasians. The INV angle in Asians is 21.6° ± 4.5°, and it is significantly larger than that of Caucasians. The reconstructed CT method has better reproducibility than the endoscopic method in measuring the INV angle. Caucasians, which has been reported to be 11.4° ± 2.6° ($p < 0.001$) [9]. This study is useful for observing the shape of INV and determining the spreader graft. It is particularly beneficial for observing the position and type of alloplastic implants in determining secondary rhinoplasty and seeing how it has a relationship with INV.

Inferior Turbinate

In the inferior turbinate, it is necessary to determine whether the bone occupies the actual volume or the venous sinusoid is enlarged along with the lamina propria to determine the surgical method. If the lamina propria is thicker than the turbinate bone, simple coblation can be applied (Fig. 5.2).

Concha Bullosa

Anomalous pneumatization of the turbinate is occasionally found. Inferior turbinate can be treated easily, but middle turbinate is following a symptomatic treatment. The author prefers a simple method for collapsing if concha bullosa found on the concave side can cause nasal obstruction after septoplasty. The medial lamina and lateral lamina can easily collapse, but in the middle turbinate, concha bullosa can be resolved with lateral laminectomy, partial turbinectomy, or concha-pexy. However, since septum and middle turbinate contact can cause rhinogenic headache, a close diagnosis is required, and accompanying sinusitis should be observed (Fig. 5.3).

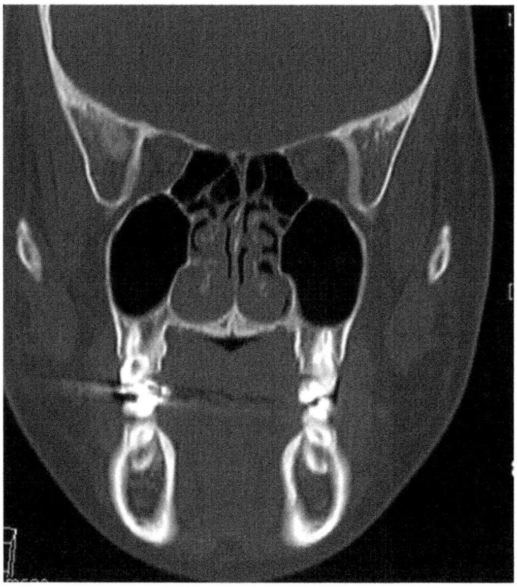

Fig. 5.2 Bilateral inferior turbinate hypertrophy: The lamina propria hypertrophied. The patient complained of severe nasal obstruction. Choanal patency is not observed

Acoustic Rhinometry

Among the objective measures, the author prefers acoustic rhinometry (AR) as an auxiliary. It is a method for viewing the cross-sectional area in the nasal cavity using acoustic reflection, and it is of sufficient value as a diagnostic aid, despite many criticisms [10].

Acoustic rhinometry is worthwhile to use as a means of getting help rather than relying on it. It is beneficial for comparing the left and right of the minimal cross-sectional area or for comparative evaluation before and after surgery. It is unreasonable to judge whether or not to perform surgery based on this. The graph is different according to the type of machine, and there may be an error in the part where the machine is inserted into the external nares, but the cross-sectional area from the inferior turbinate part forming the INV to 7 cm rear can be measured (Fig. 5.4) [11].

Even for rhinoplasty using alloplastic materials, a report recommends an examination before and after surgery using AR [12].

Many studies report on the changes before and after surgery using AR in reduction rhinoplasty, but there are few studies using AR of Asian septorhinoplasty, mainly augmentation rhinoplasty.

Case Study: A Case of CT Findings Do Not Correlate with AR

The patient with Video 5.1 complained more about nasal obstruction on the left. It is differ-

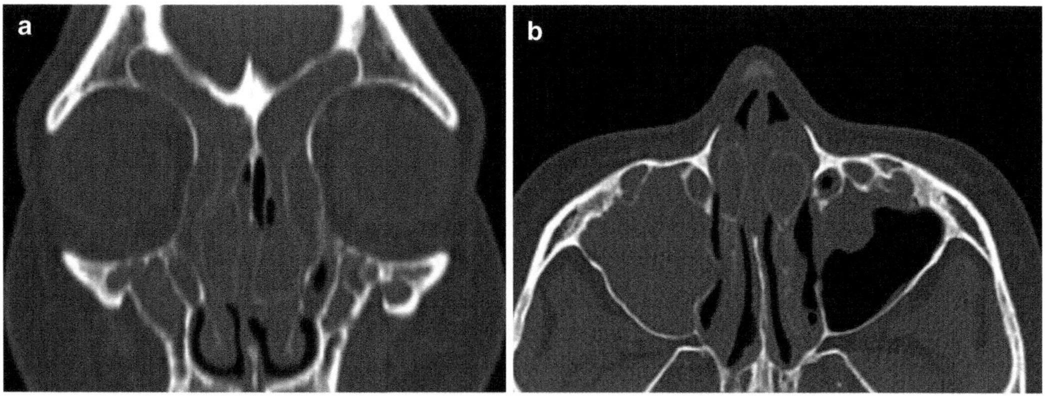

Fig. 5.3 Severe concha bullosa of the bilateral middle turbinate. (**a**) The frontal sinusitis is accompanied. (**b**) Middle turbinate concha bullosa with Rt. maxillary sinusitis and Lt. maxillary polyp

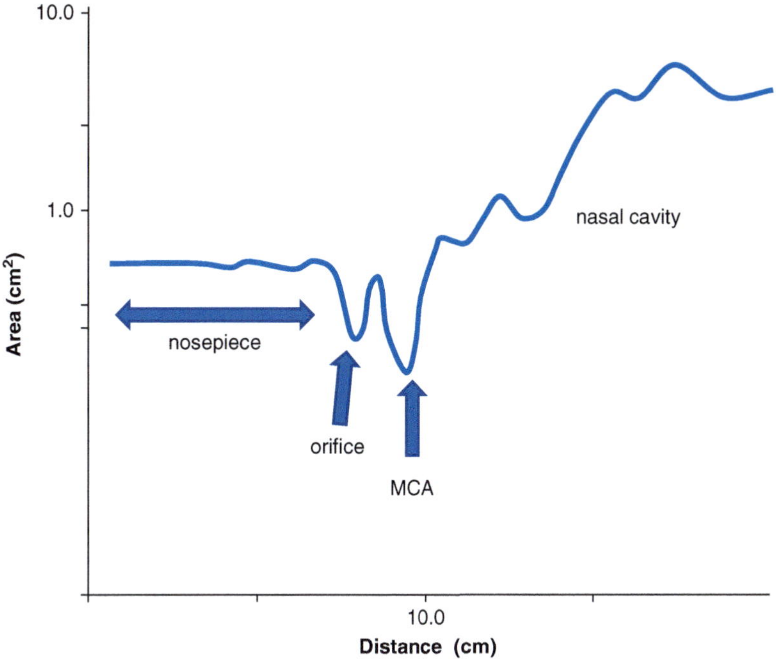

Fig. 5.4 AR: acoustic rhinometry: From the external nares, MCA exists (minimal cross-sectional area). Usually, the point is the most narrow internal valve. The picture on the left and right may change, but in general, it is interpreted as the width versus depth, the left vs. right sides, and before vs. after decongestion

ent from the findings of intranasal adhesion of the right nasal cavity. In the patient's AR, it can be found that the MCA on the left is located more anteriorly (Fig. 5.5). Since the slope of the peak is also steep in the left, it is judged that there will be more turbulence. What looks like and what the patient feels is often quite different.

Causes of Nasal Obstruction after Surgery

Intranasal Adhesion

Intranasal adhesion occurs when there is a slight wound after packing inside the nose and sticks to each other. This is the reason why gauze is not preferred as a material for nasal packing. If possible, using a more smooth surface or the recently preferred dissolving nasal packing material is a way to prevent this unwanted intranasal adhesion [13]. The author prefers Nasopore (Stryker Corporation, Kalamazoo, MI) because it has less bleeding, can be removed by suction after surgery, and results in relatively less mucosa bleeding. Severe intranasal adhesion found before surgery can be easily separated using a sharp freer elevator. At this time, the surgeon only needs to be careful with septal mucosal perforation (Fig. 5.6).

Neglected Preoperative Septal Deviation

Patients who had a septal deviation before surgery increase their concavity when heavy implants are placed at the dorsum. The cause may be due to gravity or the pressure of the tight pocket. Therefore, if the surgeon does not want the unexpected complaint of postoperative nasal obstruction, it is necessary to actively pay attention to the septum's concavity and convexity before surgery. If harvesting cartilage is required, submucosal resection inevitably leads to the weakening of the caudal septum. Therefore, it can be more easily transformed.

Aggravated Caudal Septal Deviation

Patients in the post-SMR state have a weak L-strut. At this time, the pressure applied from the implant in the tight soft tissue pocket worsens the septum's deviation. Above is a typical cause of nasal obstruction that can be seen after the Asian septorhinoplasty using implants. This situ-

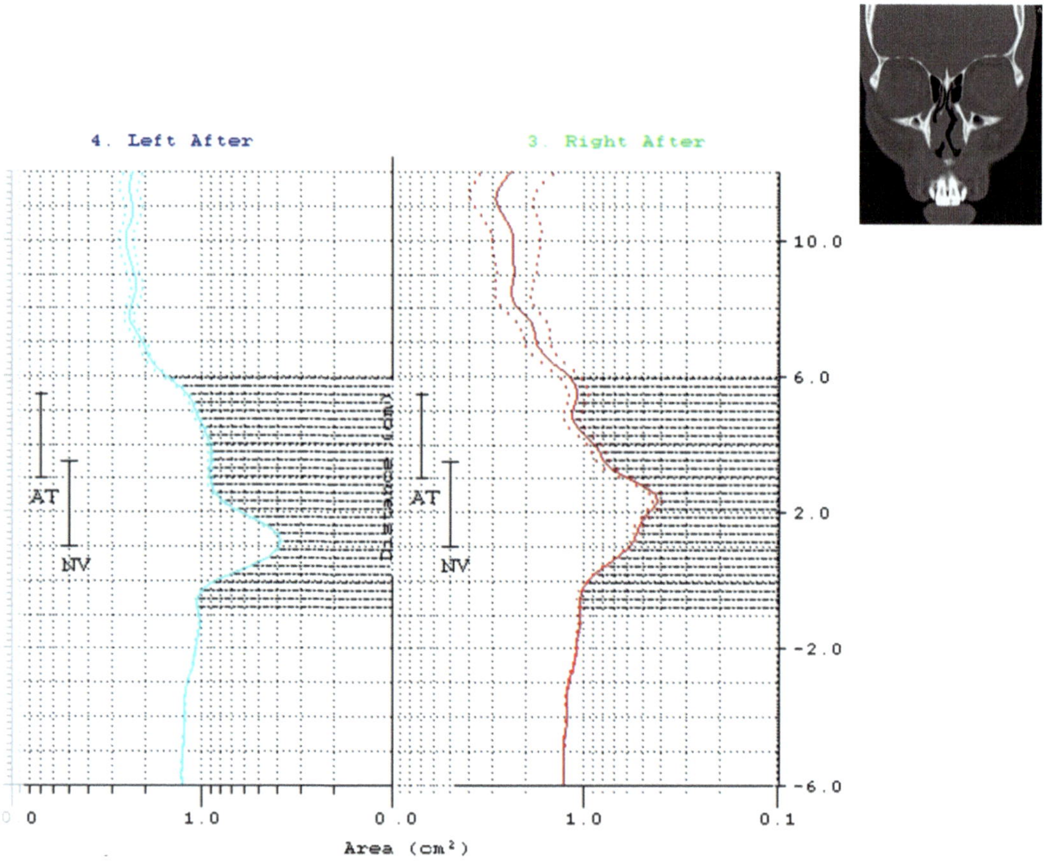

Fig. 5.5 The AR shows more anterior MCA of the left side. This is different from the findings seen on CT

ation is the most significant cause of functional deterioration and narrowing the internal nasal valve (INV).

Case Study

A 30-year-old male underwent septorhinoplasty with corrective osteotomy with the dorsal Gore-tex at another hospital 5 years before. The nasal obstruction was not severe before the operation, but after the operation, the left side became severely obstructed, and a headache occurred. A septum's convexity to the left was found in the nasoscope. The convexity of the left nasal septum was found even after decongestion. When the caudal septum was pushed with nasoscope, it recoiled again. Since the membranous septum exists, it was found that the septal extension graft was not performed (Video 5.2).

It is most important to find the caudal septum between the LLC in the middle of the surgical field, and it can be found that the convexity of the left side increases as the pocket overriding the caudal septum becomes tighter. The surgery was to securely place the caudal septum on ANS in the mid-center. Using a folded cymba concha, tongue in groove type reinforcement was performed to obtain the caudal septum's straightness (Video 5.3).

After the operation, the nasal obstruction was resolved, and the patient's headache also improved. These are the findings of the endo-

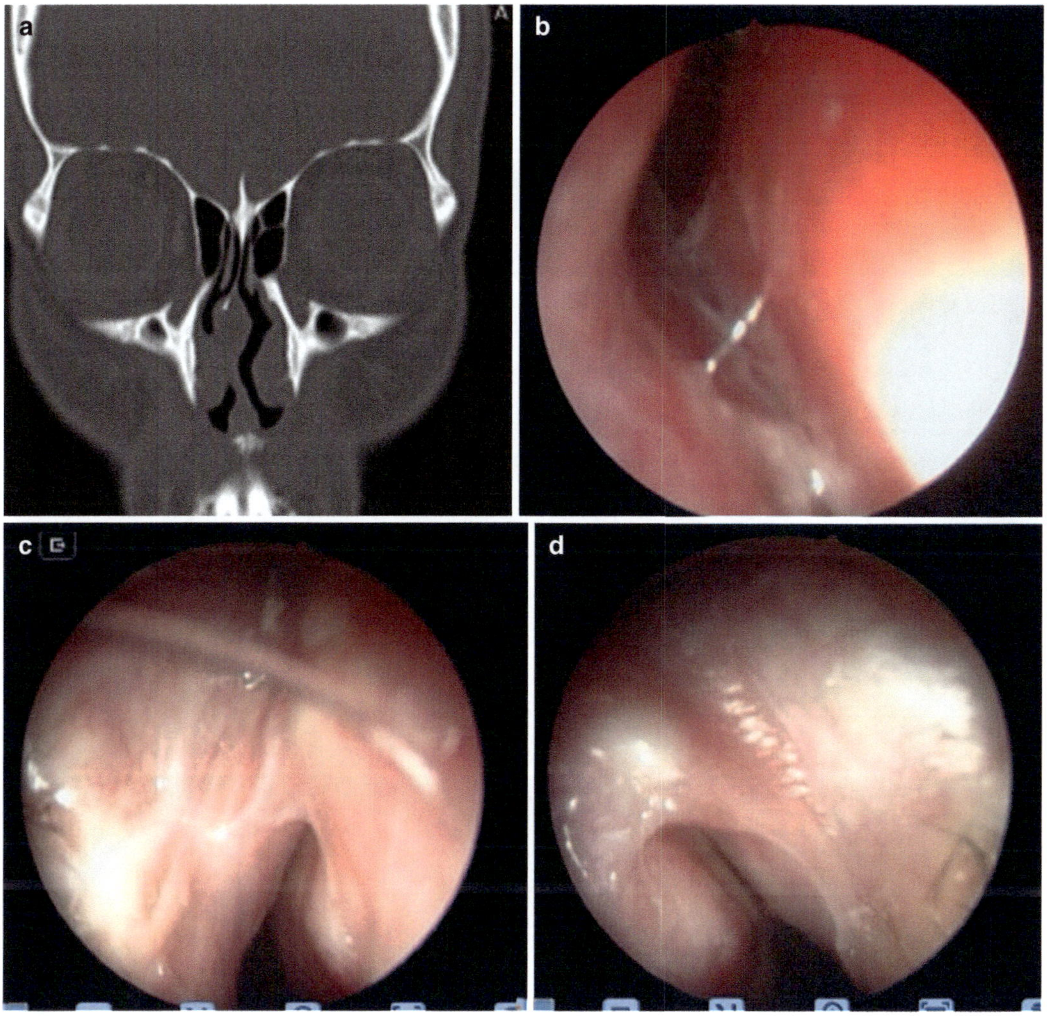

Fig. 5.6 Intranasal adhesion (**a**) CT shows Rt. side inferior turbinate attached to the septum. (**b**) The endoscopic view of the attached site was contacting and healing with each other. (**c**) The shape of Rt. the internal valve was acute, and there was synechia. (**d**) The attachment was found in the Lt. side internal nasal valve

scope after 2 years. NOSE scale also improved from 15/20 to 5/20 (Fig. 5.7).

Implant Instability over Weak Nasal Framework

Inserting the alloplastic implant into the nasal dorsum after corrective osteotomy, including the lateral osteotomy, delivers pressure to the nasal framework below, and the sinking implant can press INV.

Dorsal implanting requires the presence of a supportive cartilaginous framework. If the anterocaudal septal support is weak, the implant is easy to deviate to one side (Figs. 5.8 and 5.9). When the dorsal implant presses the INV, the INV on the pressed side or the opposite side nar-

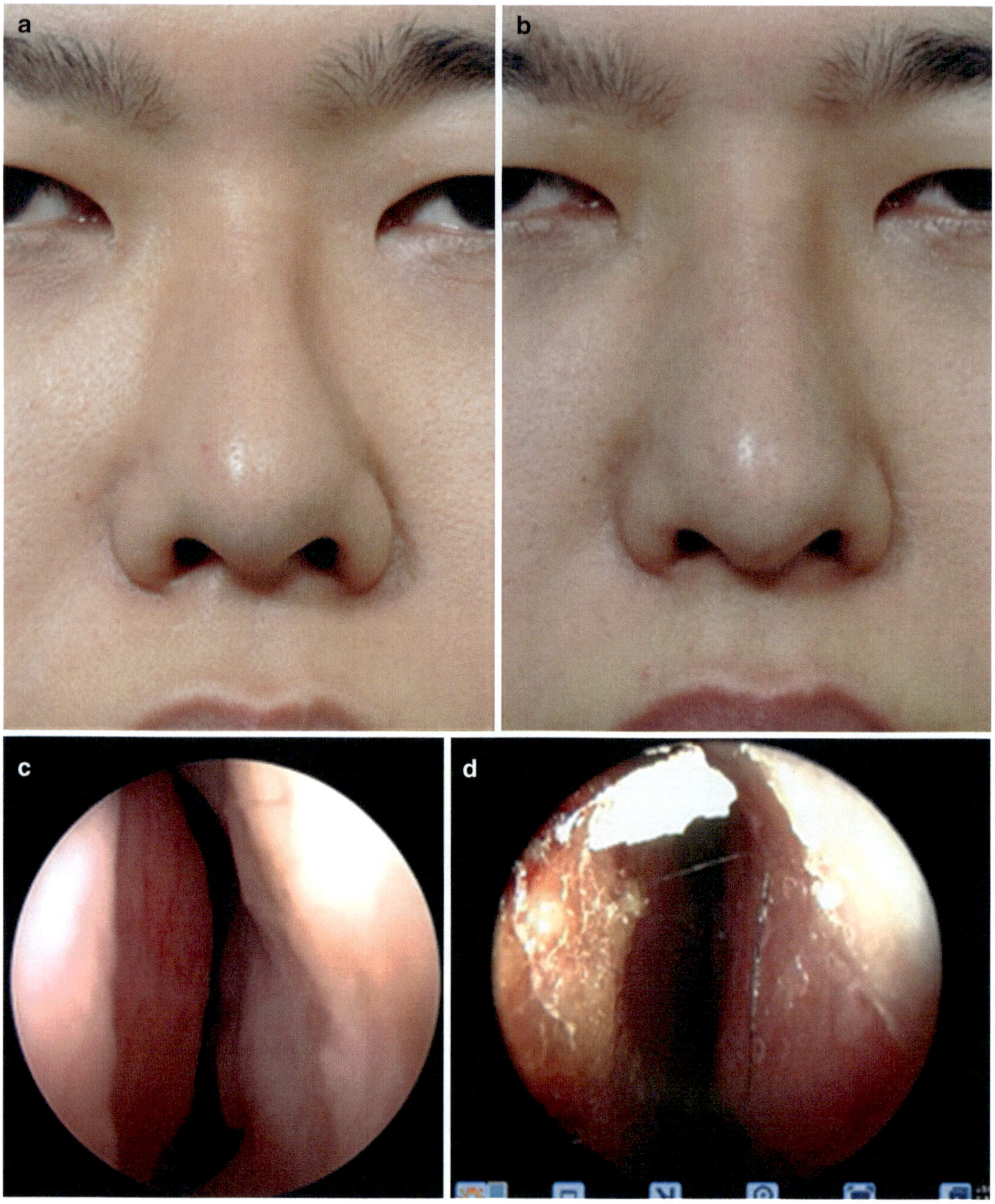

Fig. 5.7 Pre- and postoperative changes. (**a**) Preoperative AP view. (**b**) Postoperative AP view. (**c**) Preoperative Lt. nasal cavity. (**d**) Postoperative Lt. nasal cavity

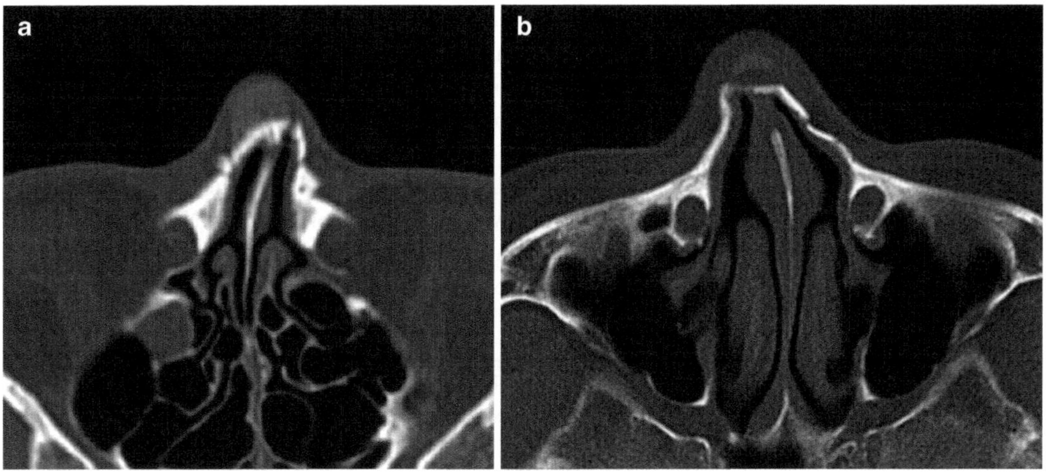

Fig. 5.8 Implant sinking on the unstable lateral wall was found. (**a**) Rt. lateral wall sinking. (**b**) Lt. lateral wall sinking

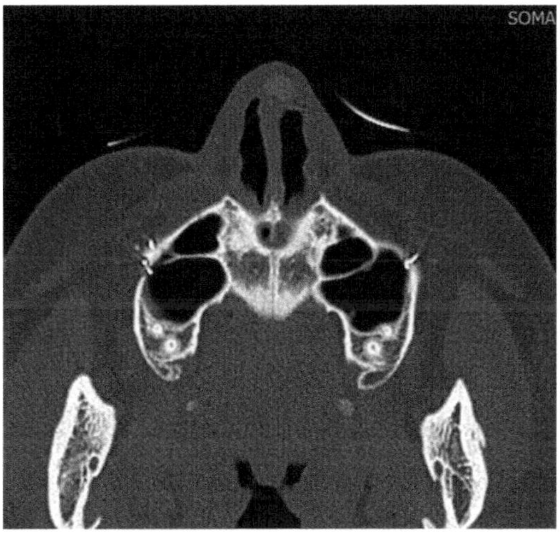

Fig. 5.9 Implant sinking on the Lt. side of ULC and INV was found. But this patient complained Rt. side nasal obstruction

rows, so it is necessary to observe what symptoms occurred in each situation.

Internal Valve Problem

Asian INV is characterized by pinching or a step ladder deformity after excessive tip projection or dorsal augmentation surgery. Most of them are not aware of an obstructive nose before surgery but the symptom aggravates after the surgery.

Patients tend to become hypersensitive to deteriorated nasal airways.

It is difficult to prove the association of nasal obstruction after surgery because meta-analysis for nasal obstruction after esthetic rhinoplasty is still insufficient.

Not all surgery will improve the symptoms, and it is essential to decide on the strategy after several interviews and long follow-ups. Surgery suitable for each cause should be chosen, and a careful surgical method should be determined after the diagnostic modalities mentioned above.

5.2 "The Tip Extension Anchoring (Suture)" Pushes down the INV

The method for stiffly anchoring lateral crus to get the tip projection excessively can have a harmful effect, which pushes down the INV when repairing above the high septum (Fig. 5.10).

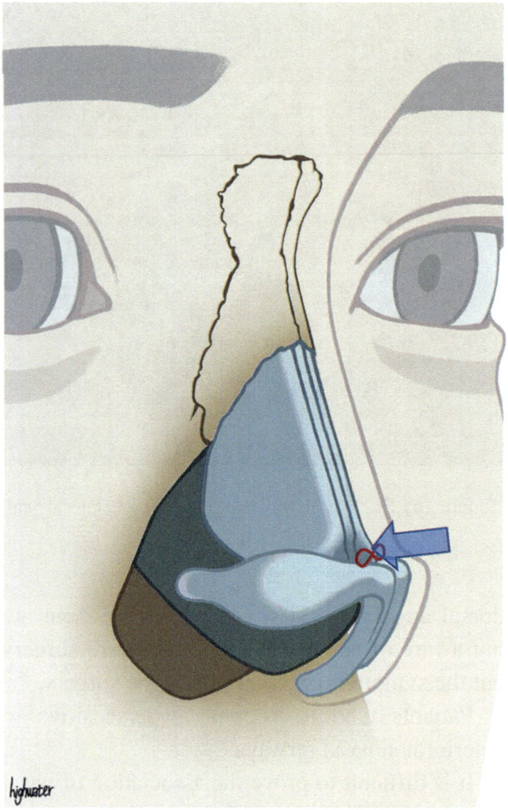

Fig. 5.10 Tip extension anchoring (suture) pushes down the INV and results in step ladder deformity

– "exaggerated tip extension anchoring (suture)" pushes down the INV.

It should be borne in mind that surgery for only the tip's projection can be a factor that degrades the entire nasal function. Most Asian rhinoplasty only pays attention to the tip's projection, and the dorsum is, of course, considered to be solved with a simple graft or alloplastic implant. Some surgeons do excessive medialization of the lateral crus for the tip projection without maintaining the angle between the long axis of the lateral crus. It has also been discovered that the long axis is located almost parallel.

For treatment, a method for increasing the height of the high septum itself should be performed by turning down the lateral crus's long axis by doing the entire tip plasty again and inserting a lateral crural spanning graft. This will be discussed again in Chap. 8.

If the anterior septum does not support the LLC, a strong force is applied to the scroll area. Moreover, the depression of INV occurs. Even if a dorsal implant is put in here, the depression will be overwhelmed.

Case Study: Exaggerated Tip by "The Tip Extension Anchoring (Suture)"

A 28-year-old female patient complained of a bulbous tip, alar flaring, and low nasal tip primarily underwent septorhinoplasty 2 months before at another clinic. SMR and right cavum concha and 3 mm silicone were used. The tip extension suture, dorsal augmentation, and alar reduction were done for the shaping. The patient complained of severe nasal obstruction and pain every time she breathed. In particular, she felt the right side tightening every time. In the surgical records, tip extension suture and derotation graft were performed for the tip projection, and the height of the tip was slightly lowered at the hospital immediately after the operation. However, she complained that nasal obstruction became more severe. She brought the pre- and postoperative CT scans. The nasal cavity was found narrowed a lot after the surgery. The INV angle is also much smaller. However, the biggest change was that the INV entrance from the external nares was abruptly lowered with a step ladder deformity (Fig. 5.11). The MCA was correlated with this deformity (Video 5.4). Although it is said that 3-mm silicone is inserted into the patient's dorsum, the cause of the sudden narrowing of the INV can be predicted that excessive tip extension anchoring occurred by pressing the upper lateral cartilage, considering the decrease in the INV angle and the increase in the tip projection.

Endoscopy: It can be seen as a typical acute angle at INV, but what stands out is that its relative position is low. However, the external dorsal

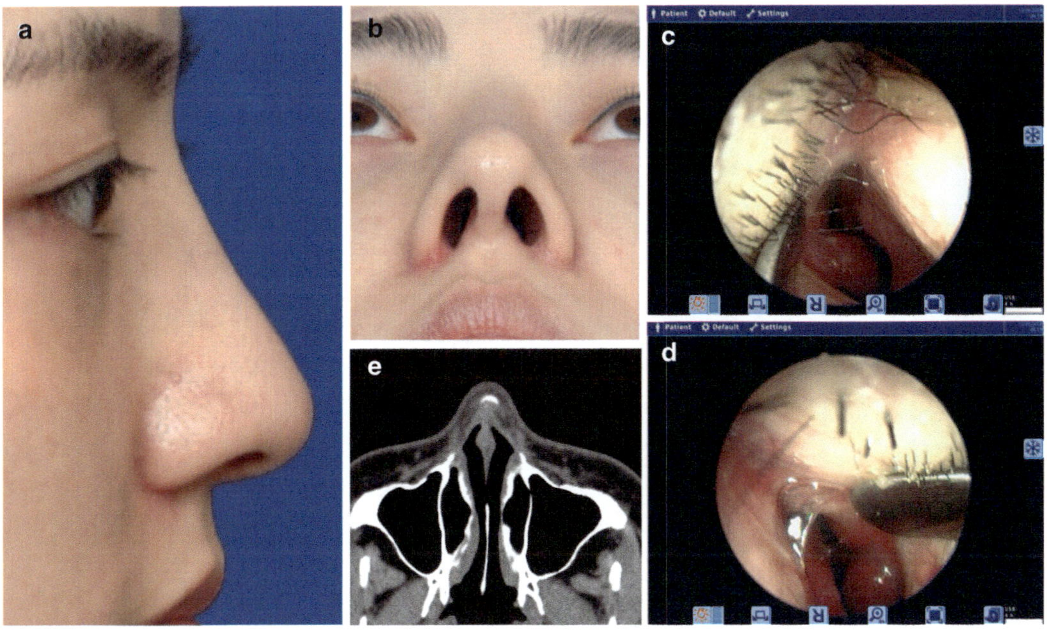

Fig. 5.11 Patient with severe nasal obstruction after septorhinoplasty: tip extension suture, derotation graft using ear cartilage, and dorsal 3 mm silicone and SMR were performed. (**a**) Postoperative lateral view. (**b**) Postoperative basal view. (**c**) Right INV angle was unfolded using a freer elevator for the inspection. (**d**) Left INV angle was unfolded for the inspection. (**e**) The nasal cavity was wide and patent without any turbinate problems

profile is smooth and high, so it can be assumed that LLC excessively projected the tip then the dorsum was augmented accordingly. Since it is only 2 months after surgery, surgery to increase the MCA in the INV area is necessary for sufficient observations.

AR: The MCA at the INV site decreased in the same way on the left and right, and the MCA on the right and left was the same. The patient complained more of obstruction on the right side (Fig. 5.12).

5.3 Aggravated Tip-Middle Vault Airway Discrepancy

As it happens in connection with the above concept, it cannot be distinguished. To respond to the tip's projection, too much a dorsal graft or thick alloplastic implant is inserted, which also affects pressing INV. This is a phenomenon that occurs during dorsal augmentation. However, in some cases, there is a phenomenon that the INV angle becomes more obtuse, thereby solving nasal obstruction. The case by case of the patient needs to be followed, and the method of resolution will differently depend on the cause.

– If the nasal framework is weak, the dorsal alloplastic implants or thick dermis graft may destroy the INV's healthy angle (Fig. 5.13).

Case Study: Too Heavy Dorsal Graft

A 45-year-old female underwent rhinoplasty 25 years ago, and 20 years ago, after failing two silicone surgeries, she underwent rhinoplasty with Gore-tex and Medpor 17 years ago. After that, nasal discharge started to appear recently, and all were removed. In addition, a dermofat graft was performed at another hospital.

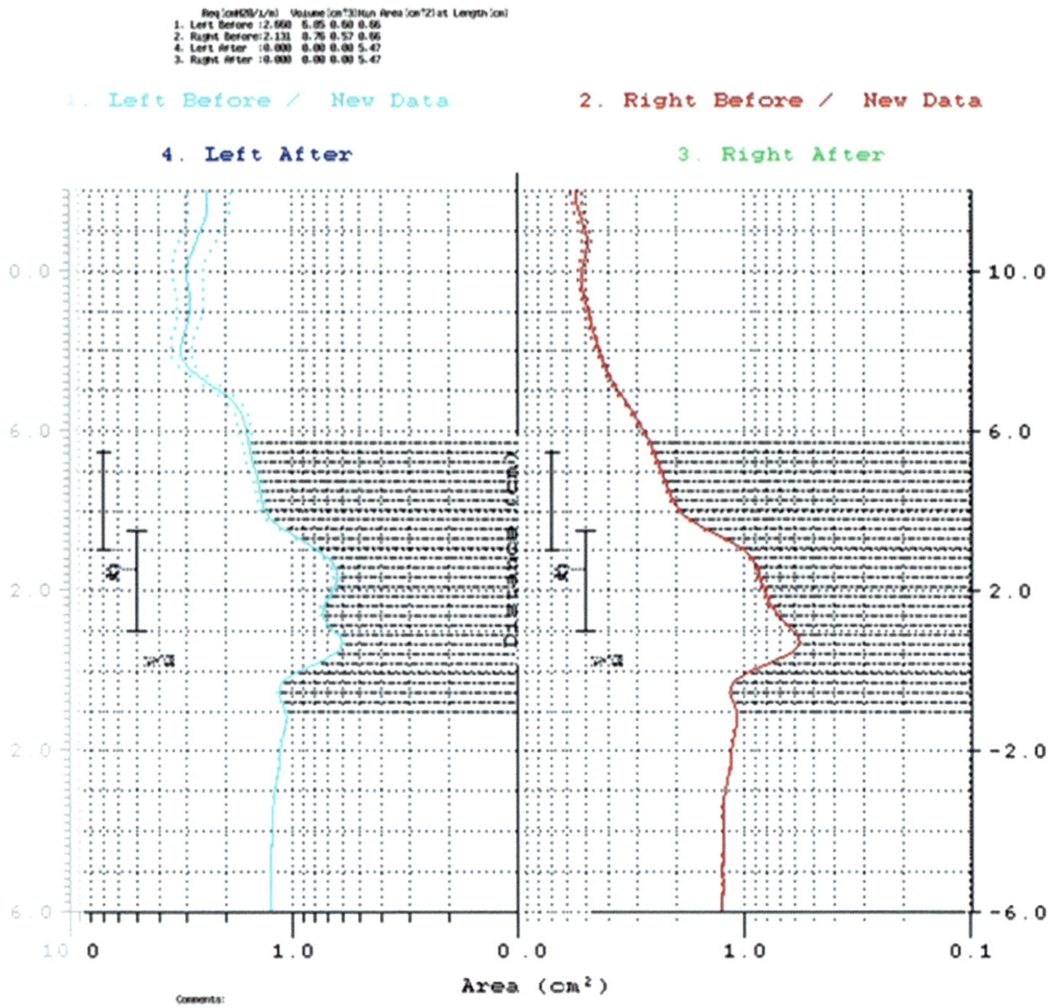

Fig. 5.12 AR showed MCA in the bilateral INV areas. Right side INV showed a stiffer notch

However, after the recent surgery, the nasal tip's asymmetry was revised 2 weeks later, and the ear cartilage batten graft inserted in the nasal tip was adjusted. At the time of referral, she was appealing for severe nasal obstruction. An excessive amount of dorsal graft was found in the pre- and postoperative axial views of CT. Since the recent surgery is dermofat, it is predicted that it will be absorbed for more than a year in the future, so the continuous observation is necessary, and if no improvement in symptoms, surgical intervention will be required. It cannot be said that the amount of the dermis is too much. The author believes that this would have been done because a large amount of absorption was expected.

Endoscopy: Severe bulging was found in the INV site ceiling, which was a dermofat graft inserted into the nasal dorsum (Fig. 5.14).

CT: When comparing the pre- and postoperative conditions, the Medpor was removed, and

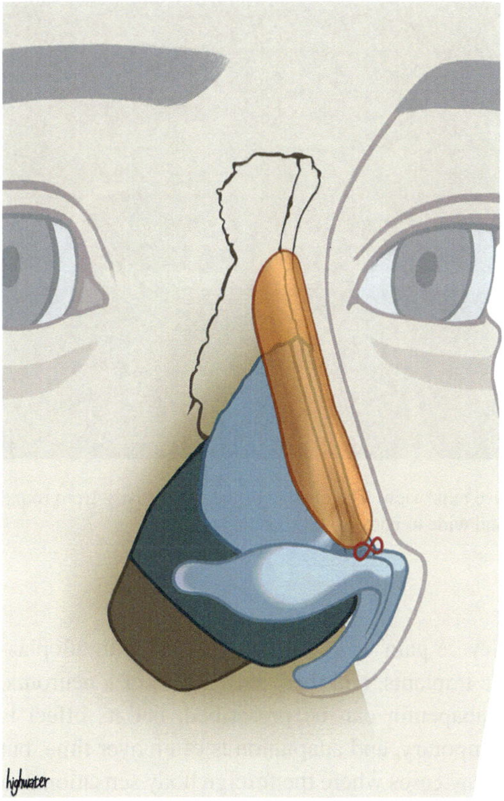

Fig. 5.13 Tip extension anchoring with dorsal onlay implant pushes down the INV and results in step ladder deformity

the ear cartilage was applied. The thickness of the dorsal graft in the INV area was increased (Video 5.5).

The dorsal contour's shape has improved with a dermofat graft, and this operation cannot be said to be wrong. I believe this would have been done because a large amount of absorption was expected.

5.4 Too Narrow INV Angle

The INV angle is too narrow, it is also related to excessive tip projection, and it can be assumed that it occurred as a result of excessive tip extension anchoring for tip projection and applying a strong strut to the tip. INV angle is less than 15°. This is the case of a typical spring graft indicated (Fig. 5.15).

Thickened Caudal Septum

When the graft applied to the columella is thick, MCA occurs from external nares before reaching INV. Therefore, care must be taken when applying rib cartilage or ear cartilage.

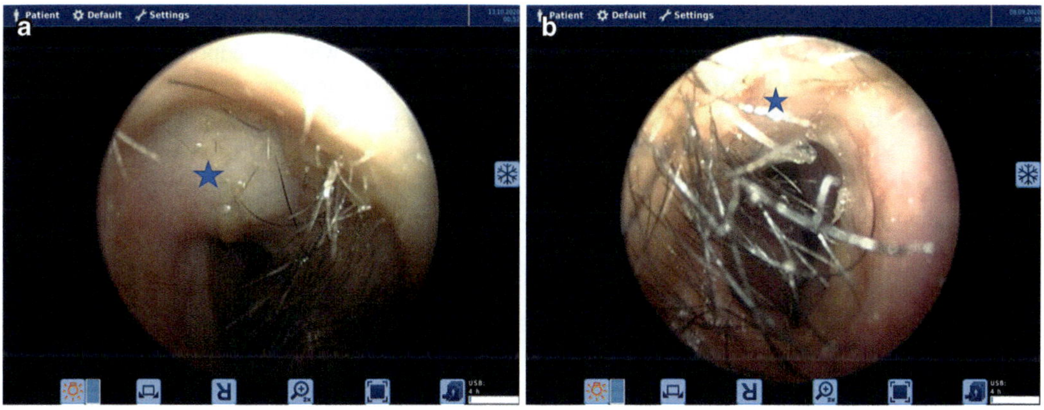

Fig. 5.14 The roof of the INV area was bulged down (the star mark), and the MCA notch was found here bilaterally. (**a**) Left side INV. (**b**) Right side INV

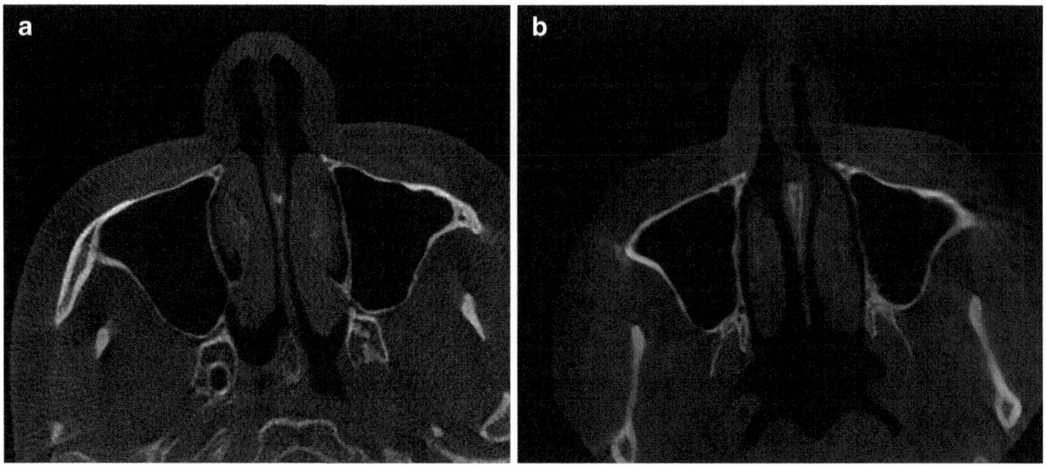

Fig. 5.15 Severe nasal obstruction after septorhinoplasty with tip extension suture and derotation graft without the dorsal implant. (**a**) Preoperative axial view. (**b**) Postoperative axial view. The change of the nasal cavity from round and wide to narrow and stiff angle

Unlike Westerners, Asians have alar flaring so that they can be relatively free from this problem. Even with severely thick columellar grafts, we can find cases where the nasal obstruction has not complained.

In the author's case, a folded cymba concha was applied to the caudal septum, and nasal obstruction complaints were found in patients with graft tilting, but there was no problem due to the thickening.

Other Combined Symptoms with Nasal Obstruction

Nasal Pain

Many Medpor users complain of nasal pain. It is proportional to the degree of stiffness at the tip of the nose, and pain when breathing should be compared with the resting pain. Sometimes it is associated with chronic nasal pain and rhinogenic headache, sometimes without.

In the case of patients who have undergone multiple surgeries, it is unknown when the pain begins. Of course, it is reported that 100% of the sensory of the skin flap returns over time [14], but in patients with more than four surgeries, the recovery is slow, and there are many cases of complaining of abnormal sensations. Severe pain was found in patients with alloplastic implants, and there were cases of a neuroma. Gabapentin can be prescribed, but its effect is temporary, and adaptation is often over time, but many cases where the foreign body sensation that has occurred once does not disappear. CT scans should be used to differentiate from pain such as rhinogenic headache, and reoperation should be selected depending on whether pain around the eyes, nasal dorsum, or tip pain.

In severe pain, the authors found that most of the cases in which Medpor was used, which is sensitive to micromovement due to strong tissue integration, and it is judged that the harness causes pain. It can be found that the pain decreases when switching to autograft.

Foul Odor

Many patients complain of a strange odor from the inside of the nose. It can be detected in patients with exaggerated transdermal suture for tip projection or acute middle to lateral crural angle. This can be found when nasal secretions or crusts are trapped between vestibules and produce foul odors or in cases where non-absorbable sutures are sometimes protruded from the tip to show local chronic inflammation. It is not the peculiar smell of chronic nasal obstruction or chronic sinusitis. It is recommended to clean the nasal tip frequently with water. If pinching is severe, securing the space under the middle crural medial crus or soft triangle of LLC reduces crust and sometimes improves symptoms.

References

1. Andre RF, Vuyk HD, Ahmed A, Graamans K, Nolst Trenité GJ. Correlation between subjective and objective evaluation of the nasal airway. A systematic review of the highest level of evidence. Clin Otolaryngol. 2009;34(6):518–25.
2. Kim CS, Moon BK, Jung DH, Min YG. Correlation between nasal obstruction symptoms and objective parameters of acoustic rhinometry and rhinomanometry. Auris Nasus Larynx. 1998;25(1):45–8.
3. Andrews PJ, Choudhury N, Takhar A, Poirrier AL, Jacques T, Randhawa PS. The need for an objective measure in septorhinoplasty surgery: are we any closer to finding an answer? Clin Otolaryngol. 2015;40(6):698–703.
4. Dadgarnia MH, Baradaranfar MH, Mazidi M, Azimi Meibodi SMR. Assessment of septoplasty effectiveness using acoustic rhinometry and rhinomanometry. Iran J Otorhinolaryngol. 2013;25(71):71–8.
5. Stewart MG, Witsell DL, Smith TL, Weaver EM, Yueh B, Hannley MT. Development and validation of the nasal obstruction symptom evaluation (NOSE) scale. Otolaryngol Head Neck Surg. 2004;130(2):157–63.
6. Kahana-Zweig R, Geva-Sagiv M, Weissbrod A, Secundo L, Soroker N, Sobel N. Measuring and characterizing the human nasal cycle. PLoS One. 2016;11(10):e0162918.
7. Suh JD, Kennedy DW. Treatment options for chronic rhinosinusitis. Proc Am Thorac Soc. 2011;8(1):132–40.
8. Lanza DC, Kennedy DW. Adult rhinosinusitis defined. Otolaryngol Head Neck Surg. 1997;117(3 Pt 2):S1–7.
9. Suh M-W, Jin H-R, Kim J-H. Computed tomography versus nasal endoscopy for the measurement of the internal nasal valve angle in Asians. Acta Otolaryngol. 2008;128(6):675–9.
10. Roithmann R, Cole P, Chapnik J, Shpirer I, Hoffstein V, Zamel N. Acoustic rhinometry in the evaluation of nasal obstruction. Laryngoscope. 1995;105(3 Pt 1):275–81.
11. Krouse J, Lund V, Fokkens W, Meltzer EO. Diagnostic strategies in nasal congestion. Int J Gen Med. 2010;3:59–67.
12. Daele JJ, Leruth E, Goffart Y. Consensus in rhinoplasty. B-ENT. 2010;6(Suppl 15):109–13.
13. Wang J, Cai C, Wang S. Merocel versus Nasopore for nasal packing: a meta-analysis of randomized controlled trials. PLoS One. 2014;9(4):e93959.
14. Bafaqeeh SA, al-Qattan MM. Alterations in nasal sensibility following open rhinoplasty. Br J Plast Surg. 1998;51(7):508–10.

6 The Various Preparations of Autologous Materials

Pearls

- Ear cartilage is the best donor cartilage that can be used with alloplastic dorsal implants.
- If enough cymba concha and cavum concha are collected from one ear, then L-Strut covering the anterior septum and caudal septum can be made.
- Deformity of the ear can be prevented by leaving a cartilage of 5 mm gap between cymba and cavum.
- Before collecting ear cartilage, a dental impression putty is used to make an embossed molding of the ear and prepare it.
- Conchal cartilage without perichondrium is brittle and fragile.
- The perichondrium on one side of the ear cartilage must be attached to the cartilage.
- The perichondrium on one side of the ear cartilage must be preserved in the skin flap.
- The superficial mastoid fascia (SMF) is not thick, but it comes out in a sufficient amount for use with a nasal tip, and it can be folded for dorsal augmentation.
- The consensus of doctors who do much dermal graft is that the dermis is absorbed until postoperative 12–18 months.
- When the absorption is considered, the dermal part is used as a double or triple layer, and the fat part is rarely used.
- If dorsal skin is too thin, a little fatty layer should be attached to the dermis. The fatty side is placed directly under the thin skin. It is suitable for shaping.
- When using sacral dermis-fat (SDF), if the fat layer is located outside the pocket, the graft appears less demarcated due to the tissue's characteristics.
- The thick SDF may appear demarcated under thin dorsal skin.

6.1 Auricular Cartilage

When cartilage graft is required in patients who do not require septal surgery, ear cartilage is the most preferred donor site in Asian rhinoplasty due to its elasticity and sufficient amount.

- In patients who do not require septoplasty, there are cases of SMR performed because of the need. In Asian rhinoplasty, this is not the best option with the dorsal alloplastic implants.
- Ear cartilage is the best donor site that can be harvested with dorsal implants.
- Surgeons who feel burdened with septal surgery should be familiar with the wise use of ear cartilage.

Supplementary Information The online version of this chapter (https://doi.org/10.1007/978-981-16-0542-0_6) contains supplementary material, which is available to authorized users.

E.-S. Dhong, M.-W. Na, *Asian Septorhinoplasty*, https://doi.org/10.1007/978-981-16-0542-0_6

Ear cartilage is the most used material in Asian rhinoplasty. It is because the septum is smaller and pliable than the Western or because more cartilage is needed after the septal cartilage is harvested. If a cartilage graft is needed in patients who do not require septal surgery, ear cartilage is the preferred donor site due to its elasticity and sufficient amount. It can be easily prepared in the same surgical field of view, so it is easy to collect, and it can be used as needed before and during surgery, and there is a donor part on the left and right. The width of the ear covering the cymba conchal cartilage was found to be 30.5 mm in African women, 32.5 mm for African men in a morphological study of 100 volunteers [1]. A study using facial computed tomography images (mid-sagittal view) of 200 Koreans reported that the mean boundary of the cartilaginous septum was 818 mm^2 [2]. Therefore, if the conchal cartilage can be harvested as much as possible without deformation of the donor site, the physical dimensions of conchal cartilage are theoretically large enough and similar to the septal cartilage. To harvest the maximum amount, Han et al. introduced a surgical technique with minimal donor site morbidity, the average size of cymba and cavum is 155.7 mm^2 and 210.2 mm^2, respectively. They could harvest the maximal amount without contour collapse leaving a helical crus of at least 5 mm [3].

However, clinically, some surgeons harvest all cymba and cavum without leaving the intermediate bridge cartilage, and depending on the situation, it can be found that patients do not complain (Fig. 6.1). Even though 5 mm bridge is left, hypertrophic and ugly scars can be created and depending on the patient's character, deformity of the ear may have complained (Fig. 6.2). The cause for the ugly scar will be covered in detail in the dissection, but the author thinks it depends on whether the perichondrium of cartilage is left or sacrificed. The author thinks that deformity can be reduced by leaving either of the perichondrium attached to one side's skin flap.

- When collecting ear cartilage, it is recommended to preserve the perichondrium on the anterior side by attaching it to the skin.
- The cartilage is harvested with the perichondrium attached on the posterior side.

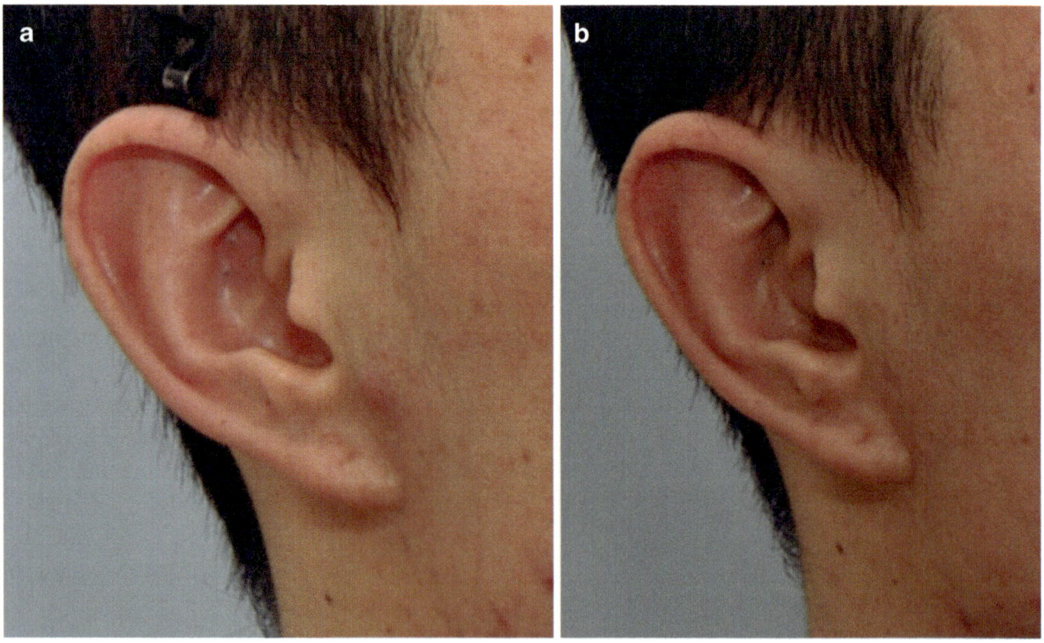

Fig. 6.1 The postoperative appearance of all patients, without the bridge between the cymba and the cavum concha, but this is not recommended. (**a**) Preoperative view. (**b**) Postoperative view

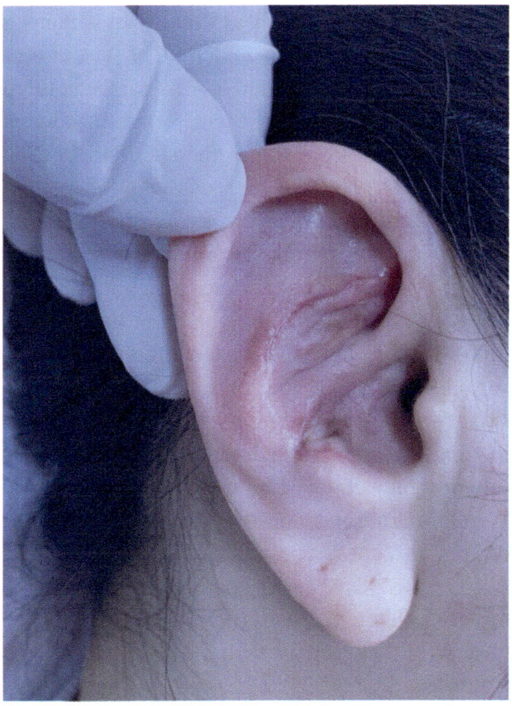

Fig. 6.2 Ugly scars; The middle bridge between the cymba concha and the cavum concha was left 5 mm, but the ugly scar remained; Both side perichondrium was harvested attached to the cartilage; the skin flap contractured after surgery

- This contributes to the stability of the skin flap on one side and the ear cartilage's stability on the other.
- If enough cymba concha and cavum concha are collected from one ear, then L-Strut covering the anterior and caudal septum can be made.

Dissection

There are two approaches for cartilage harvesting anterior incision and posterior incision. Few studies have reported on the occurrence of complications according to incision sites. Studies revealed only about the keloid or infection rate of the donor site after ear cartilage collection [4].

The author prefers the anterior approach from a direct view. According to the surgeon's skill, a posteriorly approach method leaves less scars. However, it is easy to collect the maximal width and length to separate the concavity side of the ear cartilage.

A solution containing 0.5% bupivacaine, epinephrine (1: 100,000), and hyaluronidase (50 units/100 mL) was injected at the anterior harvest site for vasoconstriction and hydrodissection. To obtain the maximum length, incisions were made as long as possible along the lower boundary of the antihelix without crossing the scaphoid. While uncovering the skin envelope, subperichondrial detachment was continued between the anterior circumcised skin and cartilage to the desired size. The antihelix and 5 mm bridge between cymba and cavum concha were preserved. The posterior skin was similarly dissected, and the posterior perichondrium was harvested and attached to the cymba concha. Then, the cavum concha was dissected in the same manner. The incision was made anteriorly at the lower border of the cavum concha. Like cymba concha, perichondrium was preserved and attached to the anterior skin.

6.2 Must Do and Must Not Do

Deformity of the ear can be prevented by leaving a cartilage of 5 mm gap between cymba and cavum concha. Collecting the entire cymba and cavum without an intermediate cartilage bridge can deform the ear width later. However, if the perichondrium is adequately preserved, there are cases where there is no significant deformity left, so choose according to the surgeon's confidence. Initially, the author preserved the anterior perichondrium attached to the skin, and then the cartilage was harvested. However, all perichondrium was attached to the cartilage for about 3 years after attending a fellow doctor's presen tation. As a result, many patients complained of severe scars during follow-up. The author hopes that readers do not commit the mistake of listening to others and changing your own beliefs. It is impossible to trust 100% of the content that others are presenting, and the presentation without a published thesis is just an empty story.

- After cartilage harvesting, the patient needs to wear an auxiliary molding for an extended time to maintain the cymba and cavum's concavity.
- Before harvesting, a dental impression putty is used to make an embossed ear model and prepare it.
- The ear embossing model is worn for more than a month after surgery.
- The perichondrium on one side of the ear cartilage must be attached to the cartilage.
- Conchal cartilage without perichondrium is brittle and fragile.
- The perichondrium on one side of the ear cartilage must be attached to the cartilage.
- The perichondrium on one side of the ear cartilage must be preserved in the skin flap.
- If perichondrium is collected from both sides, contracture of skin flap may occur.

The author uses 3M™ Express™ VPS Bite Registration Material Putty (3M, Korea) to prepare an embossed model by putting it in the ear before surgery, preparing it in sterilization in advance then applying it immediately after sealing the skin for simple dressing. Instead of this method, concavity can be maintained by tie-over dressing for 4–5 days using a bolster suture, but since it is necessary to maintain steady concavity for more than 1 month after surgery, the author uses a putty orthosis. Be careful as excessive pressure can cause pressure-sore of the skin flap.

6.3 Folded Concha: Is it Large and Stable Enough?

Folded Cymba and Cavum Concha Technique: Straightening and Stability

The biggest drawback of the conchal cartilage is its convolution and instability. The way to overcome these two points is to repair and use concavity or convexity sites [5]. Alternatively, there is a way to make the shape of the nose by using the curvature well. The author's preferred method is to obtain straightness and stability by repairing concavity sides by facing each other. The author has been using this method for 15 years, and there have been reports that recently introduced this method and the opposite method (face to face vs. back to back) [6]. For surgeons who have experienced folding directly, the method for repairing concave sides is more straightforward, and in the author's method, there is no perichondrium of this concave side, and the perichondrium is preserved on the opposite convex side. For this, it would be advantageous for the perichondrium to exist outside. For folding, 4–5 mm of cartilage in the middle can be folded without applying a longitudinal incision to obtain a more potent force. A longitudinal incision is applied to the top and bottom, except the center to obtain maximum straightness. The incision should be made in the direction that can obtain the straightest shape by observing the cartilage's shape (Fig. 6.3). Using a non-absorbable suture such as Prolene 5.0, the straightness can be obtained from 1–2 point repair at the folding point (Fig. 6.4 and Video 6.1).

Average Length and Width of Folded Cymba

The analysis of 311 intraoperative photographs of the harvested auricular cartilage revealed that

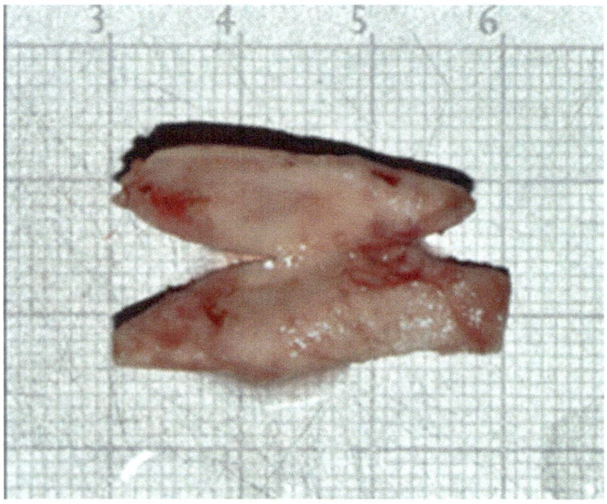

Fig. 6.3 Two longitudinal incisions were made to the mid-portion of cymba concha. More strength by folding can be achieved by leaving the middle portion

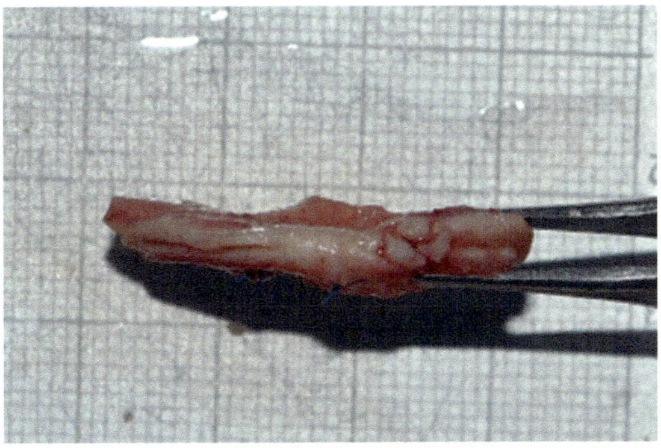

Fig. 6.4 Folded cymba concha

the mean (± SD) length of the folded cymba conchal cartilage was 24.2 ± 3.9 mm in men and 22.4 ± 3.7 mm in women. The mean width was 7.8 ± 1.9 mm in men and 7.2 ± 1.9 mm in women. This length and width are sufficient as the commonly used columella strut or spreader's length and width, making it a useful material. (data in publishing, Aesthetic surgery journal).

For Caudal Septal Extension Graft (CSEG)

Folded cymba concha or cavum concha has the advantage of being easy to apply to tongue-in-groove to anterior nasal spine (ANS) as its structural advantage.

Floating Type Columella Strut Graft

As a columellar strut, it can be used with a smaller width. That is, the maximal width mentioned above is not necessary. The authors do not prefer this method, only it is used as an auxiliary technique. The main reason is that the septal dissection is mandatory to support the caudal septum, so direct manipulation of the caudal septum is preferred. Strong coaptation between the posterior septum and ANS needs the tongue-in-groove technique. Columella strut is used as an auxiliary method.

Tongue-in-Groove Technique for CSEG

First, subperiosteal pockets were created on either side of the anterior nasal spine (ANS), leaving minimal soft tissue in the anterior pocket. While dividing both medial crura, the caudal septum was approached from ANS to the anterior septal angle, and at least 4–5 mm of the caudal edge was dissected in the subperichondrial plane. Any resection or correction of the caudal septum was performed before placing the folded concha. If necessary, a swing door procedure was performed to correct the septal tilt, and a figure of eight shaped suture was also applied between the posterior septal angle and the soft tissue part of ANS. Both columns of the folded conchal cartilage were inserted into the subperiosteal pocket with two or more transfixing sutures, and the folded cartilage was placed in the caudal septum as shown in the tongue-in-groove method [7] (Fig. 6.5). The horizontally contacted part of the conchal cartilage was sutured to the caudal septum.

Eventually, two points are under tongue-in-groove, one is ANS, and the other is the caudal septum. Various modifications are possible

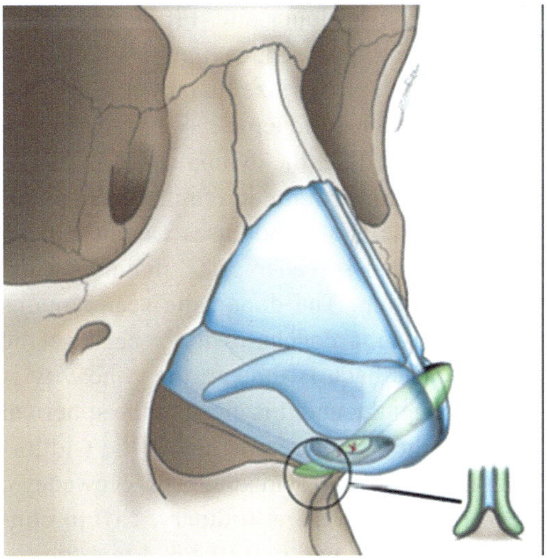

Fig. 6.5 Caudal septal extension graft: Inserting folded cymba concha by tongue-in-groove technique

depending on which part of the LLC and the CSEG tip to be repaired. When CSEG meets the anterior extended spreader graft (AESG), a de novo anterior septal angle can be created.

The Stability: Columellar Strut Vs. CSEG

To obtain the stability of the tip, the septal extension graft is more advantageous than the columella strut [8].

As mentioned earlier, the key factors determining the surgical method in Asian rhinoplasty are whether septoplasty is needed and whether alloplastic materials are used for the dorsum. Therefore, the degree of stability of the tip and the presence or absence of septal surgery are factors that determine whether to use the columella strut or CSEG. CSEG is preferred when strong tip support is required.

Cavum Concha

Along with cymba concha, cavum concha is also an excellent donor site. From experience in the anterior approach, cavum concha is harvested with a smaller size than cymba concha. If folding is done, the length is shorter, but the width is wider than the cymba concha. Taking this shape into account, determine the application location. The author uses cavum concha as an extended spreader graft, mainly on the anterior septum. The donor site scar remains less than cymba concha. This is because the tissue on the back is thicker, the concavity is relatively gentle, and it is close to the spherical shape, so the risk of contracture of the width is less than that of the cymba concha. Nowadays, when earphone wear is ordinary, cavum concha collection should preserve 3–4 mm to protect the orifice's margin that makes up external auditory meatus.

Tragal Cartilage

The third donor of the ear is tragal cartilage. This area can be accessed by retrotragal incision or incision using lateral margins. It has been reported that the size of 15 × 20 mm can be collected from here. Tragal cartilage has been used as flat cartilage [9].

However, it has no advantage over cymba or cavum concha because of the disadvantage that the amount of harvesting is less than the effort required for the incision. When the cartilage from all other places is used, it can be collected in a size of 10 × 15 mm [10]. There is no disagreement on the usefulness, a size of less than 10 mm is collected, and it also has a disadvantage in that the size is small because the marginal cartilage must be left in consideration of the inconvenience of ear phone users or projection of tragus.

The Superficial Mastoid Fascia (SMF)

The donors that can be collected for soft tissue transplantation are divided according to the dermis thickness. The thickest place is the sacral dermis, followed by the groin, but there is a disadvantage in that there is a hair-bearing. The author has also tried medial plantar but also prefers the thickest sacrum. However, there is a discomfort of having to prepare again, if necessary, during the operation. It will not be easy if the soft tissue is suddenly needed unless the operation is planned. The easiest way to access this is the superficial mastoid fascia, which is located behind the auricle [11].

Dissection

After injecting local anesthetics (0.5% marcaine, 1: 100,000 epinephrine, hyaluronidase 30 IU/mL), the area behind the ear is intended to raise a thin skin flap and leave most of the subcutaneous layer as the fascia layer. A 3–4 cm long incision made in the posterior

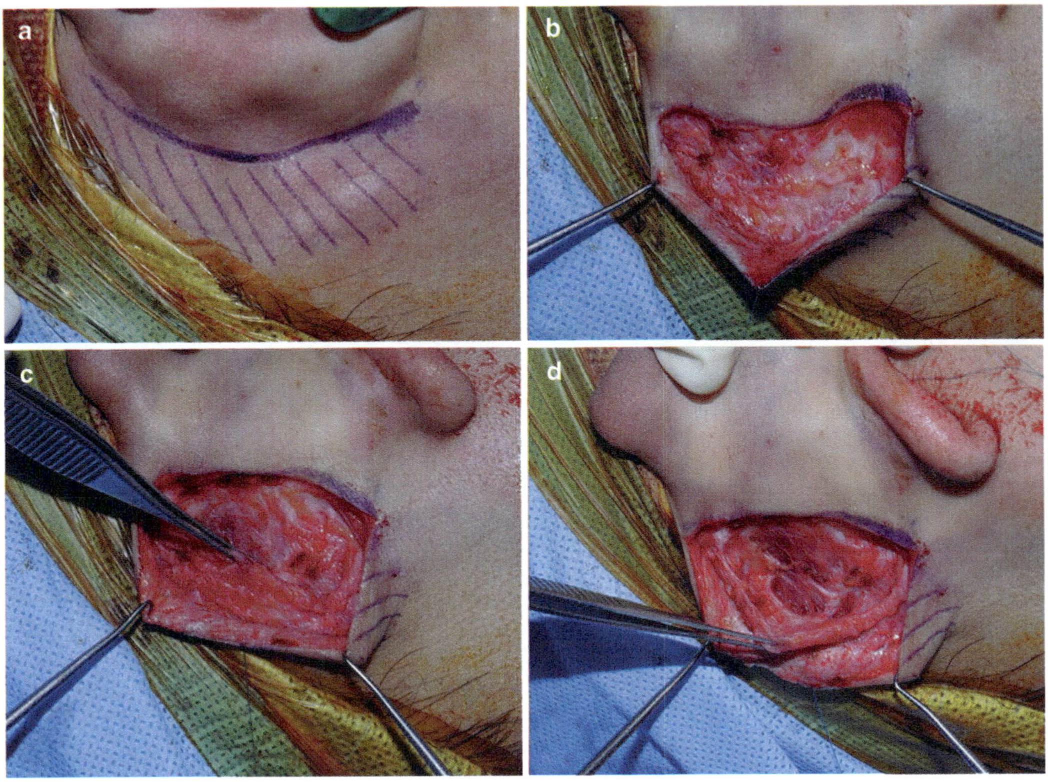

Fig. 6.6 Harvesting the superficial mastoid fascia; Clinical harvesting of the SMF from the right posterior auricular area. (**a**) Hydrodissection of the retroauricular area was done at the dashed area. (**b**) Thin skin flap measuring more than 1.0 cm wide was elevated. (**c**) Deeper dissection was performed into the incised site to find the retroauricular muscle. (**d**) The maximal SMF flap was elevated above the postauricular muscle. (Material from: Hong et al. Superficial mastoid fascia as an accessible donor for various augmentations in Asian rhinoplasty, Journal of Plastic Reconstructive & Aesthetic Surgery, 2012, Elsevier)

auricular circus placed a thin skin flap measuring a width of at least 1.0 cm. After raising the skin flap, a deeper incision is made in the incision site to locate the posterior auricular sulcus (Fig. 6.6). One or two bundles of posterior ear muscle fibers were easily found at the midpoint of the posterior incision (Fig. 6.7), and a full SMF flap was harvested over the posterior ear muscle (Fig. 6.8). The author considered this superficial subcutaneous layer of muscle as SMF. After the SMF was harvested, the skin flap was repositioned, Prolene 5.0 was used to close the incision, and a quilted suture and a light compression dressing were used to prevent hematoma (Video 6.2).

For Dorsal Augmentation

- The SMF is not thick, but it is a good material, and it comes out in a sufficient amount for use with a nasal tip, and it can be folded for dorsal augmentation (Fig. 6.9).

It is good to keep the volume by filling the diced cartilage inside the rolled SMF for more volume. Use a 1 cc syringe to seal the SMF around the periphery, and then remove the syringe and apply the space. It is a useful method of filling (Fig. 6.10). The cartilage should be minced finely. If transferring the cartilage is not easy, cut the syringe's front part to get the cartilage out.

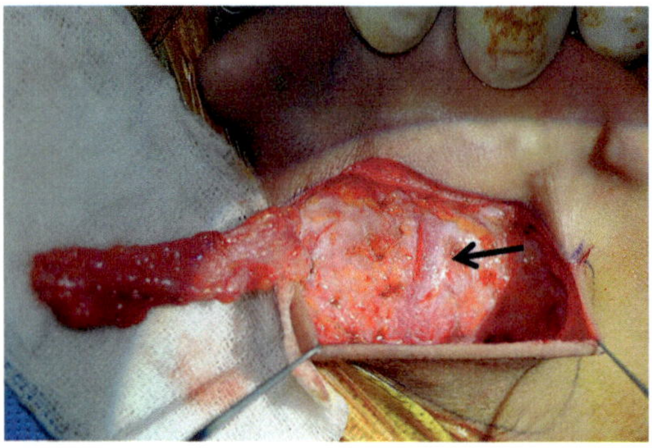

Fig. 6.7 Dissection plane and underlying posterior auricular muscle. At the midpoint of the posterior auriculocephalic sulcus, one bundle of posterior auricular muscle fibers was found (arrow). SMF flap was elevated so as not to dissect deeper than the plane of the posterior auricular muscle. (Material from: Hong et al. Superficial mastoid fascia as an accessible donor for various augmentations in Asian rhinoplasty, Journal of Plastic Reconstructive & Aesthetic Surgery, 2012, Elsevier)

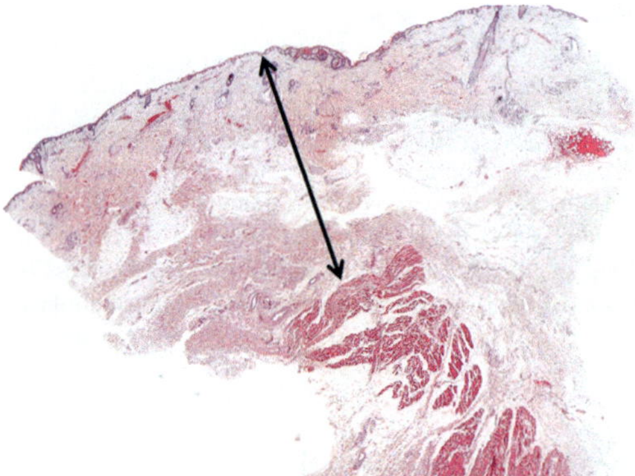

Fig. 6.8 H&E staining of transverse biopsy (×50). The histologic thickness of SMF was estimated between the skin and posterior auricular muscle plane (arrow). (Material from: Hong et al. Superficial mastoid fascia as an accessible donor for various augmentations in Asian rhinoplasty, Journal of Plastic Reconstructive & Aesthetic Surgery, 2012, Elsevier)

The Sacral Dermis-Fat (SDF)

From the early 1980s, the sacrum has been reported as the best donor site as a thick dermal graft in Korea [12]. Dr. Kim has performed more than 3000 primary and secondary nose augmentations with dermal fat grafts. He collected a

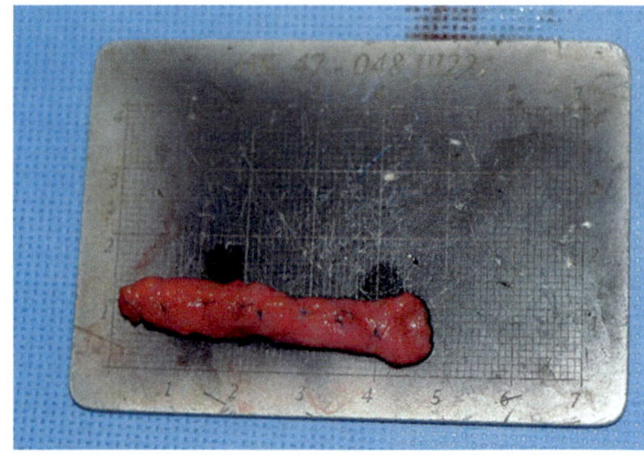

Fig. 6.9 The rolled superficial mastoid fascia

1.5 × 6.5 cm dermal fat graft between the anus and coccyx. He reported this donor tissue was denser and thicker than other areas such as the abdomen, groin area, or gluteal folds. Another study showed that the sacrum's dermis was significantly thicker ($p < 0.008$) than the other sites, and the panniculus adiposus was well developed. Moreover, they assume that dermal fat grafts harvested from the sacral region have greater viability and durability when transplanted. The sacrum is a suitable donation site for augmentation. This area boasts a thick dermis, a large number of fibroblasts and fibrocytes, dense subcutaneous tissue, and hidden scars [13]. There is no disagreement here, and the author prefers this as the first donor site when the highest dorsal projection is desired. Many doctors use the compact fold of multiple layers of the dermis.

- The consensus of doctors who do much dermal graft is that the dermis is absorbed until postoperative 12–18 months.
- When the absorption is considered, the dermal part is used as a double or triple layer, and the fat part is rarely used.
- If dorsal skin is too thin, a little fatty layer should be attached to the dermis. The fatty side is placed directly under the thin skin. It is suitable for shaping.
- When using SDF, if the fat layer is located outside the pocket (dermis-in rolling, in Chap. 7), the graft appears less demarcated due to the tissue's characteristics.
- The thick SDF dermis may appear demarcated under thin dorsal skin.

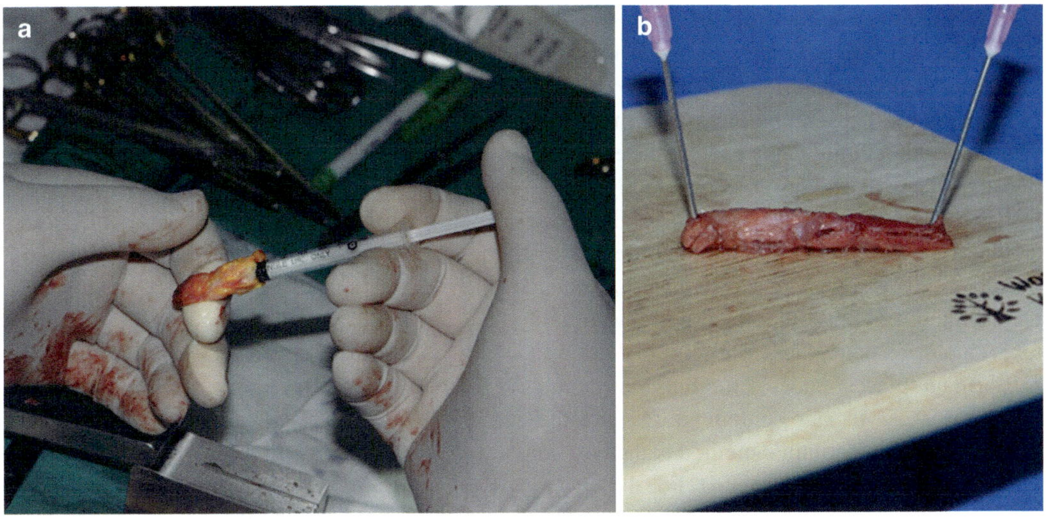

Fig. 6.10 Filling the diced cartilage inside the rolled SMF for more volume. (**a**) Use a 1 cc syringe to seal the SMF around the periphery, and then remove the syringe and apply the space. It is a useful method of filling. (**b**) Fill the cephalic portion more for the projection of Nasion

The absorption issue of autografts, including the dermis, will be covered in more detail in Chap. 7.

Harvest

The harvest is designed in the midline of the sacrum or just on the paramedian side. That is considered for a secondary harvest later.

Collect 20% longer and wider than the desired length, and keep in mind that contraction will occur immediately. The thickness is controlled using folding or molding by a triple layer. Usually, 50 mm-long and 40 mm-wide dermis yield a folded SDF of 8–9 mm wide graft. It is necessary to use a sufficient hydrodissection in the subepidermis and de-epithelization using a loop before detaching.

Septal Cartilage

The author does not use a unique method but collects septal quadrangular cartilage using a method already introduced in several textbooks. However, harvesting the septal cartilage should be determined by the priority of surgery

- The author tries not to perform SMR just because of the need for flat cartilage for the operation.
- Patients requiring septoplasty (deviated nose, hump nose, nasal obstruction) consider performing surgery only with autologous material.
- Dorsal alloplastic implant is a method of camouflage of the lower two-third of nose. Therefore, try to use it as a camouflage material.
- The nasal framework of the undersurface is better not to be destroyed.
- Putting an alloplastic implant on the top of the spreader graft, an invisible graft, if not for functional improvement, there is little evidence to do the spreader graft underneath the alloplastic implant.

The method of secondary septal surgery will be covered in detail in Chap. 11.

Rib Cartilage

Before accessing Dr. Toriumi's literature, the author used several levels of ribs. However, comparing the advantages and disadvantages of the fifth and sixth, and seventh ribs, it is advantageous to use the seventh rib for septal reconstruction because of the straightness and thickness [14]. The author entirely agrees with the explanation that the scar should no longer obligatorily match the inframammary fold if straighter rib cartilage can be obtained longer, and the risk of pneumothorax is low. It is also suitable for septal reconstruction because the upper and lower cortexes' inclusion causes less warping.

Cartilage pieces made of the only cortex are suitable for use in alar contour grafts, and the author thinks Dr. Toriumi's method is the best so far, and the evidence is sufficient. For the explanation of rib cartilage is mainly used in secondary septal surgery. It is recommended to look at Dr. Toriumi's many journals [15–17]. The authors' preferred technique for secondary septal surgery is also covered in Chap. 11.

References

1. Nyemb PM, Sankale A-A, Ndiaye L, NDiaye A, Gaye M. Morphometric study of the outer ear in young adults. Pan Afr Med J. 2014;19:355.
2. Hwang SM, Lim O, Hwang MK, Kim MW, Lee JS. The clinical analysis of the nasal septal cartilage by measurement using computed tomography. Arch Craniofac Surg. 2016;17(3):140–5.
3. Han K, Kim J, Son D, Park B. How to harvest the maximal amount of conchal cartilage grafts. J Plast Reconstr Aesthet Surg. 2008;61(12):1465–71.
4. Lan MY, Park JP, Jang YJ. Donor site morbidities resulting from conchal cartilage harvesting in rhinoplasty. J Laryngol Otol. 2017;131(6):529–33.
5. Echeverry A, Carvajal J, Medina E. Alternative technique for tip support in secondary rhinoplasty. Aesthet Surg J. 2006;26(6):662–8.
6. Sahin MS, Kasapoglu F, Demir UL, Ozmen OA, Coskun H, Basut O. Comparison of clinical results in nasal tip augmentation either via face to face or back to back technique with autogenous auricular conchal cartilage. J Craniofac Surg. 2015;26(7):2109–14.
7. Kridel RW, Scott BA, Foda HM. The tongue-in-groove technique in septorhinoplasty. A 10-year experience. Arch Facial Plast Surg. 1999;1(4):246–56; discussion 257–8.
8. Hwang N-H, Dhong E-S. Septal extension graft in Asian rhinoplasty. Facial Plast Surg Clin North Am. 2018;26(3):331–41.
9. Rabie AN, Chang J, Ibrahim AMS, Lee BT, Lin SJ. Use of Tragal cartilage grafts in rhinoplasty: an anatomic study and review of the literature. Ear Nose Throat J. 2015;94(4–5):E44–9.
10. Cochran CS, DeFatta RJ. Tragal cartilage grafts in rhinoplasty: a viable alternative in the graft-depleted patient. Otolaryngol Head Neck Surg. 2008;138(2):166–9.
11. Hong S-T, Kim D-W, Yoon E-S, Kim H-Y, Dhong E-S. Superficial mastoid fascia as an accessible donor for various augmentations in Asian rhinoplasty. J Plast Reconstr Aesthet Surg. 2012;65(8):1035–40.
12. Kim KY. Augmentation rhinoplasty using dermofat graft. J Korean Soc Aesthetic Plast Surg. 2001;5(1):33–40.
13. Hwang K, Kim DJ, Lee IJ. An anatomic comparison of the skin of five donor sites for dermal fat graft. Ann Plast Surg. 2001;46(3):327–31.
14. Toriumi DM. Dorsal augmentation using autologous costal cartilage or microfat-infused soft tissue augmentation. Facial Plast Surg. 2017;33(2):162–78.
15. Toriumi DM, Patel AB, DeRosa J. Correcting the short nose in revision rhinoplasty. Facial Plast Surg Clin North Am. 2006;14(4):343–55, vi.
16. Toriumi DM, Pero CD. Asian rhinoplasty. Clin Plast Surg. 2010;37(2):335–52.
17. Toriumi DM, Bared A. Revision of the surgically overshortened nose. Facial Plast Surg. 2012;28(4):407–16.

7 The Resorption: The Hurdle for Autogenous-Based Asian Rhinoplasty

Pearls

- Patients with too low nasion should consider using an alloplastic implant from the start.
- If the patient can wait for 12–18 months to complete the resorption, dorsal graft, including too low nasion can be grafted by autologous tissues.
- A consensus is needed between patients and doctors that the graft can be revised due to the resorption issues.
- Crushed cartilage has a significantly lower survival rate than diced cartilage. The resorption rate of diced cartilage is also high.
- Note that many methods of augmentation with micro-diced cartilage without molding can create a tremendous amount of scar tissue in unwanted areas.
- Hard scars made by micro-d iced cartilage injected without molding sometimes show a granuloma-like pattern.
- A dorsal graft of a single layer-superficial mastoid fascia is useful for obtaining a smooth dorsal line. The efficacy for augmentation is nothing more, nothing less than that.
- The long-term augmentation effect of rolled SMF is 1–2 mm. Its absorption should be con sidered more than 50%.
- The long-term augmentation effect of the rolled SDF in the same area is around 3 mm; the absorption rate is 40–50%.
- The effect of long-term augmentation of diced cartilage wrapped with SMF depends on the amount of packed cartilage, but the augmented amount should be planned with an absorption rate of 30–40%.

In Asian rhinoplasty, surgery without evidence or scientific concerns appears in many features: choosing alloplastic materials again in correcting the secondary problems resulted from previously applied alloplastic materials, applying functional spreader graft underneath ruthless thick silicone implants, harvesting conchal cartilage again in case of rib cartilage chosen as the major source of autogenous graft, and applying alloplastic materials with the belief that it will last forever.

In Asian rhinoplasty, many surgeons struggle in choosing the right autograft to get the best results.

"Resorption" is the unsolved, inextricable, imperative battle in performing "autogenous only" rhinoplasty, mostly when the grafts were applied as visible ones, and in the case of the patients' primary concern was dorsal augmentation. So the long-term results of autogenous grafts were analyzed out of 400 cases operated by the author. The categories are autogenous grafts applied on the nasal dorsum: diced cartilage only, rolled superficial mastoid fascia (SMF), diced cartilage wrapped with SMF,

Supplementary Information The online version of this chapter (https://doi.org/10.1007/978-981-16-0542-0_7) contains supplementary material, which is available to authorized users.

E.-S. Dhong, M.-W. Na, *Asian Septorhinoplasty*, https://doi.org/10.1007/978-981-16-0542-0_7

rolled sacral dermofat (SDF), and diced cartilage wrapped with rectus fascia. Autologous materials are preferred due to their high biocompatibility and low risk of infection and extrusion. However, these benefits should be balanced with concerns about graft absorption.

Moreover, in Asian rhinoplasty, which requires much dorsal augmentation, the projection from the nasal root to the tip is often the biggest goal of surgery. Therefore, the experiences of the authors below are critical in viewing Asian rhinoplasty objectively. The author prefers septorhinoplasty using the only autograft in patients who need septoplasty and have been treating patients with low nasion as an absolute indication of the alloplastic implant, so we are well aware that the largest hurdle of autograft is resorption.

7.1 Diced Cartilage

Diced Cartilage Vs. Crushed Cartilage

Crushed cartilage has a lower survival rate than diced cartilage, regardless of the amount [1]. In the author's experience, it can be found that the survival rate of crushed cartilage is very low. Even if it is troublesome, dicing the cartilage to a size of 0.5–1 mm can increase the survival of the tissue. For molding, hyaluronic acid can be sprayed for easy molding [2] (Fig. 7.1). However, the author uses Tisseel (Baxter Healthcare Corp., Deerfield, IL, USA) to mold and use it for small augmentation in the desired place. However, this use means to use the remnant without throwing it away. The authors experienced that most of these applications were absorbed. This meaning of remnant use is nothing more or less than wishing for augmentation of less than 1 mm or smoothing the dorsal profile.When micro-diced cartilage is applied without any molding or wrapping, enormous resorption and scar tissue will be encountered during revision. If a meaningful amount is needed, it is more effective to wrap it in soft tissue.

- Crushed cartilage has a significantly lower survival rate than diced cartilage.
- Diced cartilage molded with fIbrin glue is helpful for the affordable use of discarded cartilage.
- However, if meaningful augmentation is needed, wrapping it in soft tissue is good.
- Note that many methods of augmentation with micro-diced cartilage without wrapping can create a huge amount of scar tissue in unwanted areas.

Diced Cartilage Wrapped with Fascia

Probably this is one of the most used methods [3–5]. Wrapping in the deep temporal fascia is

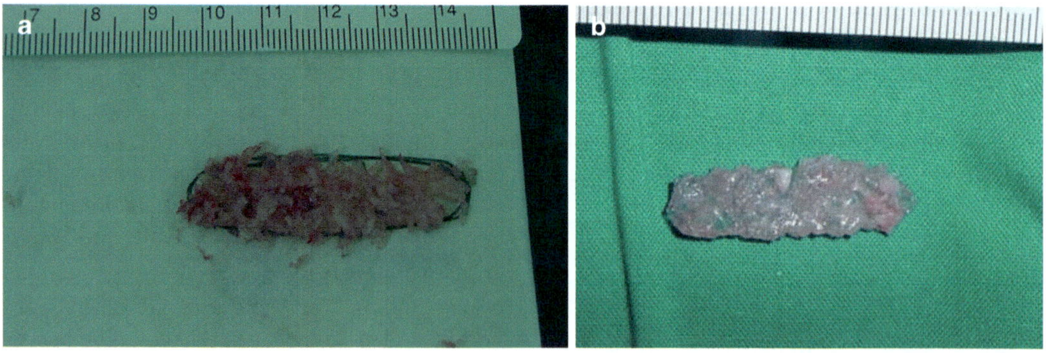

Fig. 7.1 Diced cartilage sprayed with Tisseel for molding. (**a**) Diced cartilage for the dorsal camouflage. (**b**) After applying the fibrin solution

less invading inflammatory cells than wrapping in Surgicel (Ethicon, Inc., a Johnson & Johnson company, Arlington, TX, USA), so more healthy cartilage survives [6]. The author does not prefer wrapping with Surgicel, either making an incision on the hairline during surgery. For soft tissue wrapping, superficial mastoid fascia is placed in a cartilage crusher and thinly bloomed using a mallet. Here, the author prefers the filling method using a 1 cc syringe (Chap. 6). Of course, when collecting costal cartilage, the preferred site is rectus fascia in a square shape for wrapping (Fig. 7.2).

7.2 Septal Cartilage

Septal cartilage is relatively used as strut, batten graft, and spreader graft. There is no worry about being absorbed because it is usually used as an invisible graft. The resorption is imperceptible because it is replaced by appropriate fibrous tissue. However, there are reports that the absorption rate is 12–50% in the past. Also, it is reported that even the spreader graft resorbed when its tension is severe and if it is crushed [7]. The anatomical graft or orthotopic graft does not resorb because the recipient site's remaining perichon-

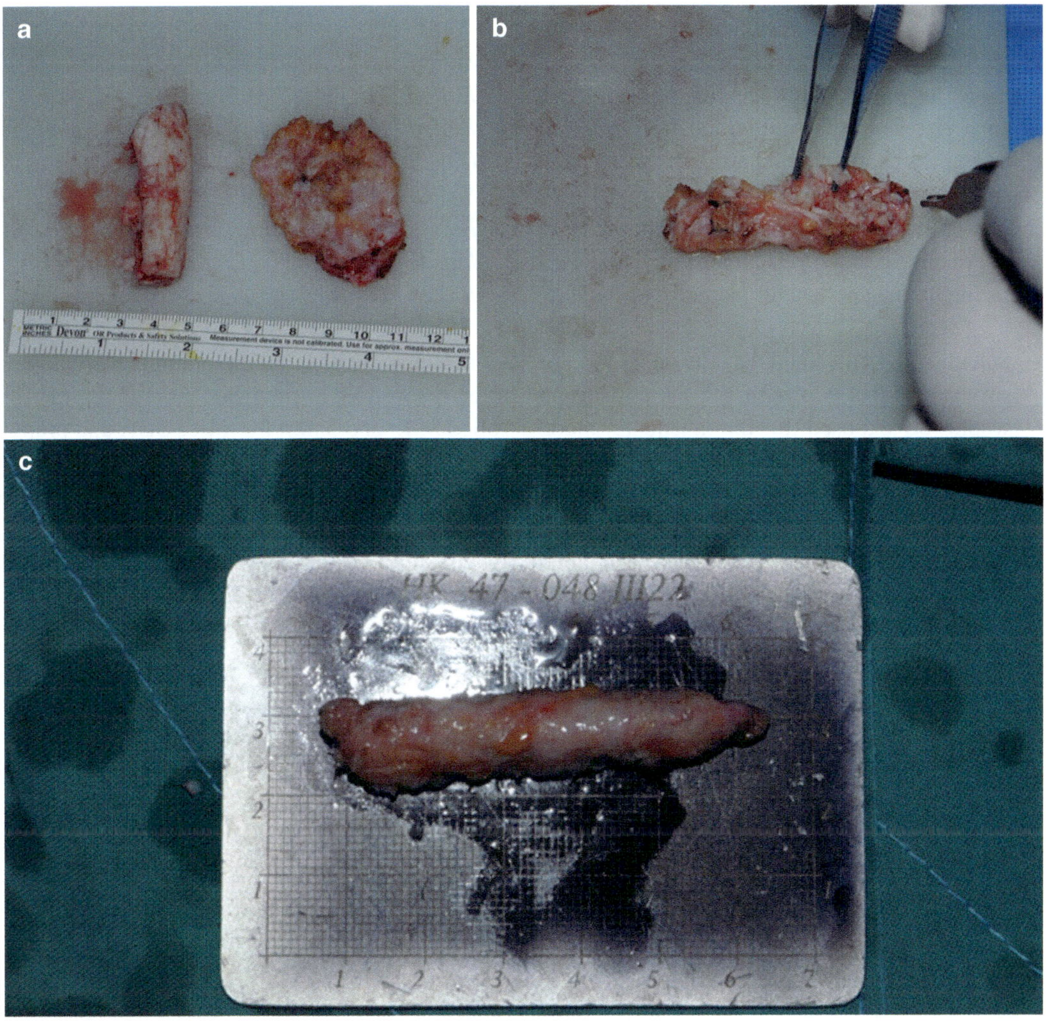

Fig. 7.2 Diced costal cartilage wrapped with rectus fascia. (**a**) Sixth rib and rectus fascia. (**b**) The remnant costal cartilages are diced and packed in the rectus fascia. (**c**) After molding for graft. (photo from other case)

drium provides an adequate blood supply. Septal cartilage cannot be harvested with perichondrium attached, so the orthotopic graft is more effective than the onlay graft.

7.3 Ear Cartilage

Like septal cartilage, ear cartilage is used in all types of rhinoplasty and is the primary choice of secondary rhinoplasty [8, 9]. In the case of secondary rhinoplasty, most of them are in SMR state, so cymba and cavum concha are the primary choices. If the septal L-strut is severely damaged and reconstruction of the nasal framework is not possible with ear cartilage, costal cartilage is used. At the time of the revision, it can be seen that most of the ear cartilages are alive, but the original size is a little smaller, and the shape of the margin is changed, indicating that resorption occurs. However, it is challenging to determine the absorption rate because it is impossible to know precisely how perichondrium was used according to the application method.

- Scientifically, it would be advantageous for survival, if the side with the perichondrium would be exposed to the adequate blood supply.
- In the author's study, when folded cymba concha is used for caudal septal extension graft, concave sides were coapted to face each other, so attaching the convex side's perichondrium would be advantageous for cartilage survival.

7.4 The Resorption Rate of Soft Tissues

The order below is from the lowest to the highest height of the target dorsum among the author's methods. There are six types of soft tissues that the author uses for dorsal enhancement. Other soft tissues include medial plantar dermis, axillary dermis, and groin dermofat graft, but each has too many disadvantages such as pain and hair-bearing, so they are not used anymore by the author. Of course, when surgery is planned with only ear cartilage, rectus fascia is not harvested only for dorsal augmentation. Rectus fascial is only used when costal cartilage is harvested.

- *Superficial Mastoid fascia (SMF)* [10].
- *Rolled SMF* (Fig. 7.3).
- *Rolled SMF filled with diced cartilage* (Fig. 7.4).
- *Sacral dermis-fat (SDF).*
- *Rolled Rectus Fascia filled with diced cartilage* (Fig. 7.2).
- *Rolled SDF* (Fig. 7.5).

In each case, the amount of targeted thickness after resorption is predicted as 1–1.5 mm for rolled SMF and 3 mm for rolled SDF, and preparations are made for surgery. The meaning of rolling is to make a tube shape by repairing both sides of the sheet and increasing the thickness twice. However, in the SDF case, due to the tissue's characteristics, the choice should be made whether placing the dermal portion inside (der-

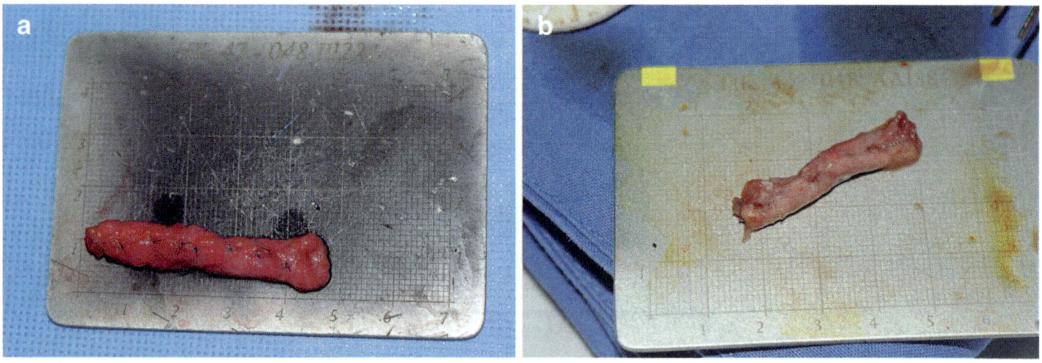

Fig. 7.3 Rolled superficial mastoid fascia. (**a**, **b**) Two different cases

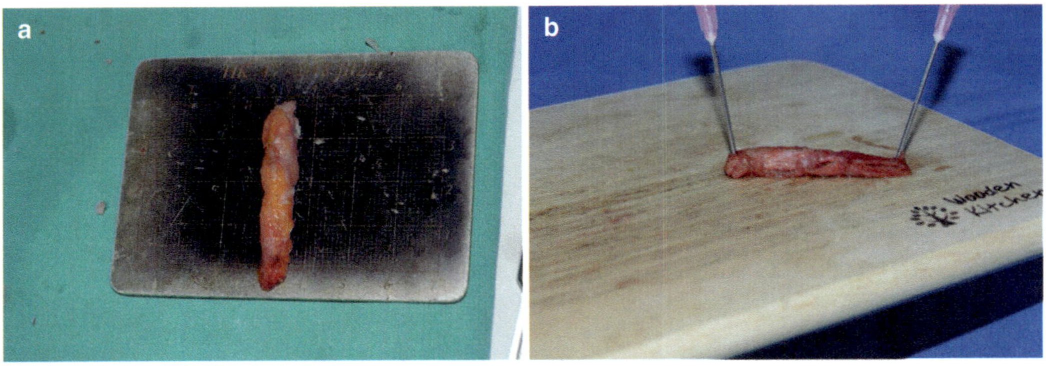

Fig. 7.4 Diced cartilage wrapped with superficial mastoid fascia. (**a**, **b**) Two different cases

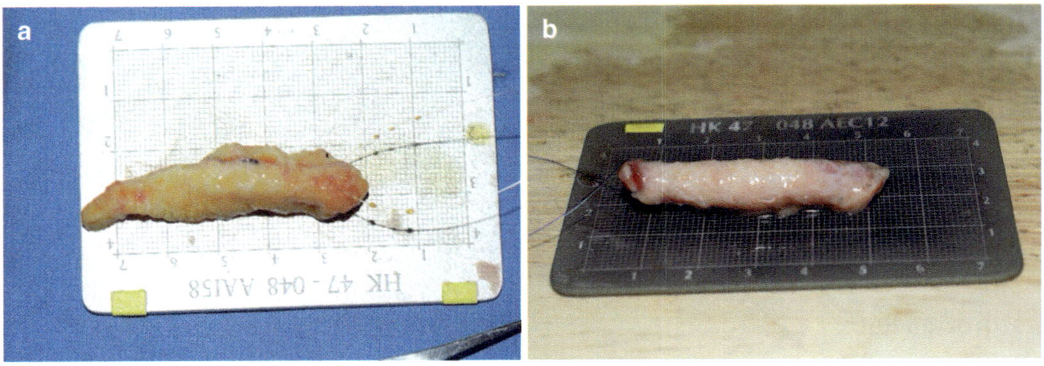

Fig. 7.5 Rolled sacral dermis-fat (SDF). (**a**, **b**) Two different cases

mis-in rolling) or outside (dermis-out rolling). The dermis-out rolling is mainly used when there is a puncture in the dorsal skin so that a uniform surface is to be placed directly under the skin and when to implement a more definite dorsal line (Video 7.1). If the remaining recipient site's skin is thin, the author selects the dermis-in rolling (fat-out rolling) technique to attenuate the graft's definition (Fig. 7.5a). Considering the dermal physiology, the dermis-out rolling, where the dermis layer contacts directly the recipient's surgical pocket, has a higher probability of rapid revascularization (Fig. 7.5b). However, since the bottom is nasal bone and the periosteum is mostly destroyed, some resorption cannot be prevented.

The dermal graft, which is located subcutaneously, is found to be hardly absorbed but rather survived at the revision surgery. The subcutaneous SDF graft is revised to move to a deeper location by elevating the nasal bone's periosteum. The demarcation is corrected by this method (Fig. 7.6).

It should be borne in mind that if the dorsal skin is too thin, the inserted SDF may be demarcated.

- Rolling method: In the case of concerning demarcation under the thin skin in reoperation, it is controlled by enrolling the thin fat layer outward (dermis-in rolling). If the subdermis of the dorsal skin is thick, it is good to use the dermis-out rolling.
- Since the dermal blood supply is critical to survival, it is suitable for the survival to use the dermis-out rolling.
- However, the author prefers to use only the dermal portion without including the fatty part due to resorption issues, and rarely uses the fatty portion.

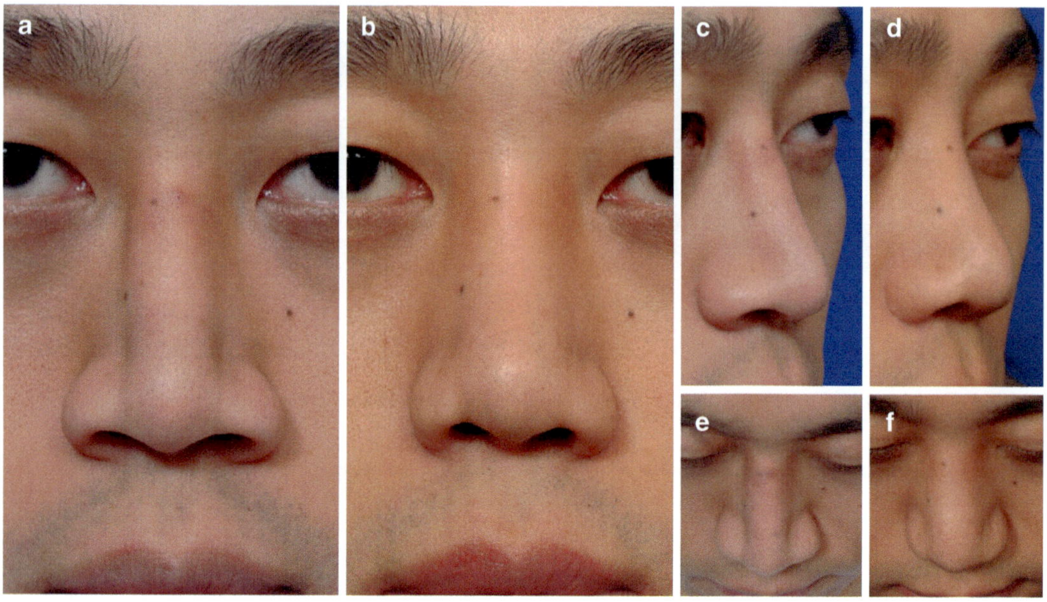

Fig. 7.6 A 34-year-old male patient underwent an SDF graft at another clinic. Demarcated SDF was corrected by changing the depth of the dissection plane from subcutaneous plane to subperiosteal plane. (**a**, **c**, **e**) Preoperative views, (**b**, **d**, **f**) Postoperative 1 year

Resorption Rate

Among the various types of autologous tissue recognition above, long-term results were obtained for the following three absorption rates. (Data in publishing, Plastic and reconstructive surgery 2021).

- ***Rolled SMF***
- ***Rolled SMF filled with diced cartilage***
- ***Rolled SDF***

One month after surgery was considered as the result of an immediate postoperative state, and the photo was used as a control. Postoperative photos of more than 1 year were used to compare as a long-term follow-up. We have recently published some of the research using two-dimensional photographs underneath three-dimensional photographs. Since a lot of past data is accumulated and written in a 2D photo, to analyze this photo objectively, two software MPS (Morpheus 3D Plastic Solution, Morpheus 3D scanner, Morpheus CO. Ltd., Seoul Korea,) and MDS (Morpheus 3D Dental Solution) was used for comparative analysis.

Usefulness of Standardized Two-Dimensional Photo Analysis

The author standardized the magnification using a baseline length adjustment for each photo. Anatomical proportions, including vertical height, were used for objective measurements: cheilion to the middle pupil line. The cheilion-mid pupil line was used as the basis for the calculation (Video 7.2). The magnification was adjusted by making each length equal. Bias in assessing the magnitude and direction of any differences found between 2D and 3D imaging software was evaluated statistically in many anthropometric points. The bias difference was calculated between the 2D and 3D imaging software measurements. For each landmark, the 3D imaging software yielded more extensive measurements on average. The average difference is 0.127 mm over the 2D imaging software. However, there were no significant differences between 2D and 3D imaging software. Therefore, it was possible to analyze past 2D pictures with modified MDS, and this standardization was possible according to this result.

How to Correct Yawing and Rolling in 2D Photographs

The author standardized the magnification using a baseline length adjustment for each photo. Anatomical proportions, including vertical height, were used for objective measurements: cheilion to the middle pupil line. The cheilion-mid pupil line was used as the basis for the calculation. To control yawing and rolling, the author standardized the two lengths of tragus-midpupil and tragus-cheilion line equal.

The Resorption Rate

To compare resorption rates, rhinion and 1/2 NR (the ½ of nasion–rhinion) projections were assessed.

In the author's surgical method, the cartilaginous dorsum and nasal tip projection were mainly projected using autogenous cartilage. The three types of autogenous grafts mentioned above were inserted from the nasal root to obtain a smooth dorsal line connected to caudally. As mentioned above, the dermal graft will survive better in the subcutaneous lower two-third of the nose, which is rich in blood supply, and it is difficult to compare the complexed surgical areas such as supratip and tip. Therefore, the author wanted to compare autologous tissue's absorption rate under the same conditions. The selected site was nasion and ½ NR (the midpoint between nasion and rhinion). Rhinion was defined here as the upper one-third point of nasion and tip defining point. All grafts were placed in the subperiosteal pocket. The results came out more than expected: "the vastness of the reabsorption."

The following is the resorption rate at 1/2NR, which is the bony dorsum's middle point among many data. If you are curious, refer to the author's journal to be published soon. It is a resorption rate expressed with a 95% confidence interval.

The resorption rate of rolled SMF at ½ NR: 50–70%.

In both three quarter and modified profile views, resorption rates were the highest and the most dramatic in the rolled SMF group: 54.8–72.8% (Figs. 7.7 and 7.8).

The resorption rate of rolled SMF filled with diced cartilage at ½ NR: 30–40%.

In both three quarter and modified profile views, The rolled SMF filled with diced cartilage showed the resorption rate as 27.3–43.3% (Figs. 7.9 and 7.10).

The resorption rate of rolled SDF at ½ NR: 40–50%.

In both three quarter and modified profile views, the rolled SD group showed the resorption rate as 37.1–51.2% (Figs. 7.11 and 7.12).

There were statistically significant resorption rate differences among the three autologous groups ($p < 0.001$).

This is a study of the upper bony dorsum's absorption rate, which is the most problematic in Asian surgery. The lowest absorption rate was SMF wrapped with diced cartilage grafted, and the highest absorption rate was rolled SMF. It is somewhat similar or different from the existing reports [11].

With the consensus among surgeons, SDF's absorption rate is thought to progress from one to one and a half years. The author also agrees that the more soft tissue graft contains, the higher the absorption rate. The more fatty tissue the graft contains, the higher the absorption rate, and absorption will proceed for more than 1 year.

- Crushed cartilage is almost completely absorbed when implanted in the nasion site.
- Diced cartilage is also absorbed, so the effect of augmentation is insignificant but remains more than crushed cartilage.
- A single-layer of SMF is useful for obtaining a smooth dorsal esthetic line at the rhinion.

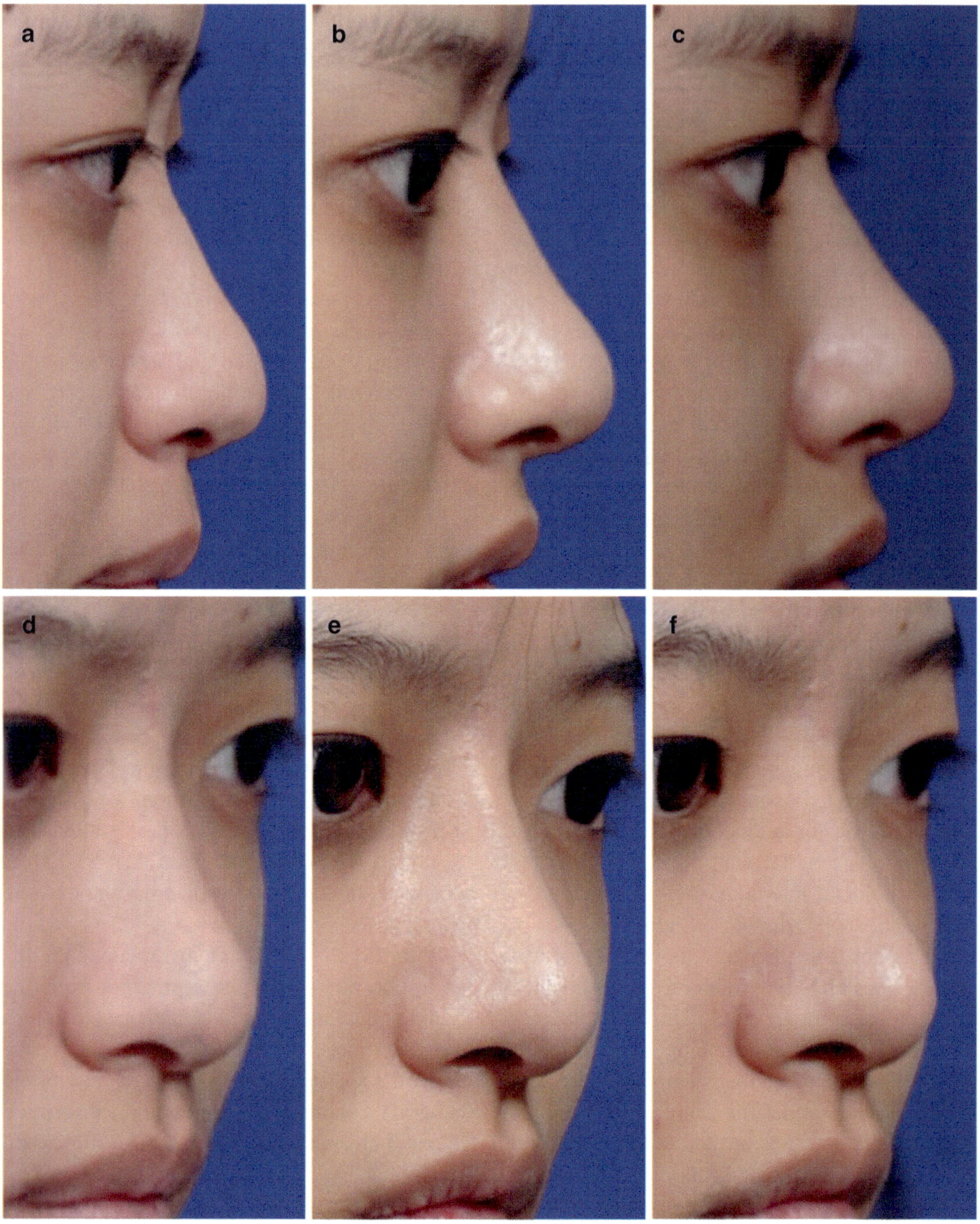

Fig. 7.7 Resorption of rolled superficial mastoid fascia (SMF). (**a**, **d**) Preoperative view. (**b**, **e**) Immediate postoperative view: postoperative 1 month. (**c**, **f**) Long-term postoperative view: 18 months postoperative

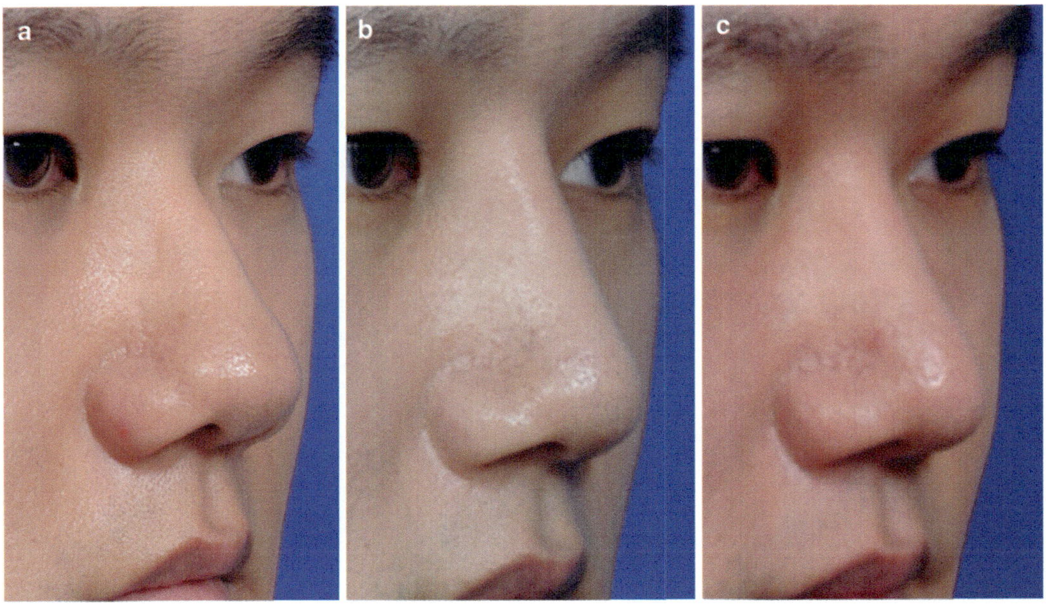

Fig. 7.8 Resorption of rolled superficial mastoid fascia (SMF). (**a**) Preoperative view. (**b**) Immediate postoperative view: postoperative 1 month. (**c**) Long-term postoperative view: 12 months postoperative

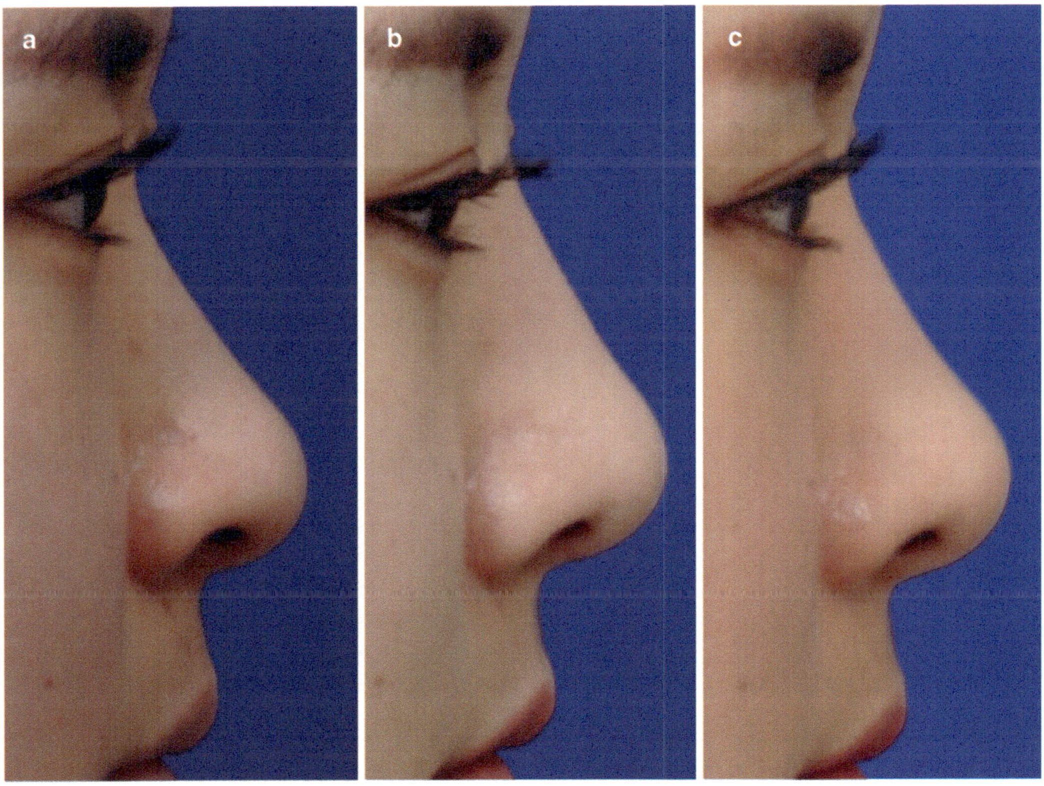

Fig. 7.9 Resorption of diced cartilage wrapped with rolled SMF. (**a**, **d**) Preoperative view. (**b**, **e**) Immediate postoperative view: postoperative 1 month. (**c**, **f**) Long-Term postoperative view: 14 months postoperative

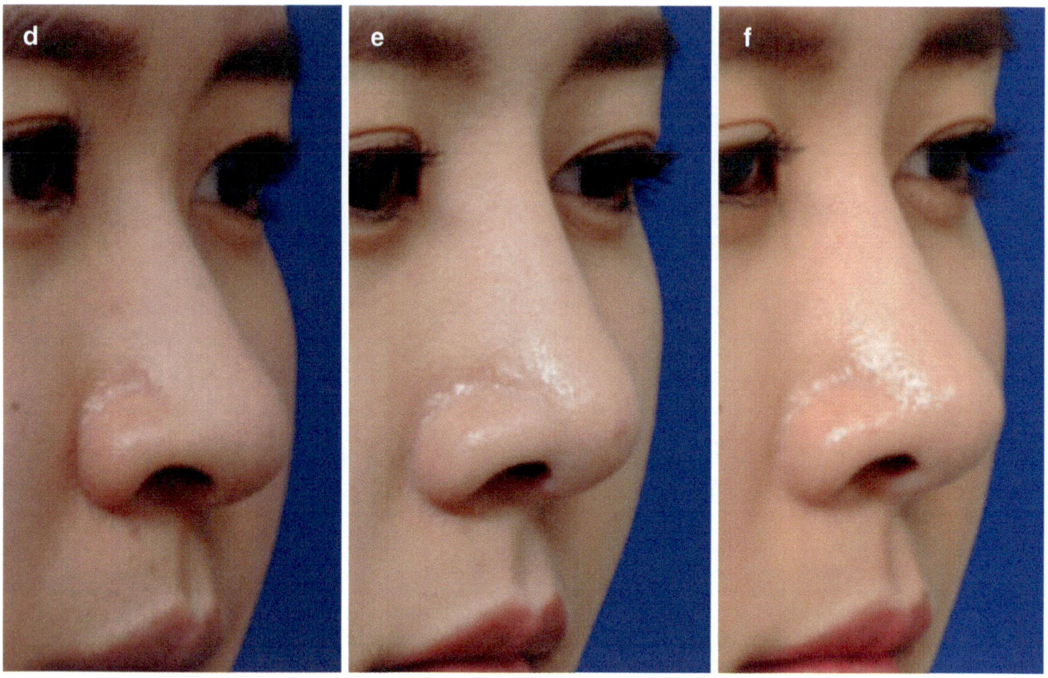

Fig. 7.9 (continued)

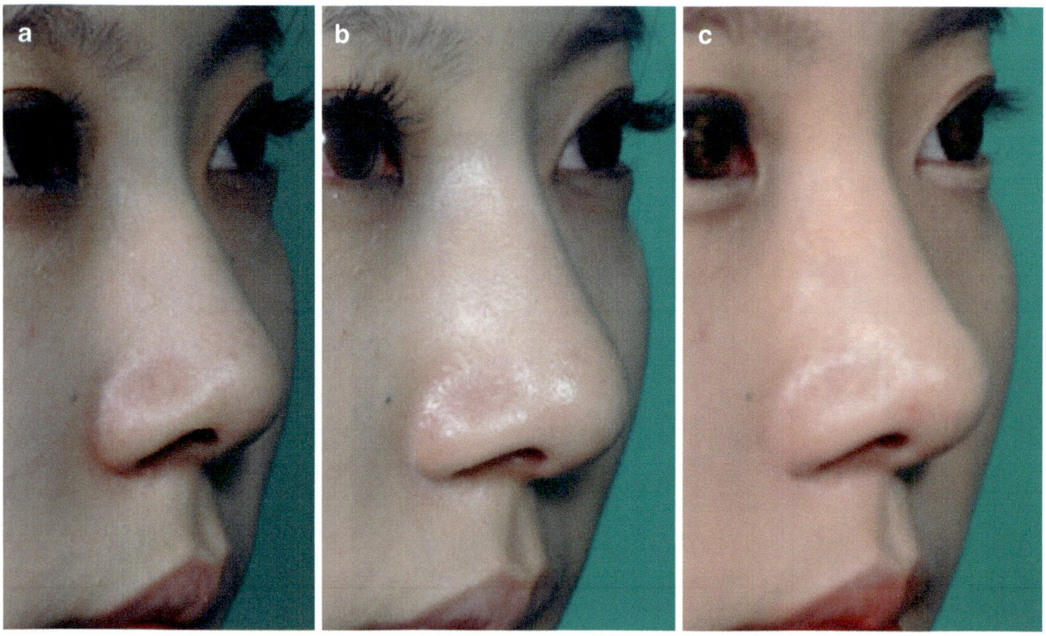

Fig. 7.10 Resorption of diced cartilage wrapped with rolled SMF. (**a**) Preoperative view. (**b**) Immediate postoperative view: postoperative fifth week. (**c**) Long-Term postoperative view: 12 months postoperative

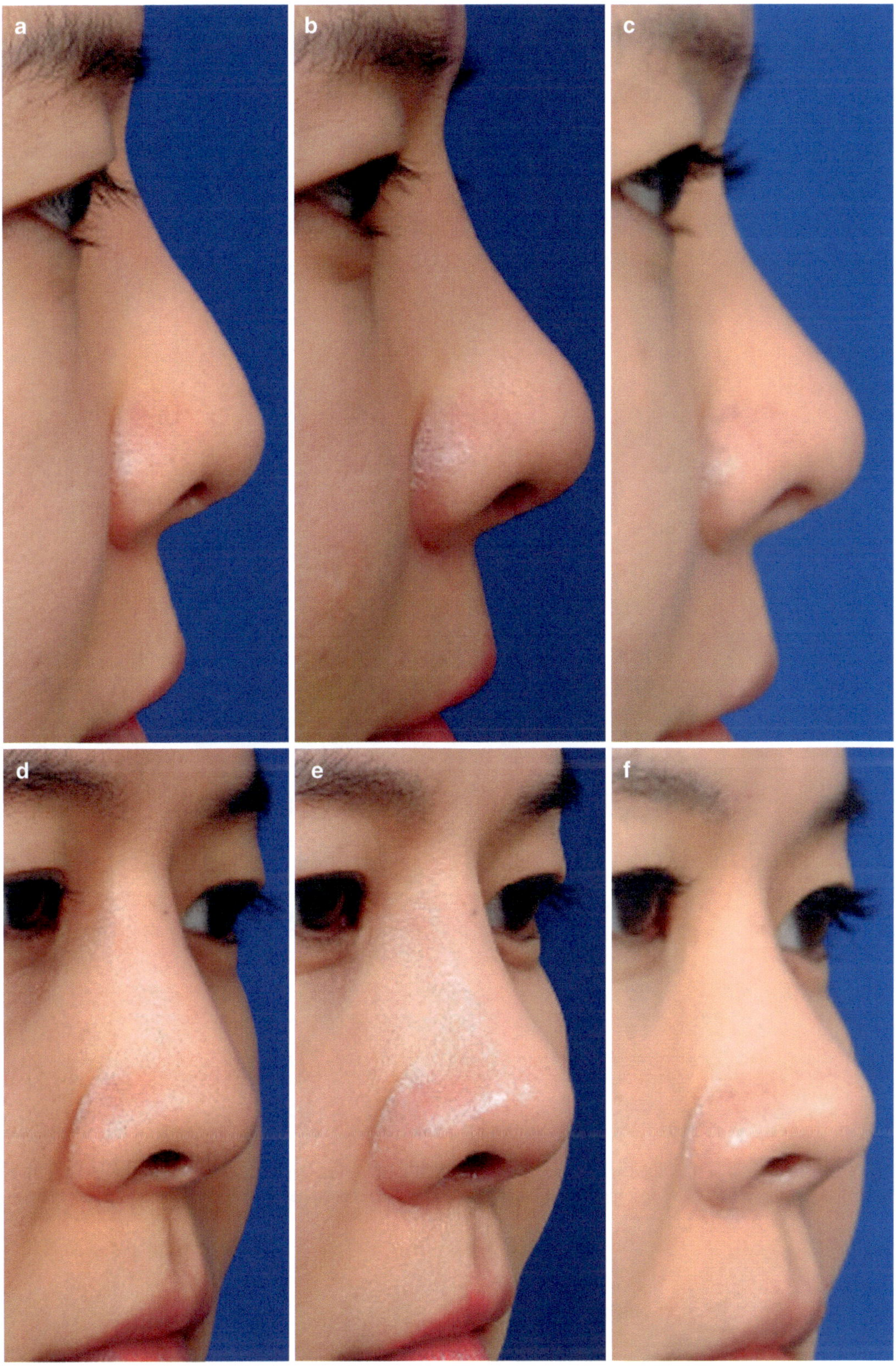

Fig. 7.11 Resorption of the rolled sacral dermis-fat graft (SDF). (**a**, **d**) Preoperative view with dorsal implant. (**b**, **e**) Immediate postoperative view: postoperative 1 month. (**c**, **f**) Long-Term postoperative view: 12 months postoperative

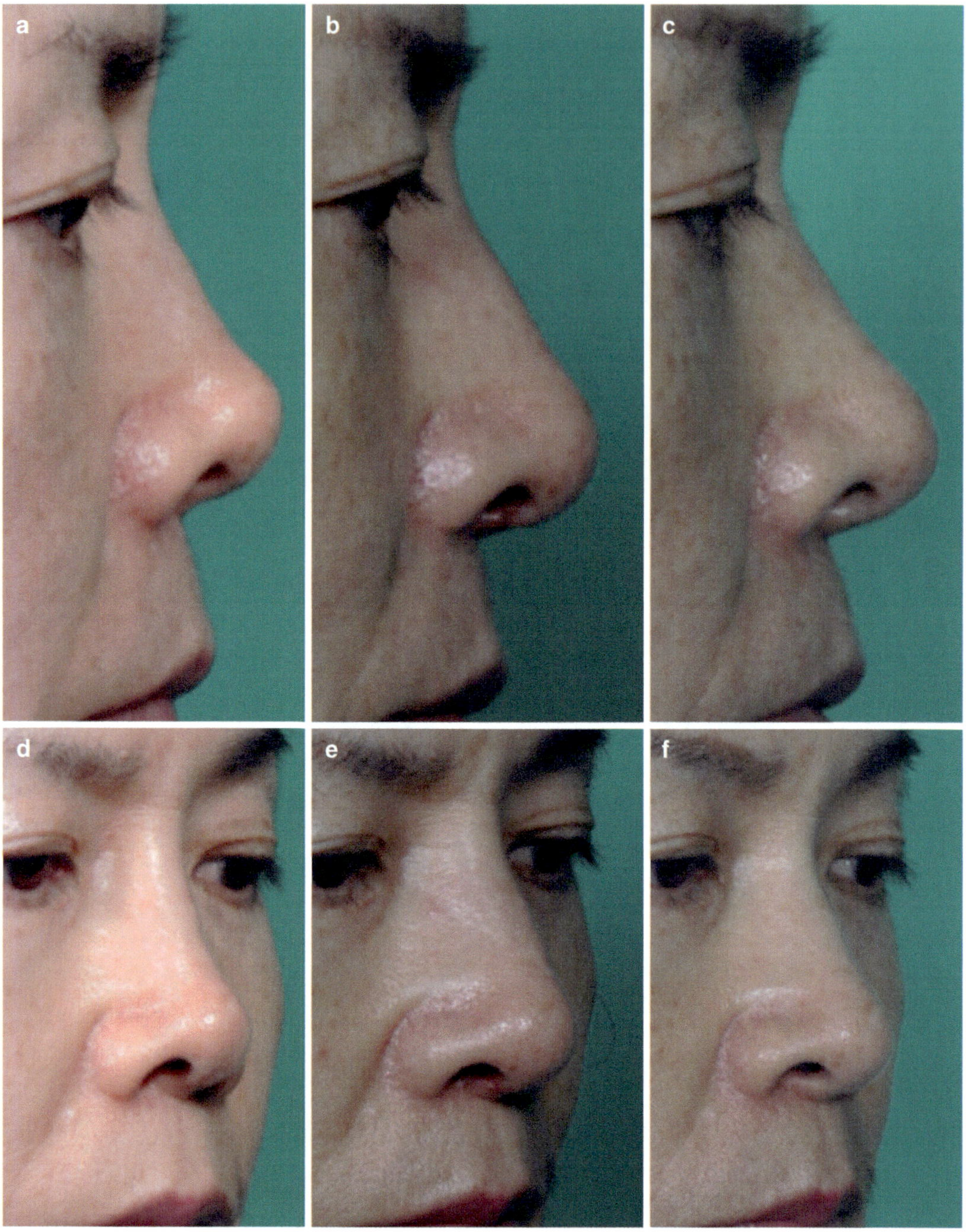

Fig. 7.12 Resorption of the rolled sacral dermis-fat graft (SDF). (**a**, **d**) Preoperative view with dorsal implant. (**b**, **e**) Immediate postoperative view: postoperative 1 month. (**c**, **f**) Long-Term postoperative view: 12 months postoperative

- Graft on the nasal bone is highly absorbed. Relatively where the perichondrium is a platform, the absorption is less.
- The long-term augmentation effect of rolled SMF is 1–2 mm in contact with bone in the bony portion of the nasion or below. Its absorption should be considered more than 50%.
- The long-term augmentation effect of the rolled SDF in the same area is approximately 3 mm. The absorption rate is regarded as 40–50%.
- The effect of long-term augmentation of diced cartilage wrapped with SMF depends on the amount of packed cartilage, but it should be planned with an absorption rate of 30–40%.

References

1. Cakmak O, Bircan S, Buyuklu F, Tuncer I, Dal T, Ozluoglu LN. Viability of crushed and diced cartilage grafts: a study in rabbits. Arch Facial Plast Surg. 2005;7(1):21–6.
2. Kazikdas KC, Ergur B, Tugyan K, Guneli E, Kaya D, Sahan M. Viability of crushed and diced cartilage grafts wrapped in oxidized regenerated cellulose and esterified hyaluronic acid: an experimental study. Laryngoscope. 2007;117(10):1728–34.
3. Daniel RK. Diced cartilage grafts in rhinoplasty surgery: current techniques and applications. Plast Reconstr Surg. 2008;122(6):1883–91.
4. Daniel RK, Calvert JW. Diced cartilage grafts in rhinoplasty surgery. Plast Reconstr Surg. 2004;113(7):2156–71.
5. Daniel RK. Rhinoplasty: dorsal grafts and the designer dorsum. Clin Plast Surg. 2010;37(2):293–300.
6. Brenner KA, McConnell MP, Evans GRD, Calvert JW. Survival of diced cartilage grafts: an experimental study. Plast Reconstr Surg. 2006;117(1):105–15.
7. Bujía J. Determination of the viability of crushed cartilage grafts: clinical implications for wound healing in nasal surgery. Ann Plast Surg. 1994;32(3):261–5.
8. Endo T, Nakayama Y, Ito Y. Augmentation rhinoplasty [Internet]. Plastic and Reconstructive Surgery. vol. 87; 1991. p 54–9. https://doi.org/10.1097/00006534-199101000-00010.
9. Toriumi DM. Augmentation rhinoplasty with autologous cartilage grafting [Internet]. Asian Facial Cosmetic Surgery. 2007. p. 229–52. https://doi.org/10.1016/b978-1-4160-0290-1.50026-x.
10. Hong S-T, Kim D-W, Yoon E-S, Kim H-Y, Dhong E-S. Superficial mastoid fascia as an accessible donor for various augmentations in Asian rhinoplasty. J Plast Reconstr Aesthet Surg. 2012;65(8):1035–40.
11. Kim H-K, Rhee SC. Augmentation rhinoplasty using a folded "pure" dermal graft [Internet]. J Craniofacial Surg. 2013;24:1758–62. https://doi.org/10.1097/scs.0b013e31828f1b5f.

8 Controlling Asian Tip: Tip Defining Point and Supratip Break

Pearls

- Asian LLC is fragile and does not have enough length, so it has limitations in making beautiful tips with its modifications.
- In many cases, the "tip tripod theory" cannot be applied. In primary rhinoplasty, the first step is to determine the position of the ideal sellion and the subnasale to determine the length of the nose accordingly.
- In secondary rhinoplasty, it is often necessary to first consider the tip position through tissue release and then perform the remaining procedures.
- Planning the tip defining point is the beginning of Asian rhinoplasty. The first step in determining the tip defining point is the interdomal suture.
- SEG has a disadvantage because the tip is tilted to one side when the nasal base is weak. Also, it is not easy to apply to secondary rhinoplasty.
- Floating type columella strut has a disadvantage. Its effect is not strong in Asian tip plasty because the amount of projection is small.
- The suture of the columella strut should be done in the area confined to the medial crura. The suture between the caudal margin of the middle crura breaks its own divergence.
- STB problems found in Asian rhinoplasty are related to alloplastic implants in many cases.
- The shield graft maintains the symmetry of the LLCs and the divergence of the middle crura and is useful for creating a tip-lobular angle.
- The anteriorly relocated high septum provides the necessary support for the positioning of the lateral crura, along with the correction of the saddle nose deformity.
- The high septal reconstruction is necessary to prevent STB deformity due to dorsal graft resorption, and STB expressed by the septum has less deformation in the long term.
- The onlay graft such as batten or derotation graft may cause convexity (supratip deformity) of STB.
- A lot of LLC's destruction or resorption is found in secondary surgery, and its strength is weak, making it difficult to obtain stability only with lateral crus. Methods such as lateral crural steal or lateral crural overlay are complicated.

Asian rhinoplasty is generally aimed into three purposes. These are lengthening the nose, enhancing the dorsum, and projecting the tip with tip plasty. Another classification uniquely exists in Asian rhinoplasty: primary vs. secondary rhinoplasty. As such, secondary rhinoplasty has an entirely different perspective. The tissue contracture is uniquely seen in Asian secondary rhinoplasty. Therefore, this chapter mainly describes general concepts, but

Supplementary Information The online version of this chapter (https://doi.org/10.1007/978-981-16-0542-0_8) contains supplementary material, which is available to authorized users.

E.-S. Dhong, M.-W. Na, *Asian Septorhinoplasty*, https://doi.org/10.1007/978-981-16-0542-0_8

we have included some pitfalls seen in the secondary nose at the end of each unit. The contracted nose will be covered again in Chaps. 11 and 12. For Asian rhinoplasty, most doctors will use a septal extension graft for extension and an alloplastic implant for augmentation. Most of the time, they will try nasal tip plasty with sutures and various grafts. Apart from that method, in this chapter, the author would like to talk about the consensus that is particularly problematic in Asian rhinoplasty or is the target of surgery. For Asians, it is difficult to obtain good results without a clear goal for the tip. The definition of the tip and soft triangle in the Western nose is clear, and the tip defining point has two highlights (Fig. 8.1). In many cases, the shape of the LLC can be observed from the external nose. Of course, some people have the same tip definition. However, a hypoplastic LLC with thick skin envelopes of Asian consists only of a smooth curve without tip definition (Fig. 8.2). It is challenging to make a beautiful tip that corresponds to the following content with a fragile LLC. The lateral crus is very short, and it is difficult to expect in East Asians that this follows Anderson's tip tripod theory [1]. Also, cartilaginous graft is required to make nasal frameworks and the tip. This is why Asian rhinoplasty has entirely different perspectives from Western one, which consisted of mainly reduction rhinoplasty. Also, a cartilaginous graft is required to make nasal frameworks and the tip.

8.1 Steps for Nasal Tip Plasty

In Asian primary rhinoplasty, the first step is to determine the position of the ideal sellion and the subnasale. That determines the total length, these two landmarks decide all. In other words, the first procedure is to decide the length with the starting point (golden point) of the nose. After that, the height of the tip is determined according to tissue resilience. Finally, the dorsal height is determined by various angles. If the nose's dorsal height is excessively projected, the tip projection will be insufficient if the tissue is not recruited. The tip projection exceeds the limit with excessive alloplastic material, causing a problem. In the case of secondary rhinoplasty, it is a little different. The resilience of the tip deteriorated. The amount of tip release determines the length of the nose.

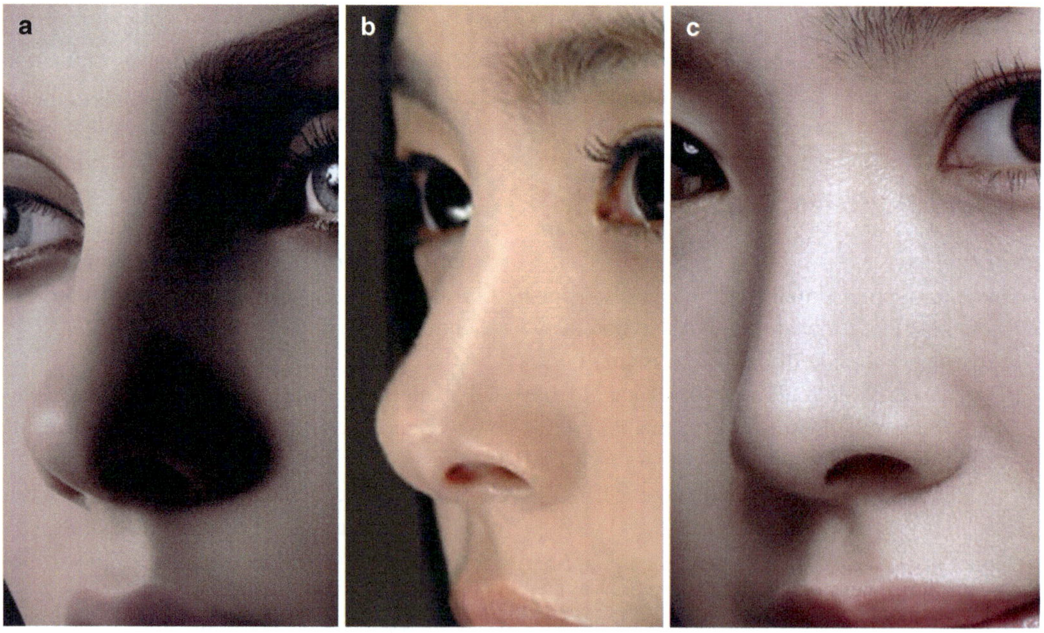

Fig. 8.1 Features of Asian nasal tip. (**a**) In Caucasian, you can find the highlight of a well-developed tip. (**b**) In the case of showing a well-developed tip definition in Asian. (**c**) Beautiful tip without definition seen in Asian

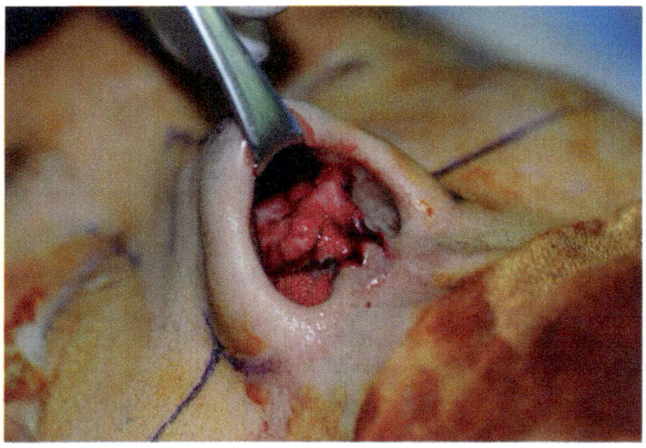

Fig. 8.2 Hypoplastic Asian nasal tip. It can be found that the development of middle crura, the medial crura is insufficient. If the cartilage is weak and subSMAS dissection proceeds, only the LLC, which is too fragile, will remain

The nose's height is automatically determined by the various ideal angles: columellolabial angle, tip-lobular angle, and nasofrontal angle. In other words, in secondary rhinoplasty, the tip position is considered first, and then performs the rest of the procedure. The amount of release determines the length of the nose and the amount of dorsal height. At this time, the modification of LLC is indispensable. In Asians, the middle crus is insufficiently developed, and the angle formed with the middle and medial crura is amorphous, so much effort is required in this part.

8.2 The Tip Defining Point

The tip defining point is the front most point of the tip projection made by two highlights of the middle crus's lateral border [2, 3]. It is the starting point of the tip plasty as the highlight of the tip of the Asian rhinoplasty. For a precise definition, a suture technique or graft is needed. If you have a weak LLC, it is difficult to obtain the desired definition with the suture technique. Tip plasty is started by the first interdomal suture on the cephalic border of the middle crus at the correct position of the tip lobule [4] (Fig. 8.3).

The tip defining point made by excessive transdomal suture applied to the lateral crus creates pinching deformity because the lateral crura and medial crural angles are too narrow. In this way, the physiology is damaged by the shape of the external nares. It can cause nasal obstruction and spoil the shape of the beautiful tip. The problem is that it also spoils the shape of the soft triangle, an essential part of the tip lobule esthetics. The following are the ways to project the tip defining point.

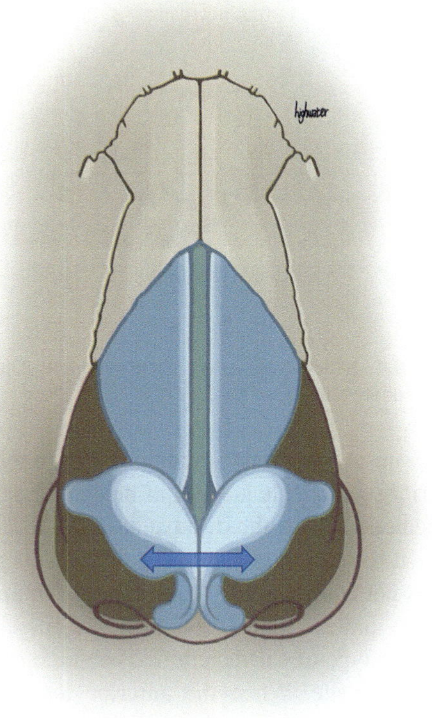

Fig. 8.3 The tip defining point: the distance between the lateral margin of caudal medial genu of middle crura

Septum-Dependent Tip Projection

A septal extension graft (SEG) is mostly used. When the caudal septum's projection is deficient, Dr. Byrd's SEG can help create a tip defining point more projected (Fig. 8.4). There are three types of SEG: direct type, batten type, and spreader type. In the author's case, the batten type is preferred, but the SEG starting from the middle of the caudal septum is not stable.

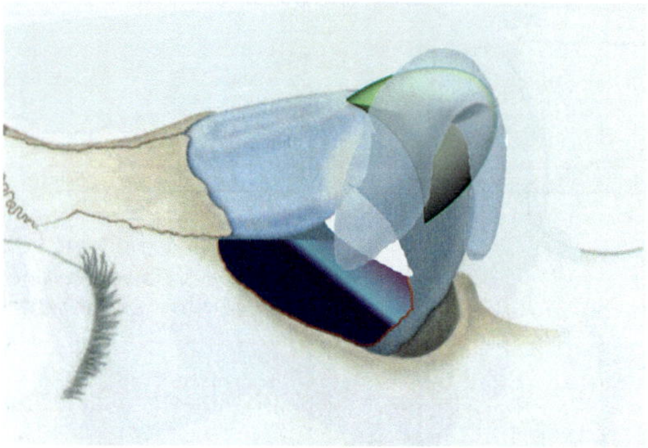

Fig. 8.4 Batten type septal extension graft: The most commonly found graft type

The nasal base constructed by ANS and the posterior septal angle is weak in many Asians. This method also has the disadvantage that the tip is tilted to one side when the nasal base is weak. It is not easy to apply to secondary rhinoplasty. Many patients underwent SMR, so there is no square type of cartilage left. The author prefers ear cartilage. When the anterior septal angle extending from the septum is directly connected to the interdomal suture, it is advantageous to place it in the cephalic portion of the middle crus when making the tip shape later. Multiple sutures in the intercrural position are performed for stability; however, the caudal border of the medial crus should be avoided (Fig. 8.5). It preserves the divergence of the medial genu on both sides of the middle crus and also preserves the divergence between the long axes of the lateral crus.

Septum-Independent Tip Projection

The representative one is the columellar strut. Floating type or fixed type can be used.

- The floating type has the disadvantage that its effect is inferior in Asian rhinoplasty because the amount of projection is small (Fig. 8.6).
- In the case of the fixed type, there is a disadvantage that a long length is required.

However, the biggest problem is that the caudal margin and repair of the medial crus or middle crus are required to obtain strong support, and the two divergence angles shown in Fig. 8.5 above are broken. When the caudal margin is coapted, the divergence of the medial genu disappears, and lateral crus is also caudally turned down. In other words, it is not easy to make beautiful infratip lobules or ideal soft triangles. For the beautiful infratip lobule, a columellolobular angle should be required, and it is difficult to make if the divergence of the middle genu is lost.

- The suture of the columella strut should be done in the area confined to the medial crura, and it is more ideal for repairing the mid-portion with the intercrural suture of the medial crura.

8.3 The Supratip Break: STB

Definition

Most Asian men want a straight dorsal line. In women, they want the subtle concavity of the part that transitions from the tip defining point to the dorsum. In the literature, the remaining convexity of this site is considered supratip deformity [5, 6]. In the primary patient, the deformity resulted from inadequate tip projection (pseudodeformation), over-projected caudal dorsum, and cephalically oriented LLC. In secondary patients, the anomaly was due to an under- or over-excised caudal dorsum, or a combination of some under the projected tip [7, 8].

From the tip defining point to STB, the subtle concavity is a part close to the straight line of lateral genu. The voluminous STB is made of the cephalic border of the lateral crus and subcutaneous fat. Convexity is worse in this area, but excessive concavity is also subject to patients' complaints. STB problems found in Asian rhinoplasty are related to alloplastic implants in many areas.

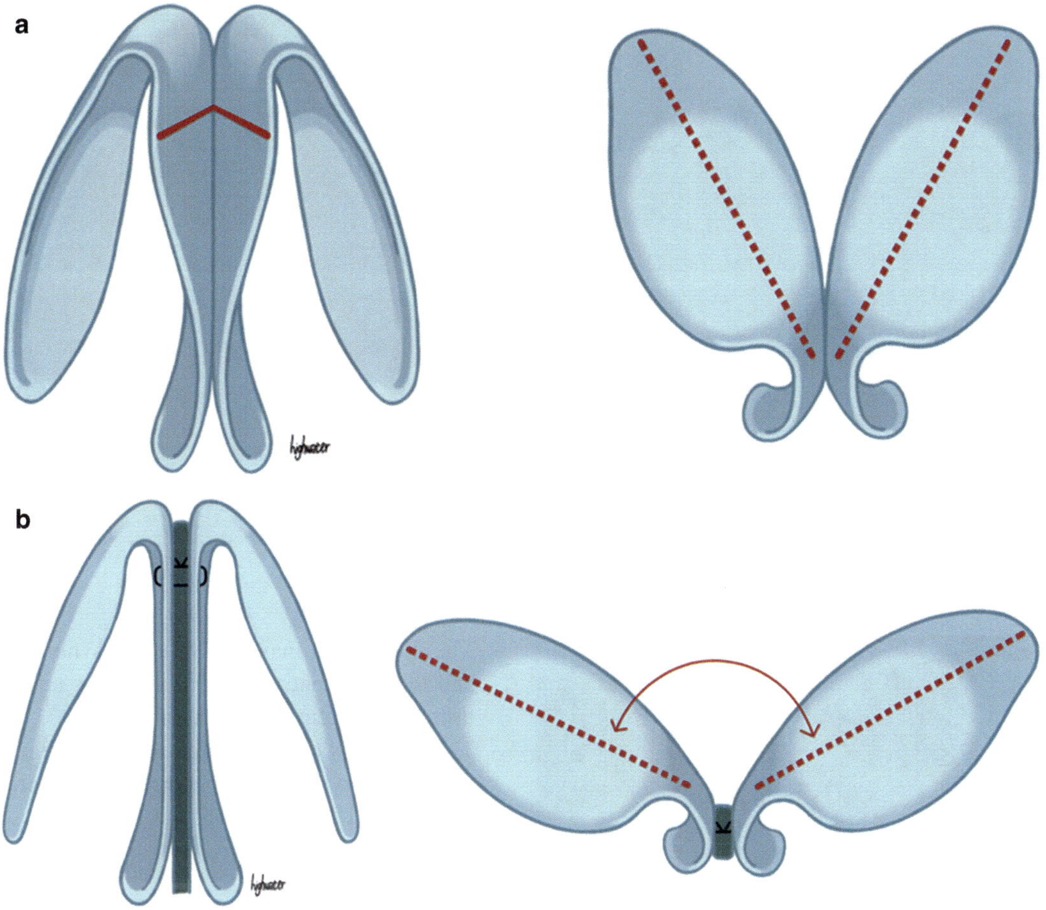

Fig. 8.5 Two divergences: middle crural divergence and the divergence of the long axis of lateral crura (**a**) Ideal feature. (**b**) The suture of the middle and medial crura's caudal margin resulted in a total break of beautiful angles. The long axis became obtuse

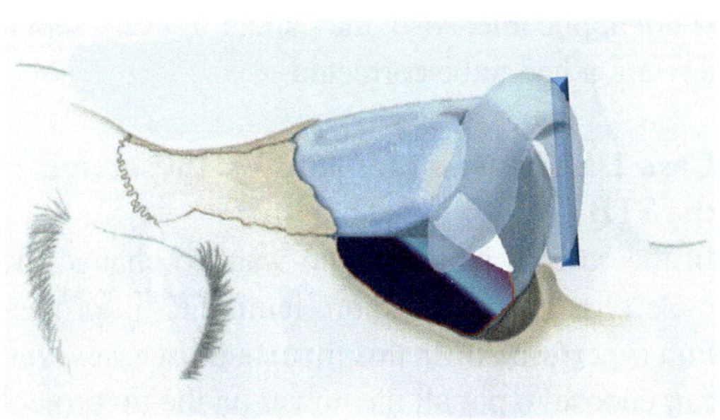

Fig. 8.6 Floating type columellar strut

8.4 My Strategy for Ideal STB in Primary Case

Case 1. Lateral Crural Deformity with Malposition

In the case of the following patients who complain of nasal obstruction with the address of nasal septal deviation, the long axis of the lateral crus is cephalically located intraoperatively, and the concavity of the STB is severely expressed because of the concavity of lateral crus (Video

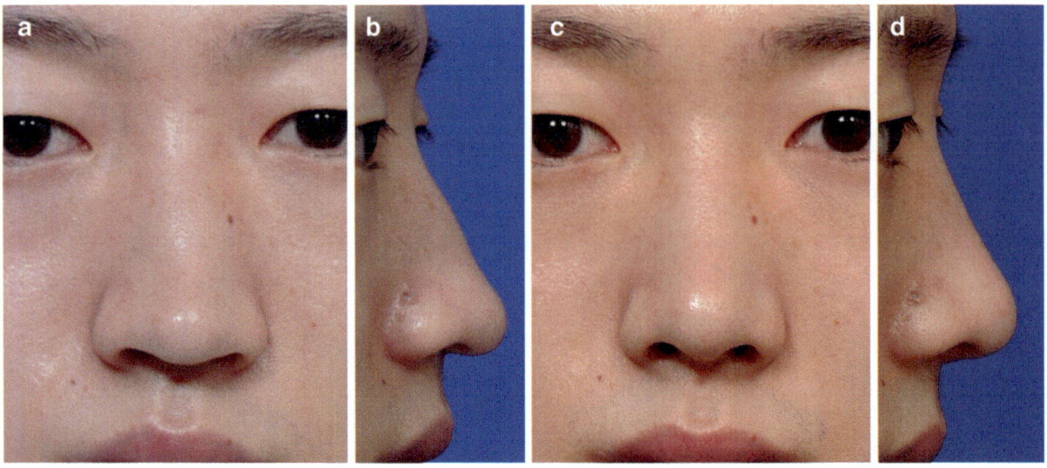

Fig. 8.7 Concave STB was corrected by lateral crural flattening and interdomal suture. And lateral crural spanning suture to the high septum after the anteriorly extended spreader graft. (**a**, **b**) Preoperative views. (**c**, **d**) Postoperative views

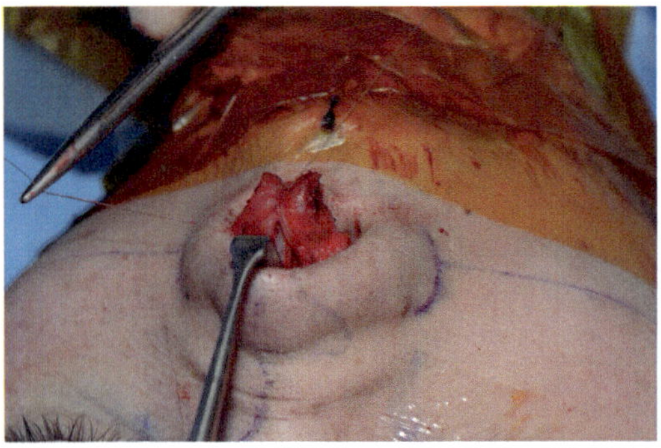

Fig. 8.8 After the key suture: the interdomal suture should be located at the cephalic portion of the middle crura

8.1). After correcting the mild hump by rasping, the lateral crus was fixed to the anteriorly extended high septum through the lateral crural spanning suture after lateral crural cephalic trim (Figs. 8.7 and 8.8).

Anterior septal reconstruction is required because fixation is required in relation to septum and LLC with lateral crural spanning suture. The septal L-strut extension will be discussed in detail later in Chap. 11 again. A shield graft was applied for the position along with the correction of the drooping of the tip.

– The shield graft maintains the tip's symmetry and the divergence of the middle crus and is useful for creating a tip-lobular angle.
– The anteriorly relocated high septum provides the necessary support to correct the lateral crus and correction of the saddle nose deformity.

Of course, the patient's saddle deformity and the concavity of the STB may be corrected using an appropriate alloplastic implant. However, in the patients' case, the augmentation of the bony dorsum is not indicated. If the skin is thin, this is not applicable. Also, the patient's severe septal deviation had to be corrected.

Case 2. Short Nasal Implant Vs. Preserving the STB

In the case of patients who want to change the male type nose to be more feminine, tip projection is performed. At this time, in most cases, you can choose to put all the power on the tip projection and camouflage the dorsum with an alloplastic material, but not using alloplastic material up to the tip is the consensus of the current Asian rhinoplasty. So many problems are caused by this short dorsal implant. These problems will be

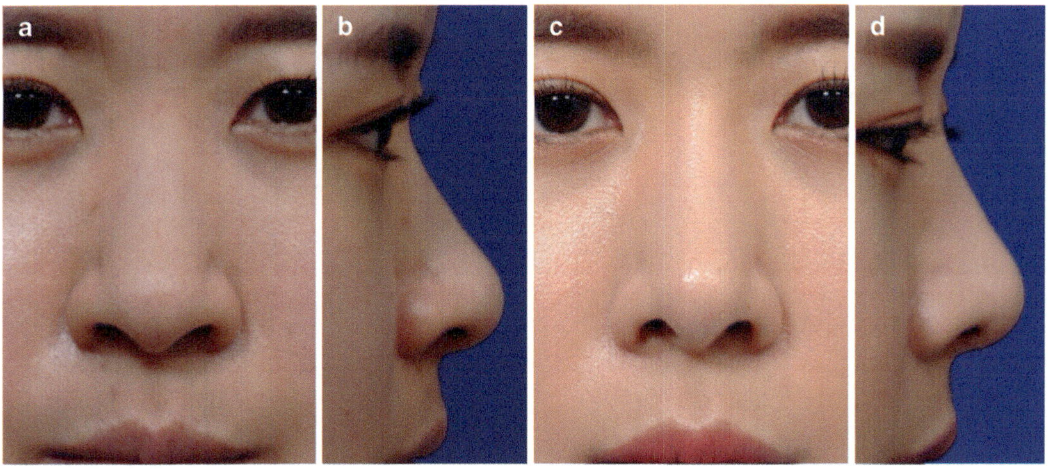

Fig. 8.9 Male type supratip bulbosity was corrected by lateral crural positioning with ideal divergence angles of LLC. Lateral crural spanning suture was applied to the high septum after the anteriorly extended spreader graft. (**a**, **b**) Preoperative views. (**c**, **d**) Postoperative views

covered in the secondary case below. In the case of using autograft without dorsal implant in the primary case, the abrupt concavity of STB can be found in the long term due to unwanted resorption, as mentioned in Chap. 7. The author recommends that the lower two-third nose is projected using cartilages as possible.

- The high septum reconstruction is required to prevent STB concavity due to resorption of dorsal graft, and supratip expressed by septum has long-term stability.
- The only graft method, such as derotation graft, may cause convexity (supratip deformity) and cause supratip deformity along with convexity. LLC, fixed to the high septum with tip projection, looks solid in the long term (Figs. 8.9 and 8.10).

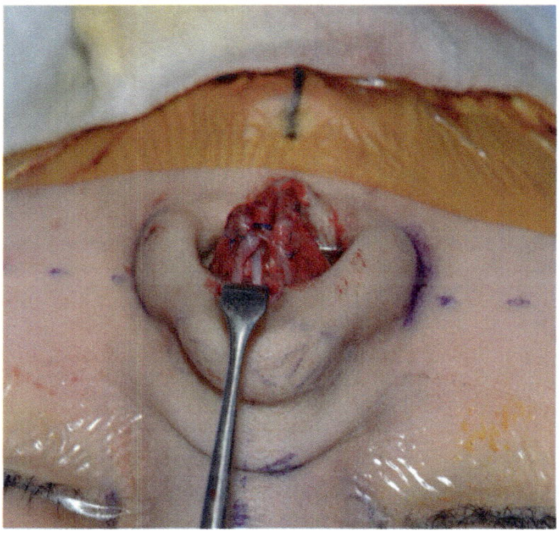

Fig. 8.10 Ideal LLC position with an apparent high septum at the supratip area

8.5 My Strategy for Restoring STB in Secondary Case

Case 1. Supratip Deformity Related to Secondary Tip Drooping

The loss of tip projection-support in the long term is the most common problem. The pseudodeformation caused by tip drooping is complicated, including scar underneath the implant, where the dead space existed between the alloplastic implant and the ULC platform (Fig. 8.11). In the case of profound tip projection, additional graft or implant molding is required to prepare for the dead space on the platform of ULC. However, the reason why the tip droops over time is complicated. The causes include loosening of suture, scar formation of applied cartilage, or the tendency of tension-loss due to depressor muscle and facial mimetic muscle (Fig. 8.12). However, most of the drooping is related to septum-non-

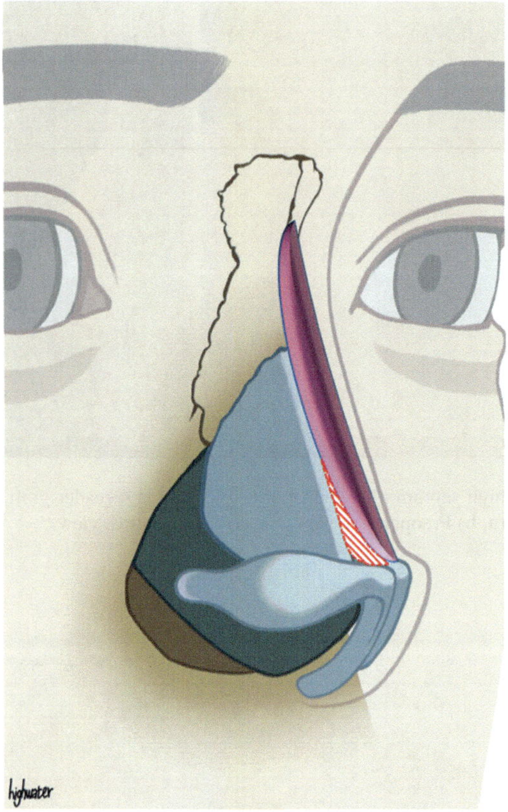

Fig. 8.11 Dead space under the alloplastic implant with the projected tip

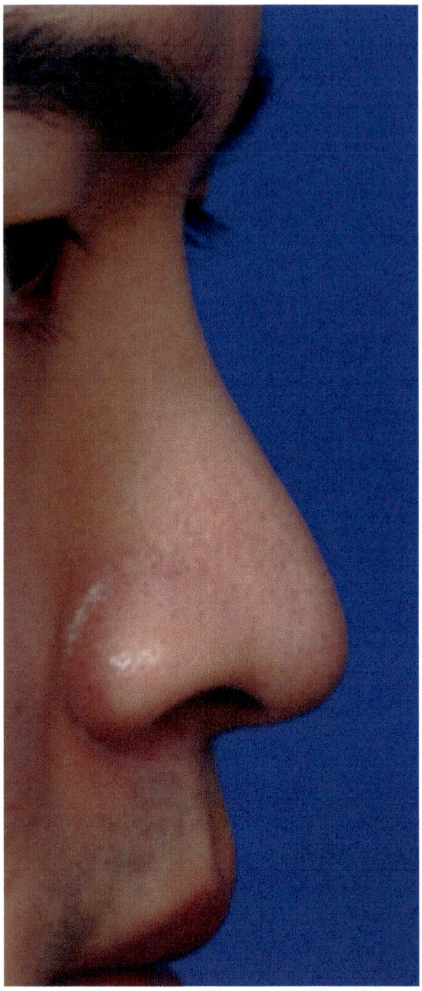

Fig. 8.12 Supratip deformity after the long-term tip drooping and dorsal silicone implant

dependency [9]. Also, there are cases where the long implant is not supported by the tip, and it is bent. Loss of tip projection-support in the long term is the most common problem. The pseudo-deformation caused by tip drooping due to this is very complicated, including scar formation underneath, such as the problem of the dead space underneath the alloplastic implant on the ULC platform (Fig. 8.11).

- Among the various methods for projecting drooped tips, LLC's own lateral crural stability method is not applicable in a secondary operation.
- A lot of LLC's destruction or resorption is found, and its strength is weak, making it difficult to obtain stability only with lateral crus (Fig. 8.13).

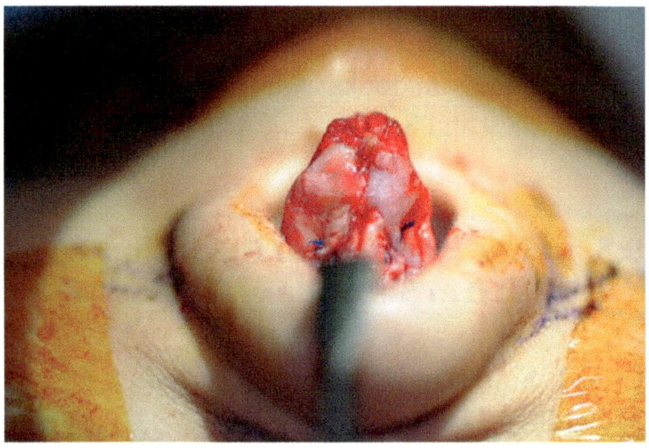

Fig. 8.13 Cartilage destruction at the right side

- Methods such as lateral crural steal or lateral crural overlay are not applicable [10].
- The author uses the lateral crural spanning suture for correcting STB as fixing the LLC to the high septum, even though it requires the reconstruction of the anterior septum. There are various reasons, the alloplastic material cannot be used, and the nasal function needs to be improved, the LLC cannot perform as much counter-clockwise rotation as desired, and the projection of the lower two-third of the nose is necessary without a dorsal graft.

Case 2. Supratip Deformity Related to Dorsal Implant

The causes of supratip deformity that can be caused by implants are diverse. The deformity of STB caused by the capsule problem caused by the dorsal implant is the most common, and it is caused by the formation of capsules and the failure of proper tip plasty without tip support. It is challenging to correct skin laxity made of capsules, and if this anterior capsulectomy cannot be completed thoroughly, the skin should naturally redrape by removing the capsule margin formed in the skin envelope with the capsulotomy in all directions (Figs. 8.14 and 8.15).

Case 3. Supratip Concavity Related to Autograft Resorption

This type is well found in patients who underwent autograft with dermis on the dorsum. The deformity occurs according to the dermis graft's resorption amount. Mainly, the dermis inserted in the bony dorsum tends to be absorbed more (Fig. 8.16 and Video 8.2). Since the findings underlying the deformity cannot be estimated using CT scan, the complex causes must be confirmed in the surgical field. Also, since the dermis graft also creates unwanted scars in the skin envelope, you must carefully score the skin flap undersurface for the dorsal skin envelope's natural redrape (Video 8.3).

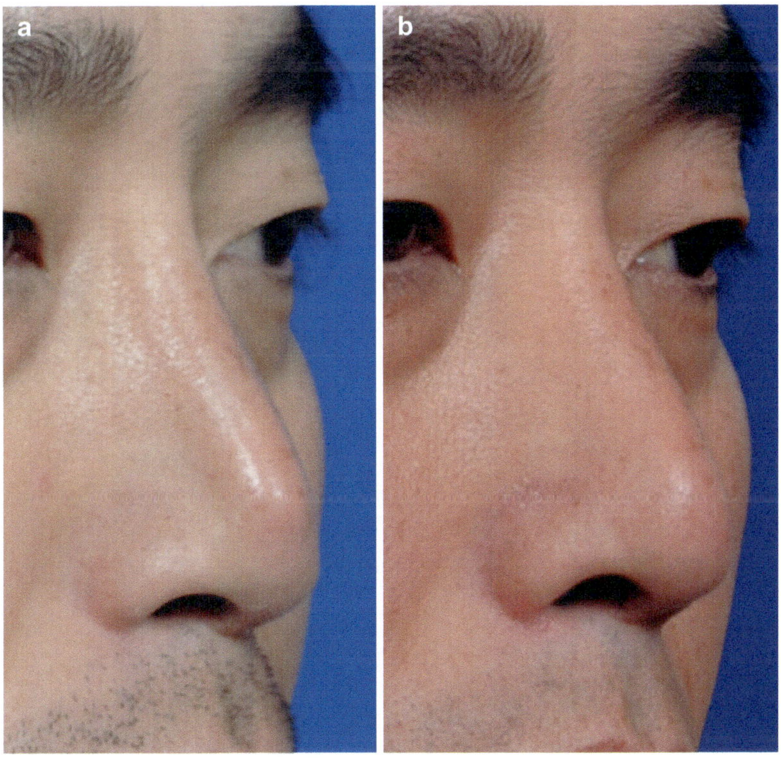

Fig. 8.14 Supratip deformity after the long-term result of Silicone implant: the skin pocket had a memory of bulbosity, so the capsular margin's scoring should be done for the redraping. (**a**) Preoperative view, (**b**) postoperative view

- Do not remove all of the previously applied cartilages. Try reusing them.
- The autologous cartilage applied with the shield graft can be used again as a middle and medial crus, and the cartilages do not need to be removed. Instead, it can be modified while attached as a reusable cartilage.
- Likewise, if there is no big problem with the septal extension graft, it is only necessary to preserve it and achieve the goal to achieve in the secondary operation.

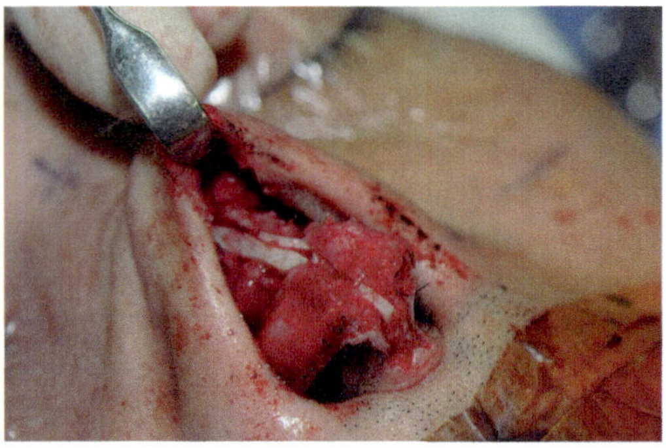

Fig. 8.15 L-strut reconstruction for the appropriate LLC positioning

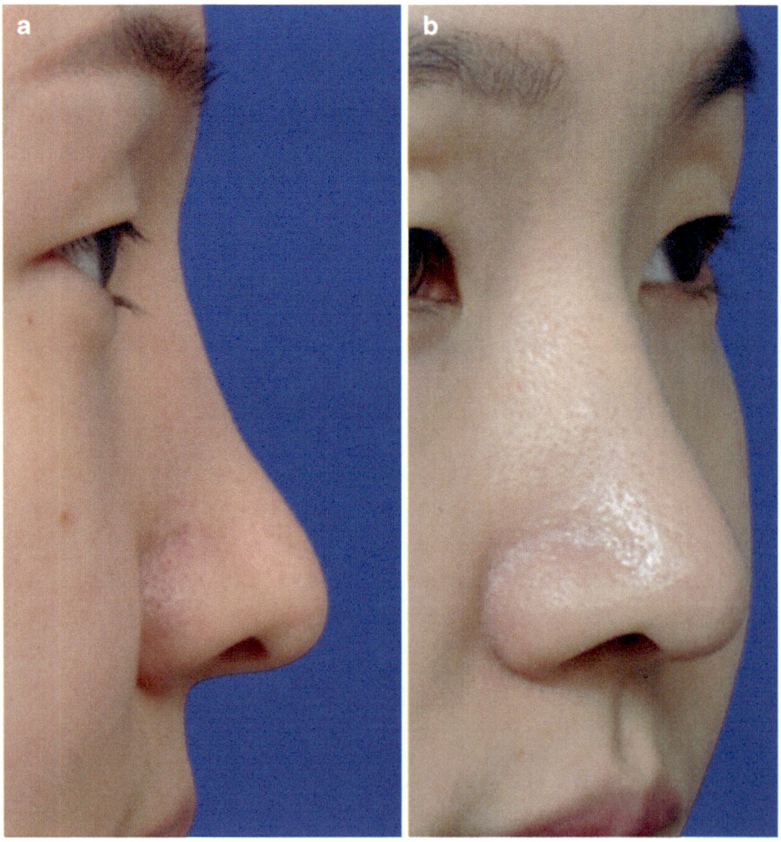

Fig. 8.16 Supratip deformity caused by irregular resorption of SDF. (**a**) Lateral view, the resorption at the bony dorsum is higher than the lower two-third. (**b**) Supratip deformity by SDF

References

1. Anderson JR. A reasoned approach to nasal base surgery. Arch Otolaryngol. 1984;110(6):349–58.
2. Toriumi DM. New concepts in nasal tip contouring. Arch Facial Plast Surg. 2006;8(3):156–85.
3. Toriumi DM, Checcone MA. New concepts in nasal tip contouring. Facial Plast Surg Clin North Am. 2009;17(1):55–90, vi.
4. Toriumi DM, Asher SA. Lateral crural repositioning for treatment of cephalic malposition. Facial Plast Surg Clin North Am. 2015;23(1):55–71.
5. Rohrich RJ, Liu JH. Defining the infratip lobule in rhinoplasty: anatomy, pathogenesis of abnormalities, and correction using an algorithmic approach. Plast Reconstr Surg. 2012;130(5):1148–58.
6. Oneal RM, Beil RJ Jr, Schlesinger J. Surgical anatomy of the nose. Otolaryngol Clin N Am. 1999;32(1):145–81.
7. Guyuron B, DeLuca L, Lash R. Supratip deformity: a closer look. Plast Reconstr Surg. 2000;105(3):1140–51; discussion 1152–3.
8. Sieber DA, Rohrich RJ. Finesse in nasal tip refinement. Plast Reconstr Surg. 2017;140(2):277e–86e.
9. Min HJ, Lee SB, Kim KS. A comparative analysis between primary and secondary nasal tip drooping. Ear Nose Throat J. 2019;11:145561319862222.
10. Foda HMT, Kridel RWH. Lateral crural steal and lateral crural overlay [Internet]. Arch Otolaryngol Head Neck Surg. 1999;125:1365. https://doi.org/10.1001/archotol.125.12.1365.

9 Controlling Asian Tip: Facet and Supra-Alar Groove

Pearls

- The soft triangle is not an object to be created but an object to be preserved.
- Since the soft triangle is made of soft tissue, it should be expressed by minimizing the dissection and reinforcing it with a structure supported behind it.
- The subdomal graft is a beneficial method in that it can obtain the desired dome angle along with the symmetry of the middle crura with a minimal amount of cartilage and secure the middle crural stability.
- The lateral crural strut graft has the most robust potency support since it can create the entire LLC angle by adjusting the lateral crus's position. However, most of the secondary operation requires the costal cartilage.
- In soft triangle correction, a resilient skin envelope is required to express the supportive graft to be considered in the primary rhinoplasty.
- Use the "sleeve-down" technique to recruit as much skin envelopes around the soft triangle as desired.
- After "sleeve-down," the nasal skin flap should be monitored well. Prostaglandin E1 and hyperbaric O_2 therapy is beneficial.
- For the definition of the supra-alar groove, the direct nasalis transverse and some complex mimetic muscles (partly LLSAN and LLS) is removed, if necessary, the fatty layer should be removed.

Supplementary Information The online version of this chapter (https://doi.org/10.1007/978-981-16-0542-0_9) contains supplementary material, which is available to authorized users.

The original version of this chapter was revised. The correction to this chapter can be found at https://doi.org/10.1007/978-981-16-0542-0_18

9.1 The "Facet"

Definition

Traditionally, facet refers to a soft triangle or soft tissue triangle. If you cut the jewel's spherical surface, you will have a beautiful surface, which is the only part of the nose that has such a surface. Just as a well-cut gemstone becomes a jewel, the soft triangle in the nose shows the beauty of the nose along with the infratip lobule (Fig. 9.1). In Western rhinoplasty, due to a well-developed LLC, the angles transferred to the middle crus [1] and well developed, so there is no big problem if these are well saved (Fig. 9.2). However, in Asian rhinoplasty, the creation of this part is challenging, and there are many reasons.

Due to the poor development of LLC, various angles of the middle crus are not well developed, the overlying skin is thick, making the inner structure difficult to express, and the amount of subcutaneous fatty tissue is thick. If the patient has a relatively voluminous tip, there is a percep-

E.-S. Dhong, M.-W. Na, *Asian Septorhinoplasty*, https://doi.org/10.1007/978-981-16-0542-0_9

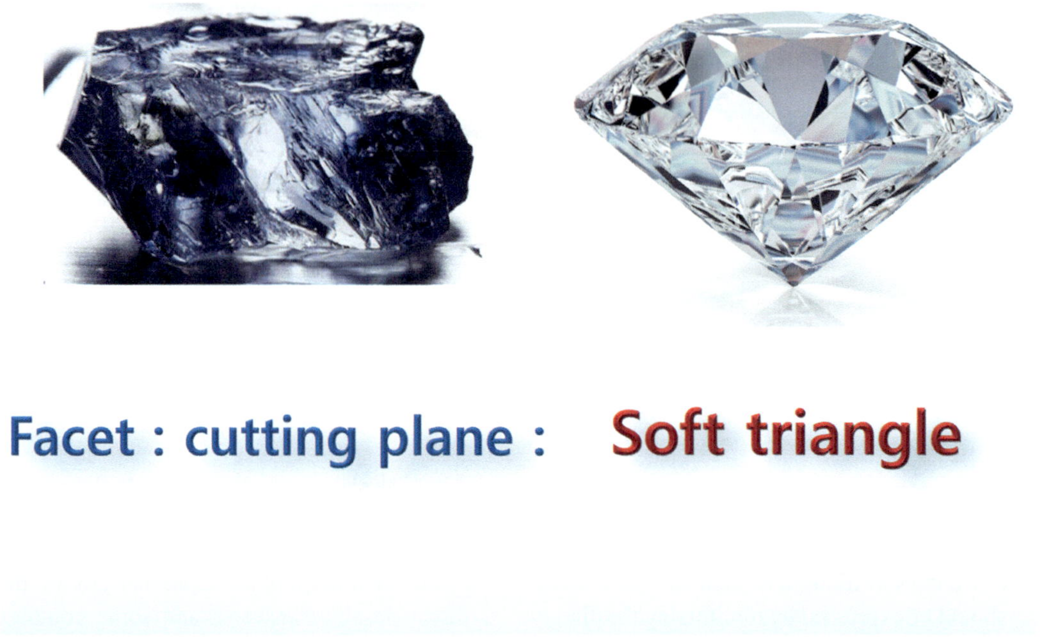

Fig. 9.1 Facet: This refers to a beautifully implemented surface by cutting an original stone and refers to a soft triangle

tion that it looks young and cute, but we need to know how to express the facet well to access the high-end result.

Anatomic Considerations

In a Cadaveric study, a study on the soft triangle revealed the safe zone for the incision. There are three zones in the soft triangle: muscle caudal to the lower lateral cartilages, an interval dermis-to-dermis contact area, and muscle interdigitating with dermis at the nostril rim [2]. Since the facet is the only body part that abut dermis to dermis, there is a characteristic that "pinch" comes well due to internal or external factors. The development of cartilage is poor, so in Asian rhinoplasty, the pinching deformity develops even though the marginal incision is well applied.

– If an implant or graft larger than the dissection pocket is contained, it may cause tension in the suture area.

According to the literature, several points are essential to preserve or make a soft triangle. First, precise marginal incision placement is the key factor. Second, LLC's internal support is needed. If existing LLCs do not have the support, various grafts can be applied, such as alar contour grafts, infratip lobular graft, and lateral crural strut graft are sufficient to create a beautiful facet. Avoiding undue tension and eradicating all dead space is indispensable during closure. Applying external supportive dressing is effective [3]. However, Asian rhinoplasty requires a graft to reinforce the weak middle crus.

Although less facet implementation is required than Western, not all patients have thicker skin. Another study categorized patients at risk of postoperative notching into three groups:

1. A narrow intermediate crus, which provided little or no caudal support
2. Adequate cartilage support but lengthy soft triangle skin
3. No anatomical problems of the soft triangle but had a wide middle crural angulation due to a cephalic orientation of the lateral crus

They believed that patients with cephalic positioning of the lateral crura are at the highest risk

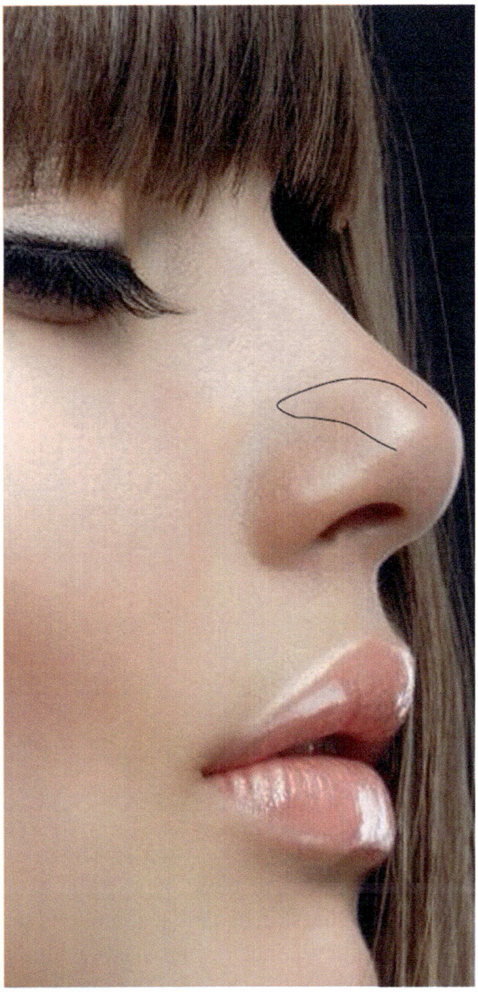

Fig. 9.2 Facet is an area of soft tissue with a unique structure under LLC's middle crura

of notching. Separating the intermediate crus cartilaginous structure from the overlying vestibular skin creates a space between two previously fused structures, causing wound healing and scarring. Moreover, they used an onlay filling graft for correction [4].

Asian primary rhinoplasty has the same problem, but with most problems, pinching is more likely to occur because the middle crus has less support. In addition to this, Asian secondary rhinoplasty must obtain the following surgical goals: (1) scar release, (2) secure soft triangle skin that can redrape, and (3) secure internal cartilaginous support. Ultimately, the supple skin's redrape is crucial because it is challenging to reconstruct after the scar is formed. Most of the alar rim graft does not affect the improvement, and it is common to correct the soft triangle along with the correction of alar retraction.

How to Preserve the Facet?

The most important thing is the correct infracartilaginous incision, also called marginal incision. Never use the rim incision. The rim incision is done only in direct ablation of the soft triangle in the cleft nose deformity (Fig. 9.3). If it is not a secondary operation, dissection of the soft triangle should be prohibited or it should be done very conservatively.

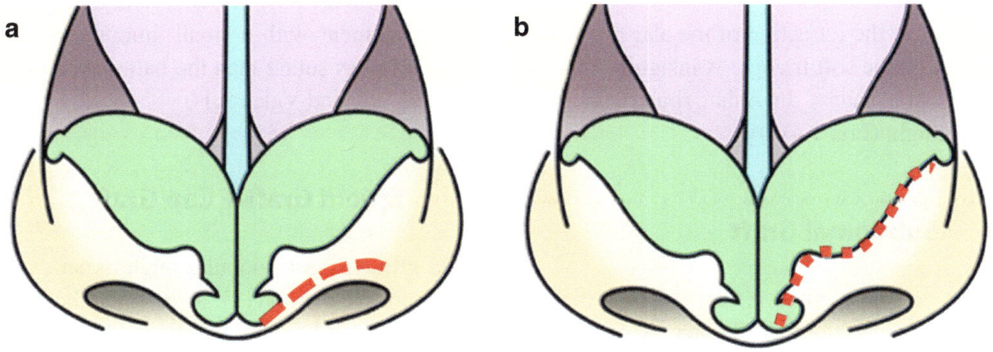

Fig. 9.3 The incision for preserving the facet must be an infracartilaginous (marginal) incision. Rim incision invades soft triangles. (**a**) Rim incision. (**b**) Infracartilaginous incision

- In many examples, soft triangles represent not objects to be created, but objects to be preserved.
- Since the soft triangle is literally made of soft tissue, it should be expressed by minimizing the dissection and reinforcing it with a structure that can support it.
- A drastic dissection can be attempted only in the secondary surgery, but the soft tissue that transitions to the alar ridges must be protected.
- In the primary and secondary surgery, the incision should be an infracartilaginous incision.
- Excessive suture tension should be avoided.

How to Create a Beautiful Soft Triangle?

As has been introduced in many other articles, the caudal support of the lateral and medial genu of the middle and lateral crus is the most important, and the corresponding sufficient skin redrape is a crucial factor. It is a subtle part that should not be too excessive or too small [1].

Among the various types of grafts that can support lateral crura, you should choose the method well depending on whether the cartilage amount is sufficient or insufficient. Below are some methods the author uses to create a beautiful angle.

9.2 Alar Rim Graft [5]

It helps solve the retraction of the alar ridge, but the effect on the soft triangle is insignificant due to the graft's nature. In Asian rhinoplasty, the effect is slight (Fig. 9.4).

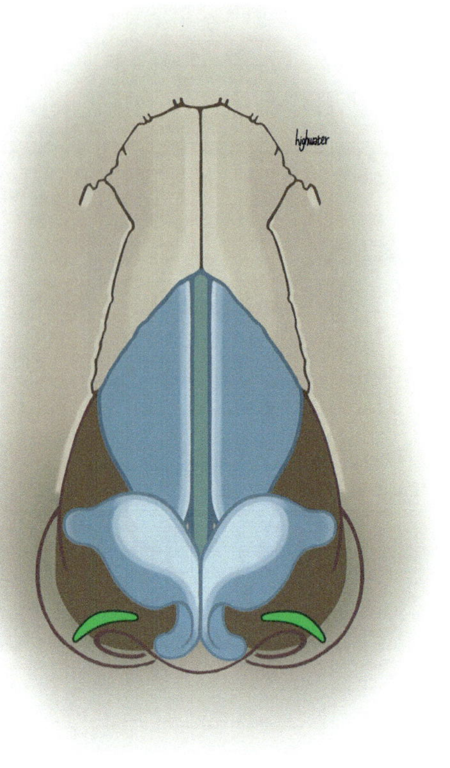

Fig. 9.4 Alar rim graft

9.3 Subdomal Graft

It is a beneficial method in that it is possible to obtain the desired dome angle and the symmetry of the middle crura with a minimal amount of cartilage and secure the middle crural stability [6, 7].

- The authors prefer this method as it is a situation where surgery with a small amount of cartilage is always required unless the costal cartilage is harvested. This technique is possible even in secondary rhinoplasty with a lot of LLC damage.

The author prefers subdomal graft because it has the advantage of natural coaptation of the cephalic portion of the middle crura, direct symmetry alignment with a small amount of cartilage, and a less suture than the batten type onlay graft (Fig. 9.5 and Video 9.1).

9.4 Shield Graft + Cap Graft

Shield graft using tip-lobular angle is an excellent supportive method [8]. In this way, the divergence of the middle crura can be saved. Moreover, simultaneously, the shape of the lobule can be created. The shape of the medial crura and symmetric LLCs can be created. To make a more sturdy middle crus, you can use an anatomic graft or cap graft on the top to reinforce the middle

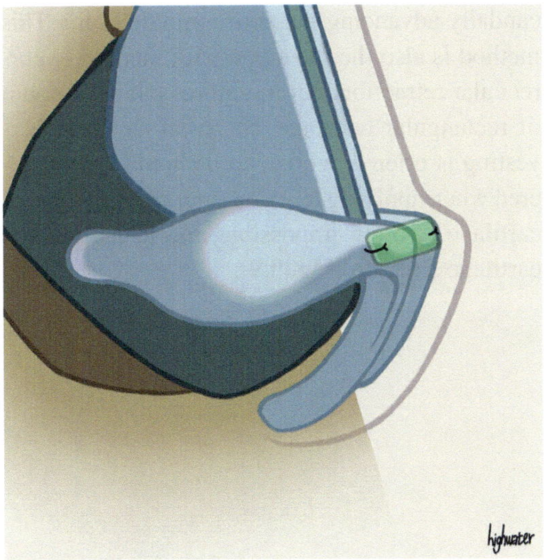

Fig. 9.5 Subdomal graft

crural support. However, without the caudal septal support, this graft alone cannot achieve tip projection, even more so when the lateral crus's strength is weak. This graft is for ideal shaping of facet and lobule rather than tip projection (Fig. 9.6 and Video 9.1).

9.5 Middle Crural Extension Graft

This method can be used when applying the double-layered conchal cartilage. If the double-layered concha position is used as a columella strut or caudal septal strut, it can be used as a method for reinforcing the middle crura by extending it from the columella strut to the middle crura. It can be used to reinforce the middle crus. It is difficult to apply with the septal cartilage (Fig. 9.7).

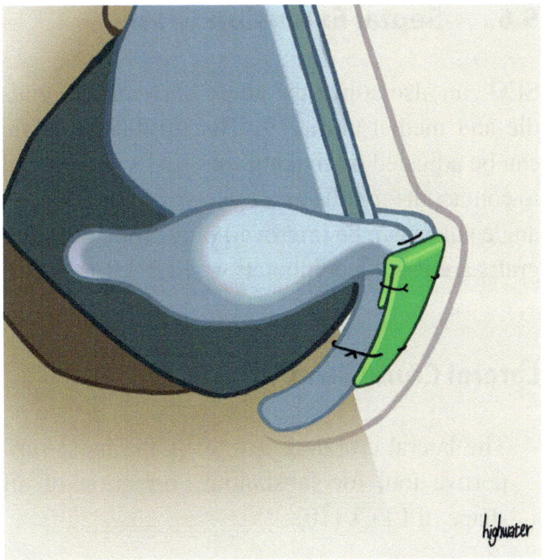

Fig. 9.6 Shield graft, the figure expresses the double-layered graft at the upper side. It is common to apply one layer

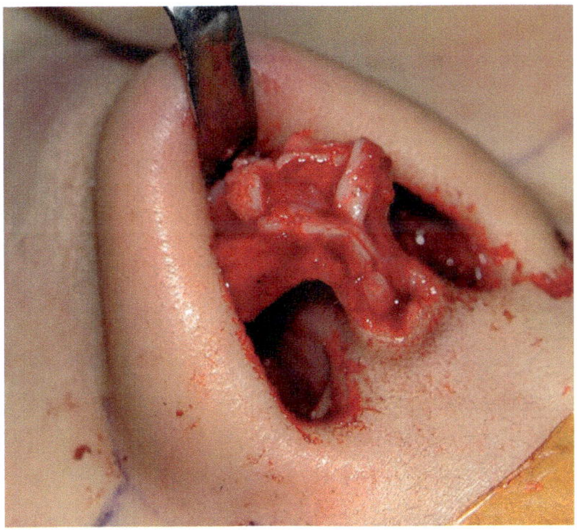

Fig. 9.7 Midcrural extension graft: Middle small rim of double conchal cartilage

9.6 Septal Extension Graft

SEG can also adjust the angle between the middle and medial crura [9]. The tip-lobular angle can be adjusted by making the SEG's caudal end to contact the middle crura. However, the soft triangle shape can be improved only when other tip grafts are used in combination (Fig. 9.8).

Lateral Crural Strut Graft

- The lateral crural strut graft is the most supportive tool for substantial correction of all shape of LLCs [10].

Therefore, there is an effect of changing the dome angle by adjusting the lateral crura and caudally advancing the entire middle crura. This method is also the most powerful method to correct alar retraction, but it requires a large amount of rectangular cartilage, so costal cartilage harvesting is often essential, so it should be considered when applying to Asian rhinoplasty. Conchal cartilage is often impossible due to the lack of cartilage strength (Fig. 9.9).

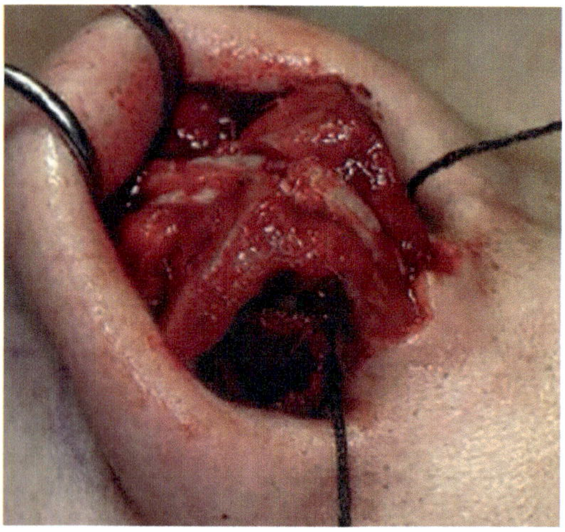

Fig. 9.8 Septal extension graft reaches to the middle crura modifying the tip-lobular angle

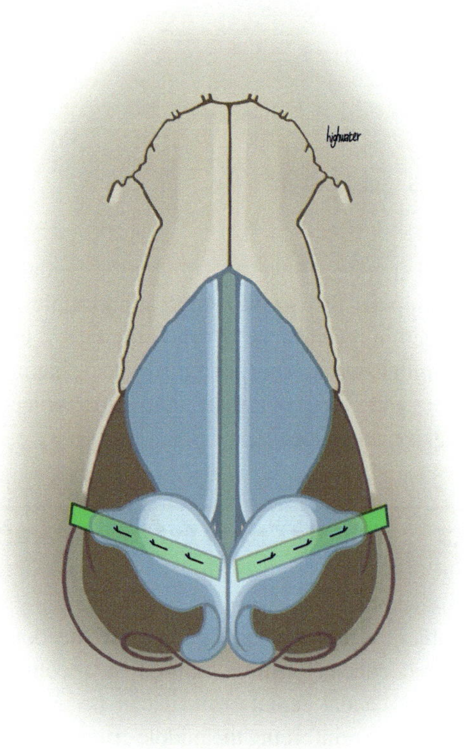

Fig. 9.9 Lateral crural strut graft

Case Study 1: Underdeveloped Middle Crura in Primary Rhinoplasty

A 20-year-old female patient was referred to the author with septal deviation and a small nose. The middle crus was underdeveloped, and the lower two-third of the nose was hypoplastic. The tip was supple and soft when the author pressed it. After structural graft, such as the caudal septal extension graft, the middle crura was reconstructed with shield graft and midcrural extension graft (Fig. 9.10).

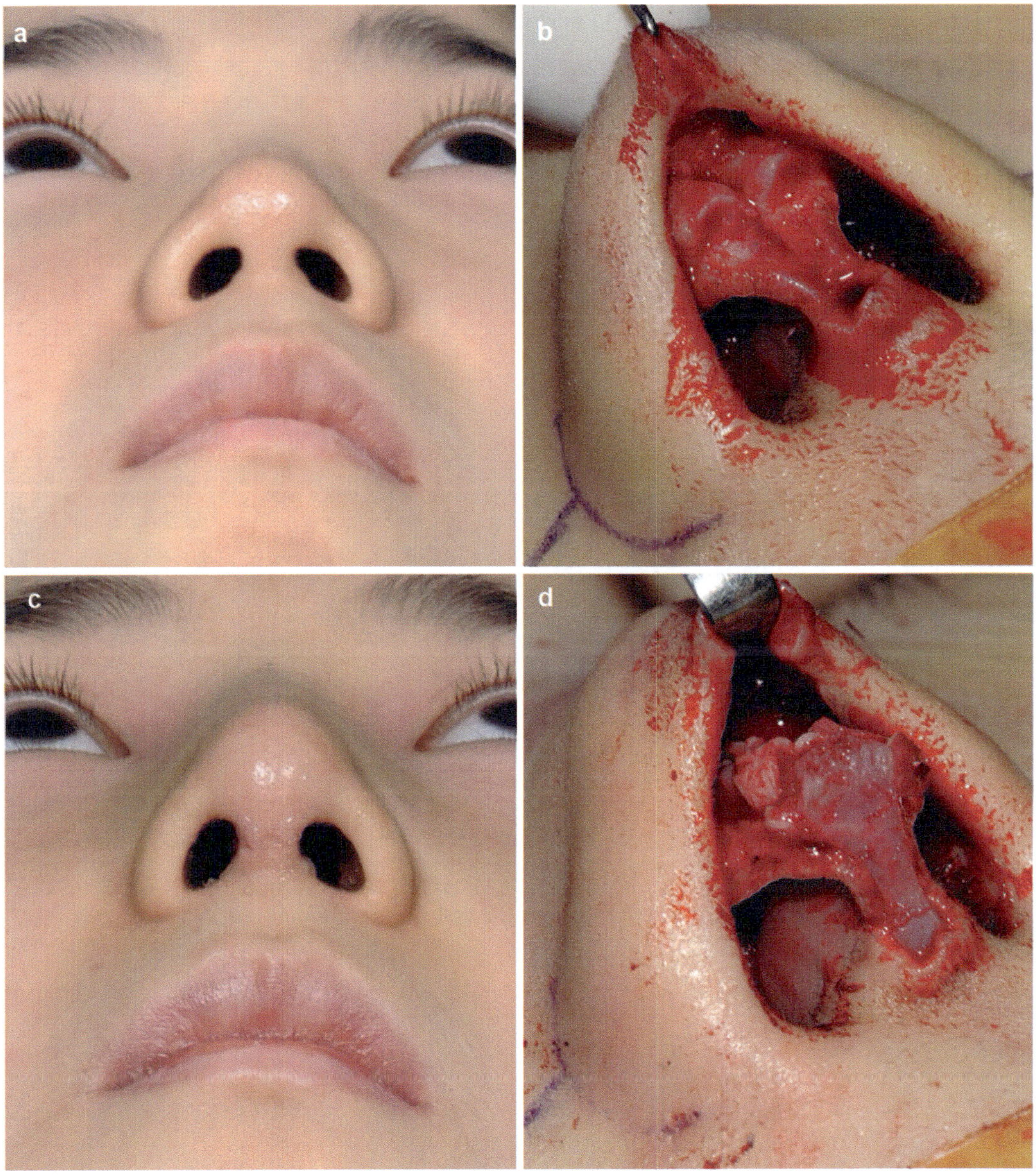

Fig. 9.10 Underdeveloped middle crura in primary rhinoplasty: reconstructed with midcrural extension graft and a shield graft. (**a**) Preoperative view. (**b**) Before the grafts. (**c**) Postoperative view. (**d**) Before closure

Case Study 2: Tortuous Middle Crura in Primary Rhinoplasty

A 19-year-old female patient was referred with a septal deviation with a mild hump nose. Cymba concha and SMF were needed to project tortuous middle crus and undeveloped medial crus. First, a septal L-strut extension graft was performed on the structural framework, a middle crural extension graft and a shield graft were applied to the tip using a concha, and an onlay graft was performed using the remaining SMF. After 2 years of long-term postoperative follow-up, a large part of the resorption of SMF was seen, but the overall balance was not broken (Figs. 9.11 and 9.12).

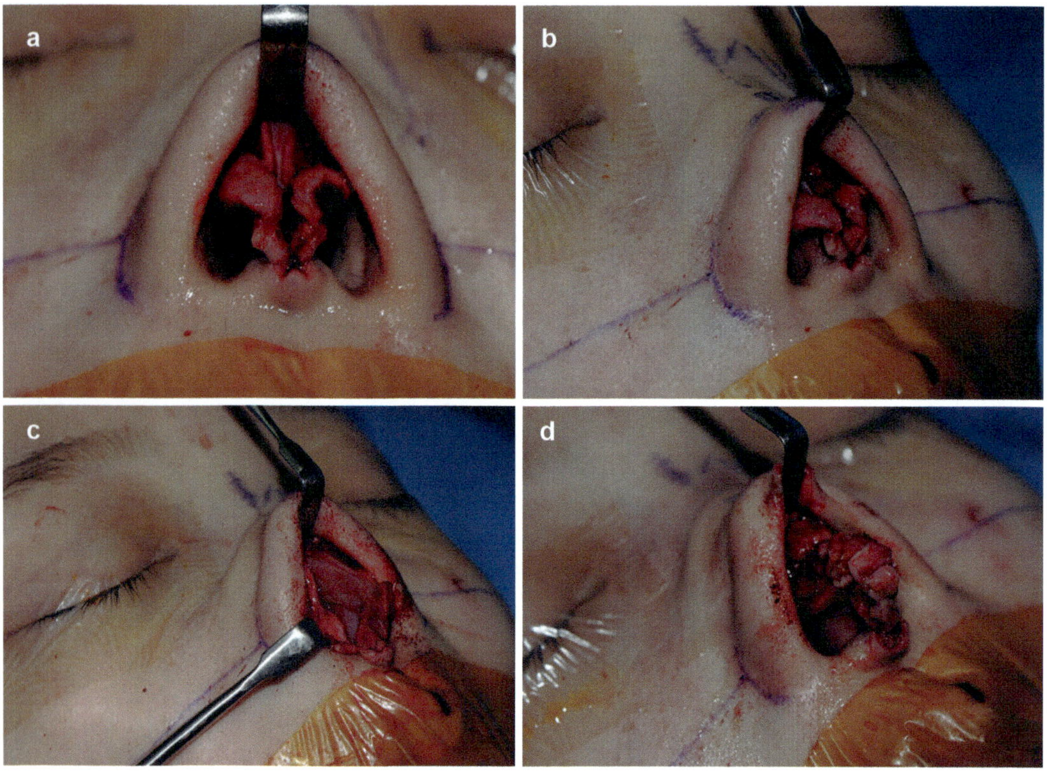

Fig. 9.11 Tortuous middle crura in primary rhinoplasty: Septal L-strut extension graft, shield graft, and a tip onlay graft using SMF (**a**, **b**) Intraoperative view before the grafts. (**c**) Septal L-strut extension graft. (**d**) Tip onlay graft

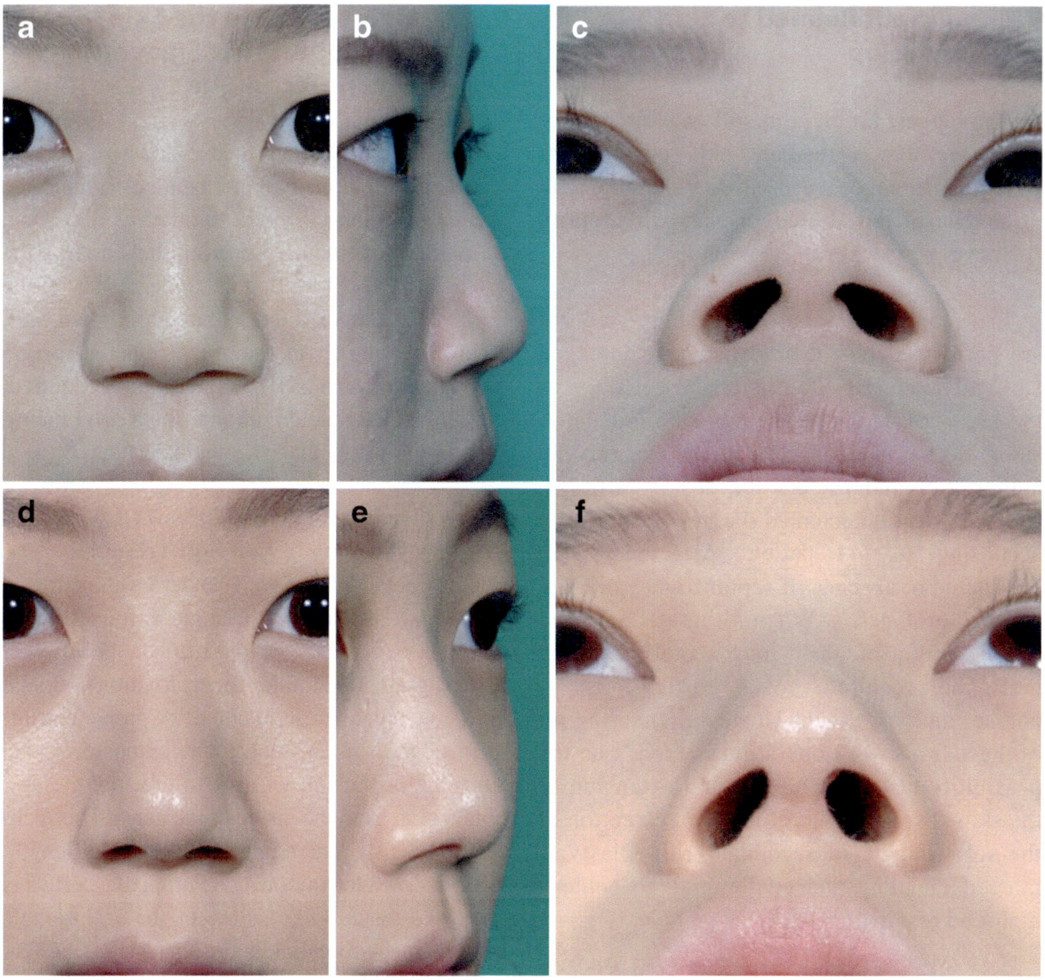

Fig. 9.12 Tortuous middle crura in primary rhinoplasty. (**a**–**c**) Preoperative views. (**d**–**f**) Postoperative view

9.7 Pitfalls Related to Skin Envelop

- The biggest problem in soft triangle correction is that a resilient skin envelope is required to succeed in all the techniques to be considered in the primary rhinoplasty above.

In secondary operation, these procedures are performed on the scar bed and damaged LLCs. The author chooses costal cartilage as the last choice. The biggest reason is to consider the hardness of the tip. Of course, the author uses and prefers the costal cartilage. However, it is selected as the next best option according to (1) patient preference, (2) destructed or absence of septal framework, (3) absence of conchas. When allografts are used at the septum or when long septal extension grafts are required, costal cartilage is, of course, the best donor. However, enabling all of these framework operations depends on the possibility of proper release and extension of the skin envelope. Therefore, the correction of the soft triangle in secondary rhinoplasty is more demanding and challenging to achieve high-end results.

9.8 How to Recruit the Skin Envelope?: The "Sleeve-Down" Technique

- The author uses the "sleeve-down" technique to recruit as many skin envelopes around the soft triangle as desired. In other words, it is a method for forcibly lowering the length of the envelope by dissecting the undersurface of the skin. Of course, if it does not come down well, bold scoring or release of the cephalic portion of the soft triangle or alar ridge is required. Here, electrocauterization using a colorado tip is used or a 15 blade scalpel is used.

Case 1: Unilateral Hypoplasia of LLC, Primary Pinching of Left Soft Triangle

The patient's left LLC is underdeveloped, and pinching of the left soft triangle is found preoperatively. Rebuild the devoid LLC on the left with batten graft (anatomic reconstruction), domal graft, and shield graft do not allow proper recruitment of the skin envelope. The author dissected the ridge of the soft triangle to take out the vestibular skin from the inside of the nares. This technique is like extending the sleeve's length: "sleeve-down technique." The immediate effect is seen, and tension-free suture of the soft triangle must be made to maintain the shape (Fig. 9.13).

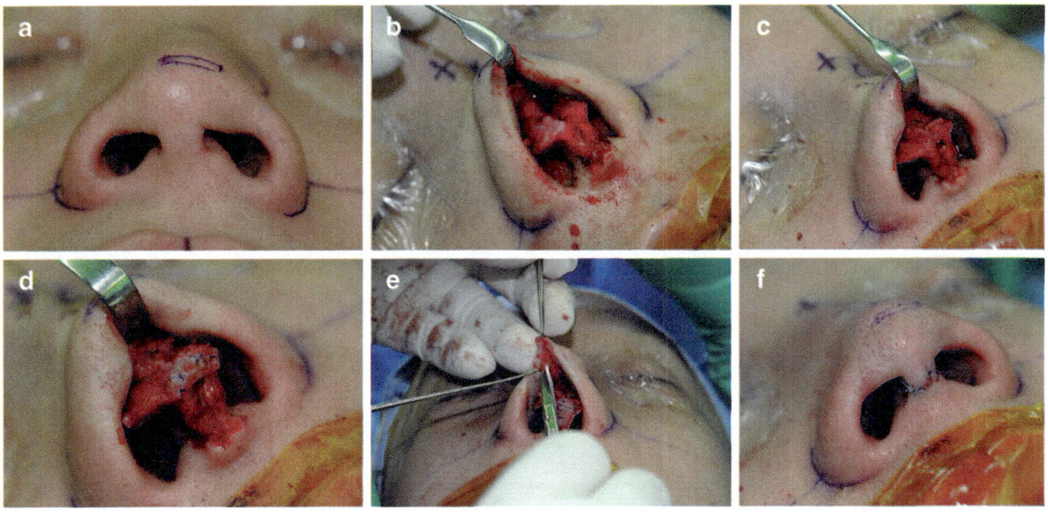

Fig. 9.13 Unilateral hypoplasia of LLC, primary pinching of the left soft triangle. (**a**) Preoperative basal view. (**b**) Intraoperative view, Lt side LLC is underdeveloped, and middle and medial crura are also hypoplastic. (**c**) Lt. LLC batten graft (anatomic reconstruction). (**d**) Domal graft (cap graft) for hypoplastic middle crura. (**e**) Sleeve-down technique after applying a short shield graft. (**f**) Immediate postoperative view

Case 2: Skin Envelope Shortage in Secondary Rhinoplasty

A 24-year-old female underwent septorhinoplasty twice using silicone and Medpor. All alloplastic materials had been removed 2 years before visiting the author. The pinching of the soft triangles on both sides was the most problematic, and septal collapse accompanied. Septal L-strut extension graft (SLEG) was performed with cymba and cavum conchas, and tip and dorsum were grafted using SDF. The shape of the soft triangle improved 2 years postoperatively.

It is more difficult to dissect the entire hard scars. As shown in Fig. 9.15, the "sleeve-down" technique may induce a temporary vascular compromise, and check for marginal bleeding. Efforts should be made to preserve the subdermal plexus as much as possible (Figs. 9.14 and 9.15).

– After "sleeve-down," the nasal tip flap should be monitored well. Prostaglandin E1, which is helpful for flap physiology, should be administered, and hyperbaric O_2 therapy, if possible.

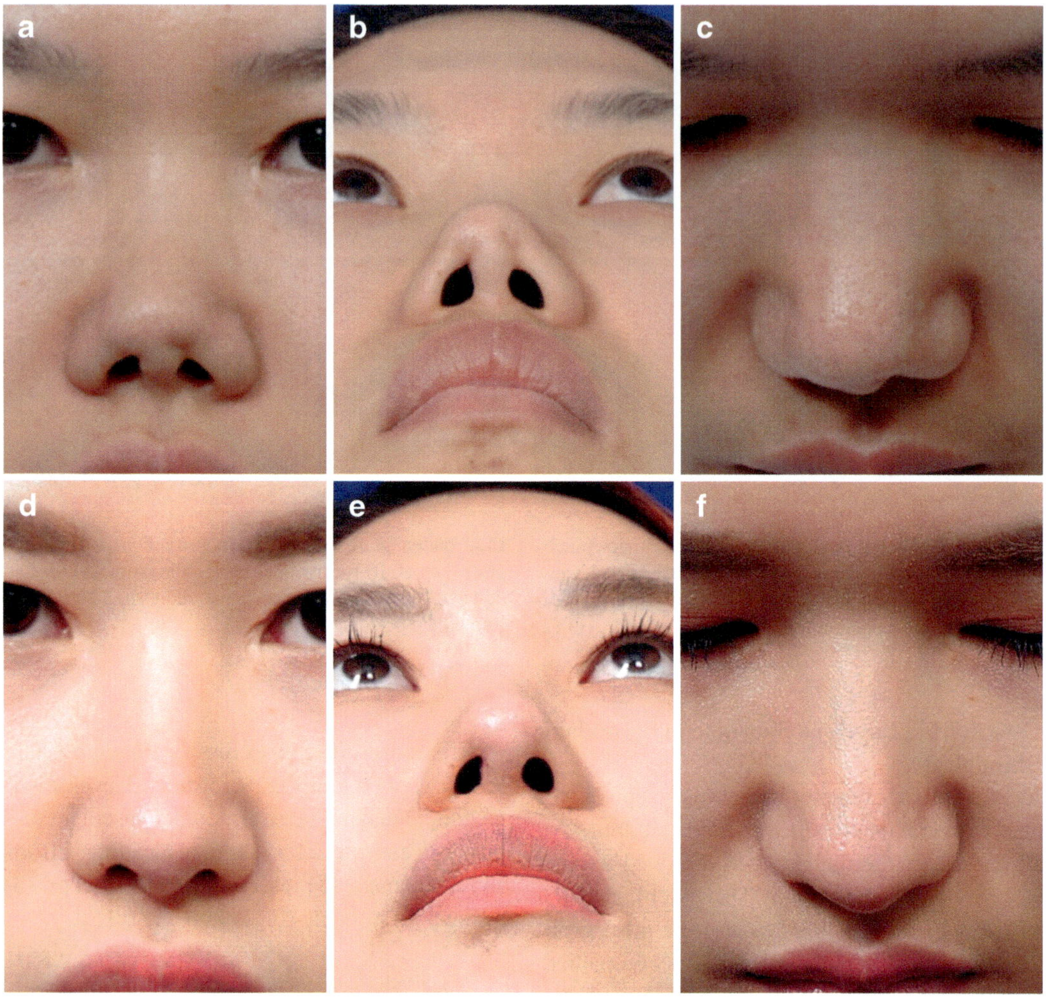

Fig. 9.14 Deformity of the soft triangle after removal of alloplastic materials. (**a**–**c**) Preoperative views. (**d**–**f**) Long-term postoperative view

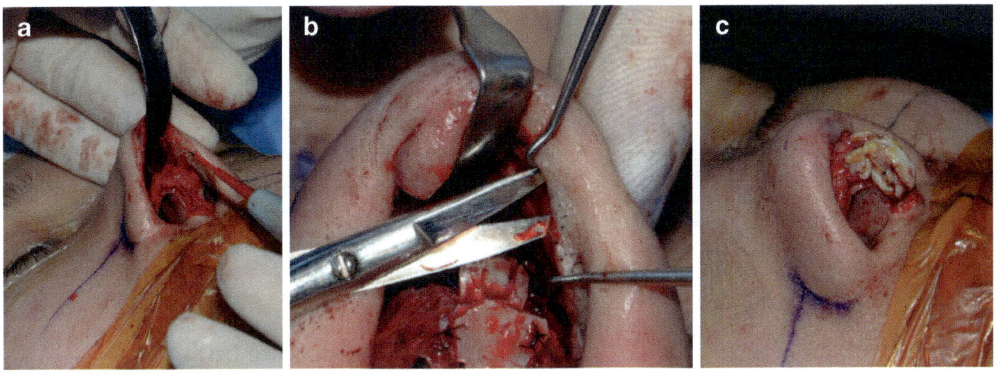

Fig. 9.15 Sleeve-down technique. (**a**) Using a fine tip of electrocauterization. (**b**) Using sharp scissors. (**c**) After the "sleeve-down," a proper amount of soft tissue should be applied

9.9 How to Reduce the Soft Triangle

When correcting the difference in the amount of soft tissue of external nares in the correction of cleft lip and nose deformity, alar rim incision is applied, or the vestibular skin is directly excised. The most reliable method is to do as many dome-lining removals as desired, and when repairing, the soft triangle skin enters the inside of the vestibule, and the total amount is reduced [11]. It is crucial never to apply direct incision to soft triangles. It is safe to remove the dome lining using the rim incision first, creating the excessive lining to be excised, which is the gap between the rim incision and the future marginal incision to be repaired (Fig. 9.16).

- Apply the rim incision first, when repairing, perform the marginal incision again. The lining removed will be the gap between two incisions, so the rim incision's position is decided by the amount to be removed.

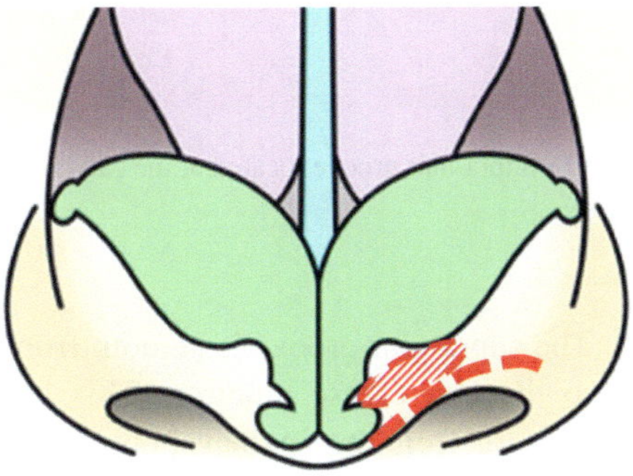

Fig. 9.16 The domal lining removal for reducing the soft triangle; the gap between the rim incision and the marginal incision is excised

9.10 The Supra-Alar Groove

Western rhinoplasty is relatively not much interested in this area. However, especially for Asian males with very thick skin envelopes, proper grooving of this area should be consid-

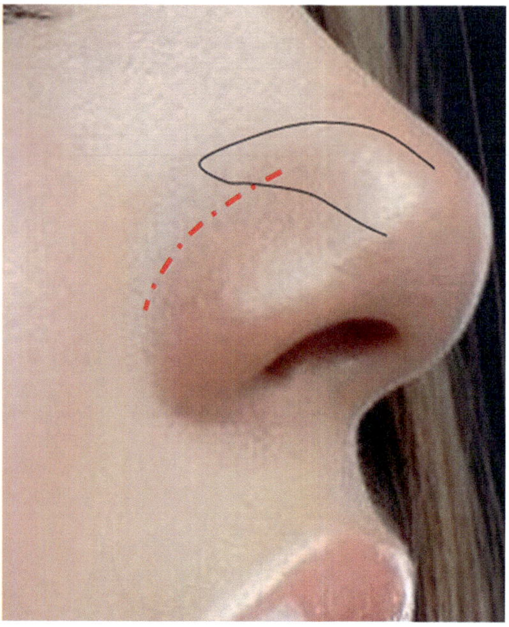

Fig. 9.17 Supra-alar groove located at the caudal area of LLC

ered. The supra-alar groove is smooth from the STB to the alar crease junction. This groove vaguely starts from the tip then shows a definite end to the alar crease junction. The shape of the lateral crus depends on the degree of cephalic rotation, but the groove is usually located at the caudal margin of the lateral crus (Fig. 9.17). This groove is intermingled with the deep levator labii superioris alaeque nasi (LLSAN) when it exists between the dilator naris vestibulars and the vertical fibers of the dilator naris anterior.

Therefore, there are several ways to sharpen this groove.

- reduce the volume of the lateral cartilage with a cephalic trim.
- make the lateral crura flat by reducing the convexity.
- reduce the soft tissue directly at that location.

How to Reduce the Bulbosity and Create the Supra-Alar Groove?

There is a method for removing the direct nasalis transverse and its alar parts from the dissected flap. The involved mimetic muscles (partly LLSAN and LLS) on the top can be removed, and if necessary, the subcutaneous fatty layer on the top is removed. Of course, it is essential to do a supra-alar stitch or firm compression dressing to eliminate dead space after removing this area. However, the dissection should be cautiously performed monitoring the vascularity and compression sore.

Case Studies: Reducing Bulbosity and Creating Supra-Alar Groove

In the case of male patients with parenthesis deformity (Fig. 9.18) and another male patient with very thick skin underwent the soft tissue reduction. When the definition of the supra-alar groove is insufficient the direct soft tissue excision can be done to reduce bulbosity (Figs. 9.19 and 9.20). However, care should be taken not to make the flap too thin, and it is necessary to check whether the pressure sore when applying the compression dressing.

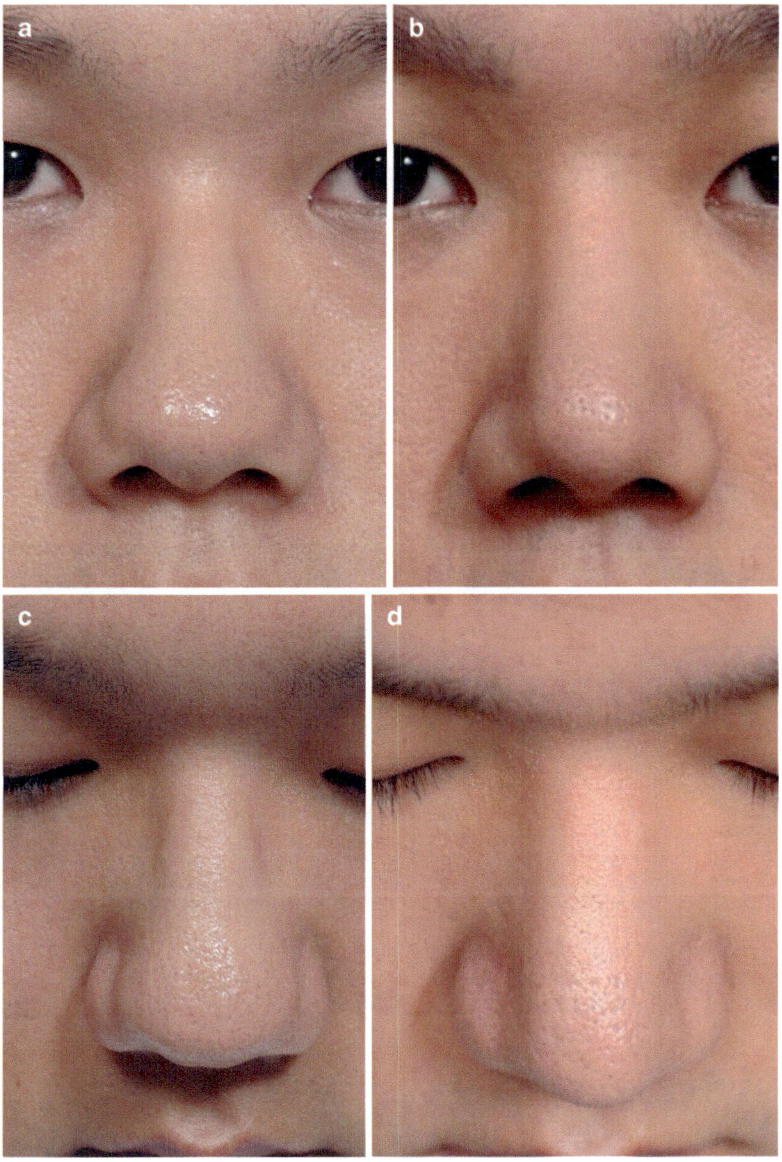

Fig. 9.18 Creating the definition of the supra-alar groove in a bulbous tip with a parenthesis deformity. (**a**, **b**) Pre- and postoperative AP views. (**c**, **d**) Pre- and postoperative bird's eye views

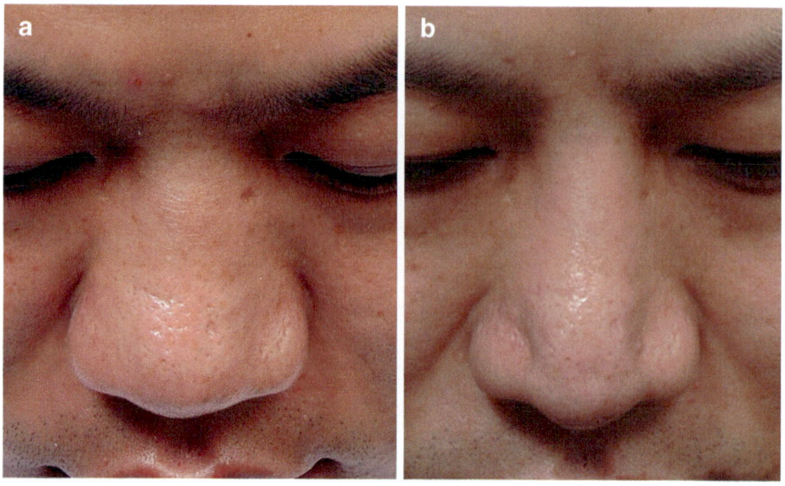

Fig. 9.19 Creating the supra-alar groove's definition in a bulbous tip with a thick skin. (**a**) Preoperative bird's eye view. (**b**) Postoperative bird's eye view

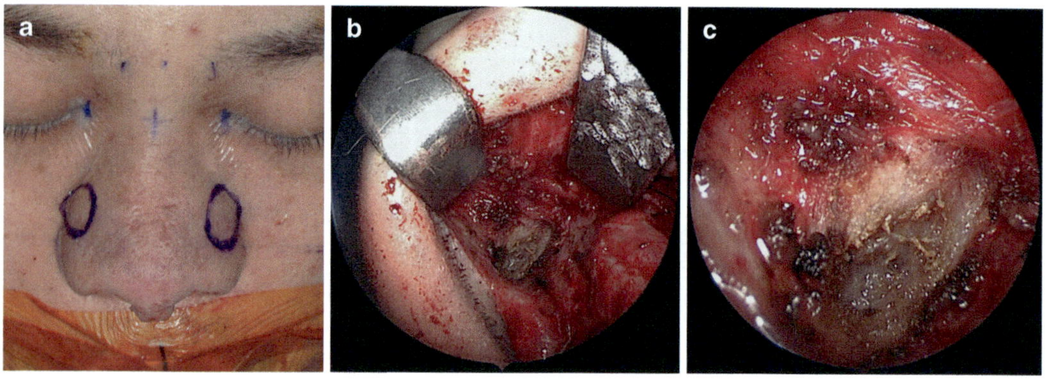

Fig. 9.20 Creating the definition of the supra-alar groove by excision of soft tissue and the muscles. (**a**) Preoperative design for excising the LLSAN and LLS. (**b**) Muscles are detached and removed. (**c**) Dermal exposure after removing the subcutaneous fat

References

1. Toriumi DM. New concepts in nasal tip contouring. Arch Facial Plast Surg. 2006;8(3):156–85.
2. Ali-Salaam P, Kashgarian M, Persing J. The soft triangle revisited. Plast Reconstr Surg. 2002;110(1):14–6.
3. Campbell CF, Pezeshk RA, Basci DS, Scheuer JF, Sieber DA, Rohrich RJ. Preventing soft-tissue triangle collapse in modern rhinoplasty. Plast Reconstr Surg. 2017;140(1):33e–42e.
4. Kayabasoglu G, Nacar A. The soft triangle: an often neglected area in rhinoplasty. Aesthet Plast Surg. 2015;39(5):659–66.
5. Fomon S, Bell JW, Berger EL, Goldman IB, Neivert H, Schattner A. New approach to ventral deflections of the nasal septum [Internet]. Arch Otolaryngol Head Neck Surg. 1951;54:356–66. https://doi.org/10.1001/archotol.1951.03750100018003.
6. Guyuron B, Poggi JT, Michelow BJ. The subdomal graft. Plast Reconstr Surg. 2004;113(3):1037–40; discussion 1041–3.
7. Guyuron B. Rhinoplasty: expert consult premium edition—enhanced online features and print. Elsevier Health Sciences; 2012. 468 p.
8. Sheen JH. Finesse in rhinoplasty. In: Symposium on corrective rhinoplasty. CV Mosby; 1976. p. 263.
9. Byrd HS, Andochick S, Copit S, Walton KG. Septal extension grafts: a method of controlling tip projection shape. Plast Reconstr Surg. 1997;100(4):999–1010.
10. Gunter JP, Friedman RM. Lateral crural strut graft: technique and clinical applications in rhinoplasty. Plast Reconstr Surg. 1997;99(4):943–52; discussion 953–5.
11. Guyuron B, Ghavami A, Wishnek SM. Components of the short nostril. Plast Reconstr Surg. 2005;116(5):1517–24.

10 Controlling Asian Tip: Infratip Lobule and ACR

Pearls

- Unlike Western classification, Asian infratip lobules can be divided into tortious middle crus, hypoplastic middle crus, asymmetric middle crus, mixed type, and secondary cases.
- Suppose the infratip lobule's shape cannot be obtained even after the interdomal suture is appropriate in the cephalic portion of the medial genu. In that case, subtle convexity can be made with a spacer graft or lobule graft.
- Most of the operations of Asian rhinoplasty are focused on enhancing the central component, the longitudinal axis of the septum, and the lengthening of the lateral component, including the alar, has received less attention.
- Extensive nasal lengthening is an operation that simultaneously causes hanging columellar and alar retraction.
- Misconfiguration of the tip-defining point ruins the entire ACR relationship.
- In the case of not harvesting costal cartilage, cartilage consumption for lengthening, and projection of the central component results in insufficient cartilage in modifying the lateral component, making this procedure impossible.
- Even a less developed LLC can solve alar retraction with proper positioning if the lateral crural spanning suture (LCSS) can be fixed to the high septum.
- If the high septum cannot be fixed, there is a method for attaching it to the septum by performing an alar spreader graft or a lateral crural spanning graft for the LLC positioning.
- The most effective method for correcting alar retraction is the lateral crural strut graft (LCSG) method.
- The method of alar base reduction does not help the practical lifting of the alar crease.
- Direct alar lift methods include resectioning the alar vestibule or detaching the alar depressor muscle. However, direct vestibular excision is more effective.
- The authors apply the LCSG method using costal cartilage, which requires total elevation from the LLC's lower mucosa in secondary rhinoplasty.

10.1 The Infratip Lobule

Definition

Infratip lobule refers to the voluminous convexity created by the middle crura descending from the tip-defining point. This angle is changed to the columello-lobular angle and transferred to the nasal base. When viewed from the side, it is an important volume that influences the entire nose's shape because it overlaps the alar base and the alar ridge above it. The tip-defining point and the lower middle crura's normal divergence are essential factors that determine the infratip lobule (Fig. 10.1).

E.-S. Dhong, M.-W. Na, *Asian Septorhinoplasty*, https://doi.org/10.1007/978-981-16-0542-0_10

Anatomic Considerations

A gentle convexity from the columella breakpoint to pronasale is created when the appropriate middle crural divergency is formed by the cephalic portions of the medial genu touching each other at the cephalic point; this is where the ideal interdomal suture located. The transition of the medial genu to the lateral genu of the middle crura is the domal segment. The lobular segment starts from the medial genu of the middle crura to the medial crura. The infratip lobule volume is adjusted by the angle formed by the left and right medial genu of the middle crura. Therefore, when the middle crus's caudal margin is repaired, the natural angle that creates the infratip lobule is lost. Instead, it is necessary to open a divergent angle with an appropriate shield graft (Fig. 10.2).

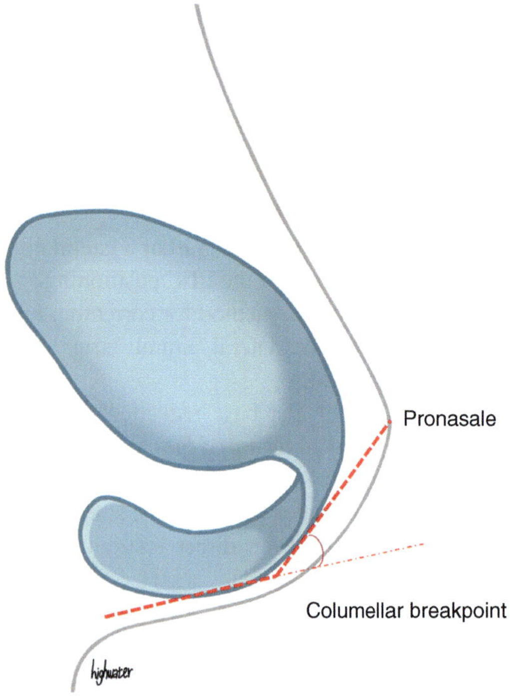

Fig. 10.1 The columello-lobular angle starts from the columellar breakpoint to pronasale

In the ideal nose, the nostril apices coincide with the midpoint of the infratip lobule. The anatomical abnormalities of the infratip lobule were divided into intrinsic and extrinsic factors, and each surgical method was well described [1].

In the Asian nose, the author has never seen a case of middle crus too wide or middle crus too long. It would be right to do an Asian classification differently. The author classified the following three intrinsic factors. However, note that in the case of hypoplastic patients, lateral crus, as well as their medial crus, are hypoplastic. It is correct to classify problematic middle crus into the following five categories (Fig.10.3).

– tortious middle crus
– hypoplastic middle crus
– asymmetric middle crus

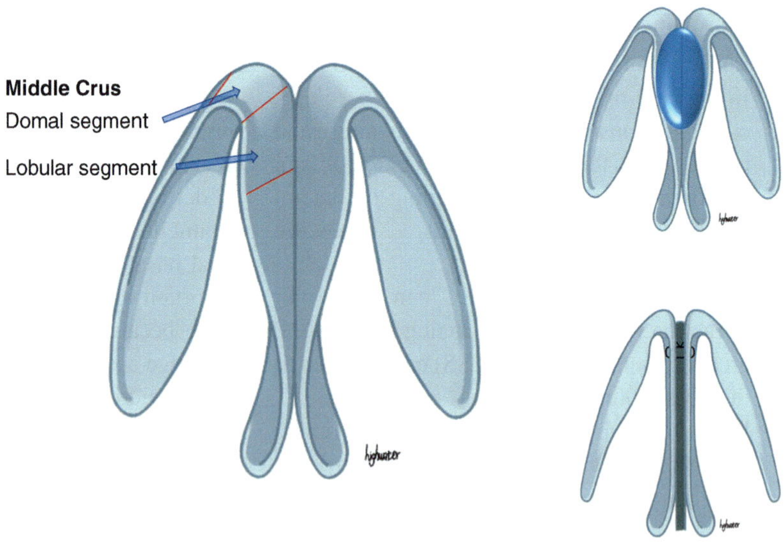

Fig. 10.2 The ideal middle crus: The lobular segment is from the middle crus' medial genu to the middle-medial crural junction. For the lobular volume, a spacer is grafted to maintain the middle crura's horizontal divergence. A columellar strut may ruin this divergence

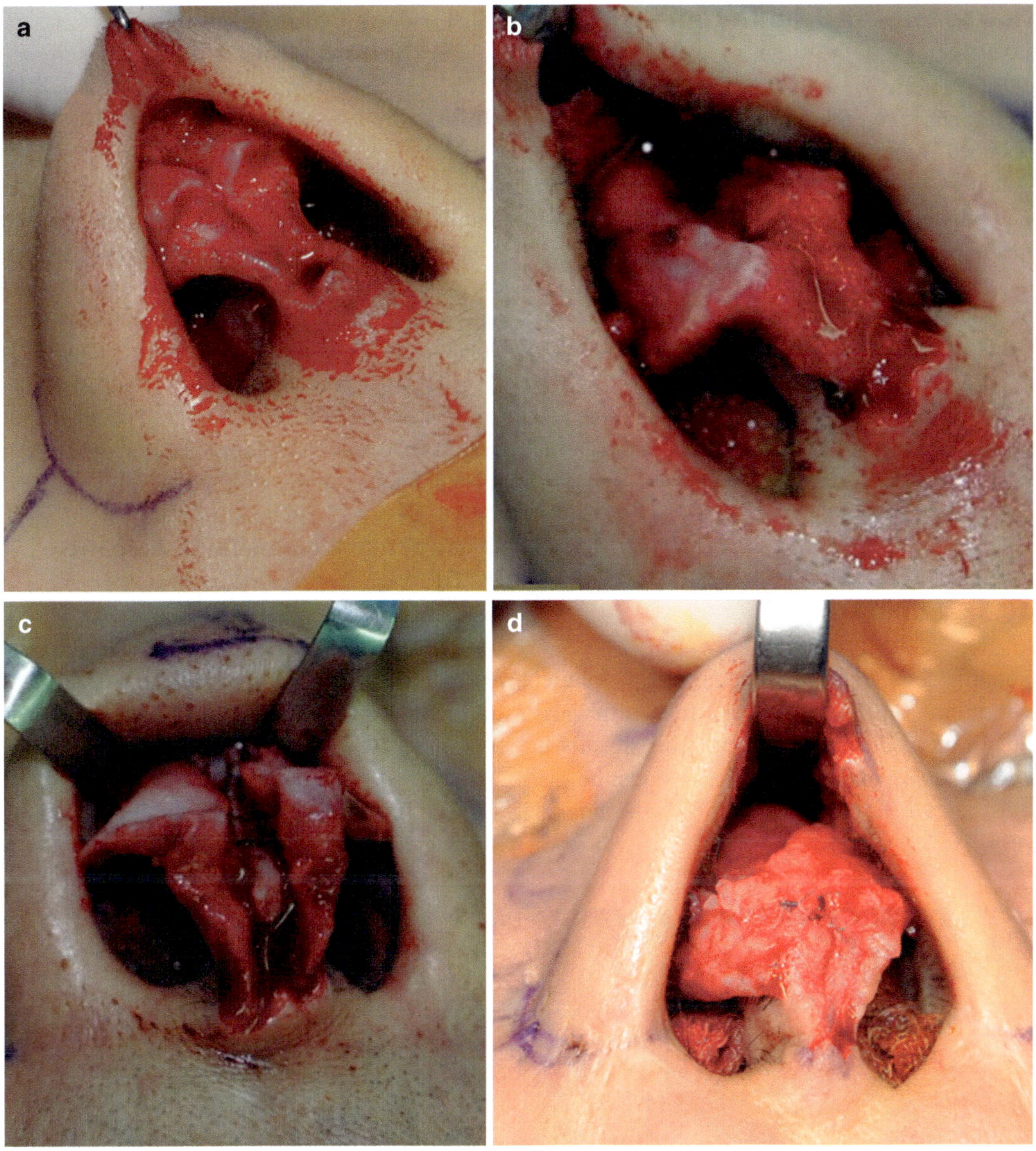

Fig. 10.3 The classification of middle crura in Asians (**a**) Hypoplastic middle crura. (**b**) Mixed type. Asymmetric + Lt. hypoplastic middle crura (**c**) Tortious middle crura. (**d**) Secondary case

- mixed type
- secondary case

The reason that the secondary case is specifically classified is that it shows different characteristics from the primary. The secondary alar-columellar discrepancy requires another level of surgery. It requires many cartilage grafts that must create something from nothing. The classification and method below were based on the primary nose. Since the secondary nose is often a total-tip-reconstruction, it is a task that requires thorough analysis and preparation of vast autogenous materials.

How to Create a Beautiful Infratip Lobule?

If the shape of the infratip lobule cannot be obtained even after the above-mentioned interdomal suture is done correctly in the cephalic portion of the medial genu, the following two methods can be used.

10.2 Spacer Graft

A spacer graft is applied between the middle and medial crura to open the divergence between the medial genu; A shield graft keeps the gap as a spacer graft (Fig. 10.2).

10.3 Lobule Graft

For the convexity of the infratip lobule, voluminous grafts can be applied with various tissues. Usually, the remaining dermis is applied using one or two layers, or just before closure, a free graft is put inside the pocket (Fig. 10.4).

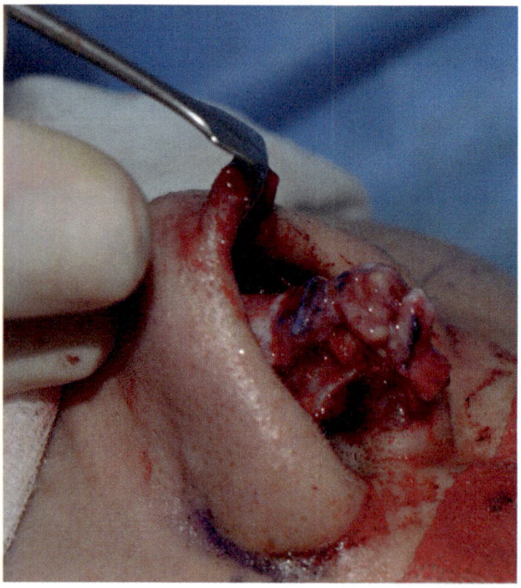

Fig. 10.4 Lobule graft using SDF remnant

10.4 Alar-Columellar Relationship: ACR

Definition

In the lateral view, the nostril's apex comes in the middle between the tip-defining point and the columellar breakpoint. The relationship between the columellar and alar is divided into hanging and retraction with the ideal alar-columellar relationship as 2 mm of columellar show [2] (Fig. 10.5). Moreover, the study concluded that graft is needed for retraction, and resection or graft is needed for hanging depending on whether it is columellar or alar (Fig. 10.6).

Cause of Alar-Columellar Discrepancy (ACD)

In Asian rhinoplasty, the cause of ACD is very complicated. Projecting the tip and extending the entire nose is defined as the operation of the central component, while the operation of the alar part is the lateral component.

- Most Asian rhinoplasty focused on enhancing the central component, which is the septum's longitudinal axis. The lengthening of the lateral component, including the alar, has received less attention.
- Extensive nasal lengthening is an operation that simultaneously causes hanging columellar and alar retraction.
- Misconfiguration of the tip-defining point ruins the entire ACR relationship.
- The wrong resting angle in the LLC's horizontal relationship will spoil the overall alar ridge's shape.

Case Study 1

A 20-year-old woman visited the author with septal deviation and a small nose. The septal deviation was corrected by swing-door procedure, and a septal extension graft was performed using conchas. The low nasion was augmented using a dorsal 3.5 mm silicone, and as shown in the picture, the length of the central component

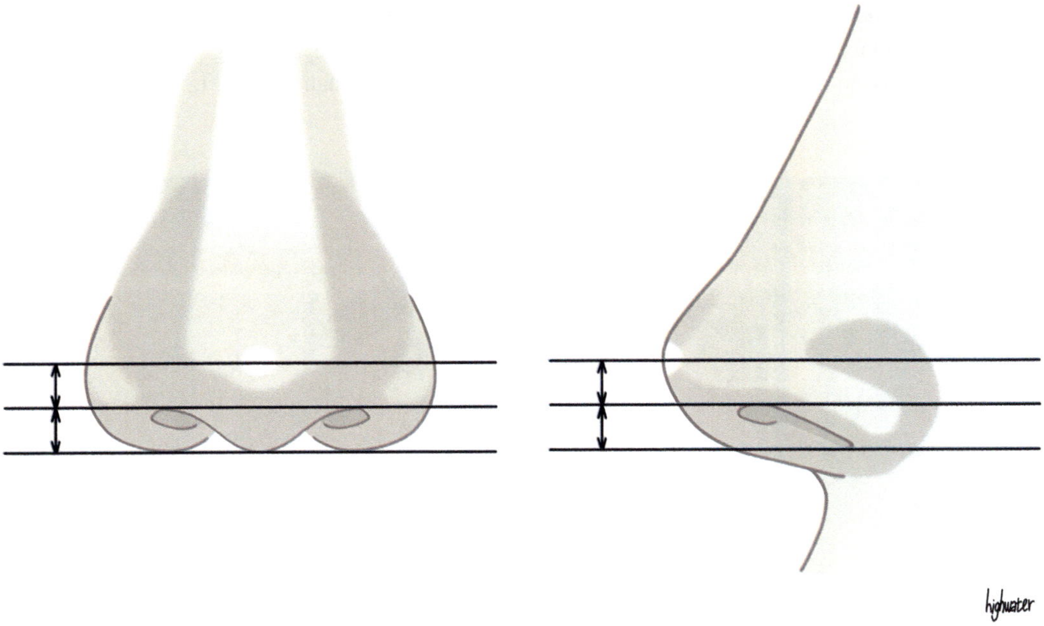

Fig. 10.5 The ideal alar rim starts at the half distance between the columellar-lobular angle and the tip-defining point [2]

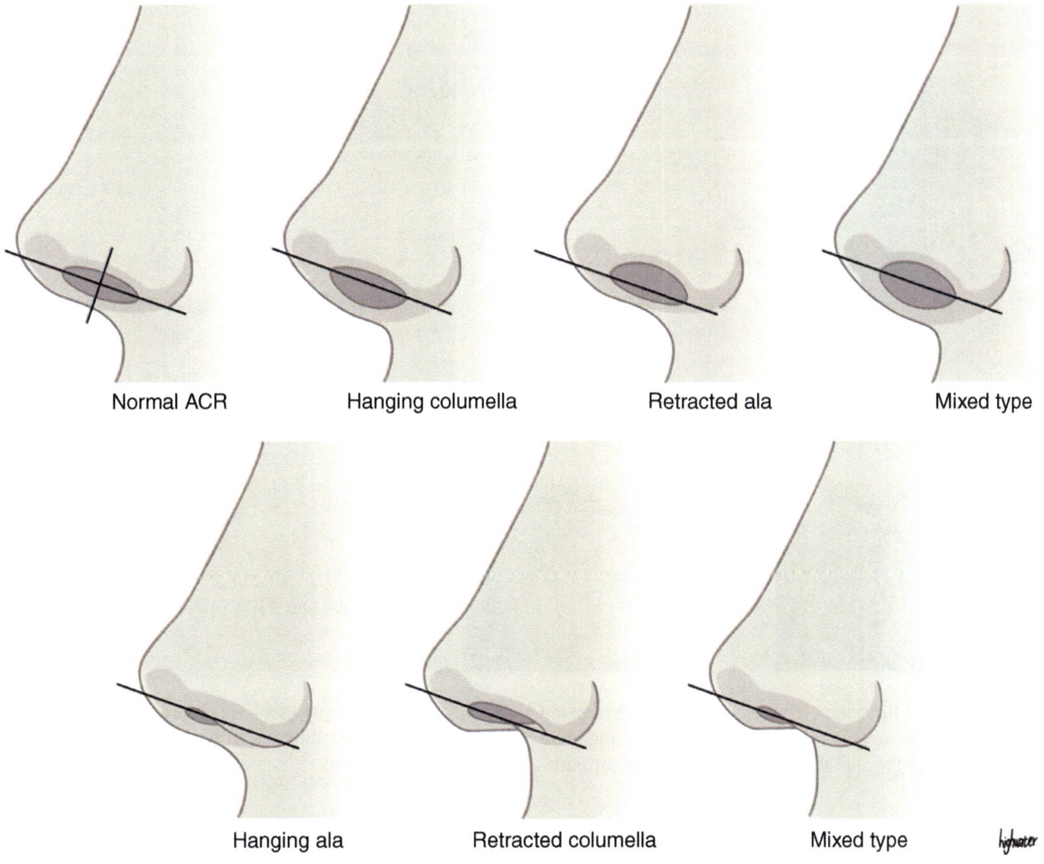

Fig. 10.6 Various types of ACR: The retraction vs. hanging [2]

was extended, and the dorsum was augmented, but there was no extension of the lateral component. There was no complaint from the patient after the operation, but the alar retraction became obvious, and the hanging of the columella appeared more than 2 mm (Fig. 10.7).

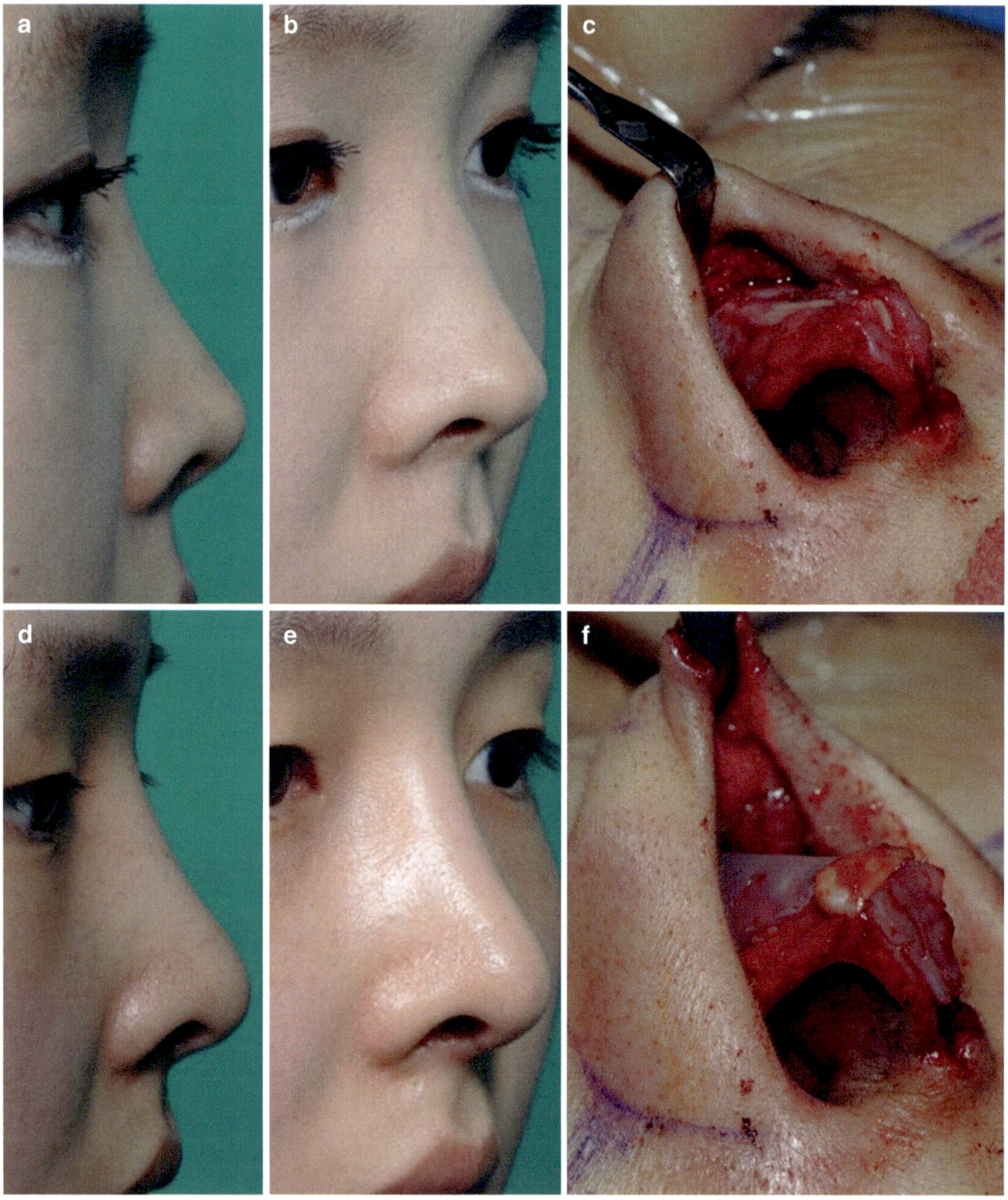

Fig. 10.7 With the perspective of ACR, septal extension graft may aggravate the alar retraction. (**a**, **b**) Preoperative views. (**c**) After the septal extension graft using ear cartilages. (**d**, **e**) Postoperative views. (**f**) Before closure, 3.5 mm silicone and shield graft were applied

- However, the cartilage was insufficient, and costal cartilage was not in the plan for modifying the lateral component, and firm slices of cartilages are indispensable.

Case Study 2

A 50-year-old male visited the author with the chief complaint of alar retraction seen from the front. Since he did not want any type of rhinoplasty, a composite graft from cavum concha for vestibular lining improved the alar retraction (Fig. 10.8).

Central Component Vs. Lateral Component Discrepancy

As shown in the above-mentioned two cases, ACR cannot be improved only by preoperative planning. Modifying ACR after lengthening the central component is required. It is necessary to consider the lateral component of ULC and LLC together after the nasal lengthening, including tip projection and caudal septal extension. In case study 1, a lateral crural strut graft would have been needed because of the underdeveloped LLCs. This would have required the costal cartilage, and the patient may have refused the surgery after being explained. Unlike secondary rhinoplasty, there are many limitations to recommending ribs as donors in Asian primary rhinoplasty.

Strategy for Lateral Component Extension

In primary rhinoplasty, since most of the harvested cartilages are spent in the central component, there are many restrictions on lowering the lateral component. The following methods are selected accordingly.

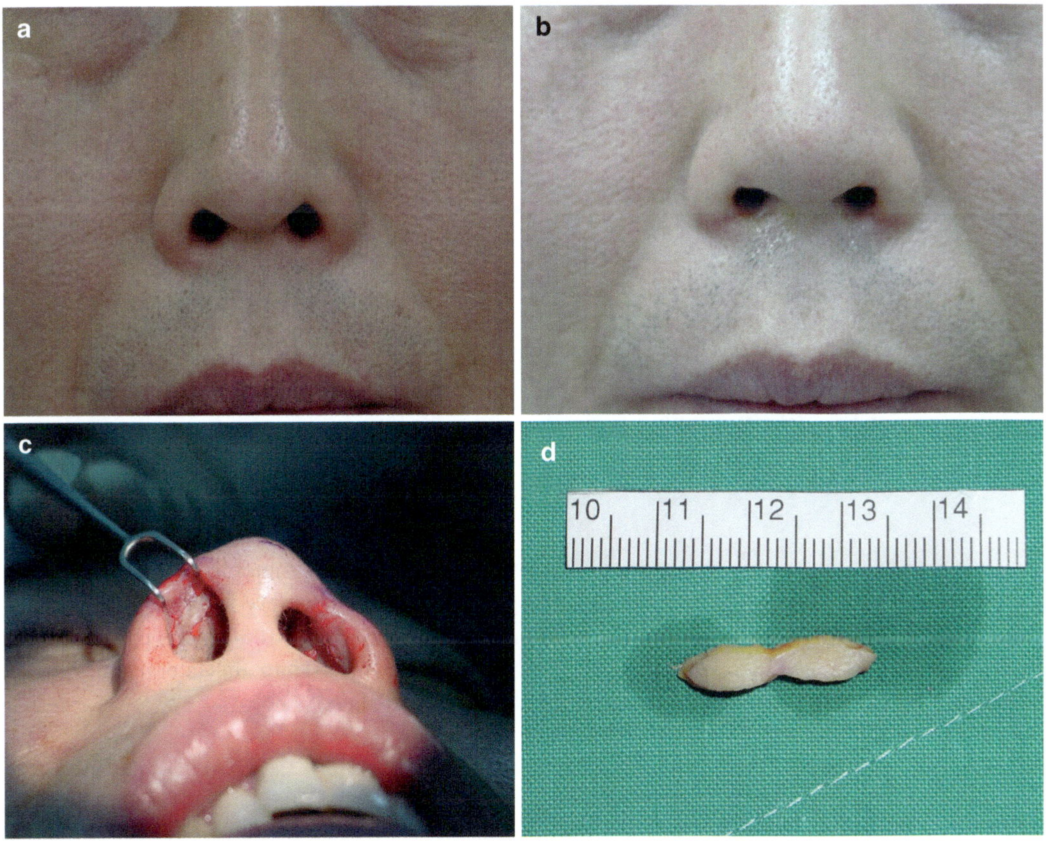

Fig. 10.8 Composite graft for the retracted alar. (**a**) Preoperative AP view. (**b**) Postoperative AP view. (**c**) Intraoperative basal view. (**d**) The composite graft was harvested from the right posterior ear

10.5 Lowering LLC by Lateral Crural Spanning Suture (LCSS)

Doing LCSS only between LLCs does not affect the position. It must be able to penetrate the high septum and lower the LLC to the desired location. LCSS can be used for reducing the bulbosity of the tip. However, LCSS is useful in the LLC positioning. If the high septum cannot be coapted together, this method will not lower the total LLC complex (Fig. 10.9). This method does not affect lowering the LLC as much as desired, but the author thinks it is a method that does not worsen the alar retraction.

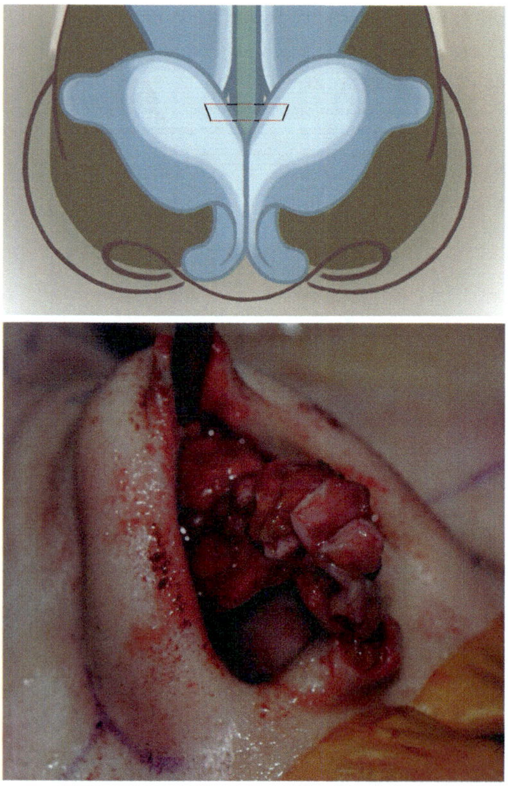

Fig. 10.9 Positioning LLC only by lateral crural spanning suture is not enough for the lowering. It is not recommended to graft excessive central components like the photo

10.6 Alar Batten Graft: Alar Extension Graft

A method was introduced to locate the nostrils downwardly applying batten graft in contact with the LLC's caudal margin [3, 4]. The entire LLC can also be lowered by performing batten graft on the scroll area at the boundary between LLC and ULC. This procedure was initially developed as surgery for internal valve collapse [5, 6]. The authors do not prefer this method because the amount of cartilage used here is too high. If the surgery of the lateral component is the main procedure, you can try. The author does not use it because of the stability issue, and the retracted alar margin does not come down in this way as much as wanted.

10.7 Camouflage of Retracted Alar Ridge

The alar rim graft and the composite graft of nasal lining introduced above is a method for improving retraction by redraping the alar ridge without moving LLC and can be used for mild alar retraction (Fig. 10.8).

10.8 Lateral Crural Strut Graft (LCSG)

The most potent LLC lowering method is LCSG [7]. It has been introduced in the literature for a long time modifying secondary rhinoplasty using costal cartilage. It can be applied as an alar contour graft according to its position [8]. However, in Asian rhinoplasty, where the central component's surgery is prioritized, it is difficult to apply due to the lack of cartilage. It is not easy to insert into the lateral side pocket with ear cartilage.

How to Recruit the Skin Envelope?: The "Sleeve-Down" Technique

- The author uses the "sleeve-down" technique to recruit skin envelopes around the alar ridge as desired.

In other words, it is a method for forcibly lowering the length of the envelope by dissecting the undersurface of the skin. Of course, if it does not come down well, bold scoring or release is needed. Electrocauterization using a colorado tip is beneficial or a 15 blade scalpel is used. These methods are the same as how to make beautiful facets in Chap. 9.

Strategy for Lifting the Alar Base: Alar Lift

Often the alar base reduction (excising the nostril sill and lateral alar base) makes the alar hanging more severe and the tip projection decreased [9].

Although the alar flaring is improved, there is no change in the alar crease junction's vertical position (Fig. 10.10). Therefore, along with alar base reduction, the vestibule skin's vertical amount should be excised and sealed in any way. Several methods are introduced, but the author prefers performing vertical wedge resection of the medial vestibule sill for reducing its internal nasal lining. If the base is not raised vertically, reducing the lateral alar flap's vestibule does not affect the alar position. Direct levator plication can be applied by dissection of the lateral sill [10].

Although the supra-alar groove's modification is described in Chap. 9, the author agrees that the alar position's vertical changed by dissecting the mimetic muscles near the alar. More simply, the elevation of the alar crease junction of 2 mm is possible even by plicating the basal cutting plane after resection of the vestibular skin. However, compared to the central component, the lateral component is affected more by facial mimetic muscles, so the effect of muscle repair is limited, and the effect will be more significant only when the vestibular lining is removed.

Case Study
A 32-year-old woman was referred to the author with nasal septal deviation, tip under projection, and alar flaring. However, a nostril sill was seen from the front, and alar retraction was accompanied. The above-mentioned method was used. The central component was extended and projected by the caudal septal extension with folded cymba concha, and an onlay graft with SMF was performed on the dorsum. Afterward, the vertical reduction of the sill was 2.5 mm during the alar base resection. It can be found that the alar crease junction was lifted after surgery (Figs. 10.11 and 10.12).

Strategy for Achieving the Ideal Resting Angle of LLC

One of the critical factors determining the alar ridge's shape is the angle between the LLC and ULC in the resting state. The left and right LLCs' symmetry can be balanced by adjusting this angle and creating an ideal alar ridge. It has been reported that 100 is the ideal angle between ULC and LLC, but Asian is different from the Western nose, so it would be correct to view this resting angle more obtuse [11] (Fig. 10.13).

Correction of Alar-Columellar Discrepancy (ACD) in Primary Rhinoplasty

The retraction is corrected by increasing with graft, and the hanging is corrected by direct excision. Below is a strategy that considers the central component and the lateral component. The ideal ACR is 1–2 mm of the columellar show below the long axis of the nostril. However, it is better to apply a more conservative amount in Asian [2].

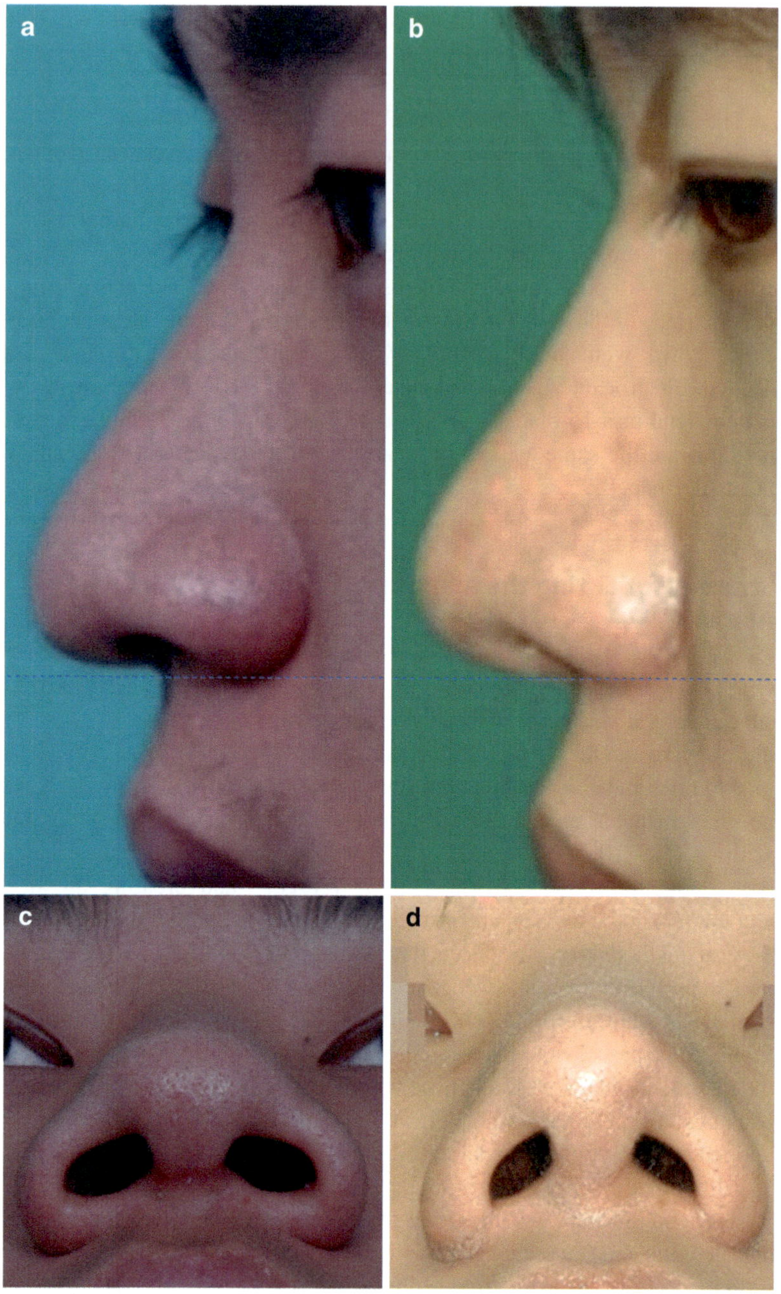

Fig. 10.10 Alar base reduction does not improve the alar hanging. (**a**, **c**) Preoperative views. (**b**, **d**) Postoperative views. Although the alar flaring is improved, there is no change in the alar crease junction's vertical position

Small Nose: Short Septum + Alar Retraction

The small nose is commonly seen in Asian, and it can be said that most LLCs are underdeveloped. Therefore, an excessive increase in the central component can worsen alar retraction (Fig. 10.7).

- Even an underdeveloped LLC can solve alar retraction with proper positioning if the lateral crural spanning suture can be fixed to the high septum.
- If it cannot be fixed to the high septum, there is a method for attaching it to the septum by performing an alar spreader graft or lateral crural spanning graft for the LLC positioning [12]

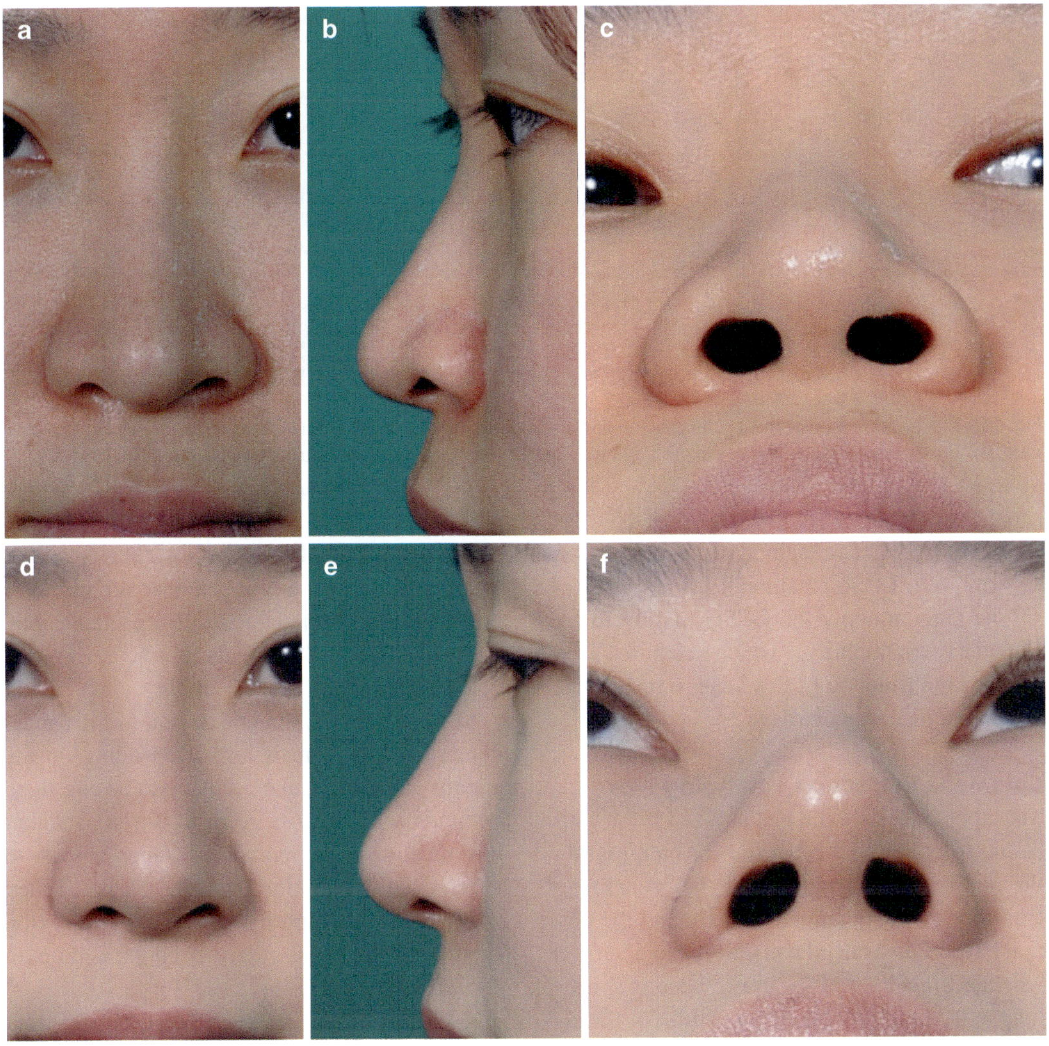

Fig. 10.11 Alar base reduction with vertical vestibular excision. (**a**–**c**) Preoperative views. (**d**–**f**) Postoperative views. Septoplasty, caudal septal extension using folded cymba, dorsal SMF graft, and alar base reduction with vertical lift was performed

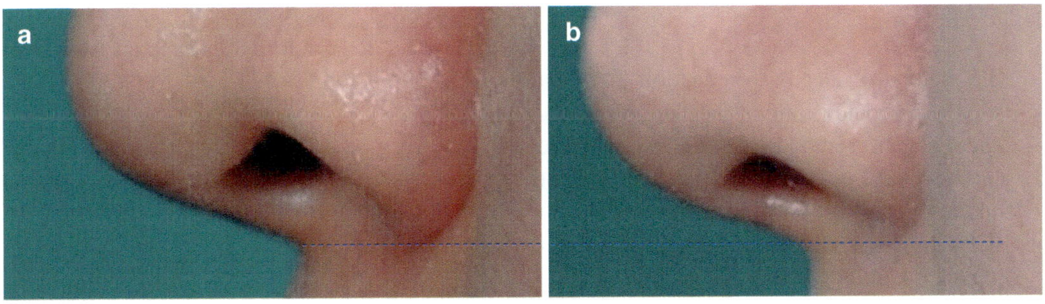

Fig. 10.12 Lateral views show improvement of alar retraction and vertical lift of alar crease junction. (**a**) Preoperative view. (**b**) Postoperative view

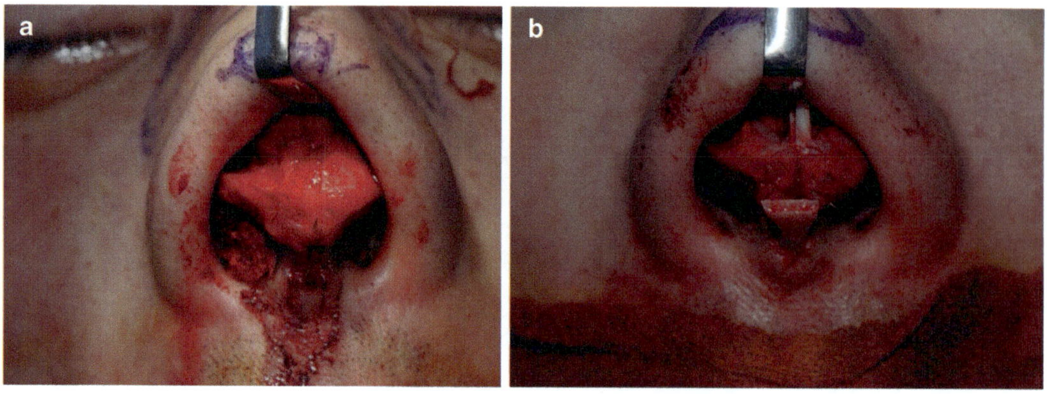

Fig. 10.13 The correction of the asymmetric resting angle between ULC and LLC. (**a**) A secondary case. Preoperative view. (**b**) Postoperative view. The costal cartilage was applied for the L-strut reconstruction and shield grafting

- The most effective method is the lateral crural strut graft (LCSG) method [7] (Fig. 9.9).
- The authors apply the LCSG mainly in secondary rhinoplasty, which requires total elevation from the LLC's lower mucosa when harvesting costal cartilage.

Columella Retraction + Hanging Alar

This appearance should be analyzed if the cause is due to columellar retraction or hanging alar, the entire nasal tip should be considered. Considering the position of the tip and the position of the subnasale, the priority is to determine whether the length of the entire nose is short or long and determine the ideal position of the columellar accordingly. The central component determines whether the alar is hanging or not. While considering ACR, the disharmony that cannot be solved by the central compart must be modified by a reduction in the lateral component.

- The method of alar base reduction does not help the practical lifting of the alar crease.
- Direct alar lift methods include resecting the alar vestibule or plicating the alar levator muscle.
- ACR is improved by increasing the tip projection and nasal length in most Asians.

Hanging Columella + Alar Retraction

Asian patients with this appearance are rare. For the hanging columella, first the caudal septal margin is removed then alar retraction is corrected with the LLC modification.

In most patients, direct excision of the caudal membranous septum is rare. Depending on the amount of quadrangular cartilage to be cut, there are times when mucosa needs to be removed, but most mucosa can be redraped. If mucosa needs to be removed, transfixion incision can be applied like Western rhinoplasty. However, transfixion incision is the most rarely used procedure in Asian rhinoplasty.

References

1. Rohrich RJ, Liu JH. Defining the infratip lobule in rhinoplasty: anatomy, pathogenesis of abnormalities, and correction using an algorithmic approach. Plast Reconstr Surg. 2012;130(5):1148–58.
2. Gunter JP, Rohrich RJ, Friedman RM. Classification and correction of alar-columellar discrepancies in rhinoplasty. Plast Reconstr Surg. 1996;97(3):643–8.
3. Toriumi DM. New concepts in nasal tip contouring. Arch Facial Plast Surg. 2006;8(3):156–85.
4. Kim HS, Roh SG. The alar extension graft for retracted ala. J Korean Soc Plast Reconstr Surg. 2009;36(1):66–74.
5. Cervelli V, Spallone D, Bottini JD, Silvi E, Gentile P, Curcio B, et al. Alar batten cartilage graft: treatment

of internal and external nasal valve collapse. Aesthetic Plast Surg. 2009;33(4):625–34.
6. Toriumi DM, Josen J, Weinberger M, Tardy ME Jr. Use of alar batten grafts for correction of nasal valve collapse. Arch Otolaryngol Head Neck Surg. 1997;123(8):802–8.
7. Gunter JP, Friedman RM. Lateral crural strut graft: technique and clinical applications in rhinoplasty. Plast Reconstr Surg. 1997;99(4):943–52; discussion 953–5.
8. Cochran CS, Sieber DA. Extended alar contour grafts: an evolution of the lateral crural strut graft technique in rhinoplasty. Plast Reconstr Surg. 2017;140(4):559e–67e.
9. Guyuron B. Dynamic interplays during rhinoplasty. Clin Plast Surg. 1996;23(2):223–31.
10. Taş S. The alignment of the nose in rhinoplasty: fix down concept. Plast Reconstr Surg. 2020;145(2):378–89.
11. Çakir B, Doğan T, Öreroğlu AR, Daniel RK. Rhinoplasty: surface aesthetics and surgical techniques. Aesthet Surg J. 2013;33(3):363–75.
12. Gunter JP, Rohrich RJ. Correction of the pinched nasal tip with alar spreader grafts. Plast Reconstr Surg. 1992;90(5):821–9.

11 Correction of the Short Secondary Nose: Dissection and the Framework Reconstruction

Pearls

- There is no rationale for using an alloplastic implant again that solves the complication caused by the alloplastic implant itself.
- The only way to secure the secondary surgery safe would be using autografts. Allografts are also unsafe substitutes.
- The addition of low concentration Hyaluronidase (50–100 unit/mL) is advantageous for a hardened scar.
- If a dorsal alloplastic implant is present, the capsulectomy range should be determined during surgery because the scar tissue around it causes the contracture.
- Depending on the thickness of the dorsal skin flap and the likelihood of compromise, you should decide whether to perform an anterior capsulectomy or not.
- If the skin is too thin to maintain vascularity, anterior capsulectomy may not be performed. At this time, it should be noted that the dorsal skin flap may not be released sufficiently.
- The posterior capsule should be removed entirely. Be careful not to communicate with the nasal cavity.
- The most crucial procedure in a short nose correction is the LLC positioning and the dorsal skin repair without tension.
- An appropriate amount of autologous cartilage should be prepared for the septal L-strut extension graft.
- In most secondary cases, there may no longer be existing septal and concha cartilages. The rib cartilage is the best and definitive source for septal reconstruction.
- The septal L-strut extension graft can be applied using folded cymba concha and folded cavum concha in most Asians.
- Dissecting the septum may be impossible in cases where the mucoperichondrium had been destroyed.
- There is severe destruction where the Medpor was applied at the septum as a spreader or septal extension graft.
- If there is severe destruction at the keystone area, stable fixation between the caudal nasal bone and the anterior grafts is needed after drill holes are made. The same principle applies to the ANS area.
- This method is applied to the septal extension graft applied to the anterior septum and the caudal septal extension graft applied to the caudal septum.

Supplementary Information The online version of this chapter (https://doi.org/10.1007/978-981-16-0542-0_11) contains supplementary material, which is available to authorized users.

E.-S. Dhong, M.-W. Na, *Asian Septorhinoplasty*, https://doi.org/10.1007/978-981-16-0542-0_11

11.1 The Secondary Rhinoplasty in Asians

A short nose is one of the biggest challenges in Asian rhinoplasty. If Asian rhinoplasty is mainly divided into two, it can be divided into primary rhinoplasty and secondary rhinoplasty. If you do secondary rhinoplasty with the strategy of primary rhinoplasty, you will be frustrated. The method of directly elongating the septum resolved the shortness and complemented the central nasal area and allowed for the next steps in the lateral side of the lower two-third of the nose.

Alloplastic Implant with SRP: Is it Safe?

There have been many reports on complication rates, such as infection in surgery using alloplastic implants, but there are few detailed studies on inflammation/infection, which cause short nose deformity. There will be a clear difference depending on the simultaneous septal surgery, only one study reported that 13.8% of 695 patients who used silicone implants had contractures requiring correction [1]. This is different from the standpoint of infection or inflammation. It can be seen as a high rate of contracture.

The septal surgery makes a considerable difference when the infection involves.

It involves two big problems. Structurally, it causes the nasal framework's collapse and chronic soft tissue contracture.

Technically, separating the upper lateral cartilage (ULC) from the anterior septum is the preferred procedure when applying septal extension grafts and spreader grafts. The mucosa area is completely separated from the nasal cavity and is well preserved, but even without communication between the incised pocket and the nasal cavity, it may not be safe to place the allogeneic implant on the widely detached platform. If an acute infection occurs after surgery, the infection around the implant can spread to the deep space, causing a severe intraseptal abscess. Most people with severe infections, whether acute or chronic develop nasal shortening due to destruction of the septal skeleton and soft tissues. Even if the capsules around the allogeneic implant are safe, the question of longevity remains. Gravity forces the homologous implant to continuously compress the platform below by adding pressure on the surrounding soft tissue (Chap. 1). Salvaging an infected nose after septorhinoplasty is entirely different from that of a relatively simple rhinoplasty. In the case of SSI or delayed infection (late-onset inflammation), the infectious soft tissue, including the capsule, can be completely excised and irrigated to save the nose. However, if the septum was dissected and grafted, nasal support may be lost, and moderate to severe malformations may remain even after complete eradication of the septal abscess (Fig. 11.1).

Bacterial biofilms result in chronic refractory inflammation and impending extraction of allogeneic implants. Further studies are needed for the growth of the mucin-producing cells or new proliferation of the endothelium. Post-inflammatory contracture is similar to breast capsular contracture. A dense layer of avascular connective tissue is formed by the aggregation of monocytes and severe fibroblasts around the capsule.

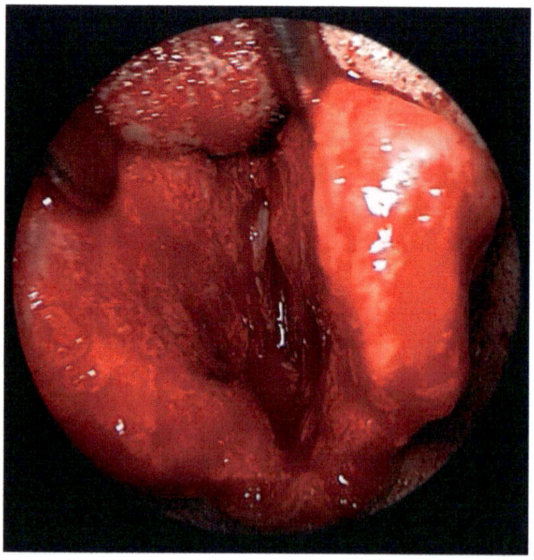

Fig. 11.1 Destruction of remaining septal cartilage after the septal abscess

- There is no rationale for using an alloplastic implant again that solves the complication caused by the alloplastic implant itself.
- The only way to secure the secondary surgery safe would be using autografts. Allografts are also unsafe substitutes.

Specific Considerations of Secondary Surgery

The biggest obstacle to surgery is that it is difficult to excise the scar tissue in detail. There is no accurate dissection plane in many cases, and if all scars are removed, a vast amount of volume is lost. All scars need to be removed when it is directly gripping the framework, and longitudinal release is not possible without release. After the scar removal, the remaining ULC and LLC's destruction or resorption can be observed (Fig. 11.2).

The Dissection

It can be said that more than 70% of the operation time is spent on proper dissection. The more complicated the dissection is, the more sharp instruments are needed, but many hard scars even do not cut well by a scalpel. Especially, such a stone-like scar is the multilayered alloderm. Sometimes the dissection is performed using a colorado microdissection tip of electrocautery.

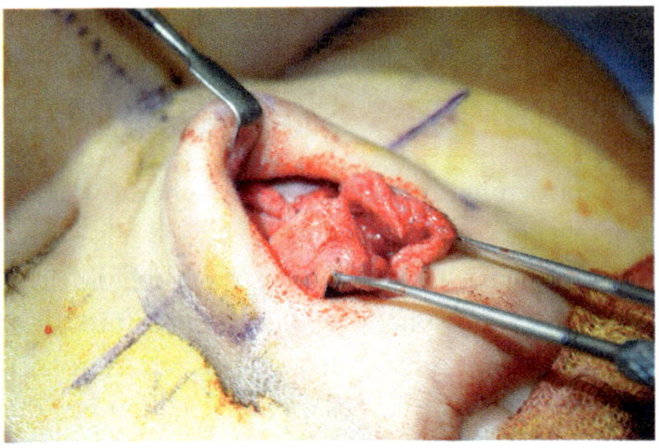

Fig. 11.2 After the scar removal, the remaining LLC's destruction was found with multiple non-absorbable sutures

- The addition of low concentration Hyaluronidase (50–100 unit/mL) is advantageous for a hard scar. This method has been used since the 1950s [2].

Its advantages are local anesthetics mixed with epinephrine quickly enter hard scar tissue; temporarily hydrodissection is facilitated; swelling caused by local anesthetics is reduced. The disadvantage is that if the pharmacological effect is maintained until the end of the surgery, it makes the thickness of the soft tissue thinner than its actual size. So the thin envelope induces overgraft more than needed. However, there are more advantages than disadvantages in dealing with hard tissues. There are cases where all of the following dissections should be performed in nine areas where severe contracture is involved. Below one to three are methods for releasing dorsal skin flaps, and the rest are methods for releasing nasal frameworks (Fig. 11.3).

- The dissection plane is the presumed sub-SMAS. However, it will be a subcutaneous plane in most secondary operations.
- If a dorsal alloplastic implant is present, the capsulectomy range should be determined during surgery because the scar tissue around it causes the contracture.
- Depending on the thickness of the dorsal skin flap and the likelihood of compromise, you should decide whether to perform an anterior capsulectomy or not.
- If the skin is too thin to maintain vascularity, anterior capsulectomy may not be performed. At this time, it should be noted that the dorsal skin flap may not be released sufficiently.
- The posterior capsule should be removed entirely. Be careful not to communicate with the nasal cavity.
- When doing the posterior capsulectomy, it is often necessary to remove all the scars, leaving only a thin intranasal mucosa.
- The most important point in a short nose correction is the LLC positioning and the dorsal skin repair without tension.

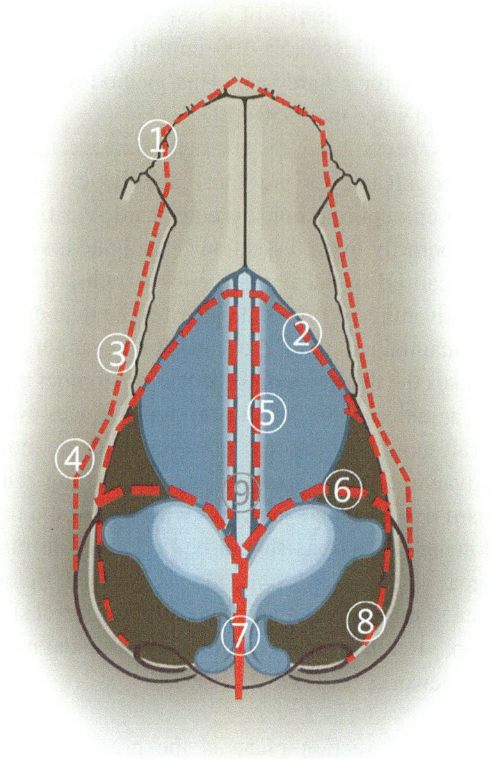

Fig. 11.3 Schematic of releasing areas in severe contracture. (1) Dissection of nasal sidewall and root. (2) Dissection between nasal bone and ULC. (3) Dissection between skin flap from the maxillary process. (4) Dissection between sidewall and maxilla. (5) Dissection between the septum and ULC. (6) Dissection between ULC and LLC (scroll area). (7) Dissection between LLC and LLC. (8) Dissection between LLC and pyriform aperture. (9) Secondary septal dissection

Dissection Above Nasal Sidewall and Root

All bone attachments of the cephalo-lateral portion of the skin flap should be released. Lateral release requires releasing part of the transverse nasalis muscle and part of the bone attachment of LLSAN. For a large amount of skin flaps to be caudally redraped, nasal root release is often essential. Temporarily, the medial canthal skin may be pulled downwardly, but this phenomenon does not cause the deformation later. The medial canthal tendon is not severed, so the mongoloid slant normalizes when swelling disappears.

Dissection Between Nasal Bone and ULC

Detaching the periosteum under the caudal nasal bone and detaching the upper part of the ULC is performed simultaneously. After dissecting this part, much release does not occur. However, since the longitudinal capsule is usually present on the top of this area, there are cases where the posterior capsule must be removed, and this area must also be released (Video 11.1).

Dissection Between Skin Flap from Maxillary Process

Like the pyriform aperture below, this part's dissection is necessary for the release and caudal extension of lateral components, including LLC.

Dissection Between Sidewall and Maxilla

It is often necessary to release the skin flap right up to the side of the LLC. Here, massive bleeding can be encountered and should be cauterized well. If you plan to do a lateral crural strut graft on this area, space should be preserved to insert the strut with partial detachment rather than complete detach.

Dissection Between Septum and ULC

This dissection must go through to reconstruct the septal framework. Care must be taken not to expose the nasal cavity. Likewise, since the strongest contracture exists in the posterior capsule area, this area must be released.

Dissection Between ULC and LLC (Scroll Area)

The most release occurs here. The scroll area is where LLC is overriding the ULC, and it is essential to release this part after the cephalic trim completely. If cephalic trim is not performed, it is challenging to release accurately, and there is a risk of exposing the nasal cavity. If you put the freer elevator in the nasal cavity and release the scroll area above, you can prevent mucosal tear and preserve mucosa as much as possible and release this area. Here you can get an extra length of 2–3 mm (Video 11.2).

Dissection Between LLC and LLC

Dissection is performed along the midline between the LLCs on both sides to find the caudal septum.

Because alloplastic material is usually contained in this area, it is often difficult to dissect. Besides, there are many cases where the middle crura's scarring is severe, or the medial crus on one side is lost. The priority is to find the caudal septum first along the midline and find the subperichondrial plane of the caudal septum. Then, if necessary, the mucoperichondrium is preserved, and the surrounding scar tissue is removed. In some cases, it may be necessary to release the perichondrium, leaving the mucosa only. Loss of mucosa in this area can cause SSI later, and in most cases, cartilage graft on the caudal septum is required, so if mucosa laceration occurs in the membranous septum, it needs to be repaired.

Dissection Between LLC and Pyriform Aperture

Pyriform ligament must be released in connection with the scar above. However, most patients' contracture rarely occurs here because this area is far from the implants and contains abundant muscles underneath.

Secondary Septal Dissection

The elevation of the bilateral septal mucosal flap has little effect on the release in the longitudinal or anterior direction. The septal mucosa to which perichondrium is attached does not have much elasticity, and this flap after infection does not stretch well. Secondary dissection of the previous SMR site is not recommended, but the dissection is possible if the dissection plane has accurately proceeded in the previous surgery.

Postoperative Re-scarring

After successful surgery, unwanted scar tissue may develop again. When the dorsal skin flap remains thin, or if a scoring incision is put on the dermal flap's undersurface, an intractable dermal scar is formed. If dermis graft was applied to the dorsum previously, more severe scar tissue might be encountered. Before redraping the dorsal skin at the end of the surgery, the author prefers to inject diluted Kenalog into the subdermis. Kenalog is effective in preventing swelling after surgery and reducing subdermal scarring (Video 11.3).

11.2 Camouflage or Restoring the Framework?

- The most important factor of planning secondary septorhinoplasty is soft tissue resilience.
- A cantilever graft can be applied to camouflage without septal surgery.
- If there is a functional problem, that is, nasal obstruction, septal surgery needs to be done.
- The cantilever graft is safe if the septal perforation is located in the anterior-caudal septum.

Specific Considerations in Septal Surgery in Asians

Septal cartilage in Asians tends to be smaller than in Caucasians. The average area of septal cartilage in Koreans was reported to be 8.18 cm^2 for men and 7.36 cm^2 for women [3].

For Koreans, the amount of septal cartilage collected was usually insufficient for various graft use. Therefore, additional cartilage grafts such as the concha and costal cartilage should be considered before surgery [4]. The septal cartilage is thinner in Asian, and submucosal resection of quadrangular cartilage also tends to weaken the nasal support. A swing door procedure performed over the maxillary and anterior nasal spine (ANS) to correct a caudal septal deviation aggravates septal instability at the base. Most Asian rhinoplasty requires two dimensions of improvement: anteroposterior and cephalocaudal extension. When the whole tip is projected, the length of the nostril should also be increased [5, 6]. However, it is impossible to even worry about this in a secondary operation. Not only the lack of donor cartilage but also because of scar tissue, the nose is often impossible to be lengthened as much as desired. In the case of the author, short nose correction is performed using the following two methods. The SLEG method has various donor cartilage options, whereas the cantilever graft has no other method than the costal cartilage. Secondary short nose deformity can be reconstructed using allograft, but this concept is excluded because the author does not have enough evidence on it. The opinion on IHCC will be discussed in Chap. 13.

Septal L-Strut Extension Graft (SLEG)

SLEG is the method that the author prefers to create a septum-dependent tip [7].

- An appropriate amount of autologous cartilage should be prepared.
- In most secondary cases, there may be no longer existing septal and concha cartilages. The rib cartilage is the best and definitive source for septal reconstruction [8].
- The septal L-strut extension graft can be applied using folded cymba concha and folded cavum concha in most Asians (Fig. 11.4).

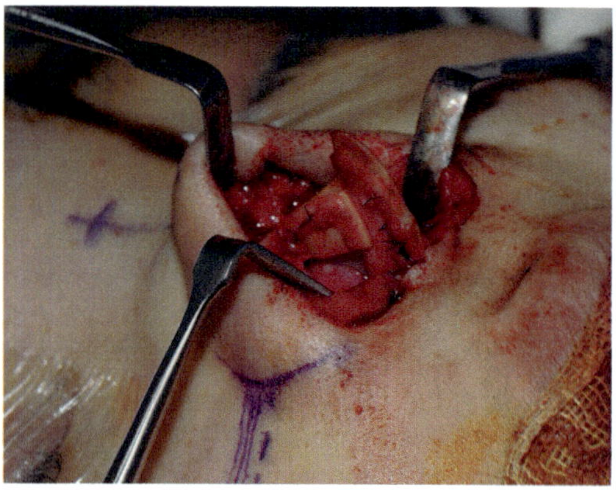

Fig. 11.4 The septal L-strut extension graft (SLEG) can be applied using folded cymba concha and folded cavum concha

- Dissecting the septum may be impossible in cases where the mucoperichondrium had been destroyed.
- There is severe destruction where the Medpor was applied at the septum as a spreader or septal extension graft.
- If there are severe destructions at the keystone area, stable fixation between the caudal nasal bone and the anterior grafts is needed after drill holes are made. The same principle applies to the ANS area.

11.3 Techniques of Septal L-Strut Extension Graft for Asians

Effective L-strut (anterocaudal) expansion requires various combinations of autologous cartilage. Sometimes the amount of septal cartilage is insufficient, making it impossible to perform effective L-strut extension. Cymba concha and cavum concha are required to perform L-strut extension. For patients with small ears, rib cartilage may be the primary option. The tongue-and-groove method also uses the septal cartilage for bilateral spreader implantation. In L-strut's caudal extension, rib cartilage provides the most source when the septal cartilage is lacking. It is most advantageous to use cymba cartilage in Asians who do not prefer tip stiffness. During the author's 20-year experience, cymba concha was used in the caudal septum for a modified tongue-in-groove technique and was useful in obtaining the tip's projection. Cymba concha, when folded, can produce 4–5 mm wide and 20 mm or longer (data in publishing, Aesthetic Surgery Journal) and are sufficient to support the medial and medial crura of the lower lateral cartilage of the Asian population (Fig. 11.5). In particular, by applying the tongue-in-groove method around ANS using a cymba concha for tip support loss after performing the caudal septum swing door technique, both projection and stability can be obtained. Additional support can be obtained by performing sutures so that the concave sides face each other during folding. It is essential to attach the cartilage mucoperichondrium of the cymba on the convex side to gain additional strength from the brittle tendency (Fig. 11.5).

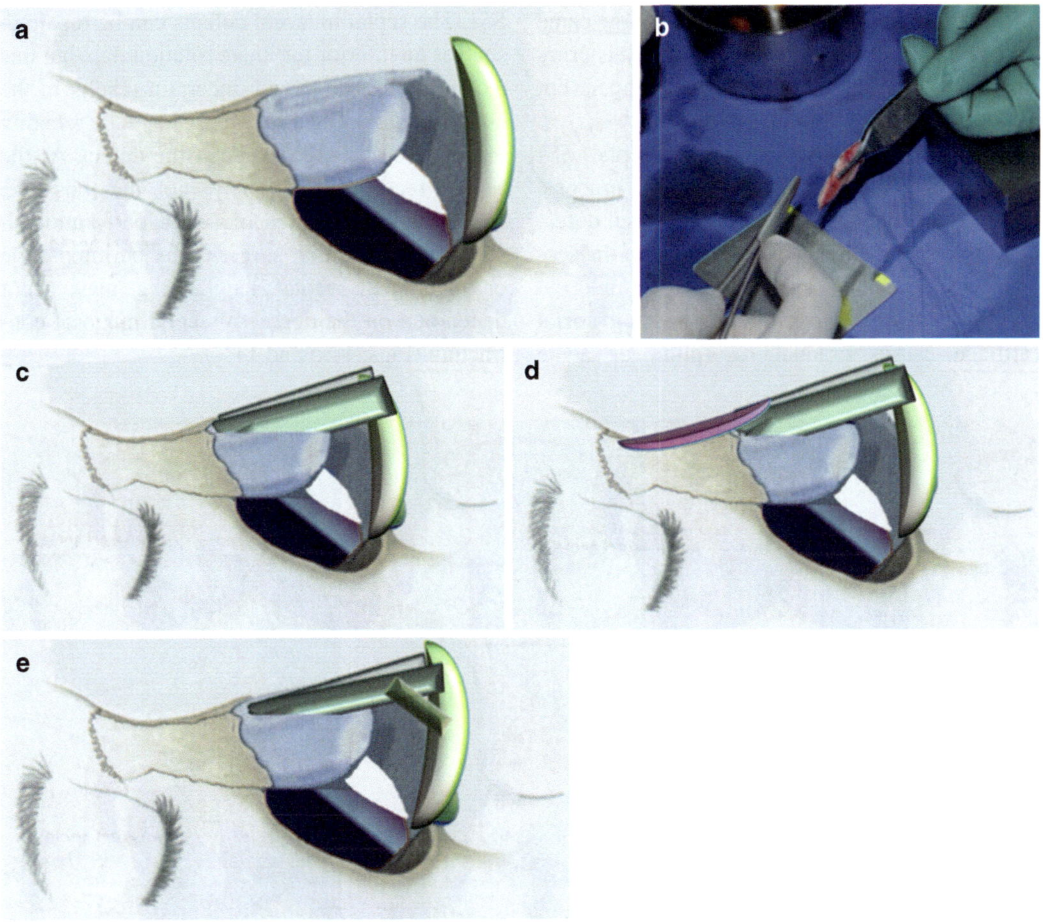

Fig. 11.5 Techniques of septal L-strut extension grafting. (**a**) Caudal SEG: folded cymba concha is sutured on both sides of the ANS for support and caudal extension, a modified tongue-in-groove technique. (**b**) Folded cymba concha: facing concave sides were sutured. Minimal continuity in the middle enhances strength. (**c**) Bilateral extended spreader graft: visible spreader grafts are applied anteriorly. (**d**) Radix graft: any type of soft tissue is grafted on the nasion to smooth the dorsum. (**e**) Rafting graft: small pieces of cartilage are applied between the anterior and caudal pillars. (Material from: Hwang and Dhong. Septal Extension Graft in Asian Rhinoplasty Facial Plastic Surgery of North America, 2018, Elsevier)

11.4 Extended Spreader Graft: Modified Tongue-and-Groove Graft

The septal cartilage is most suitable for L-strut's anterior extension. However, since most septal cartilage cannot be used in a secondary operation, conchal cartilage or costal cartilage is used. The anterior extension requires more width than other existing spreader grafts. In other words, this application can be described as a "visible spreader" graft. Simultaneously, this technique is the "modified tongue-and-groove technique" of Dr. Guyuron [9]. The anterior extension is possible from the keystone area to the tip, so the excessive anterior extension must be avoided since it leads to difficulties in obtaining a smooth line in the keystone area and requires more graft on the nasion. Multiple sutures are needed between the anterior margin of the existing septum and posterior margin of the inserted extended spreader graft (Fig. 11.5).

Case Study
A 37-year-old female patient has a history of removing late-onset inflammation after rhinoplasty using Medpor and silicone implants. She underwent septal reconstruction using sixth ribs.

Three months after the operation, discharge came out from the columella. After administering empirical antibiotics, the discharge stopped, but the volume of the tip lobule was lost.

The septal collapse caused by septal SSI causes irreversible contracture of septal mucosa. It is recommended to correct the mucosal defect first, then do the framework operation in the second stage. Cartilage exposure due to mucosal defects after framework operation using costal cartilage causes gradual resorption or acute SSI. The septal mucosal defects can be repaired, such as an inferior turbinate rotation flap, but this technique has produced uncertain results in the author's cases. The asymmetric cephalic relaxing incision can be used to repair the defect. As the septal reconstruction may not be possible, depending on the size of septal perforation, it should be noted that surgery may be impossible or incomplete septal lengthening may occur depending on the degree of septal mucosal contracture (Figs. 11.6 and 11.7).

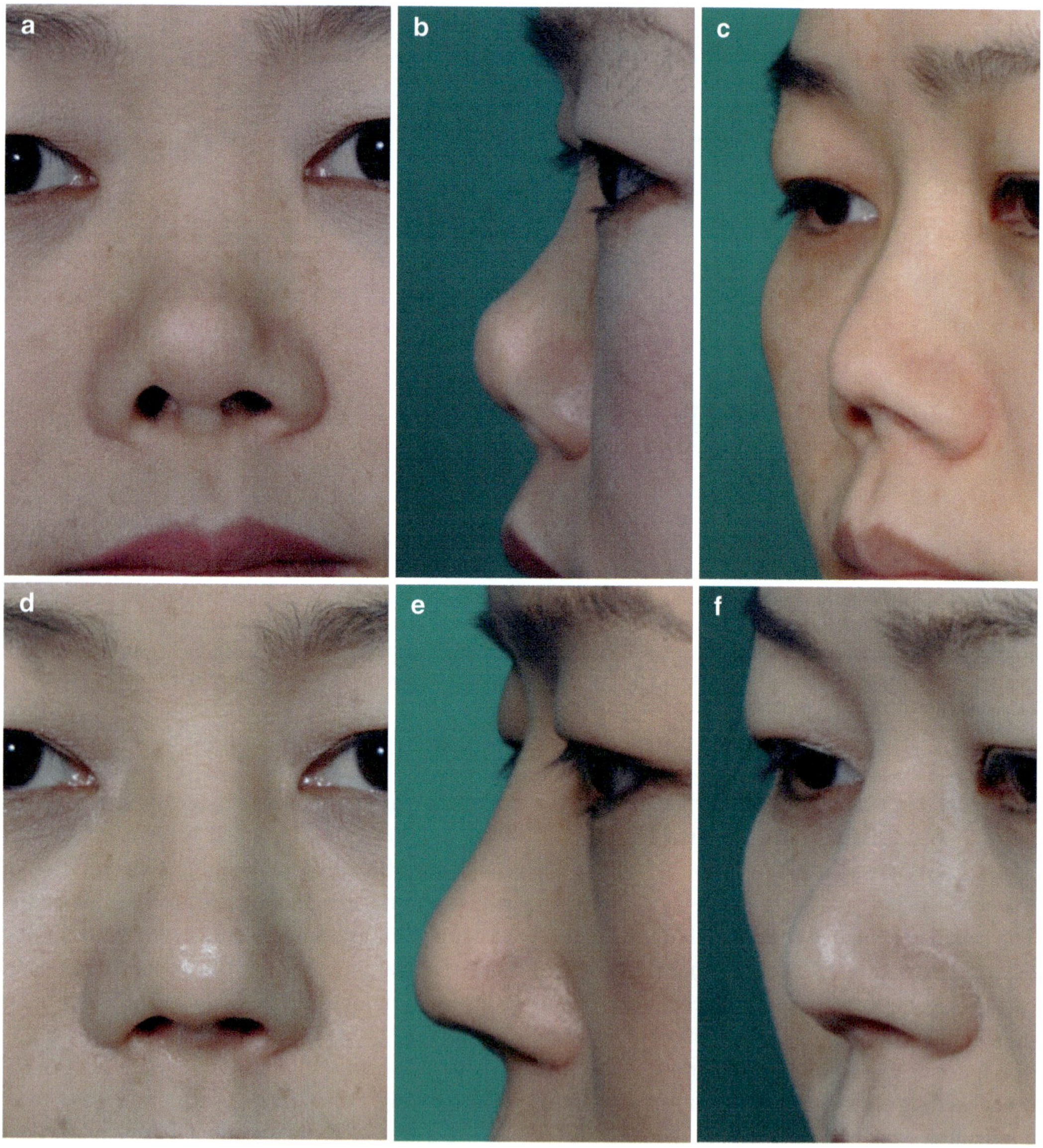

Fig. 11.6 The septal collapse caused by septal SSI causes severe contracture of septal mucosa. (**a**–**c**) Preoperative views. (**d**–**f**) Postoperative views after L-strut reconstruction

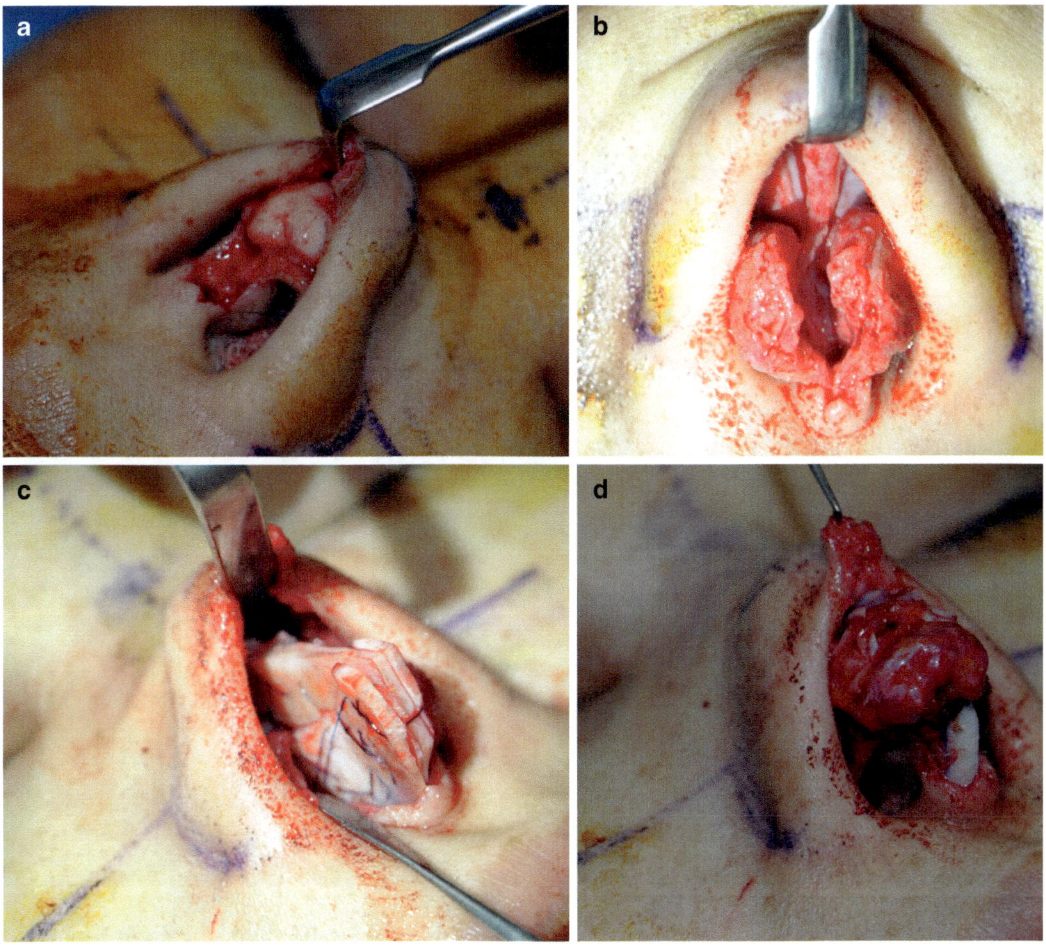

Fig. 11.7 Septal L-strut extension graft. (**a**) Intraoperative view. The vast cartilage destruction was identified under the tip allograft. (**b**) After resection of scar tissue, the nasal framework is almost lost. (**c**) Septal L-strut was reconstructed using costal cartilage. (**d**) Soft tissue was grafted on the tip

Cantilever Graft

Since long ago, rhinoplasty using rib cartilage has been performed. The cantilever graft consisting of dorsal onlay graft and columella segment was introduced 50 years ago to correct cleft lip and nose deformity in the Western operation. Surgery in a traditional cantilever graft that sustains the underlying tension, calvarial bone was introduced by nasal root integration. There are numerous reports on different techniques.

The author has also experienced secondary rhinoplasty forcibly stretching with the L framework made in this way, and it remains mostly a bad memory.

Case Study

A 22-year-old male patient visited the author to correct cleft lip and nose deformity after several previous surgeries. This patient was corrected by making an L-shaped cantilever graft using the sixth rib. The costal cartilage was carved by balanced cutting to prevent warping and waited for more than 1 hour in the saline at the time of surgery. A single K-wire was fixed on the nasal root for 7 days. After 4 months, a mild hump and a deformity of the s-shaped dorsal graft was found at the visit. After waiting for another 2 months, revision rhinoplasty underwent. The fixed L-graft was removed, and the healthy part was sliced into a small piece, and cymba concha was harvested

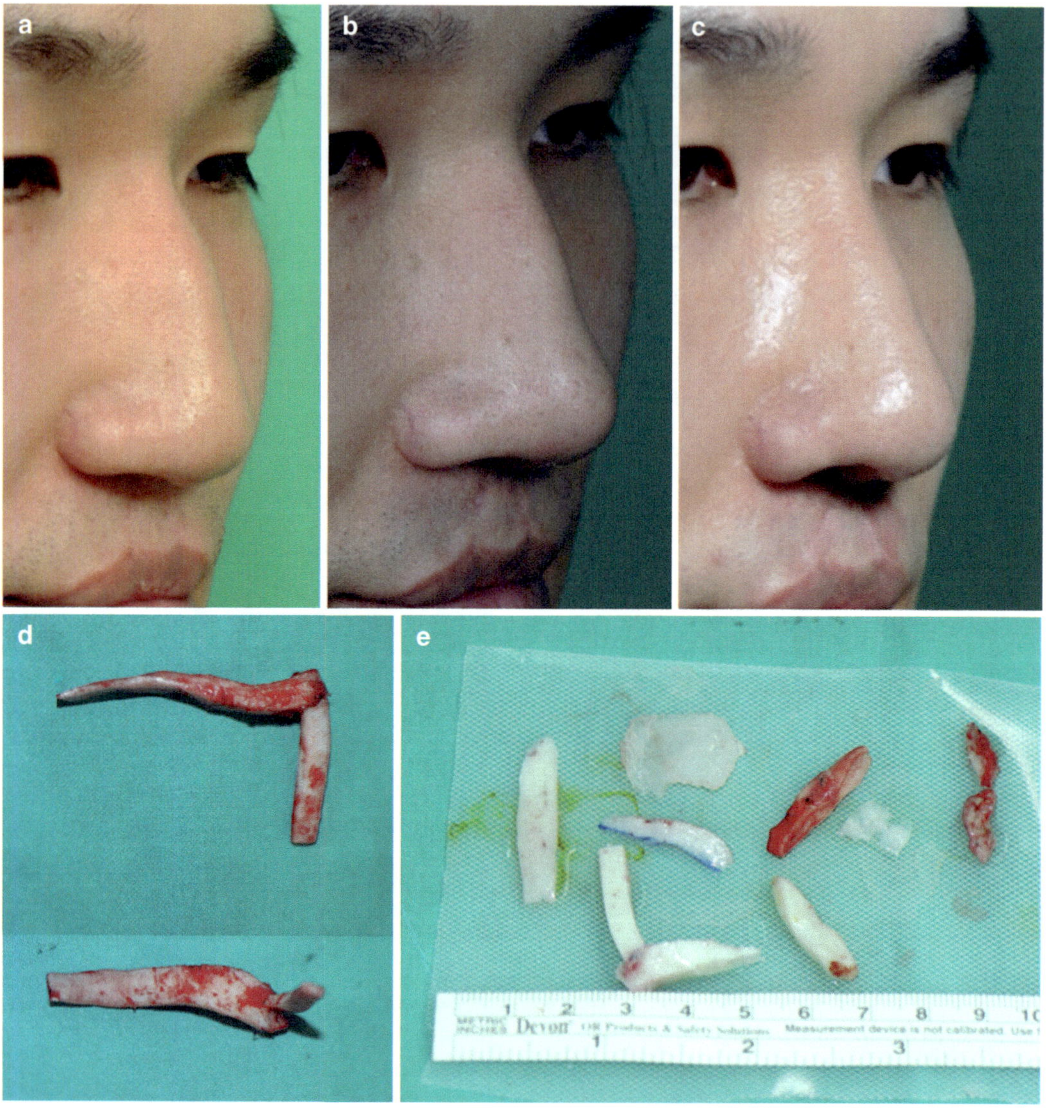

Fig. 11.8 Cantilever graft was removed because of the warping, then it was substituted by SLEG combining septal cartilage, cymba concha, and reused sliced costal cartilage. (**a**) Before the cantilever graft. (**b**) After the warping of the cantilever graft. (**c**) After the SLEG. (**d**) The warping of the costal cartilage. (**e**) Septal cartilage, cymba concha, and sliced costal cartilage

for caudal septal extension graft (CSEG). The septal surgery was performed to widen the right nasal cavity, and the posterior quadrangular cartilage dislocated to the right side was removed (Fig. 11.8 and Video 11.4).

The biggest problem with the cantilever graft is warping of the costal cartilage. In the surgery of secondary cleft lip and nose deformity, the cantilever graft can be considered first because many patients have a severe deviation of septum and vomer junction. However, the author prefers to make septum-dependent dorsum and tip with SLEG mentioned above, rather than the cantilever graft. For solid dorsal graft using rib cartilage, the author believes that Dr. Toriumi's method has the most scientific evidence. Although we have a different perspective on adipose-derived stromal cells, the author thinks the use of fatty tissue is an excellent method. This will be discussed in Chap. 13 [10].

References

1. Kim YK, Shin S, Kang NH, Kim JH. Contracted nose after silicone implantation: a new classification system and treatment algorithm. Arch Plast Surg. 2017;44(1):59–64.
2. Cottle MH, Weiss JA, Pottorff E, Herzon E. Hyaluronidase in rhinoplasty. Arch Otolaryngol. 1950;52(3):369–72.
3. Hwang SM, Lim O, Hwang MK, Kim MW, Lee JS. The clinical analysis of the nasal septal cartilage by measurement using computed tomography. Arch Craniofac Surg. 2016;17(3):140–5.
4. Kim J-S, Khan NA, Song HM, Jang YJ. Intraoperative measurements of harvestable septal cartilage in rhinoplasty. Ann Plast Surg. 2010;65(6):519–23.
5. Zelken J, Chang C-S, Chuang S-S, Yang J-Y, Hsiao Y-C. An economical approach to ethnic Asian rhinoplasty. Facial Plast Surg. 2016;32(1):95–104.
6. Dhong E-S, Kim Y-J, Suh MK. L-shaped columellar strut in East Asian nasal tip plasty. Arch Plast Surg. 2013;40(5):616–20.
7. Hwang N-H, Dhong E-S. Septal extension graft in Asian rhinoplasty. Facial Plast Surg Clin North Am. 2018;26(3):331–41.
8. Toriumi DM, Pero CD. Asian rhinoplasty. Clin Plast Surg. 2010;37(2):335–52.
9. Guyuron B, Varghai A. Lengthening the nose with a tongue-and-groove technique. Plast Reconstr Surg. 2003;111(4):1533–9; discussion 1540–1.
10. Toriumi DM. Dorsal augmentation using autologous costal cartilage or microfat-infused soft tissue augmentation. Facial Plast Surg. 2017;33(2):162–78.

12 Secondary Septal Surgery

Pearls

- Testing the hydrodissection while injecting local anesthetics into the septum is a definite method for identifying the dissectability. In case of easy infiltration, the mucoperichondrium remains, making the secondary septal dissection possible.
- If no dissection is possible, the area should be excluded from the scope of surgery. Unlike other areas, you can find a thin "no man's area."
- When the posterior septum is healthy and the deviation of the anterior septum is severe, the reverse swing door method can be applied for improving nasal function.
- Transverse K-wire fixation is helpful for the stability of the unsupported keystone area.
- Nasal bone after severe NEO fx, the decrease in intranasal cavity volume after septal collapse is expected.
- Septal collapse due to SSI in the septum after septorhinoplasty causes septal mucosal contracture. This short nose deformity is the most difficult to reconstruct.

Supplementary Information The online version of this chapter (https://doi.org/10.1007/978-981-16-0542-0_12) contains supplementary material, which is available to authorized users.

12.1 The Previous SMR State: "No Man's Land"

From the author's current perspective, the first interview with the patient at an outpatient clinic starts with whether the patient has had a history of SMR or not. Nowadays, most reoperation patients are in a post-SMR state, septal status is the most critical factor in planning the central component's strategies [1]. If patients complain about the obstructive nose, the surgeon should consider reoperation, and the revisional septoplasties revealed promising results [2, 3].

The lumination of the endoscope and gentle press by a cotton tip can be used to check the thin mucosa or measure the amount of quadrangular cartilage harvested (Video 12.1).

- A definite method for identifying the dissectability is testing the hydrodissection, which can be observed while injecting the local anesthetics. In case of easy infiltration, cartilage remains, or the mucoperichondrium remains, making it easy for the hydrodissection.
- If the mucoperichondrium is lost, the septum will not be dissected easily (Video 12.2).
- If no dissection is possible, the area should be excluded from the scope of surgery. Unlike other areas, you can find a thin "no man's land" (Fig. 12.1).

E.-S. Dhong, M.-W. Na, *Asian Septorhinoplasty*, https://doi.org/10.1007/978-981-16-0542-0_12

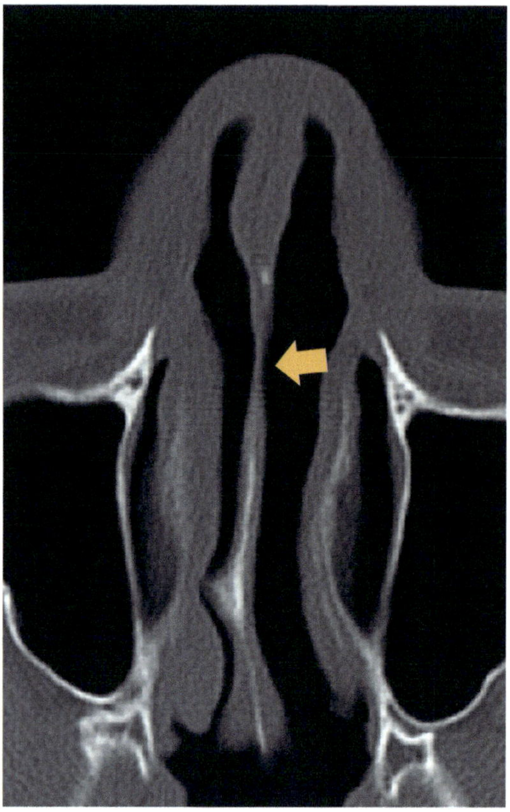

Fig. 12.1 No man's land; if the hydrodissection is not possible, do not dissect that area

12.2 The Revisional Septoplasty

Cause

The septal cartilage will grow again if mucoperichondrium is well preserved during harvesting. Adolescents with serious nasal malformation, including huge hump, have emotional problems. It is the reason for performing definitive rhinoplasty at that age. In patients who have not passed their growth period, the septal cartilage will grow again after primary septoplasty.

Anatomic Considerations

The cartilage of the previous SMR site can be harvested again. If the cartilage is regenerated, the dissection is possible. EPP can be harvested and used as a material by connecting the remaining quadrangular cartilage. Since reharvesting is insufficient, even a small piece of EPP can be useful in making the septum straight again. For the harvest of EPP, the author uses an oscillating saw and a small reciprocating saw.

Case Study

A 16-year-old male visited the author with hump nose deformity. The author persuaded the patient to delay the operation 2–3 years later, but the parents complained of a callus on his nose by self-compression due to stress and learning disabilities. Septorhinoplasty with humpectomy, medial, and lateral osteotomy was performed. Four years later, he revisited the author with septal deviation with reverse -c shape deformity. On inspection, convexity on the left side of the septum was found. The revision septoplasty was performed. After reharvesting of the septum, the spreader graft and rafter batten graft on the right side was reinforced to straighten it (Figs. 12.2 and 12.3).

12.3 Saddle Nose Deformity

Cause

- When an excessive amount of quadrangular cartilage is harvested, and the septal L-support is weak.
- When the support of the keystone area is weak.
- After the septal infection with the central contracture.
- After over-resection of the dorsal component.

Treatment

The method of camouflage with a cantilever graft is not a physiologic method. The author prefers septal reconstruction because there is an improvement in nasal physiology after surgery. Several methods of septal reconstruction according to the classification of the saddle nose have been introduced [4–6].

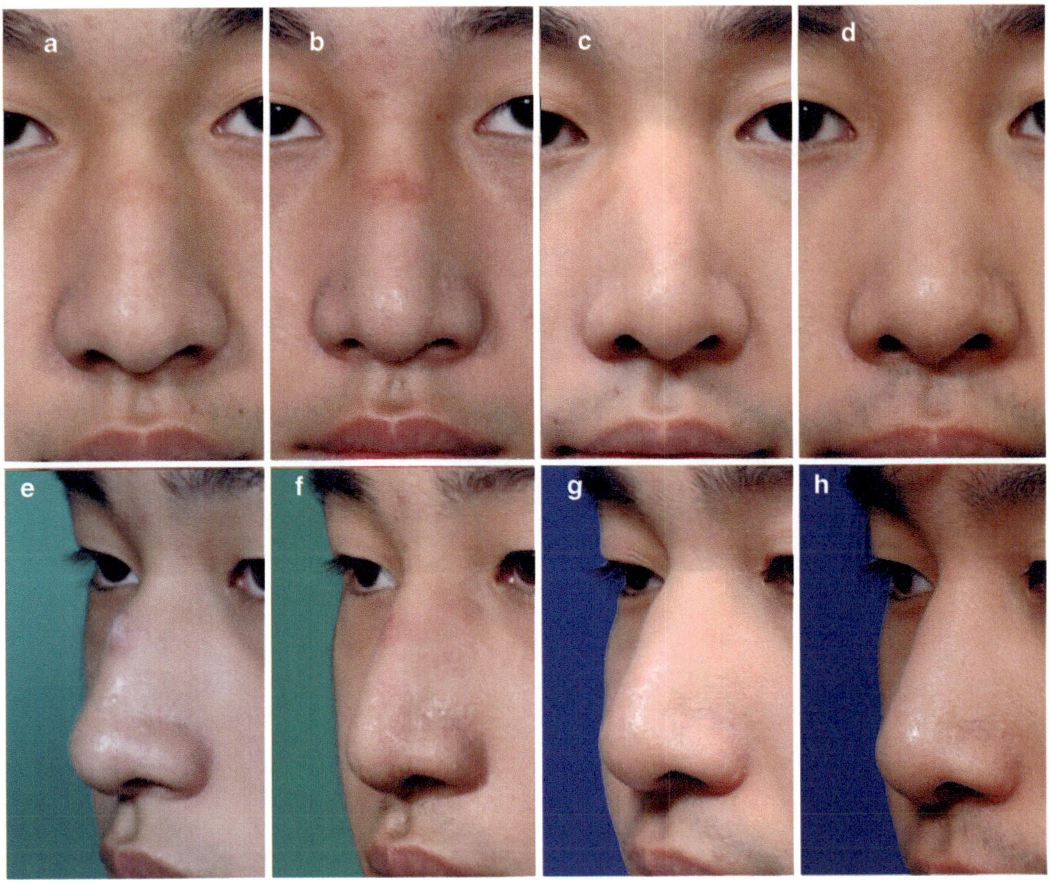

Fig. 12.2 Revisional septorhinoplasty due to the regrowth of the septal cartilage. (**a**, **e**) Preoperative view at age 16. (**b**, **f**) Postoperative view: hump reduction and septorhinoplasty. (**c**, **g**) Recurred hump and deviation at age 20. (**d**, **h**) Post-revisional septorhinoplasty

The reconstruction of the anterior septum is essential. There are only two types of donor cartilage, the costal cartilage, and the conchal cartilage. The presence of the remaining septum decides how high the extended spreader graft is to be performed anteriorly to correct the saddling. The spreader graft opens the internal valve and is an excellent way to correct the deviation of the lower two-third of the nose. It may be solved by performing a double or triple spreader graft on one side rather than a bilateral spreader graft in case of severe deviation. Of course, inferior turbinoplasty should be done considering the MCA of the internal valve on the other side. However, what is needed here is not the conventional spreader graft or the extended spreader graft for length extension, but the anteriorly extended spreader graft.

The Dorsal Margin of Anterior Extended Spreader Graft (AESG)

Should the ULC be lifted and sutured with AESG like the cartilaginous dorsum? Should the two anterior margins of the AESG directly form a cartilaginous dorsum? It is possible. Even after two margins pop out and ULC cannot catch them up, the skin is not demarcated with two lines after redraping in most Asians. However, in a female patient with a thin skin in Asians, to prevent a sharp dorsal demarcation, a layer of SMF can be

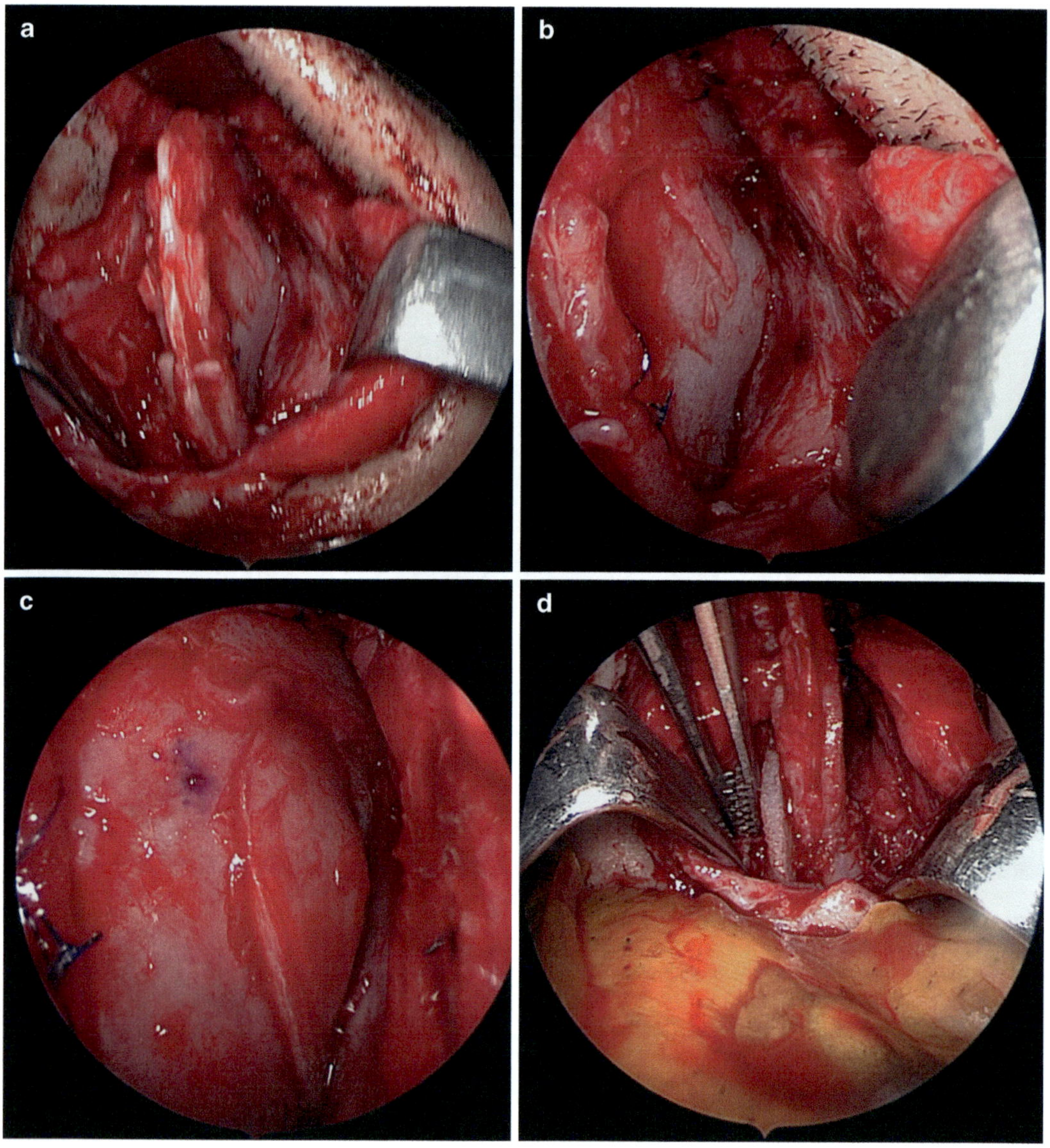

Fig. 12.3 Endoscopic views. (**a**) A previous caudal septal batten graft was found. (**b**) Left side convexity was found at the previous SMR site. (**c**) SMR has performed again. (**d**) A small piece of batten graft was applied to both sides of the caudal septum at ANS

applied to the dorsum for the smoothing of the dorsal line. If ULC does not follow, adding lateral dissection can recruit an extra length of ULC. The catch-up repair can be possible. There are obvious advantages and disadvantages to whether the donor cartilage is the concha or the costal cartilage.

Case Study 1: AESG by Conchal Cartilage
A 23-year-old male patient underwent septoplasty by an ENT doctor with a nasal septal deviation 4 years before the visit. The anterior margin and the caudal margin were found 8 mm in the surgical field. The cymba concha was used as a caudal septal extension graft, the cavum concha

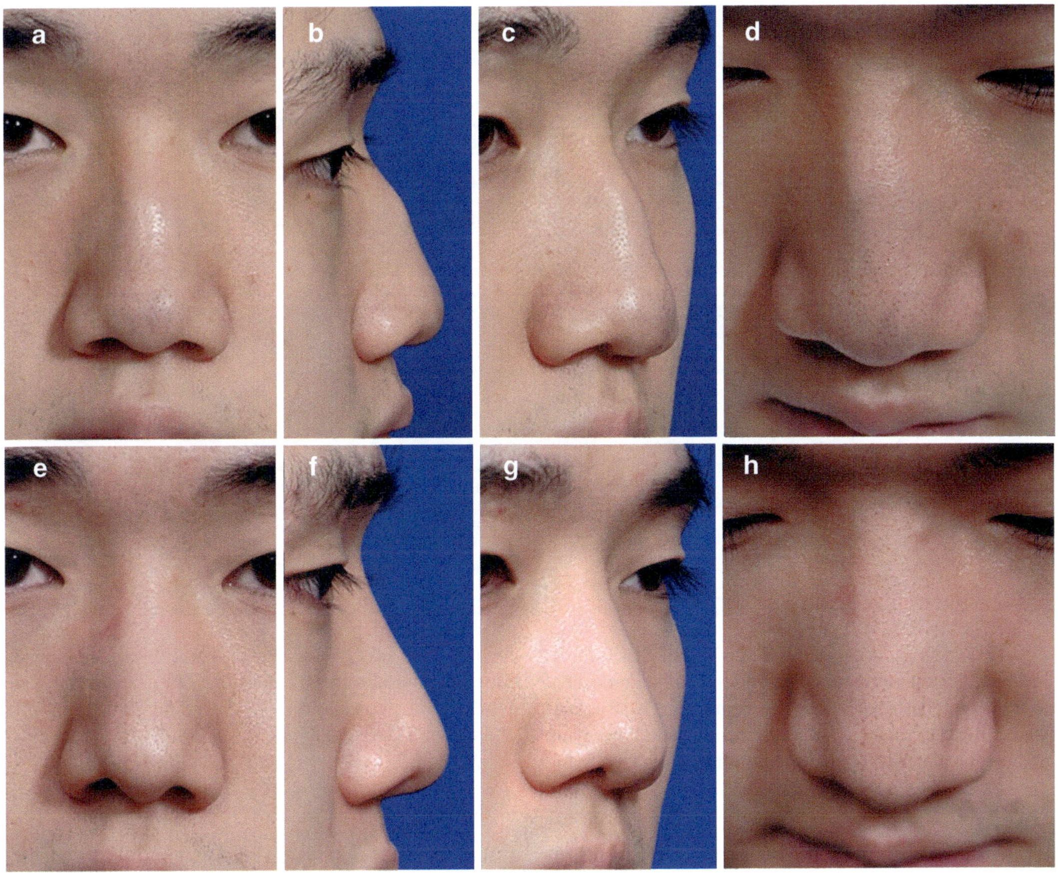

Fig. 12.4 Saddle nose was corrected by AESG using folded cavum concha. (**a**–**d**) Preoperative views. (**e**–**h**) Long-term postoperative views

was used as an anterior extended spreader graft, and a single layer of SMF was applied on the dorsum (Figs. 12.4 and 12.5).

Case Study 2: AESG by Conchal Cartilage
A 55-year-old man had a history of nasal bone fracture 20 years ago. He had been diagnosed with septal abscess 4 years ago, and I&D was done at an ENT clinic. The ear cartilages were used because he disagreed with postoperative tip hardness. One layer of SMF was implanted in the dorsum (Figs. 12.6 and 12.7, Videos 12.3 and 12.4).

12.4 Implant-Related Problems

The characteristic of Medpor and others is to destroy the septum. After removal, most of the contact site is found to be destroyed. Since the septal dissection must be performed, reconstruction after removal equals secondary septoplasty and please refer to Chap. 4 for details.

12.5 Collapsed Septum

It mainly causes the depression of the septum after trauma, such as Lefort fracture and nasoethmoid orbital fracture (NEO fracture), and the collapse of EPP and nasal bone. Also, cartilaginous collapse occurs even when the entire septal support is lost due to SSI after septorhinoplasty.

Clinical Features

In the collapsed septum, the nasal cavity is narrowed. In most patients, if the narrowed cavity is

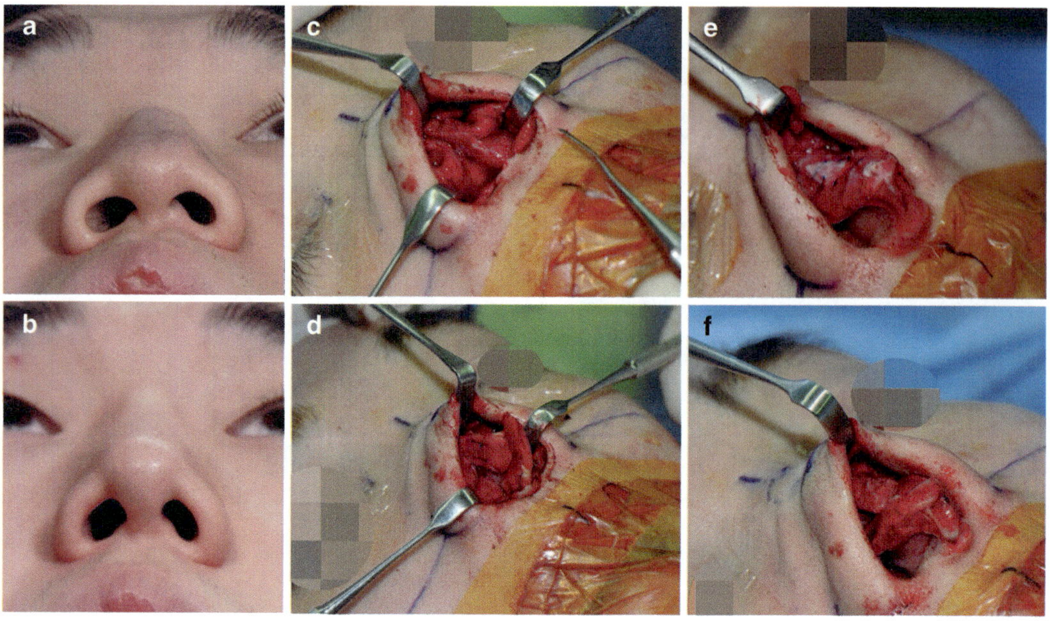

Fig. 12.5 The saddle nose with hump after SMR. (**a**, **b**) Pre- and postoperative basal views. (**c**) The anterocaudal septum was destroyed, and the remaining L-strut was weak. (**d**) After septal L-strut was reconstructed by cavum and cymba conchas. (**e**) Lateral crural spanning graft and for the long axis of the lateral crural divergence angle. Moreover, middle crural extension graft using the applied folded cymba conchal tip. (**f**) The shield graft, cap graft, and dorsal SMF were applied

not widened, there is no improvement in symptoms. In addition to doing a dorsal graft to improve the shape, it is necessary to return the depressed nasal bone to its original position to improve function. An effort may be required to return the damaged nasal bone to its original position. In severe depression of NEO fracture, reducing the nasal bone may not be possible if the bone fragment is too small or the fracture is complex. When the septum collapses, the nose's length is shortened, and the shortened soft tissue causes contracture.

Strategy

The "Key Factor": The Keystone Area

The critical role is in the keystone area. It is no exaggeration to say that the success or failure to reconstruct a collapsed septum depends on how strong a keystone area is reconstructed. In the absence of stability of the left and right nasal bones, the stability can be maintained with the transverse nasal k-wire [7]. At this time, the nasal bone's posterior sinking does not occur if the left and right sides have stability connected to the maxilla. Recently, TCC suture, which is useful for fixing the extended spreader graft near the keystone, is also useful [8]. However, the stability of the nasal bone must be premised. If this fixation becomes impossible, it is sometimes better to reshape the malunion bone by rasping and leave it in place for stability. The K-wires are retained for more extended periods, helping bone union more, but they are usually removed when skin lesions develop. If there is no stability in bilateral keystone areas, a longer spreader graft should be used. If this is not possible, cantilever graft is the answer.

The Reverse Swing Door Concept

If the collapse of the nasal pyramid is due to the impact from the front, the forceful tension of the quadrangular cartilage is applied anterior to posteriorly. The physical energy dispersed by microfracture or dislocation of the posterior

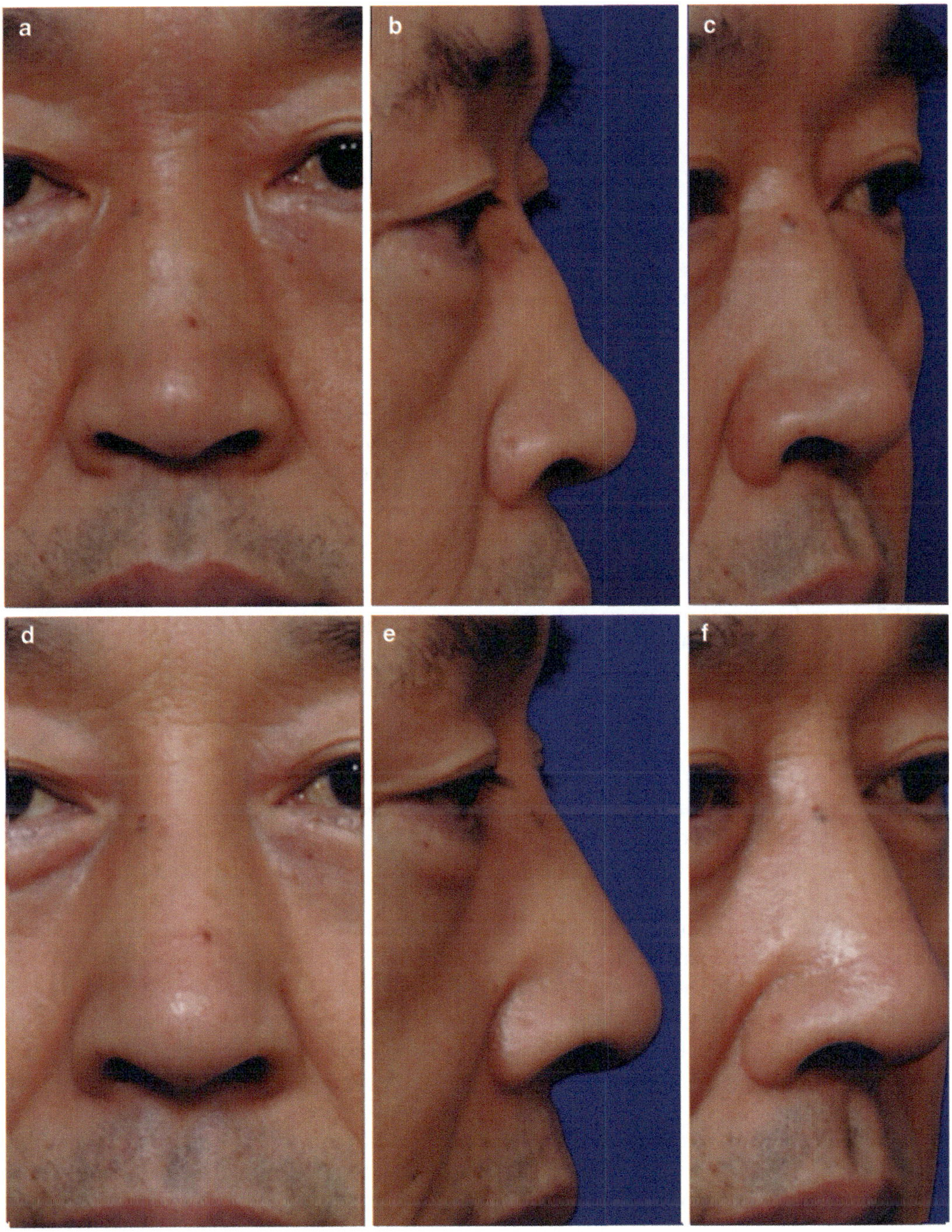

Fig. 12.6 The saddle nose after septal infection. (**a–c**) Preoperative views. (**d–f**) Postoperative views

quadrangular cartilage. As a result, septal deviation proceeds by the overgrowth of microfractures quadrangular cartilage. Most deviation corrections are performed toward preserving or straightening the anterior portion of the septum. The concept of a "swing door" procedure that releases the posterior septum tension while preserving the entire septum requires a solid premise of a keystone area's stability. In other words, all these swing door procedures are possible

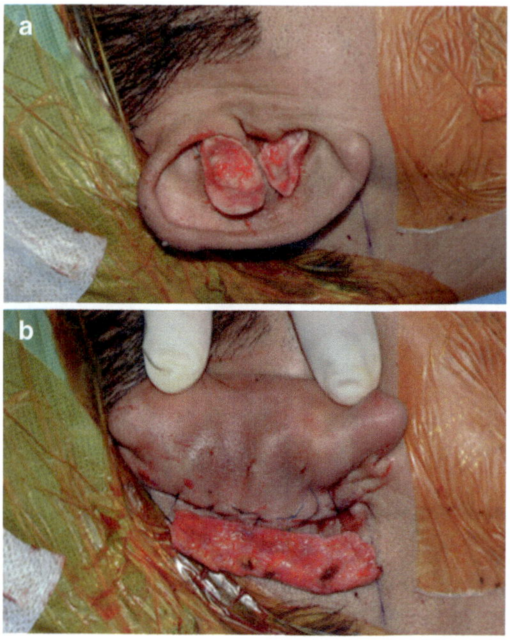

Fig. 12.7 The graft materials: Two conchas and superficial mastoid fascia. (**a**) Cymba and cavum conchas. (**b**) SMF

only when the keystone area is in good condition. Conversely, if there is no deviation of the posterior septum or if the posterior septum is sound, but the keystone area is collapsed, of course, this is very rare. The high septal deviation can be corrected by the "reverse swing door" procedure [9]. The author does not use this method for routine septal deviation correction. However, if the EPP and the septum-vomer junction are well preserved, the opposite tension release is possible using the "reverse swing door" concept [10].

Case Study 1: Old Nasal Bone Fracture
A 44-year-old man visited with an old nasal bone fracture and a nasal obstruction on the right. The camouflage method was explained, but the primary purpose was to resolve the nasal obstruction, so an operation was planned to return the nasal framework to its original shape. Relifting the depressed nasal bone was planned with the reverse swing door method of the collapsed septum. The stability of the keystone was maintained with a K-wire fixation to the right-side nasal bone, which was stable. The nasal function recovered (Figs. 12.8 and 12.9, Video 12.5).

Case Study 2: NEO Fracture
A 25-year-old woman showed septal collapse after reduction as a NEO fracture that occurred with severe laceration by in-car traffic accident. The nasal cavity was narrowed due to severe shrinkage, but the lowered nasal bone could not be advanced anteriorly. If the bony malunion was returned to its original position, too many bone defects occurred, so only the anterocaudal extension of the septum was focused after the partial reverse swing door procedure, and the rectus fascia onlay graft camouflaged the very low bony dorsum from the nasion (Figs. 12.10, 12.11, and 12.12, Video 12.6).

12.6 The Infected Nose

Unlike trauma, the collapse by infection is more complicated. The septum is sometimes preserved in the contracted nose. However, the septum is collapsed when SSI is accompanied by septal infection after SRP. The lengthening can be performed with 2–3 reoperations, but the amount is limited. The most challenging part in short nose correction is septal mucosa contracture, and in some patients, it is not possible to extend the length of the desired length. Even if the external L-framework is operated in the cantilever method, an extra composite graft may be required to correct the retracted nostril and columella. Transposition flaps from the inferior turbinate or nasolabial fold can cover the mucosal defects; however, the author does not recommend this method to young doctors who are starting their practices. The first choice should be a composite graft.

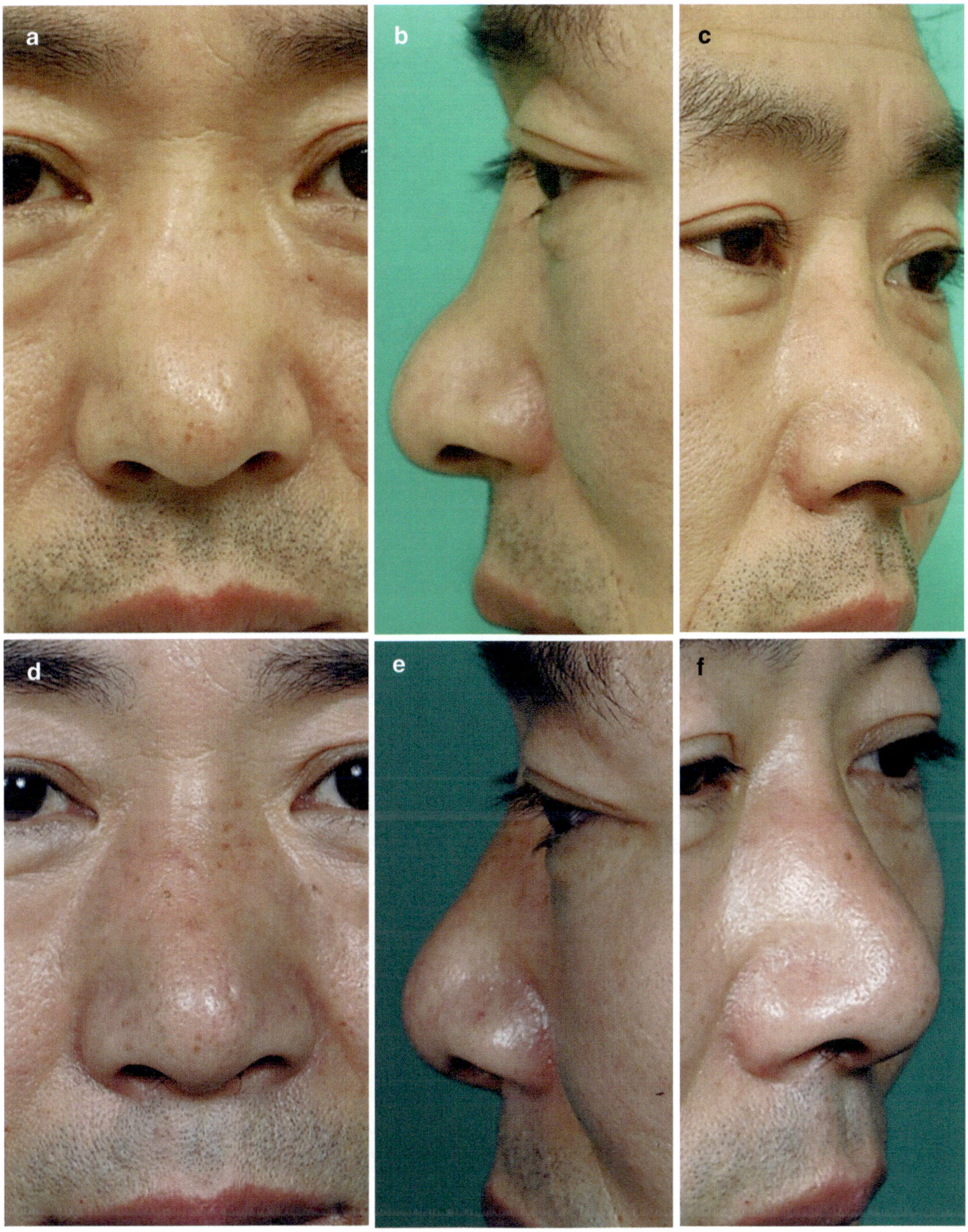

Fig. 12.8 Old nasal bone fracture was corrected by bone repositioning with the reverse swing door procedure. (**a**–**c**) Preoperative views. (**d**–**f**) Postoperative view

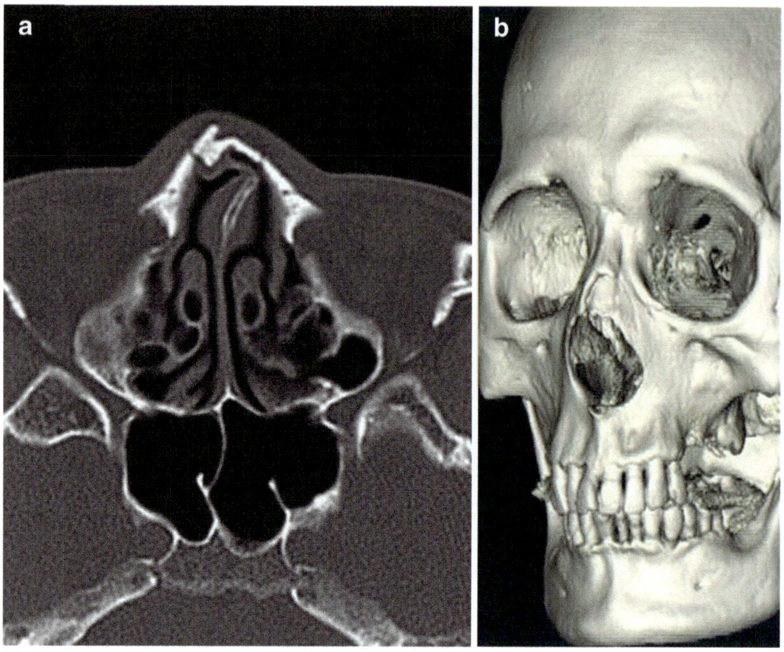

Fig. 12.9 Preoperative CT scan. (**a**, **b**) Lt. nasal bone was depressed with severe deformity at the high septum. However, the posterior septum was relatively sound

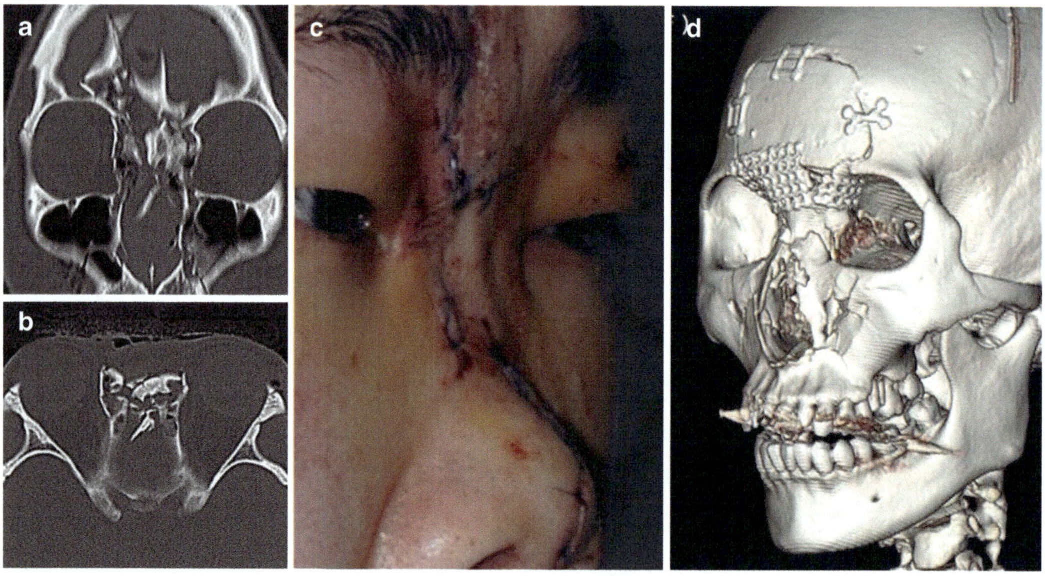

Fig. 12.10 Severe NOE fracture (**a**, **b**) Preoperative coronal and axial views. (**c**) After the key suture was done, the bony dorsum was found collapsed. (**d**) After reduction with cranialization of the frontal sinus

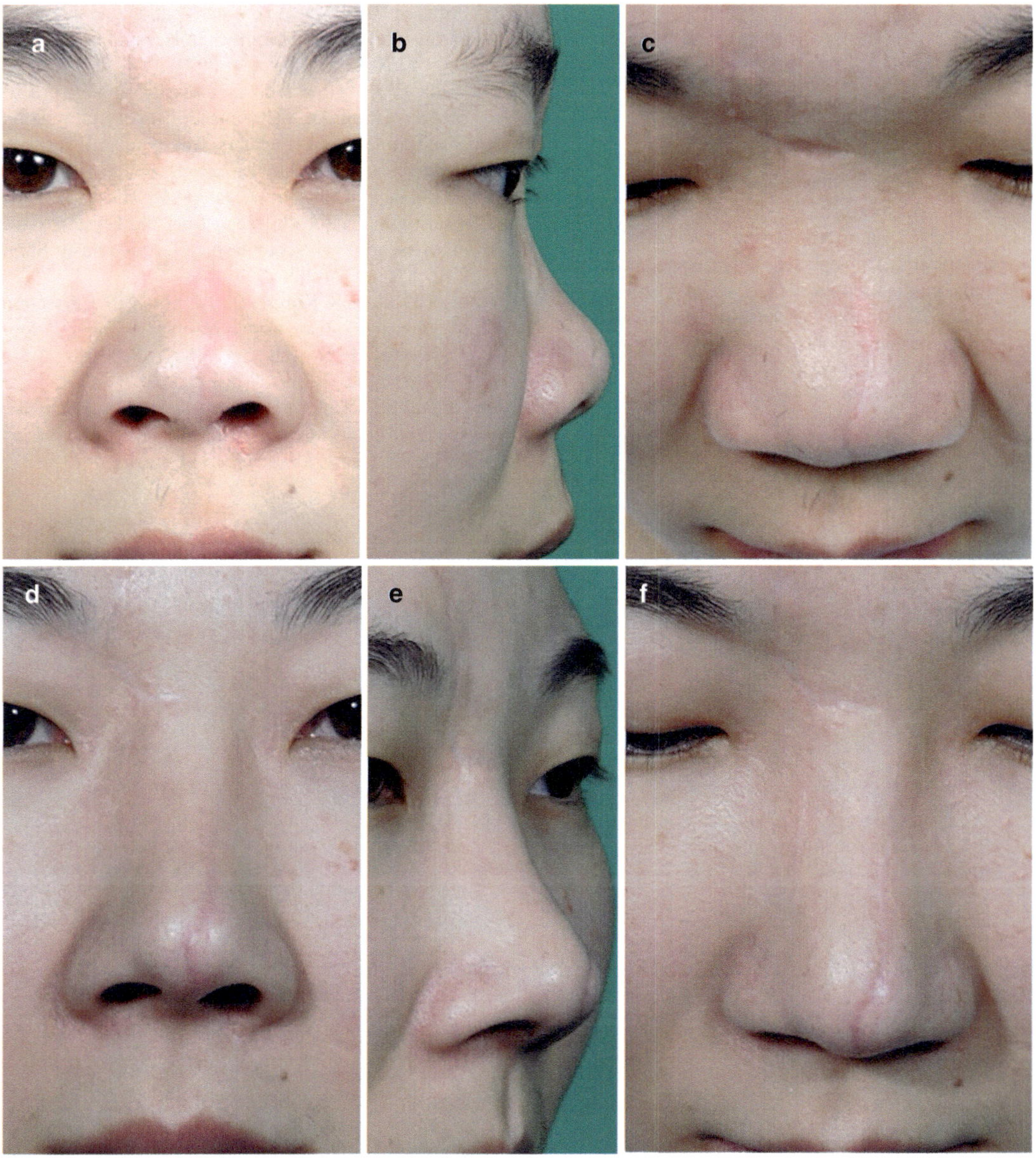

Fig. 12.11 Septal L-strut reconstruction using costal cartilage after the partial reverse swing door procedure. (**a**–**c**) Preoperative views. (**d**–**f**) Long-term postoperative views

Fig. 12.12 Intraoperative view before closure: shield graft, lobule graft using morselized costal cartilage

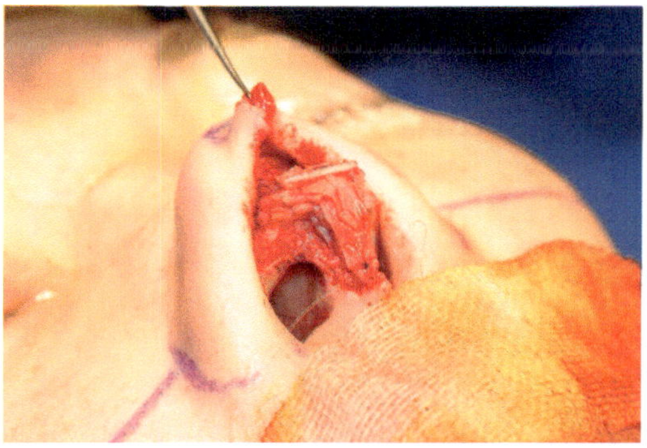

References

1. Sillers MJ, Cox AJ 3rd, Kulbersh B. Revision septoplasty. Otolaryngol Clin N Am. 2009;42(2):261–78, viii
2. Becker SS, Dobratz EJ, Stowell N, Barker D, Park SS. Revision septoplasty: review of sources of persistent nasal obstruction. Am J Rhinol. 2008;22(4):440–4.
3. Gillman GS, Egloff AM, Rivera-Serrano CM. Revision septoplasty: a prospective disease-specific outcome study. Laryngoscope. 2014;124(6):1290–5.
4. Daniel RK. Rhinoplasty: septal saddle nose deformity and composite reconstruction. Plast Reconstr Surg. 2007;119(3):1029–43.
5. Cakmak O, Emre IE, Ozkurt FE. Identifying septal support reconstructions for saddle nose deformity: the Cakmak algorithm. JAMA Facial Plast Surg. 2015;17(6):433–9.
6. Pribitkin EA, Ezzat WH. Classification and treatment of the saddle nose deformity. Otolaryngol Clin N Am. 2009;42(3):437–61.
7. Wadley JK. "How I do it"—plastic surgery practical suggestions on facial plastic surgery: correction of unstable nasal fractures by intranasal support. Laryngoscope. 1979;89(2):327–31.
8. Rezaeian F, Gubisch W, Janku D, Haack S. New suturing techniques to reconstruct the keystone area in extracorporeal septoplasty. Plast Reconstr Surg. 2016;138(2):374–82.
9. Choi JY, Lee JS, Kim JJ, Ha BJ, Shin MS. Correction of deviated nose using reverse swinging door procedure. J Korean Soc Plast Reconstr Surg. 1999;26(6):1107–11.
10. Dhong ES. Septorhinoplasty: endoscopic approach and reinforcement of nasal support line. J Korean Soc Aesth Plast Surg. 2010;16(3):111–6.

13 Think Inside the Box: Absorbable Plate, IHCC, and the Stem Cells

Pearls

- When making a framework with absorbable mesh alone, there is insufficient evidence that it can function as a long-term nasal framework only with fibrous tissue generated in the pores present therein.
- The larger or thicker the absorbable material is, the longer it takes for absorption. Therefore, there are also many tissue reactions.
- Any absorbable material is not free from infection or immune reaction.
- The adoption of PDS foil and PDS plate is relatively beneficial with the evidence and results from many rhinoplasty surgeons.
- IHCC is a nonviable biological material.
- IHCC use is not recommended as a tension-bearing frame.
- In IHCC, resorption can occur in the form of fracture, so it cannot be asserted that there is no late-onset immune reaction at all.
- The efficacy of IHCC may vary from manufacturer to manufacturer.
- It is reasonable to view IHCC as a nonviable material, which has no tissue integrity.
- However, IHCC does not form a capsule due to its biological aspect.
- Since it is applied at the last stage of Asian rhinoplasty, complications take on a more complex aspect, requiring autologous costal cartilage.
- Free fatty tissue is beneficial for soft tissue enhancement in the secondary nose.
- Also, contained preadipocytes can induce recipient-dependent neo adipogenesis.
- However, there is little evidence that SVF contains cytokines that reduce soft tissue contracture in the contracted nose or soften the contracture.
- Do not get confused, administering SVF, and administering ASCs. ASCs are the passaged plated cells.
- ASCs can also be differentiated to myofibroblast, like HDF does, depending on the surrounding wound environment, and can be the source cells of contracture.
- There is no biological in vitro evidence that neither SVF nor hASCs can improve soft tissue contracture caused by inflammation.

13.1 Absorbable Materials

The Fate of Absorbable Plate

Among the commercially available absorbable materials, there are polyglycolic acid (PGA), polylactic acid (PLA), polydioxanone (PDO/PDS), polycaprolactone (PCL), or combinations of these materials. Currently, ready-made plates for rhinoplasty include PCL mesh (TnR mesh; T&R Biofab Co., Ltd., Siheung, Korea) and PDS plate (Ethicon Inc., Johnson & Johnson, Somerville, NJ). Polymers of PLA or PGA or polymers of poly-L-lactic acid (PLLA)/hydroxy-

E.-S. Dhong, M.-W. Na, *Asian Septorhinoplasty*, https://doi.org/10.1007/978-981-16-0542-0_13

apatite (HA) are widely used in craniomaxillofacial surgery. According to the manufacturer's information, the PDS plate resorbs within 25 weeks, and its stability is maintained for 10 weeks. The biodegradation process depends on contact with body fluids, temperature, motion, molecular weight, the crystalline form and geometry of the material, and the implanted tissue [1, 2]. The absorption of PLA/PGA products is eliminated by hydrolysis and metabolism, and macrophages and giant cells absorb particles that cannot be hydrolyzed. PCL performs the same process and is decomposed into CO_2 and H_2O and absorbed. Usually, when hydrolysis occurs beyond the range of metabolism, it is said that the inflammatory reaction becomes more active [3]. The author believes that the degree of absorption varies depending on the recipient, the plate was found as particles even after 2 years postoperatively. About the complication, immune reactions have been reported, and low-grade inflammation occurred even within a few months of application. Prolonged swelling resulted in nasal obstruction, especially when applied to the septum. However, absorbable plates have been used in craniofacial surgery, and there is no lack of evidence for absorption. The belief that absorbable plates can be used for rhinoplasty is that if alloplastic materials are absorbed and disappeared eventually, there will be no problems in the long term. However, a greater belief is that the scaffold disappears, and cartilage or fibrous tissue grows into the pores, filling the pores and eventually being substituted for autologous tissue. Reports of inflammatory reactions lead to unwanted discharge, leading to an adverse immune reaction in the intraseptal or surgical pocket [4]. Also, the follow-up period was short, and there is insufficient evidence for reporting inflammatory reactions and comparative reports of infection rates [5].

All alloplastic materials have physical and chemical properties. In addition to the above-mentioned chemical properties, thick materials may cause tissue damage due to physical properties depending on the application site. There is already a lot of evidence of craniofacial surgery showing temporary compression of the bone surface (Fig. 13.1).

Two Different Concepts in Adopting Absorbable Plates

Temporary Support

PDS foil or PDS plate can be used as a cartilage stabilizer by molding fragmented cartilage on a flat plate. Many studies report that the PDS plate used with cartilage is advantageous in terms of material usage [6].

The author often uses it for flattening the tortuous ear cartilages. The author's method is to apply a chondrotomy to eliminate curvature

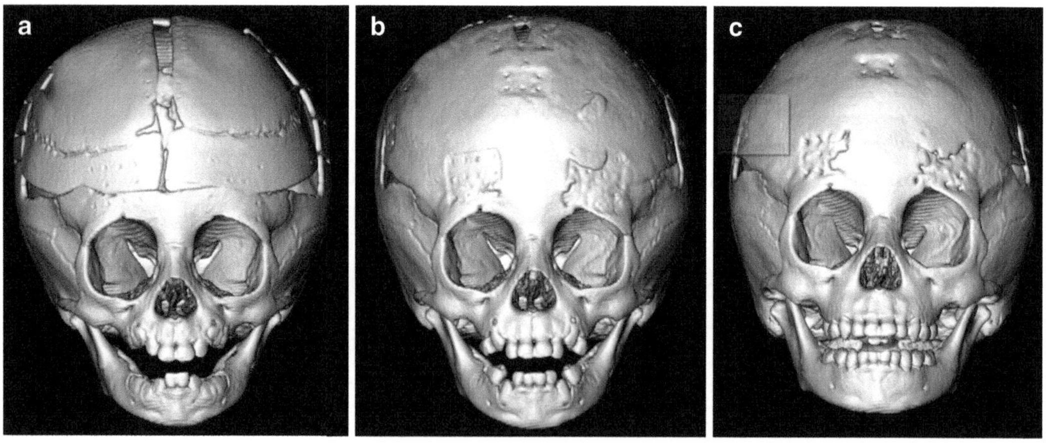

Fig. 13.1 Bone depression where the absorbable plate was applied. (**a**) Postoperative 6-month view. (**b**) Postoperative 12 months. (**c**) Even a postoperative 30-month's view shows bone depression where the absorbable plate was fixed

when folding conchal cartilage. As the number of chondrotomy increases, the cartilage's integrity decreases, and stability is lost, so it is used as the concept of the internal splint. If possible, the author tries to place the plate inside the cartilage and prohibit the PDS plate's direct exposure. The PDS plate is always used with cartilages.

Scaffold Recruiting Cartilage

The PCL mesh plate is introduced to be used for nose surgery independently. Pros explained that 50% of the absorbable mesh is made up of pores, so fibrous tissue or cartilage grows into the pores. The fibrous tissue is proliferated, and this tissue can constitute the framework. However, considering the physical properties, the evidence is needed to determine whether fibrous tissue can sustain the physical properties as a nasal framework. What is more problematic is the mechanical surface property of the plate itself. It can be predicted that multiple micropores eventually form a rough surface, and this surface can easily cause erosion to the fragile septal mucosa.

Two Different Techniques

Combining with Cartilage

Most thin PDS foils or PDS plates are introduced as a method of using cartilage, and a plate is used to mold the pieces into a big one. Eventually, cartilage fragments' survival is expected to play a supportive role by healing with neighboring cartilage fragments. If mucoperichondrium is preserved and cartilage is regenerated in the septal pocket, survival can be expected more.

Absorbable Materials Only

Below are several types of commercialized methods. The author has no experience with the three methods. The author is operating on patients with problems using the below methods.

SEG

A method for applying a PCL mesh instead of a cartilage framework for a septal extension by itself has recently emerged [5]. The plate is too thick to integrate the cartilage. Only the PCL mesh plate without attaching cartilage is used as the septal extension graft.

Tip Plasty: Soft Ball

For tip plasty, PCL in ball shape was introduced for onlaying at the tip.

Thread Tip Plasty

There are various thread names for counter-rotating the nasal tip or projecting the tip using a PDO thread cog so-called noninvasive rhinoplasty. This is a tip plasty using absorbable thread, which is the same concept as face-lift by a thread.

13.2 Pitfalls of the "Myth"

- There is a lack of evidence that the fibrous tissue generated in the pores in the absorbable mesh can function as a long-term nasal framework.
- The larger or thicker the absorbable material is, the longer it takes for absorption. Therefore, there are also many tissue reactions.
- There is no evidence that the use of absorbable materials that are not self-organized has a permanent effect. Any material is not free from infection or immune reaction.
- The adoption of PDS foil and PDS plate with evidence and results of many rhinoplasty surgeons is a relatively useful cartilage salvage method.

13.3 IHCC (Irradiated Homologous Costal Cartilage)

Is it a Viable Material?

There is only one reason to use IIHCC. Autologous material should be used, but there is a burden on the harvest.

- IHCC is considered a nonviable biologic material.

There are many reports on IHCC, and it is undeniably a convenient and useful material in that it is a material that can be useful in situations where secondary rhinoplasty or sudden cartilage is required. Compared with autologous costal cartilage, some studies show less warping and the same performance in all respects [7]. In a previous study, the author reported a resorption and fracture rate of approximately 2% in IHCC and reported a safe material. However, as experience increases, IHCC draws closer to the pessimistic conclusion that IHCC is a nonviable biological material, "a dead graft."

There is a limit to growing new cartilage, so IHCC cannot be regarded as a viable graft.

- It is not recommended to use for tension-bearing frames.
- The reason why resorption can occur in the form of fracture and viability declines over time is why it cannot be asserted that there is no immune reaction.
- The efficacy may vary from manufacturer to manufacturer.
- It is reasonable to view it as an alloplastic material that is nonviable and has no tissue integrity. However, it does not form a capsule due to its biological aspect.

Since it is often applied at the last stage of Asian rhinoplasty, complications take on a more complex aspect, which in turn requires autologous costal cartilage. When the remaining capsule from the previous silicone is not removed, the capsular contracture occurred in the later applied IHCC. Also, it is not completely free from late-onset inflammation. The reason is that it is not a viable graft. As the number of patients undergoing surgery increases, many causes are often combined. In other words, it is challenging to determine the cause of the contracture that occurred later in the case of applying IHCC as a septal extension graft.

Pitfalls of the "Myth"

- Surgery with IHCC forms no neocartilage in the long term, and tissue integration does not occur like autograft.
- IHCC is only a nonviable biologic graft and can be considered an alloplastic implant in some sense.

13.4 Human Adipose-Derived Stromal (Stem) Cells: hASCs

The author has been conducting basic research on human adipose stromal cells' biology for over 15 years and is still conducting basic research on ASCs and soft tissue contracture [8–14].

The author believes that fat graft is a useful ancillary procedure for rhinoplasty with the perspective of biological tissue recruitment. The fat graft literally injects fatty tissue directly into the tissue, so the author thinks it is a beneficial soft tissue management method. There are several reports on delivery modality, but the author thinks that direct injection or tissue-integrated graft are all excellent methods. What the author wants to discuss in this chapter is to report the harm of direct-to-consumer advertising of "the myth of stemness" [15].

- It is an act of harassing a complicated patient again. It is about stem cell treatment, which is conducted by directly charging the high cost of treatment but still lacks evidence.
- This chapter criticizes the early adoption of fatty tissue derivatives that do not benefit patients.

13.5 Direct-to-Consumer Portrayal of Stem Cell Medicine

A few decades ago, there have been pros and cons about the clinical application of new technologies. However, in-depth regulation is indeed necessary for the direct clinical application of stem cells. Although this may vary from country to country, the risk may be larger than the benefit relevantly in common [16].

Several studies have already given direct IV doses of adipose-derived stem cells [17] and even administering SVF directly as IV doses [18]. Although 10 years have passed, clinically significant effects have been reported, but no established treatment methods have appeared. There have already been reports of problems in the plastic surgery field regarding these problems [19]. A bigger problem is the reality that the high cost of treatment is charged along with this irrelevance and that this cost becomes a burden for previous surgeons. As a fellow plastic surgeon, the author feels exhausted from demanding evidence for an unscientific procedure. It is true that research reports are limited because it is illegal to inject cultured cells directly in some countries. There have been reports of sound effects by injecting stem cells into Asian contracted noses, but if you carefully read the description of stem cells, you can see that the scientific basis is insufficient [20].

The following summarizes the superficial contents of the current knowledge and the problems of early adoption of hASCs while the author has been conducting basic research on hASCs. Bench to bedside translational research requires a lot of persistence and precise in vitro data, and in vivo data must also be objective.

Counterpoints of Injecting "Adipose-Derived Stem Cells(?)" into the Contracted Nose

Contracture is one of the most severe complications after silicone-based rhinoplasty. It manifests as rigidity or hardening of the scar, deformity, asymmetry, displacement, and foreshortened nose. The causes of capsular contracture are still unclear because of the various factors contributing to it, such as hematomas, seroma, and infections. Myofibroblast displays one of the predominant cells in the capsule, and 25% of it originates from bone marrow during the inflammatory phase. Various inflammatory cytokines are responsible for the differentiation of myofibroblasts. Transforming growth factor-beta (TGF-β) plays a crucial role in differentiation, but this single factor cannot thoroughly explain differentiation. Recent studies show that interleukin-3 (IL-3) and granulocyte-macrophage colony-stimulating factor (GM-CSF) are inflammatory cytokines that contribute to the accumulation of myofibroblast-like cells, differentiation of stem cells, and stimulation of TGF-β expression. Both IL-3 and GM-CSF are produced in acute and chronic lesions within the wound and stimulate fibrosis and induce granulation tissue. Zafirlukast and montelukast are uniquely effective medicines based on clinical evidence for improving contracture, which are leukotriene receptor antagonists (LTRA) and interfere with eosinophil survival-enhancing activity (ESEA). Cysteinyl-leukotriene antagonists can inhibit dose-dependently the release of Th2 cytokines: IL-3, IL-4, and GM-CSF. In breast capsular contracture, implantation into the subglandular area, which contains a large amount of adipose tissue, often leads to a more severe degree of inflammation resulting in capsular contracture than insertion into the submuscular area, which possesses less adipose tissue. Recent studies show that human adipose-derived stem cells (hASCs) can differentiate into myofibroblasts. The hypothesis insisting that fibroblast, with hASCs, may play an essential role in capsular contracture has relevant proofs.

Human Adipose-Derived Stem (Stromal) Cells Differ from Stromal Vascular Fraction

The human adipose-derived stem (stromal) cells are different from the stromal vascular fraction. Why is it said to give stem cells while using SVF? The processed lipoaspirate (PLA) obtained by centrifuging lipoaspirate is dissolved in collagenase and then centrifuged again to obtain the stromal vascular fraction (SVF). Currently, many countries are clinically available in using SVF so far. The cells that grew by plating this SVF attached to the floor are called ASC. There is a predetermined promise for ASCs. Cells that are $CD73^+$, $CD90^+$, $CD105^+$, and simultaneously, $CD45^-$, $CD34^-$ should have been characterized [21]. If these CD markers are different, it should not be called ASC. The standard may change after the writing of this chapter, but the rules for cells' characteristics, especially the multipotent differentiation, should be kept. In the case of the sialomucin family, CD34, the representative ones that show positivity are BMSCs, hematopoietic stem cells, skeletal muscle satellite cells, keratinocyte stem cells, hair follicle stem cells, and adipogenic precursors. There was a theory that ASC was of $CD34^-$ pericyte origin [22], and there was a claim of $CD34^+$ pericyte after, but $CD34^-CD105+$ is the current consensus [23]. Later $CD106^-$, $CD36^+$ were added [24].

- A stromal cell is $CD34^+$, and a passaged ASC is $CD34^-$.
- The aqueous form of SVF is a combination of pericytes, preadipocytes, hematopoietic cells, endothelial progenitor cells, endothelial cells, and stromal cells, which are CD 34^+ $CD105^-$. Of course, SVF secretes VEGF, HGF, and bFGF, which play an essential role in wounds, and TGF-β, which will be critical in this chapter, and research on this is active.
- Many substances are involved in wound contracture in the cytokine contained in SVF.

13.6 Can ASCs Be Administered to Treat Contractures?

The causes of contracture are fibroblast and myofibroblast. In the cell's cytoplasmic skeleton, the level of expression of alpha SMA, SM 22α, or calponin can be indirectly determined. The most critical cytokine for contracture is activation of TGF. Of course, numerous cytokines are involved in contracture. Fibroblasts present in the wound are activated and transformed into myofibroblasts, as well as all types of cells (mesothelium, endothelium, epithelium) may occur metaplasia into myofibroblasts by surrounding inflammatory reactions. Related here is the inflammatory cytokine, the most important of which is TGFβ. The same mechanism works for ASCs. In other words, under the same circumstances, ASCs in chronic wounds are enough to cause tissue contracture [10]. Even ASCs' conditioned media did not antagonize the action of TGFβ, and there is no evidence to prevent myofibroblast differentiation [25]. The author is not against applying free fatty tissue graft. In a situation in which passaged ASCs can act like fibroblasts, and the role of anti-myofibroblast differentiation among the paracrine cytokines has not been proven, direct injection to the patient does not provide any evidence for prevention or treatment of contracture. The myth should be discarded.

- ASCs also show characteristics of myofibroblasts in inflammatory conditions like human dermal fibroblasts (HDF) (Fig. 13.2).
- There is no evidence that the paracrine action of ASCs prevents differentiation into myofibroblasts.

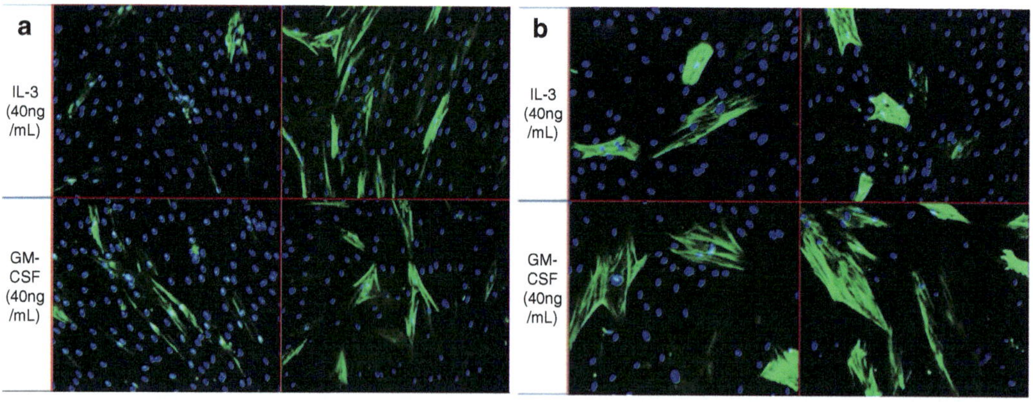

Fig. 13.2 The expression of α SMA when treated with IL-3/GM-CSF (40 ng/mL) ×400 magnification. (**a**) Human dermal fibroblast (HDF). (**b**) Human adipose-derived stromal cells (hASCs)

Pitfalls of the "Myth"

- Free fatty tissue causes soft tissue enhancement. Also, contained preadipocytes can induce recipient-dependent neo adipogenesis.
- However, there is little evidence that SVF can soften the contracted nose or relieve the contraction because it contains cytokines that cause soft tissue contracture.
- Do not assume that you are administering ASCs while administering SVF.
- ASCs can also be differentiated into myofibroblast-like HDF depending on the surrounding wound environment and can be source cells of contracture.
- There is no biological in vitro evidence that neither SVF nor hASCs can improve soft tissue contracture caused by inflammation.

References

1. Park Y-W. Bioabsorbable osteofixation for orthognathic surgery. Maxillofac Plast Reconstr Surg. 2015;37(1):6.
2. Bali RK, Sharma P, Jindal S, Gaba S. To evaluate the efficacy of biodegradable plating system for fixation of maxillofacial fractures: a prospective study. Natl J Maxillofac Surg. 2013;4(2):167–72.
3. Landes CA, Ballon A, Roth C. In-patient versus in vitro degradation of P (L/DL) LA and PLGA. J Biomed Mater Res B Appl Biomater. 2006;76(2):403–11.
4. Wang LL, Frankel AS, Friedman O. Complications of Polydioxanone foil use in nasal surgery: a case series. Facial Plast Surg. 2018;34(3):312–7.
5. Park YJ, Cha JH, Bang SI, Kim SY. Clinical application of three-dimensionally printed biomaterial Polycaprolactone (PCL) in augmentation rhinoplasty. Aesthet Plast Surg. 2019;43(2):437–46.
6. Boenisch M, Nolst Trenité GJ. Reconstruction of the nasal septum using polydioxanone plate. Arch Facial Plast Surg. 2010;12(1):4–10.
7. Alhussain OH, Alhussain GO, Rajkhan AA, Suhluli AJ, Alharbi SJ, Sherwani AA, et al. Efficacy of autologous vs. homologous costal cartilage grafts in dorsal augmentation rhinoplasty: a systematic review and meta-analysis. Ann Med Health Sci Res [Internet]. 2020;10(5). https://www.amhsr.org/articles/efficacy-of-autologous-vs-homologous-costal-cartilagegrafts-in-dorsal-augmentation-rhinoplasty-asystematic-review-and-me.pdf.
8. Moon K-C, Lee H-S, Son S-T, Lee J-S, Dhong E-S, Jeong S-H, et al. Effects of granulocyte-macrophage Colony-stimulating factor on neuronal senescence in ultraviolet irradiated skin. J Craniofac Surg. 2019;30(3):930–5.
9. Namgoong S, Lee H, Lee J-S, Jeong SH, Han S-K, Dhong E-S. Comparative biological effects of human amnion and chorion membrane extracts on human adipose-derived stromal cells. J Craniofac Surg. 2019;30(3):947–54.
10. Lee J-S, Tae S-S, Kim D-Y, Han S-K, Kim W-K, Dhong E-S. Do IL-3/GM-CSF effect on the myofibroblastic differentiation of human adipose derived stromal cells? Exp Cell Res. 2017;355(2):67–82.
11. Moon K-C, Lee J-S, Han S-K, Lee H-W, Dhong E-S. Effects of human umbilical cord blood-derived mesenchymal stromal cells and dermal fibroblasts on diabetic wound healing. Cytotherapy. 2017;19(7):821–8.
12. Gu JH, Lee JS, Kim D-W, Yoon E-S, Dhong E-S. Neovascular potential of adipose-derived stromal cells (ASCs) from diabetic patients. Wound Repair Regen. 2012;20(2):243–52.
13. Dhong E-S, Hwang N-H, Kim D-W, Rajashekhar G, Johnstone BH, March KL. Morphologic changes in photodamaged organotypic human skin culture after treatment of autologous adipose-derived stromal cells. J Craniofac Surg. 2012;23(3):805–11.
14. Hwang N-H, Jung J-E, Lee J-S, Jeong S-H, Dhong E-S, Han S-K. Effects of granulocyte macrophage Colony-stimulating factor inhibition on the skin/nerve cell model in vitro. J Craniofac Surg. 2020;31(5):1483–7.
15. Gilbody S. Benefits and harms of direct to consumer advertising: a systematic review [Internet]. Quality and safety in health care, vol 14. 2005. p. 246–50. https://doi.org/10.1136/qshc.2004.012781.
16. Ogbogu U, Rachul C, Caulfield T. Reassessing direct-to-consumer portrayals of unproven stem cell therapies: is it getting better? Regen Med. 2013;8(3):361–9.
17. Fang B, Song Y, Lin Q, Zhang Y, Cao Y, Zhao RC, et al. Human adipose tissue-derived mesenchymal stromal cells as salvage therapy for treatment of severe refractory acute graft-vs.-host disease in two children. Pediatr Transplant. 2007;11(7):814–7.
18. Riordan NH, Ichim TE, Min W-P, Wang H, Solano F, Lara F, et al. Non-expanded adipose stromal vascular fraction cell therapy for multiple sclerosis. J Transl Med. 2009;7:29.
19. Gir P, Oni G, Brown SA, Mojallal A, Rohrich RJ. Human adipose stem cells: current clinical applications. Plast Reconstr Surg. 2012;129(6):1277–90.
20. Oh YH, Seo JW, Oh SJ, Oum IT, Kim G, Kim J, et al. Correction of severely contracted nose. Plast Reconstr Surg. 2016;138(3):571–82.
21. Dominici M, Le Blanc K, Mueller I, Slaper-Cortenbach I, Marini F, Krause D, et al. Minimal criteria for defining multipotent mesenchymal stromal cells. The International Society for Cellular Therapy position statement. Cytotherapy. 2006;8(4):315–7.
22. Crisan M, Casteilla L, Lehr L, Carmona M, Paoloni-Giacobino A, Yap S, et al. A reservoir of brown adipocyte progenitors in human skeletal muscle. Stem Cells. 2008;26(9):2425–33.

23. Traktuev DO, Merfeld-Clauss S, Li J, Kolonin M, Arap W, Pasqualini R, et al. A population of multipotent CD34-positive adipose stromal cells share pericyte and mesenchymal surface markers, reside in a periendothelial location, and stabilize endothelial networks. Circ Res. 2008;102(1):77–85.
24. Bourin P, Bunnell BA, Casteilla L, Dominici M, Katz AJ, March KL, et al. Stromal cells from the adipose tissue-derived stromal vascular fraction and culture expanded adipose tissue-derived stromal/stem cells: a joint statement of the International Federation for Adipose Therapeutics and Science (IFATS) and the International Society for Cellular Therapy (ISCT). Cytotherapy. 2013;15(6):641–8.
25. Liguori TTA, Liguori GR, Moreira LFP, Harmsen MC. Fibroblast growth factor-2, but not the adipose tissue-derived stromal cells secretome, inhibits TGF-β1-induced differentiation of human cardiac fibroblasts into myofibroblasts [Internet]. Sci Rep. 2018;8. https://doi.org/10.1038/s41598-018-34747-3.

14 Pus Draining Status After Complicated Septorhinoplasty: When to Do the Secondary Rhinoplasty?

14.1 Background of Choosing this Case

When the author encounters a patient who is draining pus in an outpatient clinic, the first thought may be, "Why did the patient come to this hospital instead of where he/she has been operated?" However, the patient came to visit in a desperate condition. The doctor who performed the surgery previously might send the patient because he could not solve it. Choosing the best way to do it is to salvage both the patient and doctor in trouble. After septorhinoplasty became popular, septal extension grafts after SMR and alloplastic implants use simultaneously resulted in SSI after surgery, leaving the most severe sequelae. The pus-drainage will not improve unless alloplastic material and infected cartilage are removed. If the alloplastic implant and cartilage in the nasal framework on the undersurface are removed, will the nose's shape be maintained? Because of this fear, cartilage cannot be removed quickly, and only empirical antibiotics are used in various situations, resulting in irreversible consequences.

Pearls

- Patients with septal extension graft and alloplastic implants at the same time should be aware that it is a very urgent situation if SSI occurs after surgery.
- It is essential to be aware of any problems that may arise after removing the implant in the nose by setting the surgery's timing well.
- Once the pus is drained, all nonviable grafts must be removed. The viable graft can also be checked with the naked eye and left behind.
- SSI is a situation in which the infected tissue must be surgically removed, but it is a unique situation that requires medical control.
- Choosing the appropriate antibiotic using multiple nasal or discharge cultures is the way to succeed.
- The degree of cellulitis of columellar and dorsal skin is the criterion for determining the surgical timing. Even if the pus is drained, if the redness of the pocket skin and surrounding swelling is low, and the amount of pus in the prescribed antibiotics suddenly begins to decrease, surgery using autogenous graft may be considered. Mostly, late onset inflammation is regarded as a low-grade infection.

Supplementary Information The online version of this chapter (https://doi.org/10.1007/978-981-16-0542-0_14) contains supplementary material, which is available to authorized users.

E.-S. Dhong, M.-W. Na, *Asian Septorhinoplasty*, https://doi.org/10.1007/978-981-16-0542-0_14

- However, if SSI has occurred, active I&D should be performed first, and the flap should be monitored well. If flap swelling and rubor are severe, any graft to make the shape is not recommended.
- The framework reconstruction can be considered if the cellulitis is not severe. As it may cause more severe contracture if the framework is not considered for fear of repeated SSI.

14.2 Case Study

History

Three months before visiting the author, he underwent septorhinoplasty with a hump correction and dorsal Gore-tex implantation. SSI occurred 10 days after surgery, and the culture result was MRSA. After SSI was discovered, the wound was irrigated several times. After that, vancomycin was administered IV for 1 month at the same ENT clinic. Then, he was transferred to another university hospital. It was the fifth week postoperatively. The Gore-tex tip was partially removed, and the infected materials were removed by curettage and irrigated. However, the columella drained pus continuously after the removal, and columellar retraction was noted. He was referred to the author in the 10th week after the primary surgery.

Physical Exam and Diagnostic Findings

The first visit: A small opening was seen in the columella, and discharge was continuously drained. Vancomycin was cut, and mupirocin ointment was applied. Oral clindamycin was administered because MRSE was rediscovered in the culture performed just before the visit.

A culture study was conducted, and surgery was recommended even if there was no pus drained.

The second visit: the first visit culture was negative, and the discharge decreased after Clindamycin administration. The author recommended immediate surgery but wanted surgery after a month due to the patient's circumstances. LFT increased in liver function test.

Operation; Three weeks after the first referral to the author, surgery was performed. A total of 13 weeks postoperatively, the tertiary operation was performed.

Endoscopic Findings

Central flopping was found at the SMR status, but there was no pus pocket or perforation in the nasal septum.

A puncture confined to the columellar was found. Also, bulging of the columella on the right side was found (Fig. 14.1).

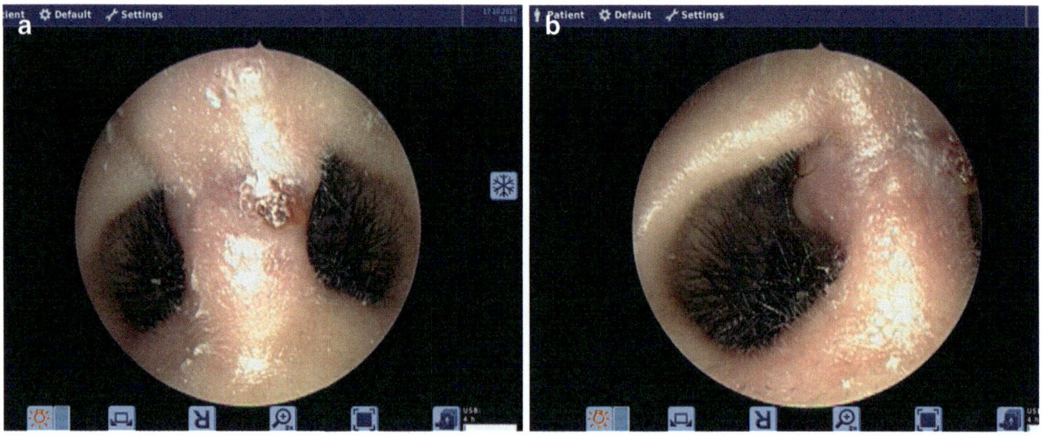

Fig. 14.1 The pus-draining anterior columellar lesion. (**a**, **b**) Close-up views

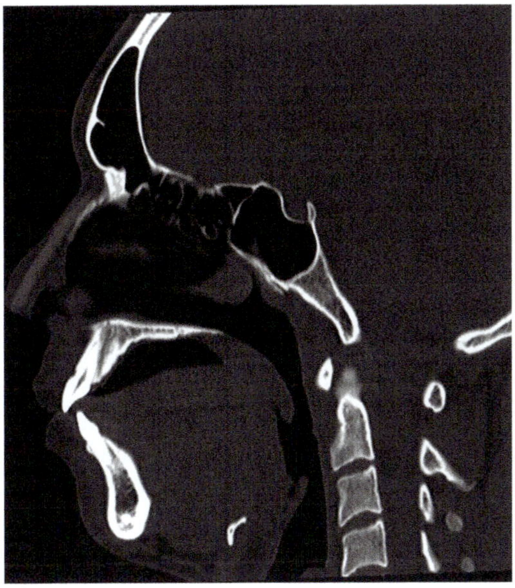

Fig. 14.2 Sagittal CT scan shows a long dorsal implant and impending protrusion

CT Scan

The alloplastic material presumed to be a long Gore-tex was up to the nasal tip, and the skin thickness of the tip was thin enough to suspect impending protrusion (Videos 14.1 and 14.2, Fig. 14.2).

Culture Study and Antibiotics

- 1st culture: no bacterial.
- 2nd culture (2 weeks after the 1st visit): Paenibacillus polymyxa (moderately).
  - Clindamycin resistant Oxacillin resistant Penicillin resistant.
  - Levofloxacin sensitive Vancomycin sensitive.
- 3rd culture (operation day): no bacterial.

Choice of antibiotics: Tarivid ointment for 7 days preoperatively and postoperatively

IV Vancomycin for 5 days peri- and postoperatively

Preoperative Surgical Planning

- The cartilage destruction of the columella is judged to be severe, which is the pus pocket.
- Since cellulitis is not severe, it was decided to reconstruct the nasal framework using a cartilage graft to solve the retracted columellar.
- The caudal septal extension will be performed first, then the extended septal extension graft will follow according to the anterior septum condition.
- The loss of dorsal height that occurs after implant removal will be reconstructed with SDF.

Intraoperative Findings

There were still unhealed columellar lesions, and incisions were made using this area. The left nasal cavity was narrower than the right side, and the lower edge of the implant was observed on the ceiling of the right nasal cavity (Video 14.3).

A mucocele-like pocket was found under the dorsal Gore-tex, showing a late-onset inflammation pattern with mucin collected (Video 14.4 and Figs.14.3 and 14.4). As a result of the lower anterior septum's dissection after removing the entire

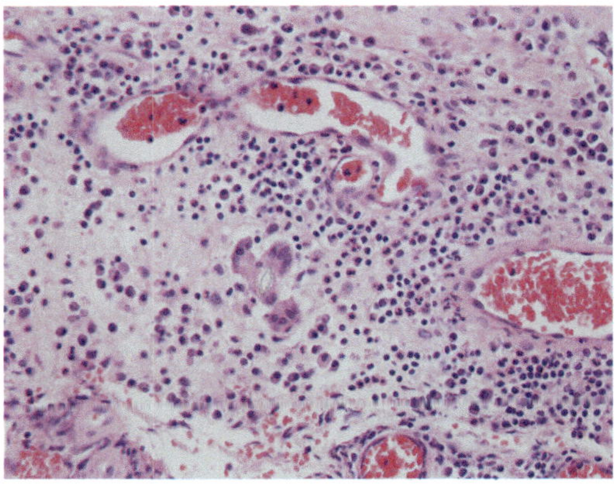

Fig. 14.3 Chronic active inflammation with granulation tissue: aggregation of inflammatory cells. (×400 H&E)

pocket, the spreader grafts on both sides, which were presumed to have been applied in surgery, were found (Video 14.5). It was decided to curettage some and leave the rest for anterior septal support. There was no history of using silicone implants in the past, but it was found that capsules were formed around Gore-tex. The caudal septum almost disappeared, but the anterior septum retained the spreader's shape, and bleeding was also found during the scrape, so it was decided to leave it after careful curettage.

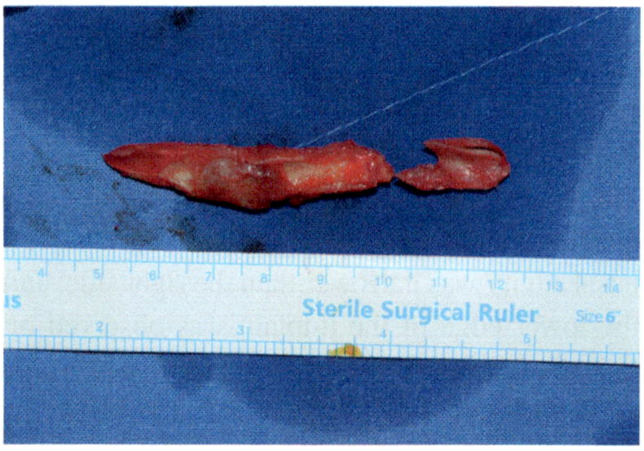

Fig. 14.4 Explanted Gore-tex and dirty capsules

14.3 Operative Strategies

- For caudal septal support, folded cymba cartilage was applied to the caudal septum (Video 14.6).
- The lateral crural spanning graft was performed on the LLC's upper part to prevent counter-clockwise rotation of the tip and increase tip support.
- The missing dorsal volume was filled with SDF.
- Operative Strategies.
- For caudal septal support, folded cymba cartilage was applied to the caudal septum.

Postoperative Results

Even though SSI appears to be well controlled with antibiotics, it can cause ongoing inflammation. Within such a short period, a typical late-onset mucin-producing pocket could be found. Since the patient did not have pus-drainage at the time of surgery, the nasal framework using a cartilage graft was possible, and the columellar retraction could be resolved (Figs. 14.5 and 14.6).

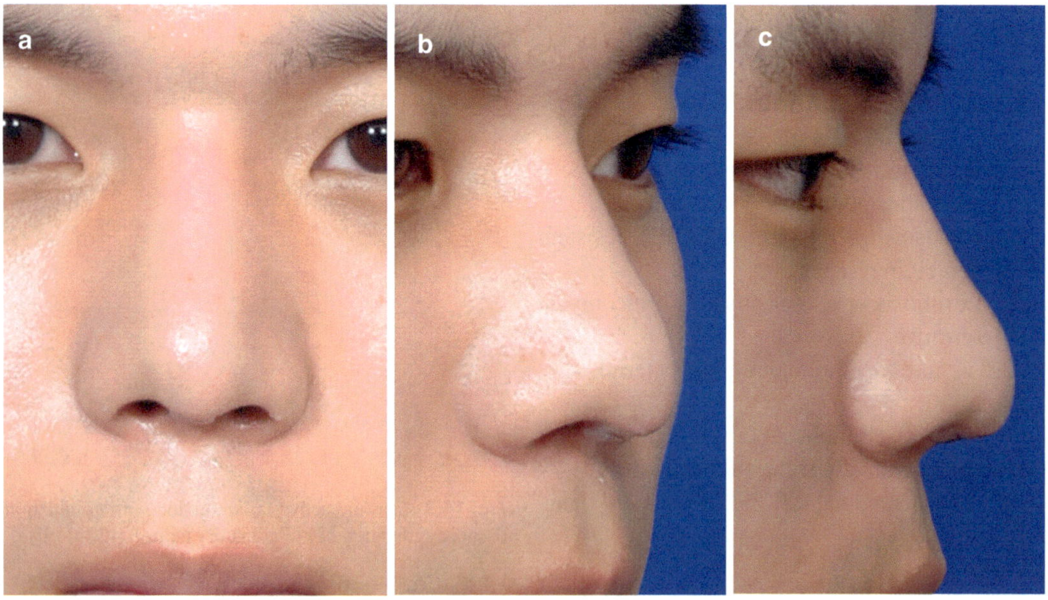

Fig. 14.5 Pre- and postoperative views. (**a**–**c**) Preoperative views. (**d**–**f**) Postoperative 2 months views

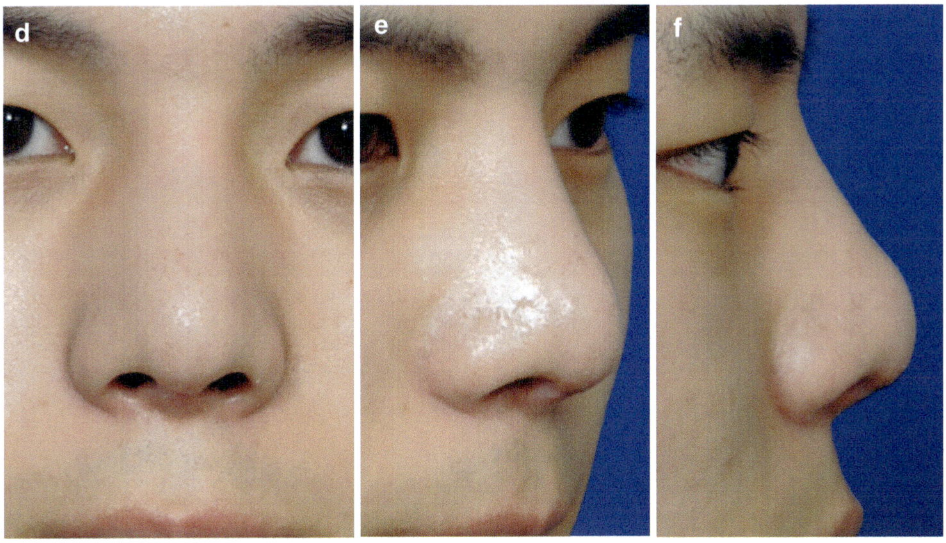

Fig. 14.5 (continued)

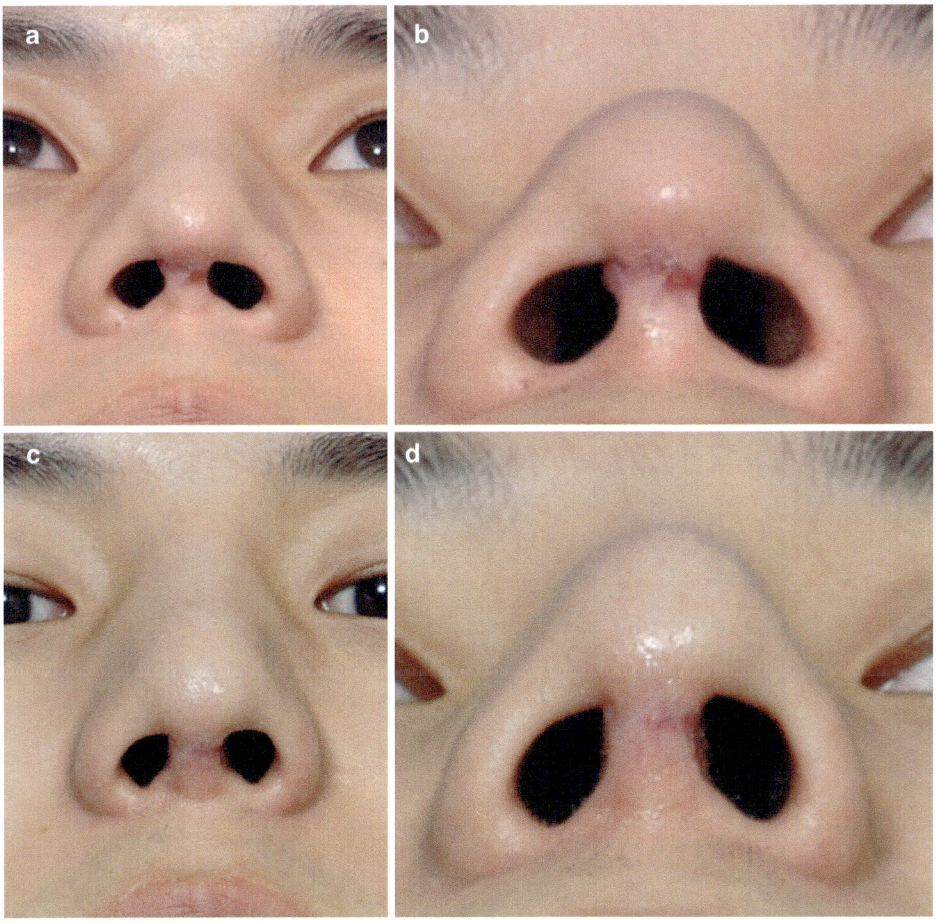

Fig. 14.6 The basal views and the columellar lesion. (**a**, **b**) Preoperative views. (**c**, **d**) Postoperative 2 months views

15 Nasal Tip Necrosis: The Midline Forehead Flap Should Be the Last Choice

15.1 Background of Choosing this Case

As the number of surgeries increases, the circulation to the nasal tip suffers. The author has experienced a few patients transferred to the author with columella necrosis after cosmetic surgery. The author also saw a patient who underwent the six different doctors' rhinoplasties, but the author thinks there is a particular reason for columellar necrosis. Vascular compromise can occur when a nonspecific mechanical trauma is applied to the tip skin or soft tissue around the LLC is not properly stretched, and excessive tension is applied. Both patients suffering from columella necrosis and surgeons are facing enormous stress and those cases become legal complaint cases. In fact, in Korea, midline forehead flaps were applied to the patients, which had become significant social issues with bad results. The problem is that the midline forehead flap is not an improper operation, but applied to a patient who has undergone nose surgery for cosmetic purposes can develop into a case that adversely affects the whole plastic surgeons or plastic surgeries in general. For recruiting soft tissue less than 0.5 × 1 cm, making a midline forehead scars ten times longer is harsh. The authors have even experienced a patient with the hair-growing columella. We have to try the most straightforward method first, and we need to share the wisdom to make sure this method does not fail, so the author has selected these patients in this chapter.

Pearls

- The midline forehead flap is a useful surgery, but it should not be chosen as the first modality of columellar necrosis caused as the complication of esthetic rhinoplasty.
- In composite graft from the ear, integral skin portion and cartilage must be attached, and perichondrium must be preserved to increase survival.
- The surgeon should know how to increase the survival rate of composite grafts.

15.2 Case Study

History

A 37 year old male patient with a bulbous nose and low nasal dorsum underwent septorhinoplasty using silicone in a private clinic.

- Four months after surgery, a silicone change was made at the same hospital, and columellar revision was made.

Supplementary Information The online version of this chapter (https://doi.org/10.1007/978-981-16-0542-0_15) contains supplementary material, which is available to authorized users.

E.-S. Dhong, M.-W. Na, *Asian Septorhinoplasty*, https://doi.org/10.1007/978-981-16-0542-0_15

- After 3 months, the silicone was changed again, and the columellar was revised using the conchal cartilage.
- Columellar necrosis occurred within 5 days after surgery.

First Choice by the Author: Composite Graft

Physical Exam and Diagnostic Findings

There was necrosis of the entire layer of columella and infratip lobule, and the wound was not open and sat down. There was no evidence of cellulitis in the skin around the necrosis (Fig. 15.1). The CT scan showed dorsal silicone and columellar alloplastic material with a white shadow (Video 15.1).

Preoperative Surgical Goals

The author chose a composite graft using conchal cartilage and attached skin as a salvaging method. Dorsal silicone was left as it is, and only the columella was reconstructed. The nasolabial perforator flap was the second choice if the composite graft was not taken, and the midline forehead flap was planned as the third option. The reason was that the patient's skin was very thick, and the forehead was relatively narrow.

Strategy for Composite Graft

- The cartilage covers the middle crura on both sides to the medial crura like the shape of the shield graft.
- The perichondrium attached to the cartilage is preserved so that the surrounding blood supply can go to the skin more smoothly.
- Hyperbaric O_2 therapy will be performed.

Intraoperative Findings

Immediately after removing the necrotic skin, discolored cartilage was seen and removed. This piece was IHCC; however, no information could be obtained (Fig. 15.2).

Most of the caudal portion of the middle crus and medial crus disappeared and after debridement. The defect became more extensive than the primary lesion.

Operation Method

- The cartilage that is larger than the range of the skin is designed (Fig. 15.3).
- As designed, it was harvested from the posterior surface of the cavum (Fig. 15.4).
- After removing the necrotic skin, the surrounding margin was debrided to make it sharper.

Result

The entire graft survived.

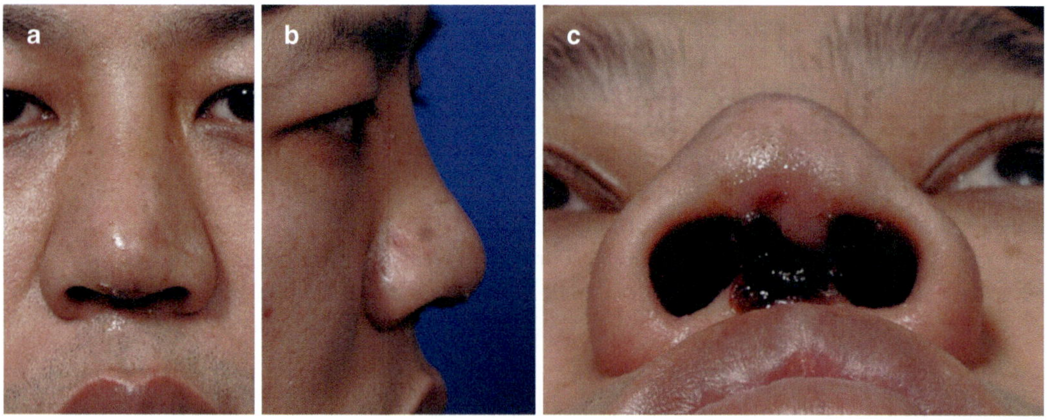

Fig. 15.1 The columellar necrosis. (**a–c**) Photos were taken at the first visit

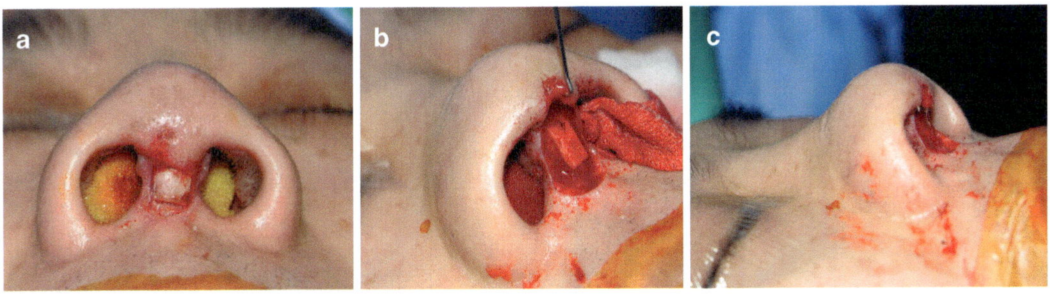

Fig. 15.2 Debridement to make a clean skin margin. (**a**) IHCC was found after removing the necrotic columella. (**b**) Margin debridement and removal of IHCC. (**c**) Wide defect remained

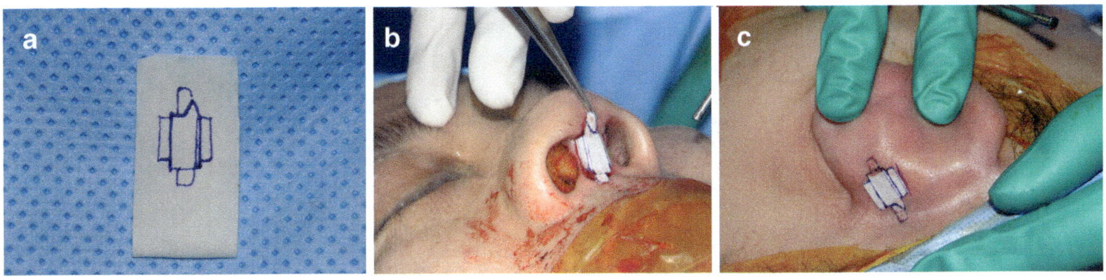

Fig. 15.3 Schematic of the composite graft. (**a**, **b**) The design and the application at the lesion. (**c**) The posterior auricular circus at the cavum concha was harvested

Secondary Operation: SRP

Physical Exam and Diagnostic Findings

Definite septorhinoplasty was performed 18 months after the last surgery.

The dorsal silicone was found, and the rigid scar tissue over the nasal tip was removed. The tip was like one big scar. Septorhinoplasty using sixth costal cartilage was planned. An L-sturt extension graft was applied for nasal lengthening. The nasal tip plasty was focused on reducing the bulbosity and creating the supra-alar groove.

Strategy for SRP

- He had a very thick skin, so costal cartilage was harvested, and a profound extension against tension was planned.
- The projection was increased at the dorsum by diced costal cartilage to be wrapped in the rectus fascia.

Intraoperative Findings

The 3.5 mm silicone was removed from the dorsum, and the very thick capsule and surrounding contracture had to be removed. The caudal septum remained, but very weak. The loss of the caudal margin of the LLC's middle crus and medial crus existed as in the first surgery, but the shield graft applied in the composite graft was integrated to form a caudal margin. This cartilage was used as the medial crura.

Operation Method

- An incision was applied using the scar on the bottom of the composite graft.
- Since it was SMR state, it was difficult to maintain the length of the nose with the remaining L-strut, so a long extended spreader graft (9 × 20 mm) was applied using a slice of the sixth rib, and a caudal septal extension graft using a slice of the costal cartilage was applied to the caudal portion (5 × 18 mm) (Fig. 15.5).

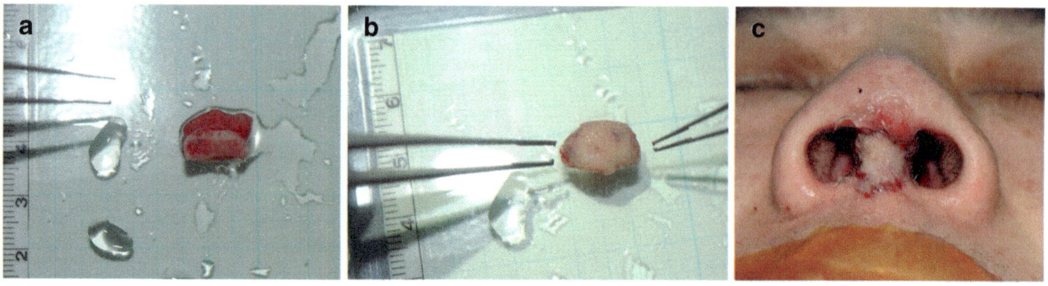

Fig. 15.4 Composite graft. (**a**, **b**) The perichondrium attached to the cartilage was preserved so that the surrounding blood supply can go to the skin more smoothly. (**c**) After the repair. The open dressing was done

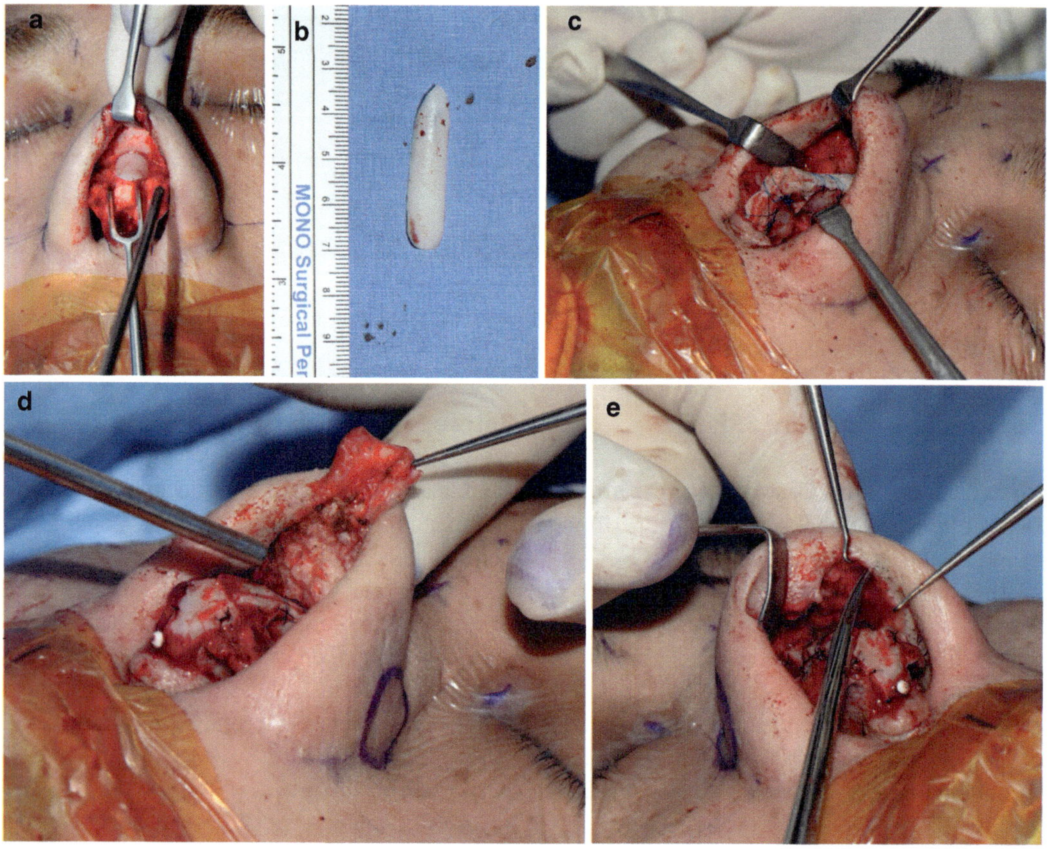

Fig. 15.5 Septal reconstruction using SLEG. (**a**, **b**) Intraoperative silicone implant. (**c**) Septal L-strut extension graft. (**d**, **e**) Sleeve down technique of dorsal skin envelope

- The loss of the caudal margin of the LLC's middle crus and medial crus existed as in the first surgery, but the shield graft applied in the composite graft was integrated to form a caudal margin. This cartilage was used as the medial crura.
- For the creation of the supra-alar groove, the LLSAN deep in the dermis and a portion of the fat layer were removed.

Result

- There was no skin loss of the composite graft.
- The overall retraction of the nose was improved, and the profile was improved.
- The columellar retraction was improved, and supratip soft tissue removal and supra-alar groove shape improvement were obtained (Figs. 15.6 and 15.7).

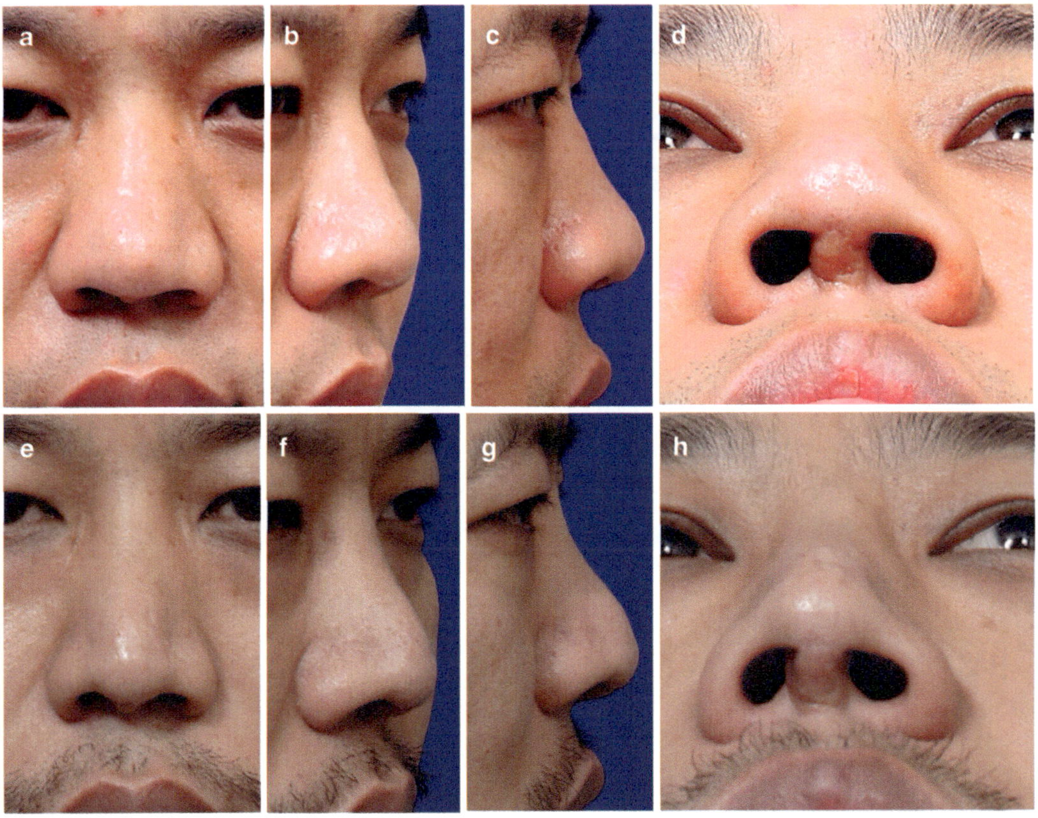

Fig. 15.6 Septorhinoplasty using costal cartilage was performed 18 months after the composite graft (**a**–**d**) Preoperative views. (**e**–**h**) Long-term postoperative views

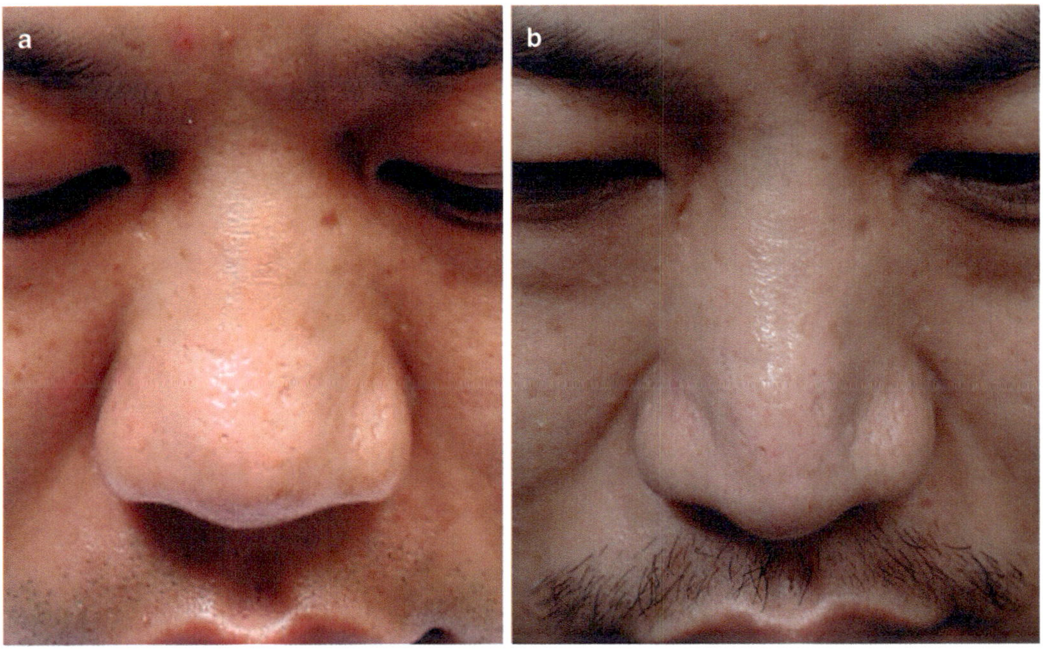

Fig. 15.7 Comparative views. (**a**, **c**) Pre- and postoperative bird's eye view. (**b**, **d**) Before the composite graft and the long-term result

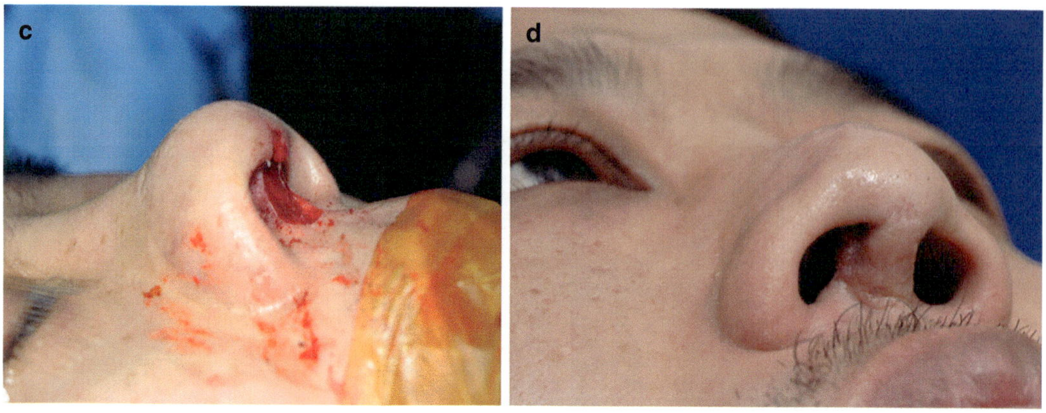

Fig. 15.7 (continued)

16 When You Encounter Very Small Septal Cartilage

16.1 Background

A common problem in Asians is that the nasal septal cartilage is collected less than expected. In old age, the amount of quadrangular cartilage decreases. It is relatively more ossified, and the amount of cartilage harvested is small. If the nose is small, or there is a history of fractures, it is possible to predict that flat quadrangular cartilage will be small. However, many Asians have a small volume of quadrangular cartilage attainable even in younger patients than the standard without any trauma history. Ossification can be detected in a CT scan in advance, but all slices of scan cannot be contained.

This patient was selected to know how to collect quadrangular cartilage wisely in an unpredicted situation.

Pearls

- When encountering unexpectedly small quadrangular cartilage, the EPP cartilage junction must be well protected.
- If the EPP-quadrangular junction is well connected, a more extended graft is available.
- EPP harvest should be performed according to a planned osteotomy.
- Osteotomy can be performed with the freer elevator, but a saw can be the alternative if it does not work well.
- A reciprocating saw and an oscillating saw should be provided.
- Efforts are made to prevent damaging the mucosal pocket.

16.2 Case Study

History

A 39-year-old man complained of nasal stuffiness on his right side and wanted to correct a reverse C-shape deformity. He had no history of trauma.

Physical Exam and Diagnostic Findings

There was no particular abnormality on physical examination.

The patient had severe nasal obstruction with a NOSE scale of 16/20.

Supplementary Information The online version of this chapter (https://doi.org/10.1007/978-981-16-0542-0_16) contains supplementary material, which is available to authorized users.

E.-S. Dhong, M.-W. Na, *Asian Septorhinoplasty*, https://doi.org/10.1007/978-981-16-0542-0_16

Endoscopic Findings

There was a protrusion suspicious of septal dislocation in the right nasal crest. Attenuation of the nasal mucosa at the nasal crest was observed. It could be suspected that lacerations existed along the maxillary crest.

The right nasal cavity looked narrower than the left, but the left EPP was also convex (Video 16.1 and Fig. 16.1).

Acoustic Rhinometry

The right MCA (minimal cross-sectional area) was measured to be 0.55, and the right nasal cavity was more obstructed (Fig. 16.2).

Preoperative Surgical Planning

- A spreader graft was planned on the patient's right anterior septum with septal cartilage.
- For the mild hump correction, only the left nasal dorsum would be rasped to obtain a straight line.

Intraoperative Findings

After the L-strut of 11 mm-width was preserved, a very small quadrangular cartilage was found.

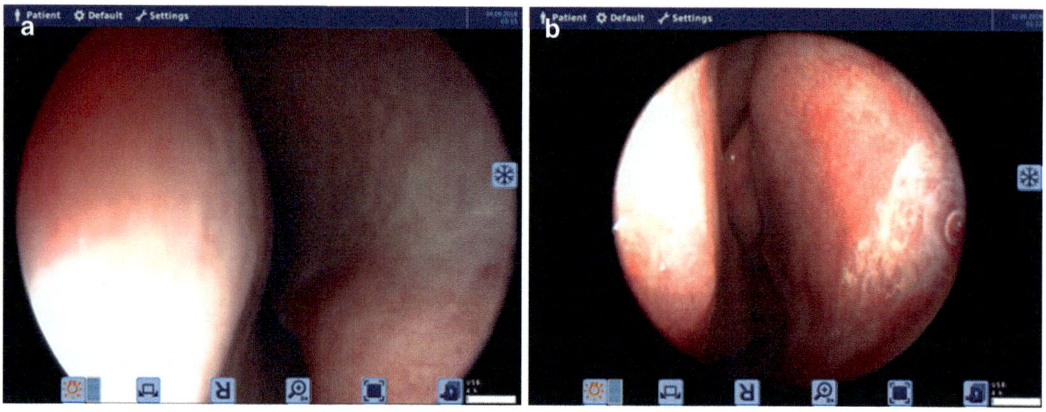

Fig. 16.1 Endoscopic views. (**a**) The right nasal cavity: septal concavity and protruded septal cartilage on the maxillary crest and vomer. (**b**) The left nasal cavity: convexity of EPP

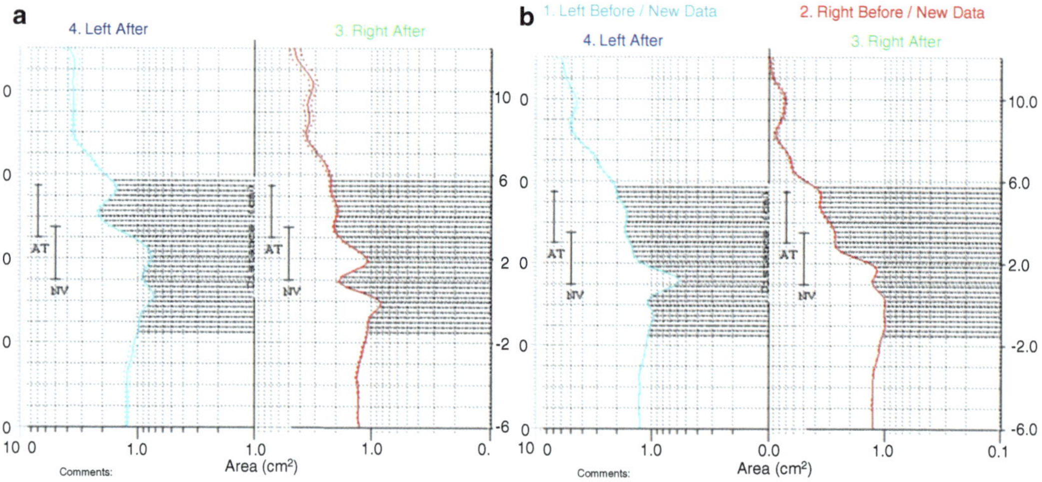

Fig. 16.2 Acoustic rhinometry. (**a**) Preoperative AR showed right MCA is located anteriorly and smaller. (**b**) Postoperatively the right curve improved. The patient NOSE score improved from 16/20 to 8/20

16.3 Operative Strategies

- Quadrangular cartilage attached with EPP (20 × 29 mm) was harvested (Fig. 16.3).
- More EPP (7 × 16 mm) was harvested and used for stabilizing the caudal septum.
- Bilateral spreader graft (9 × 26 mm) was applied (Fig. 16.4).
- A PDS plate obtained stability to integrate the anterior extended spreader graft and caudal septum (Video 16.2).
- For the correction of convexity, a mattress suture was applied to the left lateral crus (Video 16.3).
- Small columellar strut, columelloseptal suture, and tip cartilage shield graft were applied for the ideal LLC shaping (Video 16.4 and Fig. 16.5).
- Bilateral out fracture of inferior turbinate was performed (Video 16.5).
- Bilateral coblation of inferior turbinate was performed (Video 16.6).

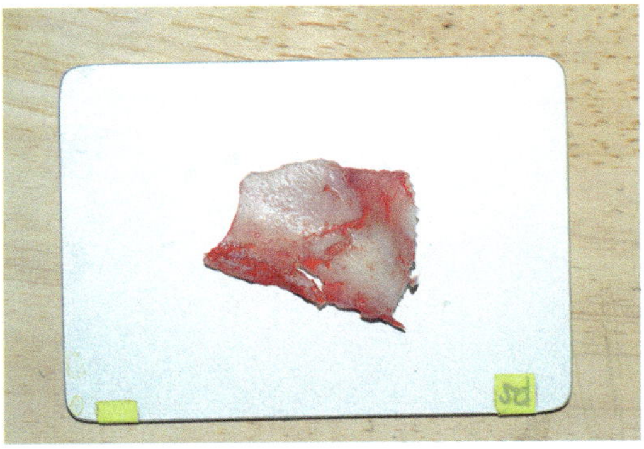

Fig. 16.3 Harvested septal cartilage (20 × 29 mm). This was cut into two spreader grafts

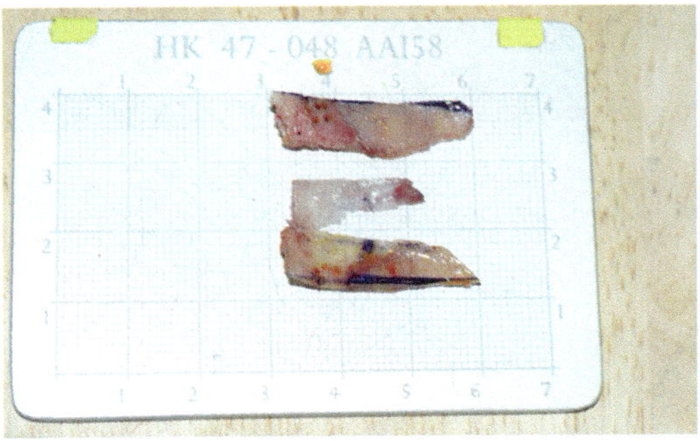

Fig. 16.4 Cartilage with bone segment was ready for the bilateral spreader graft. Multiple drill holes were made for the suture. (center) A bone piece harvested from EPP (7 × 16 mm) was prepared for the small caudal batten graft

Postoperative Results

- The NOSE scale decreased from 16 points to 8 points.
- The curve on the AR on the Rt side improved (Fig. 16.2).
- The stuffy nose disappeared. He smells better and sleeps better (Video 16.7).
- The reverse C-shape deviation was corrected (Figs. 16.6 and 16.7).

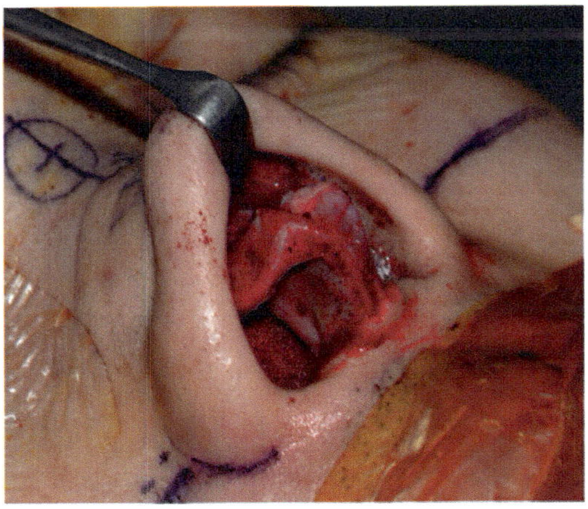

Fig. 16.5 The feature of the LLCs: Small columellar strut graft and short shield graft

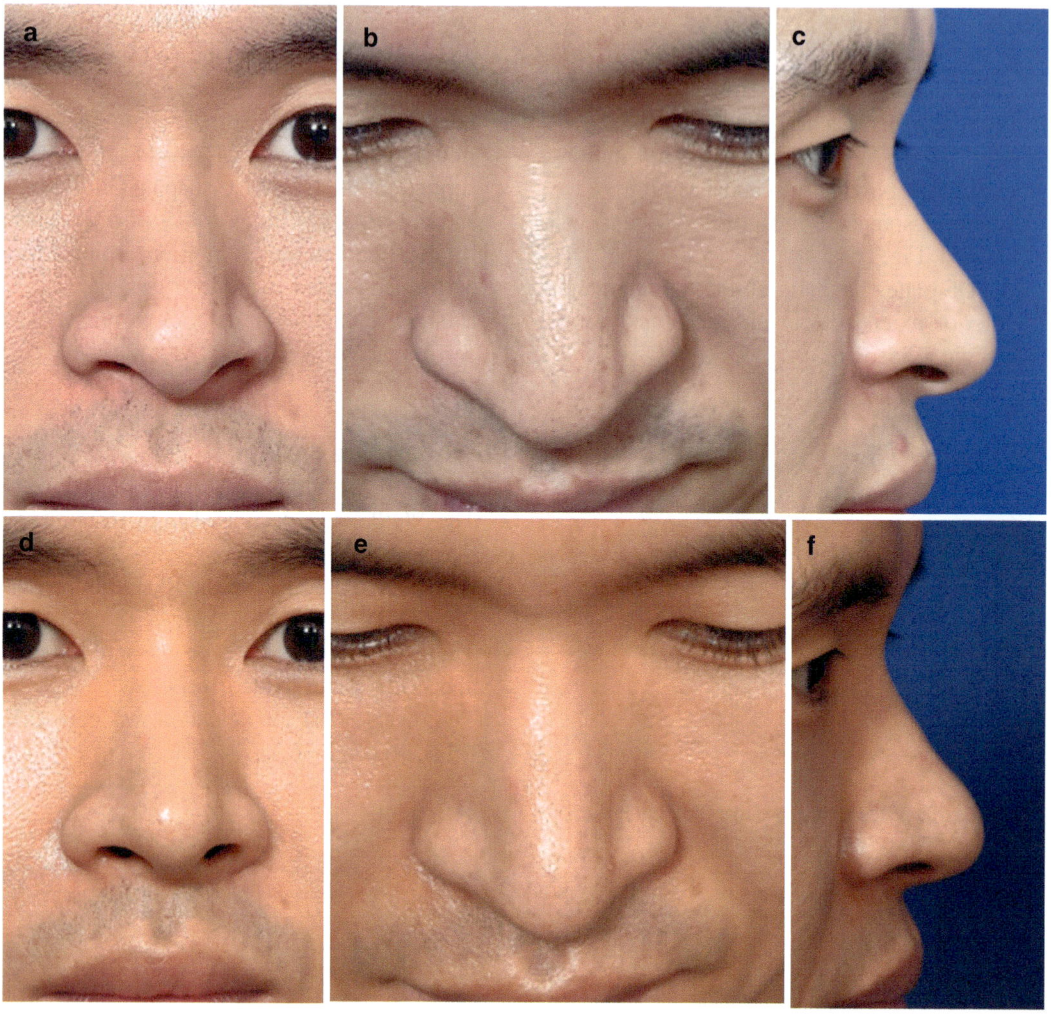

Fig. 16.6 Pre- and postoperative views. (**a–c**) Preoperative views. (**d–f**) Long-term postoperative views

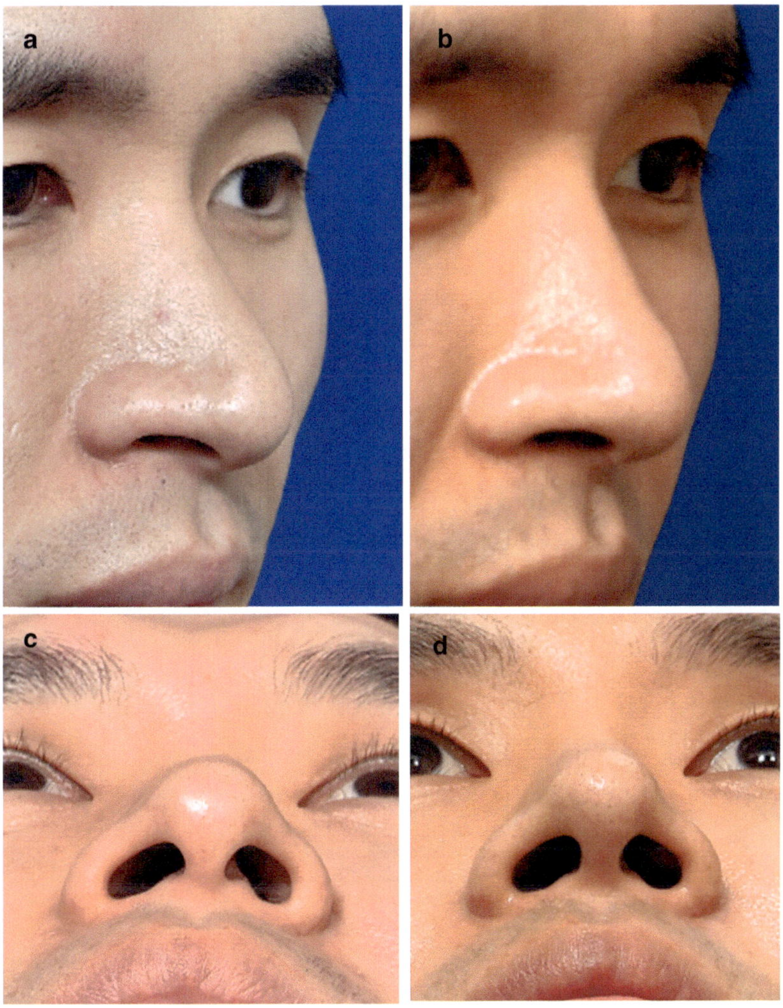

Fig. 16.7 Pre- and postoperative views. (**a**, **c**) Preoperative views. (**b**, **d**) Long-term postoperative views

Hypoplastic Lower Two-Third Nose: Camouflage Vs. Reconstruct the Framework

17

17.1 Background of Selecting this Patient

This feature accounts for many patients of Asian rhinoplasty. The bony dorsum is appropriately projected, whereas the height of the cartilaginous dorsum is relatively low. Whether the clinical manifestation is a saddle nose or a hypoplastic lower two-third nose without a saddle, there is likely a septal deviation or septal depression. If there is a deviation or tilt of the septum or a defect, the cartilaginous dorsum is usually very low. In these patients, choosing a dorsal alloplastic implant is not a good option. Dead space will be created in the lower part of the implant, even though it fits the nasion. Conversely, many surgeons do resect the bony dorsum to fit the upper one-third nose. The author prefers to perform only by increasing the lower two-third nose. This method can express the dorsum and tip as septum-dependently. In the author's choices, costal cartilage is the last resort of choice. The costal cartilage has already been introduced as a novel technique several times, and the author agrees that there is no better way than that. However, the author prefers septal reconstruction to solid costal cartilage onlay graft. If septal surgery is not possible, the camouflage method will be a second strategy. The author disagrees with the notion that patients complain of discomfort with the stiff nasal tip, which other Asian surgeons are concerned about. However, various Asian problematic noses can only be reconstructed by costal cartilage. If some membranous septum is left, the nasal tip can be movable on a long term. The autologous costal cartilage is the last scone of the rhinoplasty surgeon and is a treasure trove that allows multiple surgeons.

Pearls

- If the lower two-third of the nose is hypotrophied, the upper one-third of the nose may look rather large. In this situation, the right plan will be only enhancing the hypoplastic portion. Surgeons should imagine the original state of the nose.
- The long extended spreader graft's success in the correction of the over-resected nose is the stability of the rhinion region.
- The soundness of the anterocaudal margin of the lateral nasal bone plays an important role in the success of the surgery.
- Anterior projection of more than 3 mm is not easy by applying separate L-strut extension graft using conchal cartilage.
- More projection is possible only by costal cartilage.

Supplementary Information The online version of this chapter (https://doi.org/10.1007/978-981-16-0542-0_17) contains supplementary material, which is available to authorized users.

E.-S. Dhong, M.-W. Na, *Asian Septorhinoplasty*, https://doi.org/10.1007/978-981-16-0542-0_17

17.2 Case Study

History

First Operation

A 26-year-old female patient with a hump nose and deviation underwent septorhinoplasty with corrective osteotomy and SMR, dorsal graft with alloderm, and IHCC at a private clinic. After that, the dorsum was too high, and the deviation recurred.

Revision at the Private Clinic

Alloderm removed and first fat injection 3 months after surgery. Two months later, she received the second fat injection. Another month later, she received third fat injection.

Tertiary Operation at a Different Clinic

Three months later, IHCC was removed at another private clinic through cosmetic dissatisfaction such as tip asymmetry, and secondary rhinoplasty was performed using bilateral conchal carriage and SDF. After 2 days of operation, SDF was removed due to inflammation. After the last operation, a severe saddle nose occurred, and she visited the author 1 year and 3 months later.

Physical Exam and Diagnostic Findings

At the first examination, the tip felt hard, and there was no movement at all. The dorsal skin adhered to the underneath tissue. After a three-month follow-up, she took Zafirlukast and continuously massaged the nose. The skin, including the tip and dorsum, was observed to become soft (Video 17.1).

17.3 Nasal Swab Study

Zafirlukast was prescribed, and culture studies were conducted periodically during the follow-up period. Follow-up every 2 weeks and six culture studies were conducted. When MRSA was first identified, mupirocin ointment was applied, and then it was not identified. MRSE was cultured in the last culture before surgery. Tarivid ointment was applied to the nasal cavity for 1 week before surgery. Ciprofloxacin was selected and used for 4 days from the day of surgery, and the culture performed immediately before surgery was negative. Antibiotics were continuously used without changing.

Endoscopic Findings and CT Scan

The ceiling of the nasal cavity was found low from external nares to INV. She did not complain of a stuffy nose. A CT scan showed over-resected dorsum and showed deformity in which the open roof was not closed at all (Video 17.2).

17.4 Acoustic Rhinometry

From the entrance to INV, it did not show a sudden MCA. Nose score was 7/20.

Preoperative Surgical Goals

- The anterior septum was reconstructed with a thin slice of costal cartilage. With this spreader graft, the cartilaginous dorsum was projected.
- Bone fixation was attempted to fix the weak rhinion area.

Strategy for the Operation

- The skin was very thin. The solid dorsal graft would cause excessive tension in the nasal tip skin.
- A solid dorsal graft was not required because she did not want the projection of the nasion area.
- However, considering the overall dorsal line, it was judged that the augmentation of 2 mm of the bony dorsum was necessary.
- More than two suitable ear cartilages were left, but a long spreader graft was needed, so

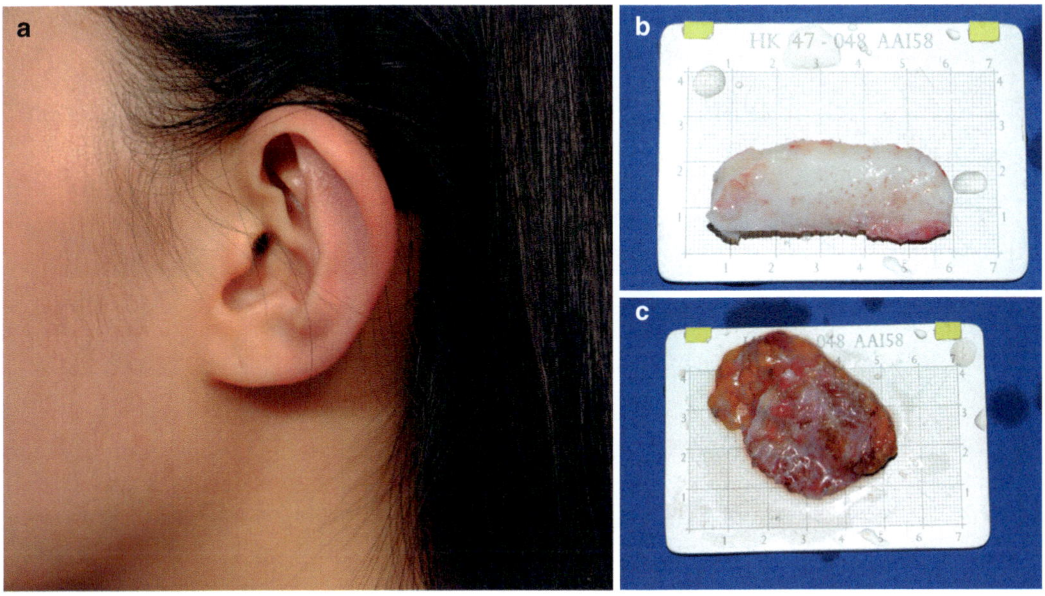

Fig. 17.1 The materials of the operation. (**a**) The ear cartilage was already harvested from the left cymba and cavum concha. (**b**) Sixth costal cartilage. (**c**) The rectus fascia

the author decided to use costal cartilage (Fig. 17.1).

- A long extended spreader graft was required to improve the inverted V deformity.
- The lateral wall of the nasal bone was relatively palpated, but the lateral osteotomy would not be performed.

Intraoperative Findings

- The ossification of costal cartilage was found.
- Although the anterior septum was almost lost, detachment of the left and right mucoperichondrium was possible successfully.
- The lateral nasal bone in the rhinion site was partially destroyed.

17.5 Operation Method

- Extended spreader graft was performed using costal cartilage of long slices (9 × 25 mm).
- Two layers of caudal septal extension graft were also applied to the caudal septum (6 × 18 mm).
- To prevent warping, coaptation was performed using multiple sutures.
- Except for the two 5.0 nonabsorbable sutures, only PDS 4.0 and 5.0 were used.
- For a smooth dorsal line, partially rolled rectus fascia was grafted onlay to the dorsum (Video 17.3). The bony dorsum area over the nasion, the fascia was rolled, but the lower two-third area was not rolled.

17.6 Result

- After surgery, inverted V deformity disappeared, but some deformity reappeared after the dorsal resorption.
- But the saddle nose deformity was improved.
- She did not appeal for nasal obstruction after septal reconstruction.
- Vast resorption of dorsal rolled rectus fascia occurred.
- The author persuaded secondary insertion of dorsal onlay graft, but she did not want a revision. The dorsal esthetic line was agreeable with the patient.
- Severe warping has not occurred (Figs. 17.2, 17.3, 17.4, 17.5, and 17.6).

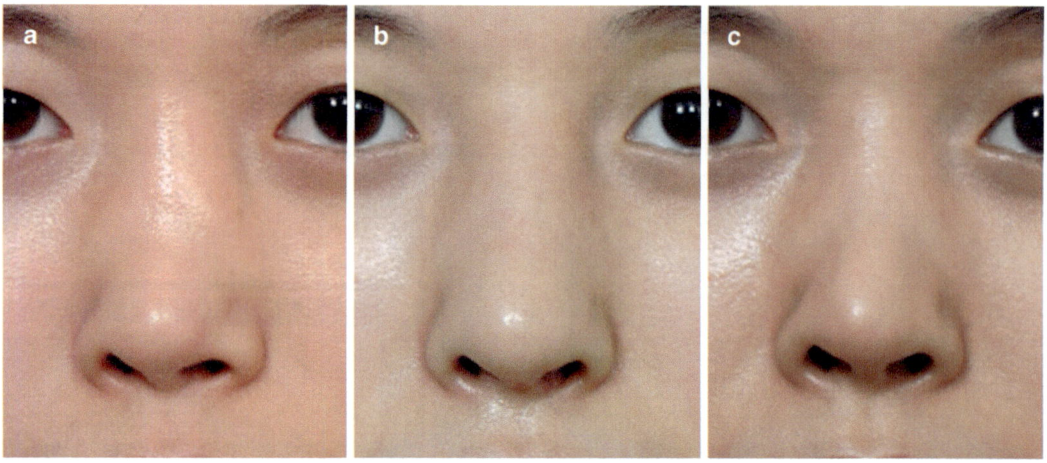

Fig. 17.2 Pre- and postoperative AP views. (**a**) Preoperative view. (**b**) Postoperative 6 months view. (**c**) Postoperative 18 months view

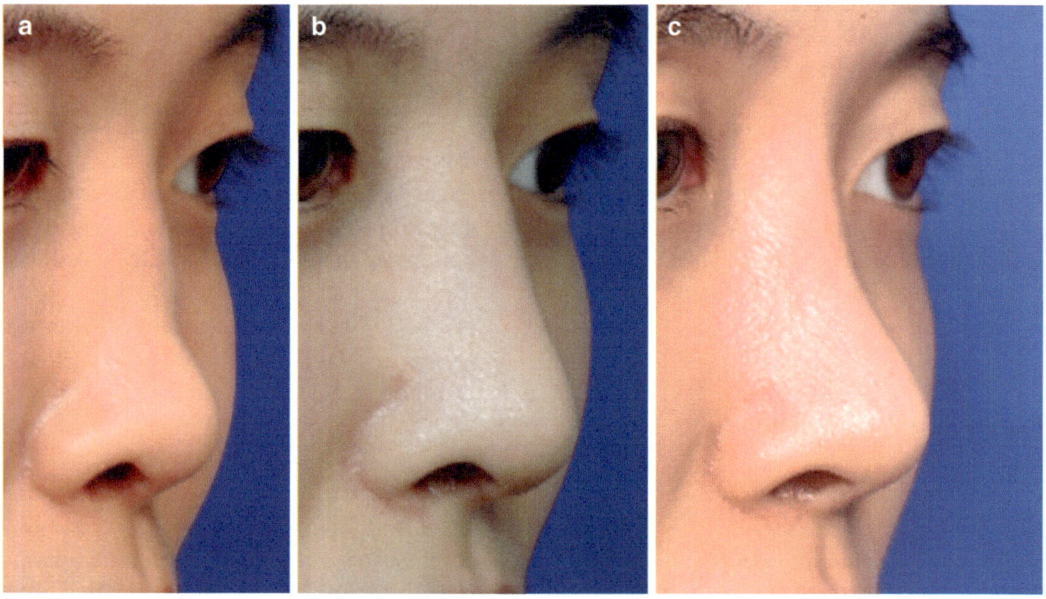

Fig. 17.3 Pre- and postoperative quarter views. (**a**) Preoperative view. (**b**) Postoperative 6 months view. (**c**) Postoperative 18 months view

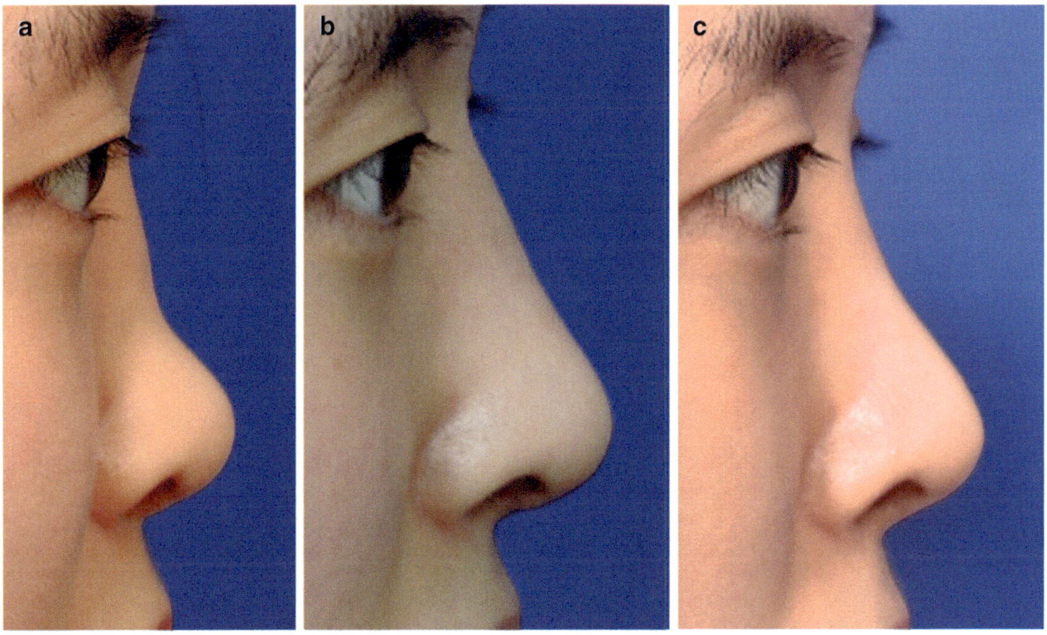

Fig. 17.4 Pre- and postoperative lateral views. (**a**) Preoperative view. (**b**) Postoperative 6 months view. (**c**) Postoperative 18 months view

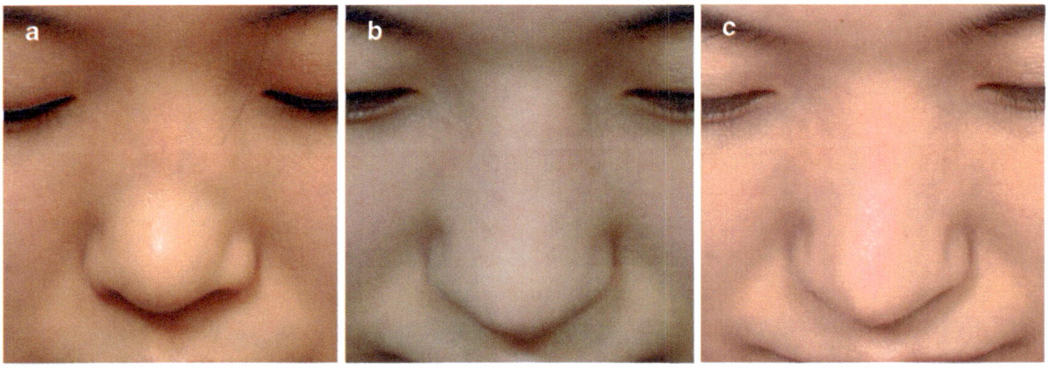

Fig. 17.5 Pre- and postoperative bird's eye views. (**a**) Preoperative view. (**b**) Postoperative 6 months view. (**c**) Postoperative 18 months view

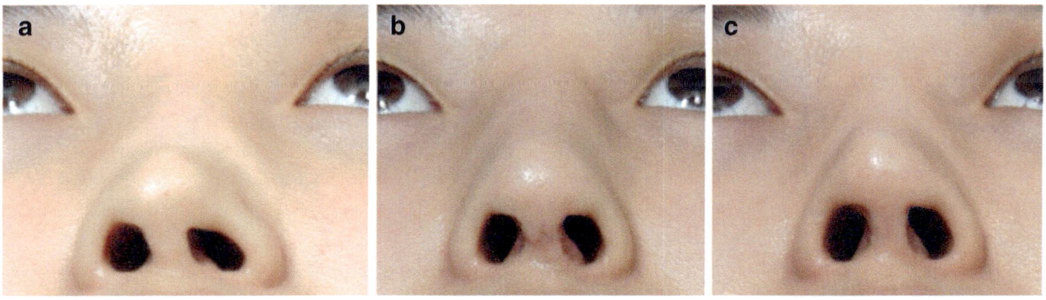

Fig. 17.6 Pre- and postoperative worm's eye views. (**a**) Preoperative view. (**b**) Postoperative 6 months view. (**c**) Postoperative 18 months view

Correction to: Controlling Asian Tip: Facet and Supra-Alar Groove

Correction to:
Chapter 9 in: E.-S. Dhong, M.-W. Na, *Asian Septorhinoplasty*,
https://doi.org/10.1007/978-981-16-0542-0_9

In chapter 9, Figures 9.6, 9.7, 9.8, 9.10, and 9.11 were incorrectly published. This has now been corrected by replacing them with the correct figures.

The corrected figures and their captions are printed below:

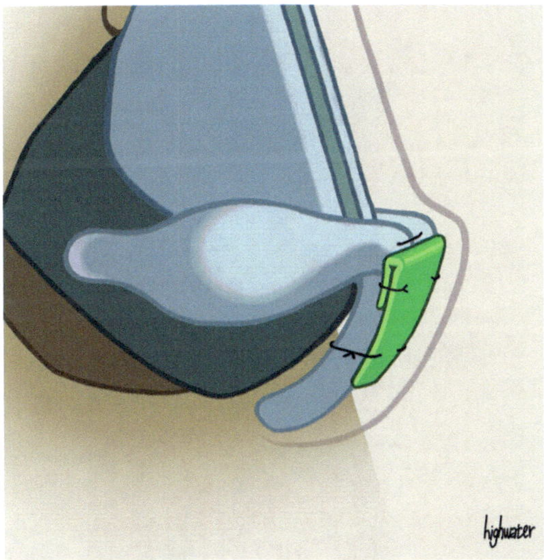

Fig. 9.6 Shield graft, the figure expresses the double-layered graft at the upper side. It is common to apply one layer

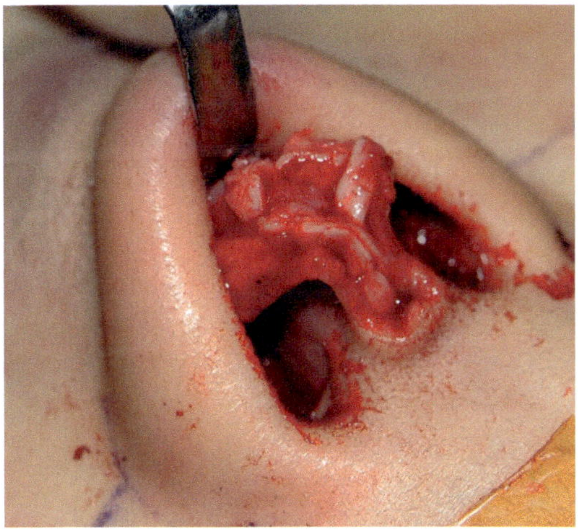

Fig. 9.7 Midcrural extension graft: Middle small rim of double conchal cartilage

The updated version of this chapter can be found at https://doi.org/10.1007/978-981-16-0542-0_9

E.-S. Dhong, M.-W. Na, *Asian Septorhinoplasty*, https://doi.org/10.1007/978-981-16-0542-0_18

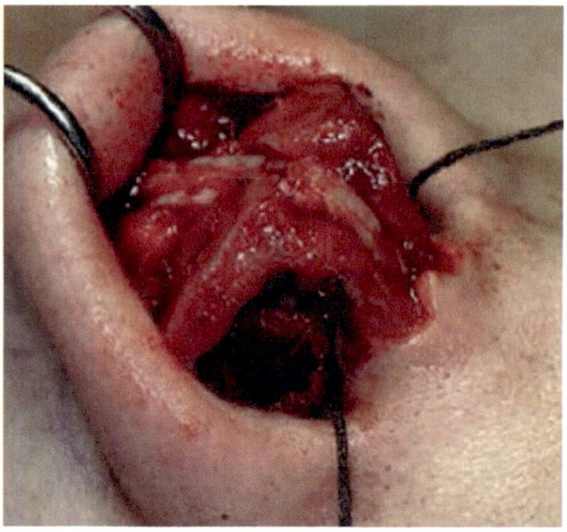

Fig. 9.8 Septal extension graft reaches to the middle crura modifying the tip-lobular angle

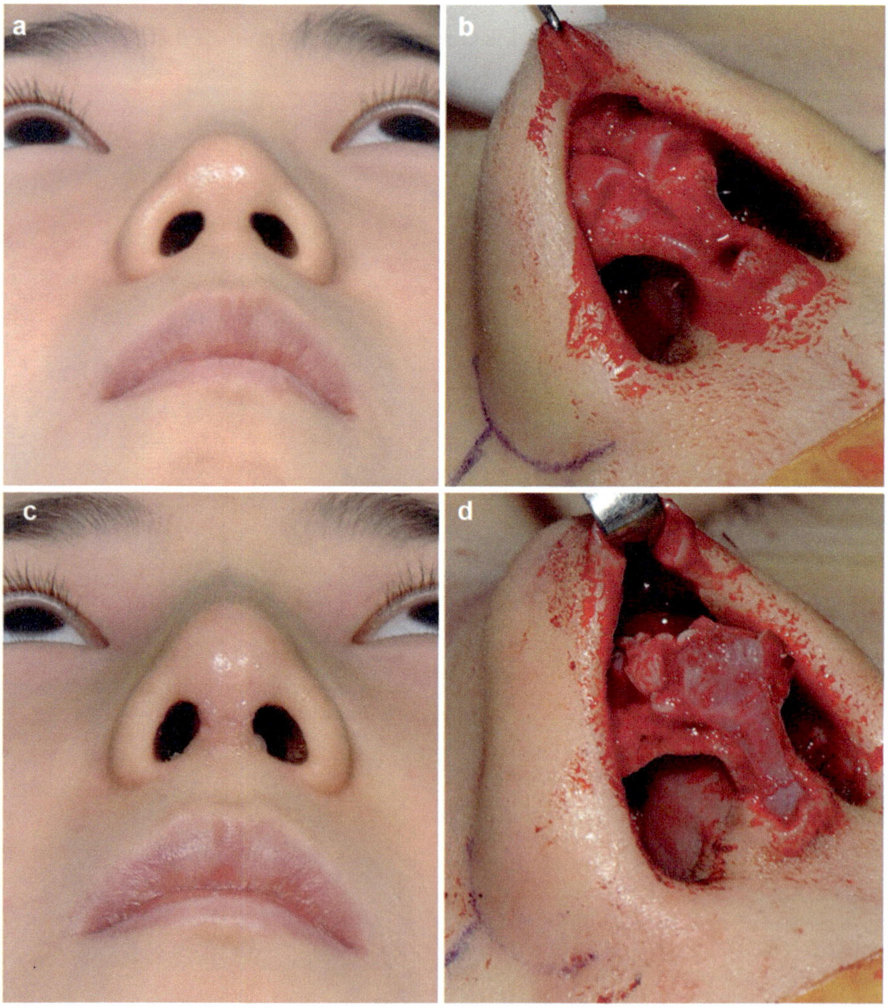

Fig. 9.10 Underdeveloped middle crura in primary rhinoplasty: reconstructed with midcrural extension graft and a shield graft. (**a**) Preoperative view. (**b**) Before the grafts. (**c**) Postoperative view. (**d**) Before closure

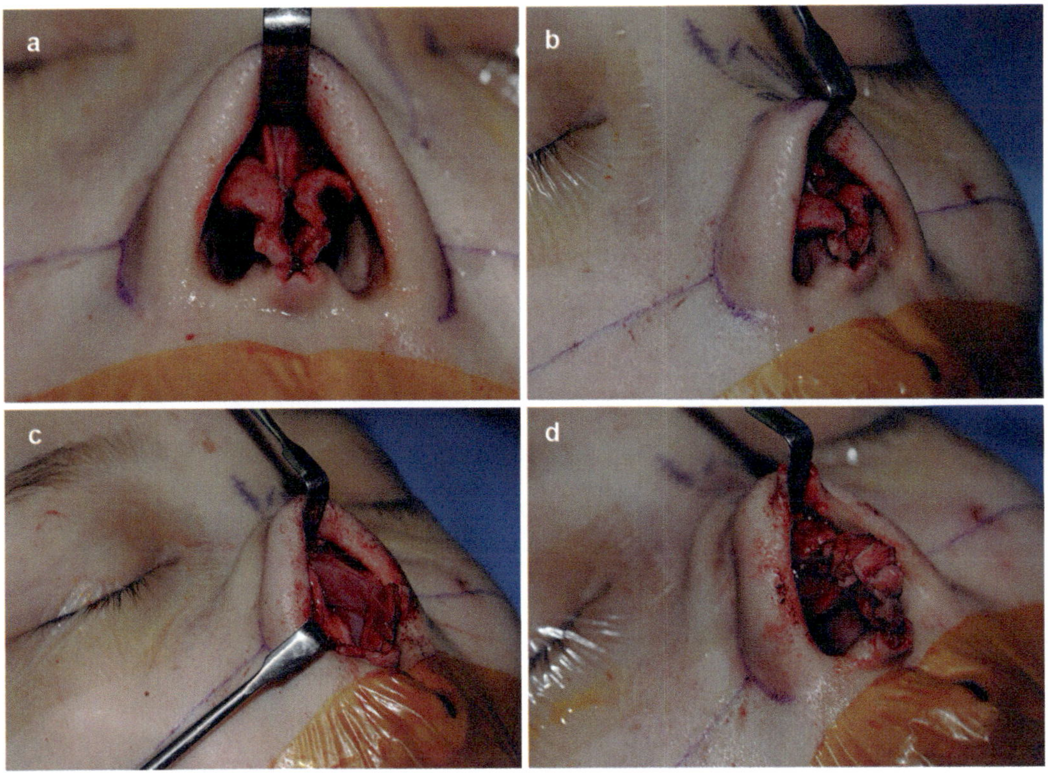

Fig. 9.11 Tortuous middle crura in primary rhinoplasty: Septal L-strut extension graft, shield graft, and a tip onlay graft using SMF (**a**, **b**) Intraoperative view before the grafts. (**c**) Septal L-strut extension graft. (**d**) Tip onlay graft

GPSR Compliance

The European Union's (EU) General Product Safety Regulation (GPSR) is a set of rules that requires consumer products to be safe and our obligations to ensure this.

If you have any concerns about our products, you can contact us on ProductSafety@springernature.com

In case Publisher is established outside the EU, the EU authorized representative is:

Springer Nature Customer Service Center GmbH
Europaplatz 3
69115 Heidelberg, Germany

Batch number: 10732823

Printed by Printforce, the Netherlands

Betätigungsorientierte Ergotherapie bei Morbus Parkinson

Springer Nature More Media App

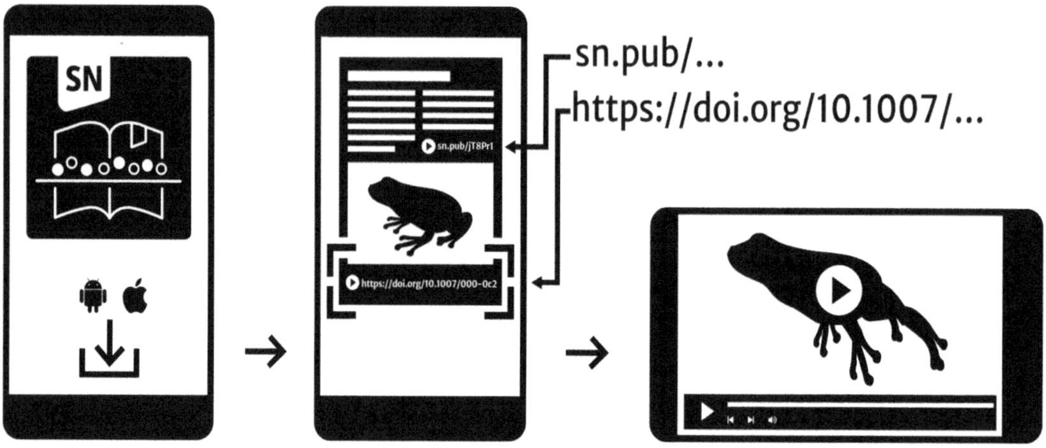

1.
Download

2.
Scan Link

3.
Enjoy Video

Amy Orellana

Betätigungsorientierte Ergotherapie bei Morbus Parkinson

Springer

Amy Orellana
Stuttgart, Deutschland

Die Online-Version des Buches enthält digitales Zusatzmaterial, das berechtigten Nutzern durch Anklicken der mit einem „Playbutton" versehenen Abbildungen zur Verfügung steht. Alternativ kann dieses Zusatzmaterial von Lesern des gedruckten Buches mittels der kostenlosen Springer Nature „More Media" App angesehen werden. Die App ist in den relevanten App-Stores erhältlich und ermöglicht es, das entsprechend gekennzeichnete Zusatzmaterial mit einem mobilen Endgerät zu öffnen.

Ergänzendes Material zu diesem Buch finden Sie auf http://link.springer.com.

ISBN 978-3-662-62582-8 ISBN 978-3-662-62583-5 (eBook)
https://doi.org/10.1007/978-3-662-62583-5

Die Deutsche Nationalbibliothek verzeichnet diese Publikation in der Deutschen Nationalbibliografie; detaillierte bibliografische Daten sind im Internet über http://dnb.d-nb.de abrufbar.

Planung/Lektorat: Eva-Maria Kania

Springer ist ein Imprint der eingetragenen Gesellschaft Springer-Verlag GmbH, DE und ist ein Teil von Springer Nature.
Die Anschrift der Gesellschaft ist: Heidelberger Platz 3, 14197 Berlin, Germany

Vorwort

Die einzigartige Stärke der Ergotherapie liegt in der betätigungs- und klientenorientierten sowie kontextbezogenen Arbeit. Nur so kann man der Individualität eines Menschen, der großen Vielfalt seiner Lebenswelt und dem extrem breiten Spektrum der Symptome bei M. Parkinson gerecht werden.

Wir Ergotherapeutinnen sind dazu ausgebildet, genau hinzusehen, den Menschen als Ganzes zu erfassen und ihn als Teil seiner Lebenswelt wahrzunehmen. Die Anwendung von ergotherapeutischen Modellen, das Assessment von Klientenzielen und die Durchführung einer Betätigungsanalyse sind passende Werkzeuge, um ergotherapeutisch in die Intervention zu starten. Kombiniert man dies mit aktuellen Erkenntnissen aus Studien zur Verbesserung der motorischen und psychischen Parkinson-Symptome, und kennt man auch die modernen technischen Hilfsmittel und Wohnraumanpassungen, ist eine umfassende Therapie gewährleistet.

Ich freue mich die Gelegenheit zu haben, meinen Kolleginnen umfangreiche Informationen und Ideen an die Hand zu geben, um den Klienten in Zukunft eine wirklich individuell angepasste ergotherapeutische Intervention bieten zu können. Der Grundgedanke ist, keine vorgefertigten Therapiemethoden zu liefern. Vielmehr finden Therapeutinnen hier eine Mischung aus fundierten wissenschaftlichen Erkenntnissen, Grundkonzepten zur Behandlung von M. Parkinson und konkreten Beispielen, wie beides in die Praxis umgesetzt werden kann. Mit diesen Werkzeugen wird die Therapeutin befähigt, einen auf die besondere Situation des Klienten passenden Therapieplan zu erstellen.

Weil ich eine gendergerechte Sprache wichtig finde und den Lesefluss aber nicht abbremsen will, habe ich gewählt, in jedem Kapitel abwechselnd Klient plus Therapeutin und anschließend Klientin plus Therapeut zu schreiben. Alle anderen Charaktere sind gemischt, wie im Leben (Ärztin, Angehöriger, Physiotherapeutin …).

Im Verlauf des Buches ist mal der Begriff „Klient", mal der Begriff „Patient" zu finden. Ich differenziere die Bezeichnung, je nachdem wie ich den Menschen wahrnehme. Geht es eher um den leidenden Kranken, erscheint meines Erachtens „Patient" passend, geht es um einen selbstwirksamen Menschen, trifft „Klient" besser zu.

Die Erkrankung „Morbus Parkinson" hat viele Bezeichnungen, z. B. „parkinsonsche Krankheit", „Parkinson", „MP". Ich habe mich auf „M. Parkinson" und „Parkinson-Erkrankung" beschränkt.

Mit dem allergrößten Respekt beende ich gerade den Prozess des Buchschreibens – Respekt für meine Klienten, die mit dieser komplexen Krankheit, Morbus Parkinson, leben. Immer wieder aufs Neue erlebe ich den kurzen Moment des Staunens, wenn aus einem starren Gesicht plötzlich ein breites Grinsen herausbricht. Wie viel positive Kraft viele Betroffene versprühen, obwohl die Liste der Einschränkungen lang ist. Mit anderen Klienten, deren klaren Blick auf das Leben ich häufig sehr bewundere, führe ich bewegende Gespräche.

Die meisten Menschen mit M. Parkinson können sich nicht mehr auf ihren Körper verlassen. Er zittert und stockt, bremst und beugt sich. Und trotzdem wird in der Ergotherapie gelaufen, gekocht und geschrieben – mit Cues, Repetitionen und fokussierter Aufmerksamkeit. Vielen herzlichen Dank an alle meine Klienten: beginnend mit dem ersten Klienten, mit dem ich zu Beginn meiner Arbeit ein Anziehtraining gemacht habe, bis zu denen, die sich für diese Publikation fotografieren ließen.

Ich empfinde Respekt für alle Wissenschaftlerinnen, Ärzte, Mit-Therapeutinnen und Kollegen anderer Fachrichtungen. Durch die Recherche für dieses Buch habe ich eine nicht endende Menge an Studien, Büchern, Leitlinien und Artikeln gefunden, ein Beitrag interessanter und faszinierender als der andere: Immer im Streben danach, die bestmögliche Unterstützung für die Klienten zu bieten. Besonders sticht hier ein Netzwerk an Wissenschaftlern und Therapeutinnen aus den Niederlanden hervor, die u. a. erstklassige ergotherapeutische Leitlinien für die Behandlung von M. Parkinson entwickelten (Sturkenboom et al. 2011).

Ich freue mich sehr, dass ich die Gelegenheit bekommen habe, auf den folgenden Seiten die Evidenz der Forschenden mit der Erfahrung aus der Praxis von zahlreichen Kolleginnen zusammenzubringen. Denn glauben Sie mir, ein Buch schreibt man nicht alleine! Auch wenn ich die Worte getippt habe.

Ohne Martina Hoch wäre ich niemals an den Punkt gekommen, ein Buch zu verfassen. Als meine Mentorin, Cheerleaderin und Freundin findet sich ihre Handschrift zwischen den Zeilen vom ersten bis zum letzten Kapitel. Sie ist unersetzlich! Danke auch Gunda Wolter, die mich auf die Idee gebracht hat und Florian Bracker, Ruth Hamilton, Christina Harms, Tony Seidl, Dr. Tim Vanbellingen, Stefanie Völler und vielen anderen für zahllose anregende Gespräche und Tipps aller Art.

Meinen Korrekturlesern Charlotte Bracker, Dr. Heinz Herbst, Martina Hoch, Maxie Karius, Alexandra Steibler, Dr. Claude Vaney und Gunda Wolter danke ich dafür, dass sie mir andere Sichtweisen, ergänzendes Wissen, Verbesserungen und ihre kostbare Zeit gegeben haben. Andreas Vogt danke ich für das wirklich ansprechende und gut durchdachte Design unseres Schaubildes „Perfect fit" in Kap. 4, welches er unermüdlich mit Martina Hoch und mir abstimmte.

Vielen Dank an die Mitarbeiter des Springer Verlags. Besonders an Eva-Maria Kania, sie ist die geduldigste Editorin der Welt und hat mich stets darin unterstützt, den Überblick über dieses Projekt zu behalten und im weiteren Verlauf dann Frau Niesel, die mir die Details der formalen Strukturierung optimal vermittelt hat. Meine eifrigen Fotografen Alistair Gill, Dalia,

Jade, Mateo und Juan Orellana, Alexandra Steibler und Catherine Suter haben mir geholfen, das Buch mit Leben zu füllen. Und dem unbekannten Mädchen mit Blumen in den Haaren, das an IHREM Einschulungstag MIR einen schönen Tag wünschte und damit meinen trüben Tag erhellte … Danke!

Ich wünsche allen Kolleginnen viel Spaß beim Lesen und vor allem beim Anwenden. Ich freue mich auf Rückmeldungen und Austausch.

Inhaltsverzeichnis

Teil III Assessmentphase

Teil IV Interventionsphase

Über die Autorin

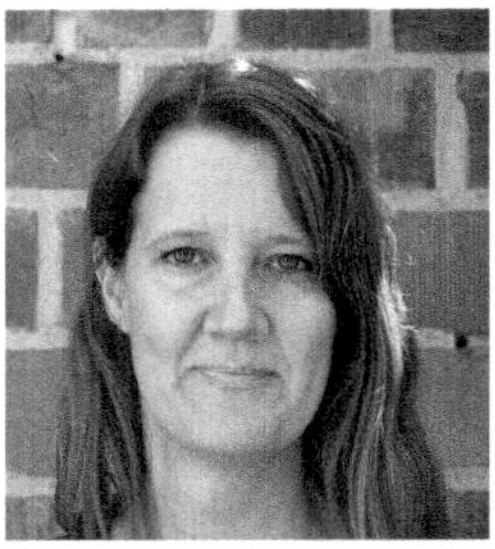

Amy Orellana ist begeisterte Ergotherapeutin mit langjähriger Erfahrung in vielfältigen Settings – Klinik, ambulante Rehabilitation, Praxen und als Selbständige –, jedoch immer in der Neurologie. Seit sie ihre Arbeit auf Klientenzentrierung umgestellt hat und sich auf Betätigung fokussiert, erfährt sie die Fülle der Sinnhaftigkeit ihres Berufs. Es ist für sie inspirierend zu sehen, wie Klienten ihre Probleme benennen, um anschließend selbstwirksam ihre Ziele zu formulieren und dann anzupacken.Sie freut sich, die Erkenntnisse aus der Praxis und Wissenschaft als Dozentin und Autorin sowie bei Vorträgen weiterzugeben. Der ständige Austausch mit einer Reihe von Fachkollegen sowie mit Betroffenen und ihren Angehörigen ist ihr sehr wichtig, um auf dem Laufenden zu bleiben und aus deren Erfahrungsschatz zu lernen. Frau Orellana ist immer an Neuem interessiert und bringt ihr Wissen gerne in innovative Projekte ein.

Teil I

Medizinische Grundlagen

1 Idiopathisches Parkinson-Syndrom

1.1 Hintergründe und Ursachen

Die komplexe Parkinson-Erkrankung mit ihren vielfältigen motorischen und nicht-motorischen Symptomen schreitet unaufhaltsam fort. Deshalb fordert sie den Betroffenen und seine Wegbegleiter, zu denen oftmals auch Ergotherapeutinnen gehören, kontinuierlich heraus. Die Lebensqualität wird von vielen Patienten als erheblich herabgesetzt eingestuft. Neben den Kardinalsymptomen Akinese, Tremor und Rigor rücken zunehmend auch die nicht-motorischen Symptome wie Depression, Apathie und Demenz in den Fokus klinischer Untersuchungen und gewinnen somit auch an Bedeutung in der medizinischen und therapeutischen Versorgung.

Ein immer größer werdender Anteil der Gesellschaft erkrankt jährlich an Morbus Parkinson (M. Parkinson). Dies hängt hauptsächlich mit der demografischen Entwicklung in der westlichen Welt zusammen. Durch den größeren Anteil alternder Menschen nimmt auch der Anteil der Menschen zu, die am idiopathischen Parkinson-Syndrom (IPS) erkranken. M. Parkinson ist nach Alzheimer die zweithäufigste neurodegenerative Erkrankung und tritt damit immer mehr ins Bewusstsein der Gesellschaft.

Prävalenz

In Deutschland sind laut der DPG (Deutsche Parkinson Gesellschaft e. V.) ca. 250.000 bis 280.000 Personen von M. Parkinson betroffen. Wissenschaftlerinnen gehen davon aus, dass sich die Anzahl der Menschen mit der Diagnose „Morbus Parkinson" zwischen 2020 und 2030 verdoppeln wird. Dies wird größtenteils durch die demografische Entwicklung bedingt; neuere Auswertungen der Daten weisen darauf hin, dass wahrscheinlich weitere, bisher unbekannte, äußere Faktoren die Zunahme der Krankheit begünstigen. Im Durchschnitt sind Patienten bei Diagnosestellung 60 Jahre alt. Mit zunehmendem Alter nimmt die Erkrankungswahrscheinlichkeit zu: Bei über 85-Jährigen ist die Erkrankungswahrscheinlichkeit fünf Mal höher als bei 60-Jährigen. Doch auch jüngere Menschen um die 40 Jahre können die Diagnose „Morbus Parkinson" erhalten, dies betrifft etwa 5 % der Menschen mit der Parkinson-Erkrankung.

Ätiologie

Die Ursache für IPS ist noch ungeklärt, deshalb heißt es **idiopathisches** Parkinson-Syndrom. Es spielen vermutlich eine Bandbreite unterschiedlicher Faktoren eine Rolle. Als größter Risikofaktor gilt das Alter. Die Wahrscheinlichkeit einer Erkrankung nimmt mit dem Alter zu.

Es gibt einen geringen genetischen Zusammenhang, mit 10–15 % Wahrscheinlichkeit einer Erkrankung bei familiärer Krankheitsgeschichte. Außerdem scheinen Umweltfaktoren einen auslösenden Effekt zu haben. IPS tritt regional

A. Orellana, *Betätigungsorientierte Ergotherapie bei Morbus Parkinson*,
https://doi.org/10.1007/978-3-662-62583-5_1

unterschiedlich stark auf. So ist in Europa, Nord- und Südamerika ein gehäuftes Auftreten feststellbar, im Gegensatz zu Asien, Afrika und den Arabischen Staaten.

Pestizide, Herbizide, Lösungsmittel (Trichlorethylen) und Schwermetalle konnten in einigen Studien mit M. Parkinson assoziiert werden. So stellten die Wissenschaftler*innen bei ländlich lebenden Menschen ein etwas erhöhtes Erkrankungsrisiko fest. Regelmäßiger Kaffeekonsum scheint einen schützenden Effekt zu haben und auch Raucher scheinen eine etwas geringere Erkrankungswahrscheinlichkeit zu haben, doch der kausale Zusammenhang ist nicht endgültig nachgewiesen. Forschungsergebnisse zu den Ursachen der Parkinson-Erkrankung sind noch uneindeutig und stehen häufig sogar im Widerspruch zueinander.

Pathophysiologie

Die pathologischen Abläufe im Körper eines Menschen mit Parkinson sind in den letzten Jahren gut untersucht worden, sodass diverse neue Erkenntnisse gewonnen werden konnten. Trotzdem sind die neuropathologischen Mechanismen nur zum Teil geklärt. Die meisten motorischen Symptome entstehen durch einen Dopaminmangel. Dieser kann wiederum auf den Untergang der Dopamin-produzierenden Zellen der Substantia nigra zurückgeführt werden. Wird das Gehirn von Menschen mit M. Parkinson *post mortem* untersucht, können in zahlreichen Nervenzellen sog. Lewykörperchen gefunden werden. Das sind abnormale Ansammlungen eines pathologisch gefalteten Proteins, dem α-Synuclein (siehe Abb. 1.1).

Braak et al. (2003) und Hawkes et al. (2007) stellten aufgrund Untersuchungen der α-Synucleine die Hypothese auf, dass M. Parkinson durch einen unbekannten Auslöser zunächst im Riechnerv und im Dünndarm beginnt und sich von dort entlang des Vagusnervs über Jahre nach oben bis zum Gehirn ausbreitet. Dabei wird α-Synuclein von Nervenzelle zu Nervenzelle übertragen. Der genaue Mechanismus der Übertragung ist unbekannt. Im Gehirn angekommen, gibt es laut Braak und Kollegen eine vorhersagbare topografische Sequenz, in der sich das Synuclein im gesamten Gehirn ausbreitet: beginnend im peripheren Nervensystem, über den unteren Hirnstamm, dann den oberen Hirnstamm, weiter über das Mittelhirn, in der sich auch die Substantia nigra befindet, später über den Mesokortex und als letztes zum Neokortex (siehe Abb. 1.2).

Diese genaue Abfolge konnten weitere Forscher nicht immer bestätigen. Es ist jedoch nachgewiesen, dass sich die Erkrankung nicht nur in der Substantia nigra manifestiert, sondern im gesamten Gehirn, und darüber hinaus im vegetativen Nervensystem und dem Verdauungstrakt. Die umfassende Beteiligung der einzelnen Gehirnabschnitte und des vegetativen Nervensystems erklärt die Komplexität des Krankheitsbildes und seines Verlaufs. Es begründet nicht nur die motorischen Symptome (Zelluntergang in der Substantia nigra – Dopaminmangel – Akinese, Rigor), sondern auch die vielfältigen nicht-motorischen Symptome (Verdauungsstörungen durch Beteiligung des N. vagus, Riechstörung durch Angriff auf den Riechnerv, Demenz durch Abbau der subkortikalen Strukturen, Schlafstörungen in REM-Phase – Hirnstamm …).

Die Ärzte, meist Neurologen, stellen die Diagnose „Morbus Parkinson" nach dem klinischen Bild. Das heißt, dass, obwohl meist schon Jahre vorher einzelne unspezifische Symptome auftreten (Riechstörung, REM-Schlaf-Verhaltensstörung, Verstopfung, Depressionen), die Diagnose erst gestellt werden kann, wenn die motorischen Symptome deutlich werden (Bradykinese, Rigor, Tremor).

Die motorischen Symptome sind auf den Dopaminmangel in der Substantia nigra zurückzuführen und treten erst auf, wenn ca. 80 % der Dopamin-produzierenden Zellen untergegangen sind. Davor kompensiert das Gehirn die Funktionsstörungen durch eine Überaktivierung des Kortex. Wie im Gehirnschnitt in Abb. 1.3 deutlich erkennbar ist, ist der pathologische Prozess sichtbar. Die Substantia nigra (schwarze Substanz) ist im gesunden Gehirn durch die hohe Dichte an dopaminergen Neuronen schwarz gefärbt, im Gehirn eines Parkinson-Betroffenen verliert dieser Bereich seine Farbe.

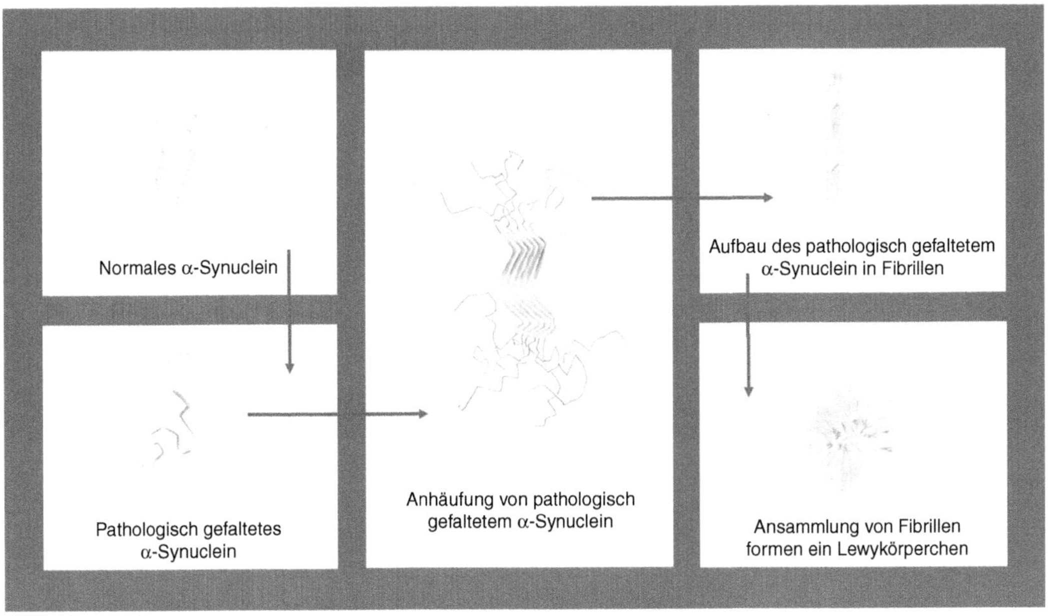

Abb. 1.1 Entstehung von Lewykörperchen durch die Ansammlung pathologisch gefalteter α-Synucleine

Abb. 1.2 Ausbreitung von Lewykörperchen vom peripheren Nervensystem über die Medulla oblongata, das Pontine tegmentum, das basale Mittel- und Vorderhirn, den Hypothalamus, den Thalamus, den Mesocortex und Allocortex bis zum Neocortex. (Abbildung mit freundlicher Genehmigung von Anthony E. Lang)

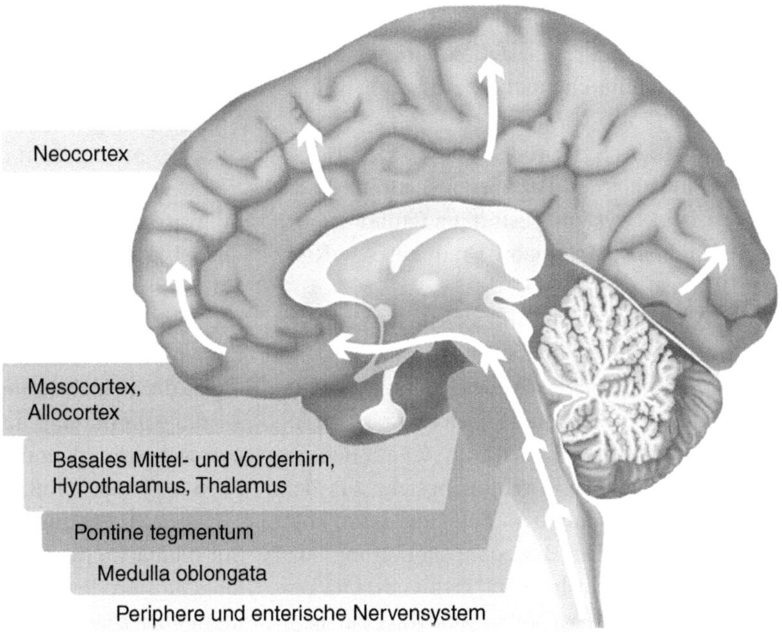

► Der M. Parkinson beginnt schon Jahre vor der Diagnosestellung. Einzelne unspezifische Symptome können rückblickend mit der beginnenden Erkrankung in Zusammenhang gebracht werden, doch erst, wenn ca. 80 % der Substantia nigra untergegangen ist, treten die Parkinson-typischen Symptome auf.

Dopamin ist ein Neurotransmitter, welcher viele Funktionen im Gehirn erfüllt. Er trägt zum

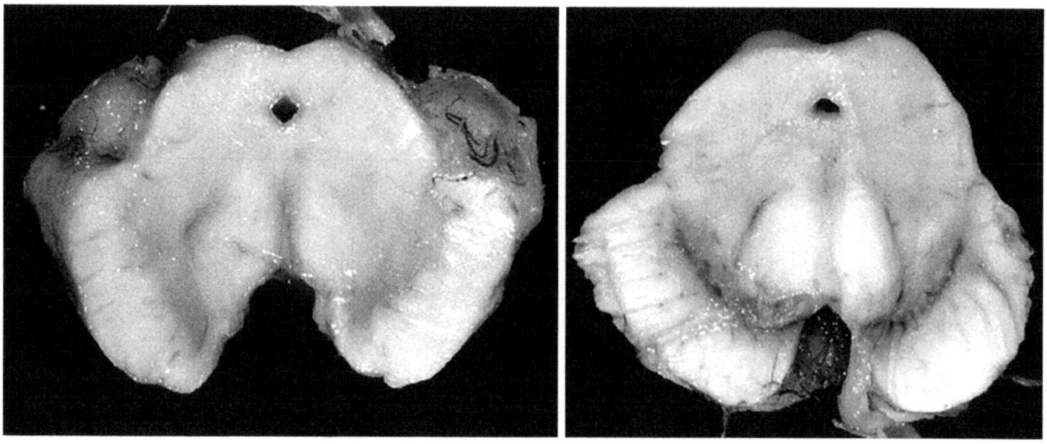

Abb 1.3 Links: pathologische Veränderung entfärbte Substantia nigra. Rechts: gesundes Gehirn mit typischer schwarzer Färbung des Kerngebiets, Substantia nigra. (Mit freundlicher Genehmigung von D.P. Agamanolis, An illustrated interactive course for medical students and residents, www.neuropathology-web.org)

Glücksempfinden bei und motiviert als „Belohnungshormon" zum Bewegen und Lernen. Außerdem wirkt Dopamin vasodilatatorisch (gefäßerweiternd) und spielt bei der Verdauungsregelung eine Rolle. Zusätzlich wirkt es bei der Bewegungsinitiierung und -koordination mit.

Nigrostriatales System

Beim idiopathischen Parkinson-Syndrom ist das nigrostriatale System gestört und führt zu den drei Kardinalsymptomen: Bradykinese, Rigor und Tremor.

Im Mittelhirn sitzen die Basalganglien – zu diesen gehört u. a. die Substantia nigra, deren Zellen Dopamin bilden. Außerdem ist in den Basalganglien das Striatum (Streifenkörper) zu finden, welches im Gehirnschnitt tatsächlich gestreift aussieht. Das Striatum besteht aus dem Nucleus caudatus und dem Putamen. Beim komplexen Ablauf der Bewegungsinitiierung sind verschiedene Gehirnbereiche involviert. Das nigrostiatale System hat dabei sowohl eine hemmende, als auch eine enthemmende – also initiierende Rolle.

In Abb. 1.4 wird die motorische Schleife dargestellt. In der Großhirnrinde – genauer gesagt, vom motorischen Kortex und dem prämotorischen Kortex – wird ein Bewegungsplan erstellt (Bewegungsvorbereitung). Dieser wird über afferente Nervenbahnen mit dem Neurotransmitter Glutamat zur Substantia nigra weitergeleitet. Von der Substantia nigra führen Nervenbahnen als sog. nigrostriatale Bahn weiter, deren Neurotransmitter Dopamin ist. Auf diesem Weg hemmt die Substantia nigra das Striatum. Das Striatum hat (wenn es nicht gehemmt wird) einen hemmenden Effekt auf motorische Impulse. Diese komplexe motorische Schleife hemmt also die Inhibition und wirkt so bewegungsinitiierend. Dieser Bewegungsimpuls wird über den Thalamus zum Kortex geleitet, der über das Rückenmark die Muskelaktivität einleitet. Das nigrostriatale System regelt die Feinabstimmung der Motorik, die Bewegungsinitiierung, automatisierte Bewegungen und wahrscheinlich die lokomotorischen Reaktionen auf externe Reize.

Beim M. Parkinson ist die Verbindung von der Substantia nigra zum Striatum defizitär, da die Dopamin-produzierenden Zellen der Substantia nigra absterben. Ohne diesen wichtigen Neurotransmitter findet keine Hemmung des Striatums statt. Deswegen tritt das hemmende Attribut des Striatums in den Vordergrund und es zeigen sich die charakteristischen Krankheitszeichen des M. Parkinson: Bradykinese – bis hin zu Akinese, Freezing und der erhöhte Grundtonus, der Rigor.

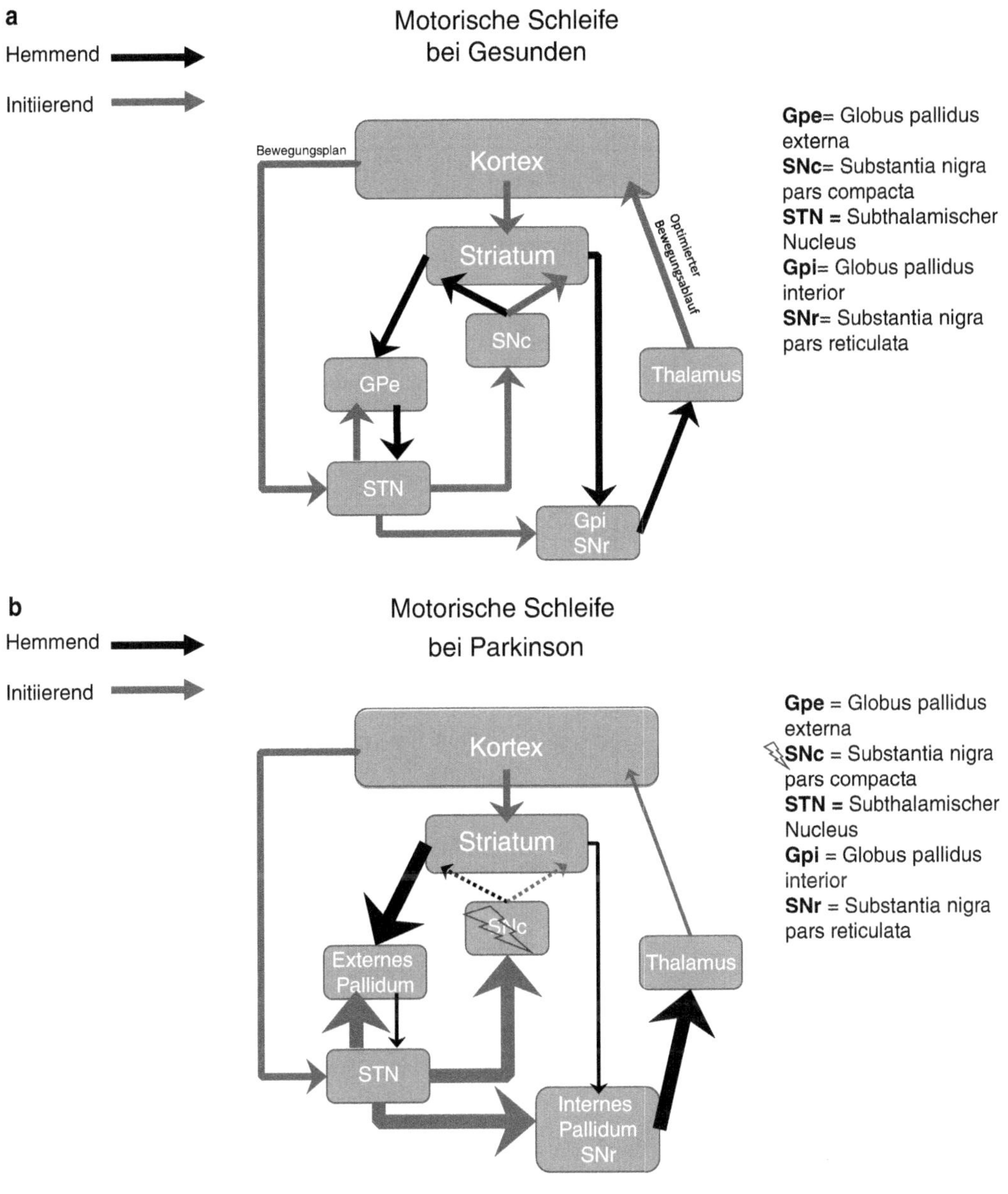

Abb. 1.4 Motorische Schleife

1.2 Stadieneinteilung

Der M. Parkinson ist eine degenerative Erkrankung mit progredientem Symptomverlauf. Der Verlauf der Krankheit ist von Mensch zu Mensch unterschiedlich.

- Sowohl die Schwere der Erkrankung als auch die Zusammenstellung der Symptome sowie die Geschwindigkeit, mit der sie voranschreitet, variiert stark, sodass kein Klient dem anderen gleicht.

Schon Jahre vor dem Auftreten der ersten motorischen Symptome, leiden die meisten Patienten an nicht-motorischen Symptomen wie Depressionen, Riechstörung, Verstopfung und Schlafstörungen mit REM-Schlaf-Verhaltensstörung. Die motorischen Symptome beginnen normalerweise unilateral. Im späteren Verlauf wird auch die kontralaterale Seite betroffen, wobei die Symptome auf der zuerst betroffenen Seite meist die schwerer ausgeprägten bleiben. Mit dem Eintreten der motorischen Symptome kann die Diagnose gestellt werden.

Stadien nach Hoehn und Yahr

Zur Einteilung in Stadien der Erkrankung und um die Schwere der Erkrankung einschätzen zu können, wird die Hoehn und Yahr-Skala (siehe Tab. 1.1) verwendet. Obwohl nicht alle Patienten die Stadien identisch durchlaufen und die nicht-motorischen Symptome außer Acht gelassen werden, ist sie eine international anerkannte Einteilung und bietet eine gute Richtlinie.

Krankheitsprogression

Die Geschwindigkeit, mit der die Parkinson-Erkrankung voranschreitet, variiert stark von Patient zu Patient. Um einen groben Anhaltspunkt zu geben, kann die Tabelle zur Krankheitsprogression genutzt werden, in der gezeigt wird, dass die Progression von einem Stadium zum nächsten im Durchschnitt 2–2,5 Jahre dauert.

Hoehn und Yahr-Stadium	Mittlere Zeit vom Krankheitsbeginn
II	2,9 Jahre
III	5,5 Jahre
IV	7,5 Jahre
V	9,7 Jahre

Krankheitsprogression nach Hoehn und Yahr-Stadien im „Off" (Marttila und Rinne 1977).

Es wurde lange davon ausgegangen, dass die Krankheit von Patienten mit Tremor als Erstsymptom etwas weniger schnell fortschreitet. Mehrfach zweifelten Wissenschaftler dies jedoch an.

Tab. 1.1 Stadien nach Hoehn und Yahr

Stadieneinteilung nach Hoehn und Yahr	
Stadium	Beschreibung
1	Unilaterale Symptomatik, mit minimaler oder keiner funktionellen Einschränkung.
2	Bilaterale Symptomatik oder Beteiligung der Mittellinie, ohne Einschränkung der Balance.
3	Erste Anzeichen für eingeschränkte Stellreflexe, Unsicherheit beim Drehen und Retro- oder Propulsion. Leichte bis mittlere funktionelle Einschränkungen, im Alltag jedoch noch selbständig.
4	Voll ausgeprägte stark behindernde Symptomatik. Patient kann noch ohne Hilfe Stehen und Laufen (evtl. mit Hilfsmittel), ist jedoch deutlich beeinträchtigt.
5	Hilfsbedürftig beim Aufstehen aus Bett oder Rollstuhl.

Heute geht man von anderen Faktoren aus, die die Schwere und Geschwindigkeit beeinflussen. In einer Studie konnten Fereshtehnejad et al. (2015) drei nicht-motorische Faktoren identifizierten, die die Wahrscheinlichkeit eines schwereren Verlaufs und einer rapiden Progression erhöhen. Wurden **orthostatische Hypotonie**, **REM-Schlafverhaltensstörungen** und **kognitive Defizite** diagnostiziert, war der Verlauf wesentlich schwerer und schneller fortschreitend. Standen hingegen die motorischen Symptome im Vordergrund, war die Prognose besser.

Betroffene und Angehörige haben eine große Angst vor einem besonders schweren Verlauf oder einem frühen Tod durch die Parkinson-Erkrankung. Beim IPS sind nur 5 % der Erkrankten im späteren Verlauf der Erkrankung auf einen Rollstuhl angewiesen oder bettlägerig. Am idiopathischen Parkinson-Syndrom stirbt man nicht, sondern an dessen Sekundärfolgen wie z. B. Pneumonie(durch Schluckstörung). Die Lebenserwartung von Menschen mit dem idiopathischen Parkinson-Syndrom liegt, dank heutiger Medikamente, nur minimal unterhalb der von Nicht-Betroffenen. Die atypischen Parkinson-Syndrome haben jedoch meist schwerere Verläufe mit einer schlechteren Prognose.

1.3 Kardinalsymptome

Der M. Parkinson ist durch ein großes Spektrum an verschiedenen Symptomen gekennzeichnet. Die Diagnosestellung erfolgt immer aufgrund der klinischen Symptomatik. Die detaillierten Symptombeschreibungen sind in Kap. 14 zu finden. Hier ein kurzer Überblick:

Die drei Kardinalsymptome des M. Parkinson sind:

- Bradykinese (oft als Akinese bezeichnet),
- Rigor,
- Tremor.

Es muss zwingend eine Bradykinese und mindestens eines der weiteren Kardinalsymptome feststellbar sein, um die Diagnose sicherzustellen.

Bradykinese
Das auffälligste Merkmal der Parkinson-Erkrankung ist die Bewegungsarmut. Die Motorik der Betroffenen ist verlangsamt und weniger ausladend. Vor allem die unbewusste spontane Motorik ist reduziert, was sich in der Mimik, Gestik und dem Armpendeln beim Laufen zeigt. Der Klient wirkt von außen oftmals matt und ausdruckslos.

- Akinese = A-kinese = keine Bewegung
- Bradykinese = Brady-kinese = verlangsamte Bewegung
- Hypokinese = Hypo-kinese = Unterbewegung (weniger ausladend)

Für eine ausführliche Beschreibung der Bradykinese siehe Abschn. 14.1.1.

Rigor
Der erhöhte Muskeltonus im gesamten Körper, der für die Parkinson-Erkrankung typisch ist, wird Rigor genannt. Bei passiver Mobilisation ist ein wächserner Widerstand spürbar, die Betroffenen nehmen den Rigor als konstante Tonuserhöhung wahr, der jede Bewegung bremst. Dadurch wirken Bewegungen zäh und die Haltung ist vornübergebeugt. Für eine ausführliche Beschreibung des Rigor siehe Abschn. 14.2.1.

Tremor
Bei etwa 70 % der Menschen mit M. Parkinson tritt ein Tremor auf. Der Parkinson-typische Tremor ist der einseitig beginnende Ruhetremor. Es kann jedoch auch Halte- und Bewegungstremor oder eine Kombination auftreten. Der Parkinson-Tremor hat im Gegensatz zum essentiellen Tremor eine langsame Frequenz und größere Amplitude. Für eine ausführliche Beschreibung des Tremors siehe Abschn. 14.3.1.

1.4 Weitere motorische Symptome

Posturale Stabilität
Durch das fehlende Zusammenspiel von Stellreflexen, Aufrichtung und Kraft in der unteren Extremität resultiert eine erhöhte Stand- und Gangunsicherheit. Die posturale Instabilität tritt meist im späteren Krankheitsverlauf auf und führt zu akuter Sturzgefahr. Für eine ausführliche Beschreibung der Posturalen Stabilität siehe Abschn. 14.4.1.

Automatisierte Bewegungen
Bei zahlreichen Betätigungen im Alltag werden automatisierte Bewegungen benötigt, um zwei oder mehr Bewegungsabläufe gleichzeitig durchzuführen. Die Durchführung von automatisierten Bewegungen ist bei Menschen mit M. Parkinson eingeschränkt. Die Bewegungen werden ungenau und es kommt zu Freezing-Episoden. Für eine ausführliche Beschreibung der Einschränkung von automatisierten Bewegungen siehe Abschn. 14.5.1.

Dystonie
Eine Dystonie kann sich als Primärsymptom oder als Folge einer Langzeiteinnahme von L-Dopa im Rahmen der Parkinson-Erkrankung

manifestieren. Dabei treten unwillkürliche Kontraktionen der quergestreiften Muskulatur auf, die zu Haltungsanomalien, verzerrter Mimik und verdrehten Bewegungen und Fehlstellungen führen kann. Meist ist eine Verschlechterung der Dystonie mit Abnahme der Medikamentenwirkung festzustellen. Für eine ausführliche Beschreibung der Dystonie siehe Abschn. 14.6.1.

Haltungsanomalien – Kamptokormie, Pisa-Syndrom, Anterocollis

Bei der Parkinson-Erkrankung sind häufig verschiedene Haltungsanomalien feststellbar, dazu gehören die Kamptokormie, das Pisa-Syndrom und der Anterocollis.

Kamptokormie

Die Kamptokormie ist eine stark ausgeprägte Rumpfkyphose von mindestens 45°, evtl. mit einer Seitneigung kombiniert. Sie ist nur in der aufrechten Körperposition sichtbar, im Liegen ist sie vollkommen reversibel. Für eine ausführliche Beschreibung der Kamptokormie siehe Abschn. 14.7.1.

Anterocollis

Tritt eine starke Flexion im Nacken auf, spricht man von Anterocollis (auch Antecollis). Die Ursachen sind noch ungeklärt. Für eine ausführliche Beschreibung des Anterocollis siehe Abschn. 14.7.2.

Pisa-Syndrom

Bei einer seitlichen Achsenabweichung ab 10° spricht man vom Pisa-Syndrom. Die Ursachen sind nicht abschließend geklärt, eine knöcherne Veränderung wie bei der Skoliose ist nicht der primäre Auslöser. Für eine ausführliche Beschreibung des Pisa-Syndrom siehe Abschn. 14.7.3.

1.5 Kognitiv/psychische Symptome

Übersicht

James Parkinson beschrieb schon vor 200 Jahren die motorischen Symptome der Erkrankung sehr genau. Die nicht-motorischen Symptome wurden lange Zeit unterschätzt. In den letzten 20 Jahren sind die nicht-motorischen Symptome, im Englischen non-motor symptoms oder NMS, vermehrt in den Fokus gerückt. Dies hat auch mit der Veränderung von Denkmustern im Gesundheitswesen zu tun – weg vom Hierarchiedenken, mit dem Arzt als Überfigur – hin zu Klientenzentrierung, mit dem Menschen im Mittelpunkt. Befragt man nämlich jene Menschen, die es am besten wissen, die Klienten selbst, welche Symptome sie am meisten einschränken, werden zuerst die nicht-motorischen Symptome genannt.

Untersuchungen kommen zu den Ergebnissen, dass 98,6 % der Menschen mit M. Parkinson nicht-motorische Symptome haben. Im Durchschnitt haben Morbus-Parkinson-Patienten acht verschiedene NMS, die, wie auch die motorischen Symptome, in den Off-Phasen verstärkt auftreten.

Die nicht-motorischen Symptome können in drei Untergruppen eingeteilt werden (Tab. 1.2).

Psychische Symptome

Die vielschichtigen psychischen Symptome mit ihren komplexen Ursachen und Zusammenhängen stellen ein lange Zeit unterschätztes Gebiet für die Medizin und Therapie von M. Parkinson dar.

Tab. 1.2 Nicht-motorische Symptome bei M. Parkinson

Kognitiv/psychisch	Vegetativ	Sensorisch/Schmerz
Demenz	Dranginkontinenz	Dysästhesien
Depressionen	Schweißausbrüche	Akathisie
Ängste/Phobien	Dyspnoe	Restless-Legs-Syndrom
Fatigue	Orthostatische Hypotension	Hyposmie
Apathie	Sexuelle Dysfunktion	Schmerzen
Schlafstörungen	Seborrea	
Exzessive Tagesschläfrigkeit	Blasen Dysfunktion	
Psychotische Episoden mit visuellen Halluzinationen	Obstipation	

Stress

Der Auslöser von Stress bei Menschen mit der Parkinson-Erkrankung variiert stark. Dazu gehören z. B. Zeitdruck, Angst vor Stürzen, Sorge um die Arbeit, belastete Partnerschaft … Der Stress führt oftmals zu vermehrter Anspannung, welche die Parkinson-Symptome wiederrum verstärkt. Dadurch entstehen beim Klienten negative Gedanken, die wieder zu mehr Stress führen. Dies nennt man „negativer Stresszirkel“. Für eine ausführliche Beschreibung von Stress siehe Abschn. 14.8.1.

Kognitive Einschränkungen/Demenz

Etwa 48–80 % der Menschen mit M. Parkinson entwickeln im Laufe der Erkrankung eine Demenz. Dabei sind vor allem Aufmerksamkeit, Merkfähigkeit, Exekutivfunktionen und räumlich visuelle Wahrnehmung auffällig. Eine Demenz hat einen stark negativen Einfluss auf die Lebensqualität der Betroffenen. Für eine ausführliche Beschreibung von Demenz und kognitiven Einschränkungen siehe Abschn. 14.9.1.

Depressionen

Depressionen treten häufig bei Parkinson-Betroffenen auf (ca. 40 %). Sie können als Reaktion auf die Diagnosestellung, abnehmende Funktionen oder reduzierte Lebensqualität auftreten (reaktive Ursache) oder ein Primärsymptom des M. Parkinson sein. Typische Kennzeichen einer Depression sind Gefühle von innerer Leere und Hoffnungslosigkeit, Müdigkeit, Gereiztheit und Suizidgedanken. Für eine ausführliche Beschreibung von Depression siehe Abschn. 14.10.1.

Ängste/Phobien

Ängste und Phobien erscheinen im Zusammenhang mit dem idiopathischen Parkinson-Syndrom gehäuft. Vor allem treten soziale Phobien auf, als Angst vor sozialen Situationen, in denen die Symptome des Betroffenen in der Öffentlichkeit offensichtlich sind. Folglich ist meist ein sozialer Rückzug zu beobachten. Für eine ausführliche Beschreibung von Ängsten siehe Abschn. 14.10.1.

Fatigue

Die Fatigue (auch Erschöpfungssyndrom) ist von einer totalen geistigen, psychischen und/oder körperlichen Erschöpfung gekennzeichnet, bei der die Betroffenen eine extreme Energielosigkeit verspüren und folglich inaktiv bleiben. Für eine ausführliche Beschreibung der Fatigue siehe Abschn. 14.11.1.

Apathie

Klienten, die von Apathie betroffen sind, wirken nach außen passiv. Emotionen, Interesse und Motivation sind reduziert, ohne dass eine Niedergeschlagenheit vorliegt. Dies führt zu teilweise langanhaltender Inaktivität, wenn von außen keine Aufforderung erfolgt (s. Tab. 1.3). Für eine ausführliche Beschreibung von Apathie siehe Abschn. 14.12.1.

Tab. 1.3 Übersicht zur Abgrenzung unterschiedlicher nicht-motorischer Symptome bei M. Parkinson

	Fatigue/ Erschöpfungssyndrom	Exzessive Tagesschläfrigkeit	Apathie	Depression
Unaushaltbare Müdigkeit, überwältigende Erschöpfung, Energielosigkeit	Stark ausgeprägt	tendenziell	tendenziell	tendenziell
Besserung nach Schlaf oder Erholung		✓		
Desinteresse an Aktivität			✓	✓
Niedergeschlagenheit				✓

Schlafstörungen
Die meisten Menschen mit der Parkinson-Erkrankung sind von Schlafstörungen betroffen (ca. 80 %). Häufiges nächtliches Aufwachen und Schwierigkeiten wieder einzuschlafen, ausgelöst durch unterschiedliche Einflussfaktoren wie Restless-Legs-Syndrom, Schmerzen und Medikamentenwirkung, prägen das Symptom und führen zu exzessiver Tagesschläfrigkeit. Für eine ausführliche Beschreibung von Schlafstörungen siehe Abschn. 14.13.1.

RBD (REM-Schlaf-Verhaltensstörung)
RBD steht für Rapid Eye Movement-sleep-behaviour-disorder (REM-Schlaf-Verhaltensstörung), bei der Träume aktiv ausgelebt werden, da die Muskeln im Schlaf nicht erschlaffen. Dieses Symptom ist eines der Frühsymptome für das idiopathische Parkinson-Syndrom. Für eine ausführliche Beschreibung der RBD siehe Abschn. 14.13.2.

Exzessive Tagesschläfrigkeit
Ursache für exzessive Tagesschläfrigkeit können Schlafstörungen oder eine ungünstige Medikamenteneinstellung sein. Betroffene fühlen sich häufig müde und müssen tagsüber Schlafpausen einlegen. Für eine ausführliche Beschreibung der exzessiven Tagesschläfrigkeit siehe Abschn. 14.13.

Psychotische Episoden mit visuellen Halluzinationen
Die Psychose bei IPS ist ein Oberbegriff für ein klinisches Spektrum. Dazu gehören verschiedene kognitive Störungen, Wahrnehmungsstörungen, Halluzinationen (meist visuell), Wahnvorstellungen, Verwirrtheit und paranoide Wahrnehmungsverarbeitung. Für eine ausführliche Beschreibung der Bradykinese siehe Abschn. 14.14.1.

1.6 Vegetative Symptome

Das vegetative Nervensystem reguliert die Funktion der inneren Organe und Gefäße und kann beim M. Parkinson von zahlreichen Einschränkungen betroffen sein. Dazu gehören:

- Dranginkontinenz
- Hautveränderungen
- Vermehrtes Schwitzen
- Seborrhoische Dermatitis
- Fettige Haut
- Dyspnoe
- Orthostatische Hypotension
- Sexuelle Dysfunktion
- Verstopfung

Für eine ausführliche Beschreibung der verschiedenen vegetativen Symptome siehe Abschn. 14.15.1.

1.7 Sensorische/ Schmerzsymptome

Dysästhesien
Es können Hypästhesien oder Parästhesien, meist im Zusammenhang mit dem Restless-Legs-Syndrom beobachtet werden. Für eine ausführliche Beschreibung von Dysästhesien siehe Abschn. 14.16.1.

Akathisie
Akathisie ist eine starke Unruhe, die die Betroffenen ständig in Bewegung hält. Für eine ausführliche Beschreibung von Akathisie siehe Abschn. 14.16.1.

Restless-Legs-Syndrom
Beim Restless-Legs-Syndrom empfinden die Betroffenen eine Unruhe mit Parästhesien in den Beinen, welches nur durch aktive Bewegung gelindert wird.

Hyposmie
Als eines der ersten Frühsymptome des IPS tritt häufig eine Hyposmie (Riechstörung), schon Jahre vor Diagnosestellung auf. Patienten können Gerüche nur reduziert wahrnehmen und nicht gut unterscheiden.

Schmerzsyndrome
Schmerzen, vor allem im Rücken, sind bei Parkinson-Betroffenen häufig anzutreffen. Die Ursachen sind vielfältig, z. B. Rigor, Dystonie und Bewegungsmangel. Für eine ausführliche Beschreibung der Schmerzsyndrome siehe Abschn. 14.17.1.

Dysfunktion der sensomotorischen Integration und Propriozeption
Die Verarbeitung von sensomotorischen und propriozeptiven Reizen ist bei den meisten Menschen mit M. Parkinson gestört, was zu ungenauer Motorik und nicht vollständigen Aufrichtung des Oberkörpers führt. Für eine ausführliche Beschreibung der Dysfunktion der sensomotorischen Integration und Propriozeption siehe Abschn. 14.18.1.

Literatur und weiterführende Literatur

Balleine B, O'Doherty J (2010) Human and rodent homologies in action control: corticostriatal determinants of goal-directed and habitual action. Neuropsychopharmacology 35:48–69. https://doi.org/10.1038/npp.2009.131

Braak H, Del Tredici K, Rüb U, de Vos R, Jansen Steur E, Braak E (2003) Staging of brain pathology related to sporadic Parkinson's disease. Neurobiol Aging 24(2):197–211. https://doi.org/10.1016/s0197-4580(02)00065-9. PMID: 12498954

Brown R, Jahanshahi M (1995) Depression in Parkinson's disease: a psychosocial viewpoint. Adv Neurol 65:61–84. PMID: 7872153

Deuschl G, Bain P, Brin M (1998) Consensus statement of the movement disorder society on tremor. Ad Hoc Scientific Committee. Mov Disord 13(Suppl 3):2–23. https://doi.org/10.1002/mds.870131303. PMID: 9827589

Deuschl G, Oertel W, Reichmann H (2016) Leitlinien für Diagnostik und Therapie in der Neurologie Idiopathisches Parkinson-Syndrom Entwicklungsstufe: S3 Kurzversion, DGN, Marburg

Fereshtehnejad S, Romenets SR, Anang JBM, Latreille V, Gagnon J, Postuma RB (2015) New Clinical Subtypes of Parkinson Disease and Their Longitudinal Progression: A Prospective Cohort Comparison With Other Phenotypes. JAMA Neurol 72(8):863–873. https://doi.org/10.1001/jamaneurol.2015.0703

GBD (2016) Parkinson's disease collaborators. Global, regional, and national burden of Parkinson's disease, 1990–2016: a systematic analysis for the Global Burden of Disease Study 2016. Lancet Neurol 17(11):939–953. https://doi.org/10.1016/S1474-4422(18)30295-3. Epub 2018 Oct 1. PMID: 30287051; PMCID: PMC6191528.

Hacke W, Mair J, Berg D (2019) Neurologie. Springer, Berlin, S 47–51, 96, 589–604

Hawkes CH, Del Tredici K, Braak H (2007) Parkinson's disease: a dual-hit hypothesis. Neuropathol Appl Neurobiol 33(6):599–614. https://doi.org/10.1111/j.1365-2990.2007.00874.x. Epub 2007 Oct 24. PMID: 17961138; PMCID: PMC7194308

Hemmerle AM, Herman JP, Seroogy KB (2012) Stress, depression and Parkinson's disease. Exp Neurol 233(1):79–86. https://doi.org/10.1016/j.expneurol.2011.09.035. Epub 2011 Oct 6. PMID: 22001159; PMCID: PMC3268878

van Hilten J, Weggeman M, van der Velde E, Kerkhof G, van Dijk J, Roos R (1993) Sleep, excessive daytime sleepiness and fatigue in Parkinson's disease. J Neural Transm Park Dis Dement Sect 5(3):235–244. https://doi.org/10.1007/BF02257678. PMID: 8369103

Hoehn MM, Yahr MD (1967) Parkinsonism: onset, progression, and mortalityNeurology 50(2):318 and 16 pages following. https://doi.org/10.1212/wnl.50.2.318. PMID: 9484345.

Joshi N, Singh S (2018) Updates on immunity and inflammation in Parkinson disease pathology. J Neurosci Res 96(3):379–390. https://doi.org/10.1002/jnr.24185

Kidron D, Melamed E (1987) Forms of dystonia in patients with Parkinson's disease. Neurology 37(6):1009–1011. https://doi.org/10.1212/wnl.37.6.1009. PMID: 3587617

Konczak J, Corcos D, Horak F, Poizner H, Shapiro M, Tuite P, Volkmann J, Maschke M (2009) Proprioception and motor control in Parkinson's disease. J Mot

Behav 41(6):543–552. https://doi.org/10.3200/35-09-002. PMID: 19592360.

de Lau L, Giesbergen P, de Rijk M, Hofman A, Koudstaal P (2004) Breteler M (2004) Incidence of parkinsonism and Parkinson disease in a general population: the Rotterdam Study. Neurology Okt. https://doi.org/10.1212/01.WNL.0000140706.52798.BE

Lemke M, Ceballos-Baumann A (2002) Depression bei Parkinson-Patienten: diagnostische, pharmakologische und psychotherapeutische Aspekte. Dtsch Arztebl 99(40):A-2625/B-2237/C-2100

Marttila RJ, Rinne UK (1977) disability and progression in Parkinson's disease. Acta Neurol Scand 56:159–169. https://doi.org/10.1111/j.1600-0404.1977.tb01420.x

Mazzoni P, Hristova A, Krakauer J (2007) Why don't we move faster? Parkinson's disease, movement vigor, and implicit motivation. J Neurosci 27(27):7105–7116. https://doi.org/10.1523/JNEUROSCI.0264-07.2007. PMID: 17611263; PMCID: PMC6794577

Menza M, Dobkin R, Marin H, Bienfait K (2010) Sleep disturbances in Parkinson's disease. Mov Disord 25(Suppl 1):S117–S122. https://doi.org/10.1002/mds.22788

Radakovic R, Abrahams S (2018) Multidimensional apathy: evidence from neurodegenerative disease. Curr Opin Behav Sci 22:42–49. https://doi.org/10.1016/j.cobeha.2017.12.022

Redgrave P, Rodriguez M, Smith Y, Rodriguez-Oroz MC, Lehericy S, Bergman H, Agid Y, DeLong M, Obeso JA (2010) Goal-directed and habitual control in the basal ganglia: implications for Parkinson's disease. Nature reviews. Neuroscience 11(11):760–772. https://doi.org/10.1038/nrn2915

Richard I, Justus A, Kurlan R (2001) Relationship between mood and motor fluctuations in Parkinson's disease. J Neuropsychiatr Clin Neurosci 13:35–41

Shetty A, Bhatia K, Lang A (2019) Dystonia and Parkinson's disease: what is the relationship? Neurobiol Dis 132. https://doi.org/10.1016/j.nbd.2019.05.001

Spillantini M, Schmidt M, Lee VY, Trojanowski J, Jakes R, Goedert M (1997) α-Synuclein in Lewy bodies. Nature 388:839–840. https://doi.org/10.1038/42166

Sturkenboom I, Thijssen M, Gons-van Elsacker J, Jansen I, Maasdam A, Schulten M, Vijver-Visser D, Steultjens E, Bloem B, Munneke M (2008) Guidelines for Occupational Therapy in Parkinson's Disease Rehabilitation Nijmegen. ParkinsonNet/NPF, The Netherlands/Miami

Tarakad A, Jankovic J (2019) Essential Tremor and Parkinson's disease: exploring the relationship. Tremor Other Hyperkinet Mov (NY). https://doi.org/10.7916/D8MD0GVR. PMID: 30643667; PMCID: PMC6329774

Visanji NP, Brooks PL, Hazrati LN, Lang AE (2013) The prion hypothesis in Parkinson's disease: Braak to the future. Acta Neuropathol Commun 1(2). https://doi.org/10.1186/2051-5960-1-2

Yoritaka A, Shimo Y, Takanashi M, Fukae J, Hatano T, Nakahara T, Miyamato N, Urabe T, Mori H, Hattori N (2013) Motor and non-motor symptoms of 1453 patients with Parkinson's disease: prevalence and risks. Parkinsonism Relat Disord 19(8):725–731., ISSN 1353-8020. https://doi.org/10.1016/j.parkreldis.2013.04.001

2 Einteilung der Parkinson-Syndrome

Die Parkinson-Syndrome werden in drei Gruppen unterteilt, je nach Bekanntheit der Ursache.

- Primäre Parkinson-Syndrome
  - IPS, idiopathisches Parkinson-Syndrom
  - hereditäre Parkinson-Syndrome (erblich)
- Sekundäre (symptomatische) Parkinson-Syndrome
- Atypische Parkinson-Syndrome

2.1 Primäre Parkinson-Syndrome

Idiopathisches Parkinson-Syndrom (IPS)
Das idiopathische Parkinson-Syndrom wird mit „IPS" abgekürzt. Idiopathisch heißt, dass keine Ursache bekannt ist. Dieses Syndrom wird auch Morbus Parkinson, M. Parkinson und Parkinson'sche Krankheit genannt und ist weitaus am häufigsten (ca. 80 %). Für weitere Informationen zu Hintergründen und Ursachen, Stadieneinteilung, Kardinalsymptomen, weiteren motorischen und nicht-motorischen Symptomen (siehe Kap. 1).

Hereditäre Parkinson-Syndrome
Meist tritt M. Parkinson ohne erkennbaren familiären Hintergrund auf, nicht immer wird sicher herausgestellt, ob eine hereditäre (erbliche) Form zugrunde liegt oder nicht. Erbliche Formen der Parkinson-Erkrankung treten nur sehr selten auf. Dabei gibt es unterschiedliche genetische Muster.

Entweder vererbt ein Mensch die genetische Veränderung autosomal-dominant. In diesem Fall wird die genetische Veränderung an die Hälfte Kinder weitergegeben, alle Merkmalsträger erkranken auch an M. Parkinson. Anderenfalls wird die Parkinson-Erkrankung autosomal-rezessiv vererbt. Das bedeutet, dass beide Eltern des Kindes das Gen in sich tragen müssen, damit die Erkrankung beim Kind auftritt. Hat nur ein Elternteil das veränderte Gen, wird es an das Kind weitergegeben, es kommt jedoch nicht zum Ausbruch der Krankheit. Hereditäre Parkinson-Syndrome lösen oftmals schon in jungen Jahren Symptome aus, meist vor dem 50. oder sogar 40. Lebensjahr.

2.2 Sekundäre Parkinson-Syndrome

Bei den sekundären Parkinson-Syndromen gleichen die Symptome denen des IPS, die Ursache ist jedoch bekannt, siehe Tab. 2.1.

A. Orellana, *Betätigungsorientierte Ergotherapie bei Morbus Parkinson*,
https://doi.org/10.1007/978-3-662-62583-5_2

Tab. 2.1 Mögliche Ursachen für sekundäre Parkinson-Syndrome

Name	Ursache
Vaskulär bedingtes Parkinsonoid	Apoplex, Durchblutungsstörung im Gehirn
Medikamentöses Parkinson-Syndrom (medikamentöses Parkinsonoid)	Nebenwirkung nach Einnahme von Medikamenten wie Neuroleptika, Blutdruckmittel, Anti-Arrhythmica, Mittel gegen Brechreiz, Lithium und Kalziumantagonisten (nach Absetzen des Medikaments meist symptomfrei)
Metabolische Genese	• Stoffwechselkrankheit: Unterfunktion der Schilddrüse, schwere Systemerkrankung der Leber und Niere, Morbus Wilson, Hypoparathyreoidismus • Raumfordernder Prozess: Gehirntumor, Normaldruckhydrozephalus
Posttraumatisches Parkinson-Syndrom	Gehirnverletzung
Toxisches Parkinson-Syndrom	Akute oder chronische Vergiftung z. B. durch Kohlenmonoxid, Pflanzenschutzmittel, Blei, Mangan, Heroinersatzstoff (Meperidin MPTP)
Entzündliches Parkinson-Syndrom	Nach Gehirnentzündung z. B. bei AIDS

2.3 Atypische Parkinson-Syndrome

Im Rahmen anderer neurodegenerativer Erkrankungen können atypische Parkinson-Syndrome auftreten. Für Ärzte ist es nicht immer leicht, die korrekte Diagnose zu stellen, da die Symptome sich mit denen des IPS überschneiden. Es ist jedoch entscheidend, die atypischen Parkinson-Syndrome zu unterscheiden, da sie oftmals schwerwiegender verlaufen und schneller fortschreiten. Außerdem ist die medikamentöse Behandlung, die beim IPS angewandt wird, bei den atypischen Syndromen häufig wirkungslos.

▶ Atypische Parkinson-Syndrome verlaufen oft schwerwiegender und schreiten schneller fort als das idiopathische Parkinson-Syndrom. Dies ist bei der Planung der ergotherapeutischen Intervention zu bedenken.

Progressive Supranukleare Blickparese (PSP)
Die häufigste Form der atypischen Parkinson-Syndrome ist, mit ca. 6 % der Menschen mit Parkinson-Symptomen, die PSP. Typische Anzeichen dieser Erkrankung sind frühe, herausragende posturale Instabilität mit häufigen Stürzen, supranukleare vertikale Blickparese (Unfähigkeit den Blick nach unten, später auch nach oben zu richten) und eine schwere Demenz.

Menschen mit PSP zeigen eine Reihe an weiteren, teils schweren Symptomen, wie starke faziale Bradykinese, Dysarthrie, progressive Dysphagie, visuelle Einschränkungen, Apathie, Depressionen, Enthemmung, emotionale Instabilität und Perseveration. Die Lebenserwartung liegt bei etwa 5–8 Jahren nach Diagnosestellung. Eine multidisziplinäre Therapie wird empfohlen, um das komplexe Krankheitsbild adäquat zu behandeln.

Multisystematrophie (MSA)
Die Multisystematrophie entsteht durch neuronalen Verlust in zahlreichen Gehirnarealen und beinhaltet folgende Bereiche: Putamen, Substantia nigra, Pons, Nucleus olivaris inferior, Zerebellum sowie präsynaptische sympathische Neuronen im Rückenmark.

Die Multisystematrophie hat zwei Erscheinungsbilder, die durch einen unterschiedlich starken Zelluntergang in bestimmten Gehirnarealen ausgelöst werden. Überwiegen die Parkinson-Symptome, wird von MSA-P gesprochen, bei überwiegend zerebellaren Symptomen von MSA-C. Beim MSA-P zeigen sich klassische Parkinson-Symptome mit raschem Voranschreiten und autonomen Defekten (orthostatische Hypotonie, erektile Dysfunktion, Blasenfunktionsstörung). Beim MSA-C steht eine Ataxie im Vordergrund, mit milden Parkinson Symptomen und kognitivem Abbau. Beide Erscheinungsbilder sind von frühen Schlafstörungen, autonomen Defekten und respiratorischen Dysfunktion geprägt, nach wenigen Jahren benötigt die Mehrzahl der Betroffenen einen Rollstuhl.

Die Krankheit schreitet schnell voran, die Lebenserwartung liegt bei ca. 6–9 Jahren nach Diagnosestellung. Bei einer MSA kann die medikamentöse Therapie mit L-Dopa anfangs einen positiven Effekt zeigen. Allgemein ist eine kompensatorische Therapie durch verschiedene Berufsgruppen angezeigt.

Lewy-Körper Demenz

Die Lewy-Körper-Demenz wird mit DLB abgekürzt (aus dem Englischen *dementia with Lewy-bodies*) und ist eine früh auftretende, schnell fortschreitende Demenz. Die Klinik zeichnet sich durch Parkinson-Symptome, die zeitgleich mit der Demenz auftreten, fluktuierende Kognition und Wachheit sowie wiederholt auftretende visuelle Halluzinationen aus. Zusätzlich treten Gangunsicherheiten, Stürze, Synkope, vorrübergehender Bewusstseinsverlust, Paranoia, Depressionen und REM-Schlaf-Verhaltensstörung auf.

Die medikamentöse Therapie ist symptomatisch. Es werden parkinsonreduzierende Medikamente, wie L-Dopa, mit Medikation für Demenz-assoziierte Psychosen ausbalanciert, da sie gegensätzlich wirken können. Eine gut abgestimmte Zusammenarbeit von Pflege und sämtlichen Therapeuten ist wichtig, um den Menschen mit dieser schweren Erkrankung gerecht zu werden.

Kortikobasale Degeneration (CBD)

Die CBD zeigt ein recht variables Bild. Eine deutliche Asymmetrie ist kennzeichnend, die die CBD von anderen neurodegenerativen Erkrankungen abgrenzt. Asymmetrisch eingeschränkte Motorik einer Hand und der Finger, frühe Bradykinese, Frontalhirnsyndrom, Tremor und Rigor sind die häufigsten Symptome. Zusätzlich können auch folgende Symptome auftreten: Ruhe-/Aktionstremor, Dystonie der Extremitäten mit Kontrakturen als Folge, motorische Apraxie, Sprechapraxie, Myoklonien (unwillkürliche Zuckungen), sensorische Einschränkungen, frontotemporale Demenz, posturale Instabilität, Gangunsicherheit und weitere Symptome. Die Lebenserwartung liegt bei durchschnittlich sieben Jahren nach Diagnosestellung.

Da eine effektive medikamentöse Behandlung fehlt, ist bei der CBD ein multidisziplinärer therapeutischer Ansatz zur Erleichterung des Alltags, unterstützt durch Sport und aktive Bewegung früh in der Erkrankung, empfehlenswert.

Literatur und weiterführende Literatur

Herting B, Reichmann H (2016) Parkinsonsyndrome: Fallstricke bei der Diagnose. Dtsch Arztebl 113(15):4. https://doi.org/10.3238/PersNeuro.2016.04.15.01

McFarland NR (2016) Diagnostic approach to atypical Parkinsonian syndromes. Continuum (Minneapolis, Minn) 22(4 Movement Disorders):1117–1142. https://doi.org/10.1212/CON.0000000000000348

Sturkenboom I, Thijssen M, Gons-van Elsacker J, Jansen I, Maasdam A, Schulten M, Vijver-Visser D, Steultjens E, Bloem B, Munneke M (2008) Guidelines for occupational therapy in Parkinson's disease rehabilitation. ParkinsonNet/NPF, Nijmegen/Miami

3 Medikamentöse Therapie und Operationen

3.1 Medikamente und Nebenwirkungen

Es wird heute schon früh mit der Medikamentengabe begonnen. Diese haben meist eine derart positive Wirkung, dass Patienten über Jahre ein nahezu uneingeschränktes Leben führen können. Durch die reduzierte Dopaminausschüttung ersteht ein relativer Überschuss an Acetylcholin (siehe Abb. 3.1). Um dem entgegenzuwirken, werden Medikamente gegeben, die in Dopamin umgewandelt werden (L-Dopa), den Übertritt durch die Blut-Hirn-Schranke erleichtern (Dopa-Decarboxylase-Inhibitoren), die Dopaminrezeptoren stimulieren (Dopaminagonist) und den Abbau von Dopamin verhindern (MAO-B-Hemmer, COMT-Hemmer) (siehe Abb. 3.2).

Medikamente
Folgende Medikamentengruppen sind Usus in der Behandlung von M. Parkinson.

- Levodopa (s. Abb. 3.3)
  Um den Dopaminmangel im Gehirn auszugleichen, wird Levodopa (auch L-Dopa genannt) verabreicht, eine Vorstufe von Dopamin, da Dopamin die Blut-Hirn-Schranke nicht passieren kann. Dabei wird eine möglichst niedrige, aber ausreichend wirksame Dosis Levodopa eingesetzt, um das Auftreten motorischer Komplikationen zu verzögern.
  Effekte von Levodopa:
  - Reduziert Muskelsteifigkeit
  - Verbessert Bradykinese
  - Reduziert Tremor
- Dopa-Decarboxylase-Inhibitoren (z. B. Benserazid oder Carbidopa) mit Levodopa kombiniert.
  Effekte von Dopa-Decarboxylase-Inhibitoren
  - Decarboxylase Hemmer haben die Funktion, den peripheren Abbau von Levodopa zu verhindern.
  - Levodopa muss immer in Kombination mit Decarboxylase-Hemmern gegeben werden.
- Dopaminagonist
  Wird in der Regel als Monotherapie bei über 70-Jährigen eingesetzt und stimuliert die Dopaminrezeptoren im Gehirn.
  Effekte von Dopaminagonisten:
  - Sie verbessern die Bradykinese, den Rigor und Tremor.
  - Sie verzögern das Auftreten von Fluktuationen.
- COMT-Hemmer (Entacapon, Tolcapon) und MAO-B-Hemmer (Selegin, Rasagilin)
  COMT-Hemmer und MAO-B-Hemmer haben ähnliche Aufgaben, beide:
  - Verhindern den Abbau von Levodopa durch COMT und MAO-B.
  - Damit wird die Wirkung von Levodopa unterstützt und verlängert.

A. Orellana, *Betätigungsorientierte Ergotherapie bei Morbus Parkinson*,
https://doi.org/10.1007/978-3-662-62583-5_3

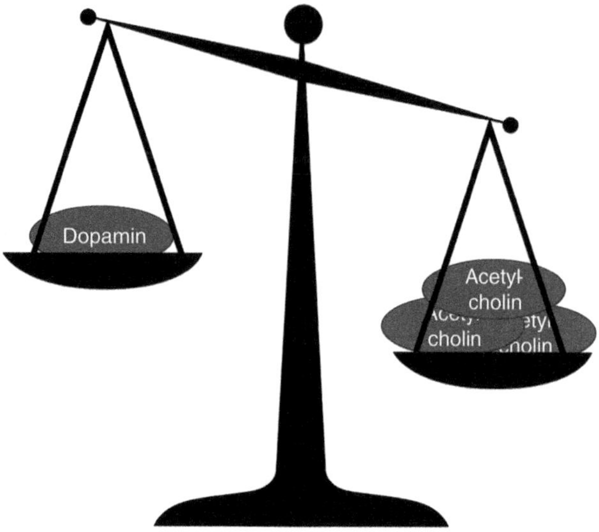

Abb. 3.1 Die verminderte Dopaminausschüttung führt zu einem relativen Überschuss an Acetylcholin

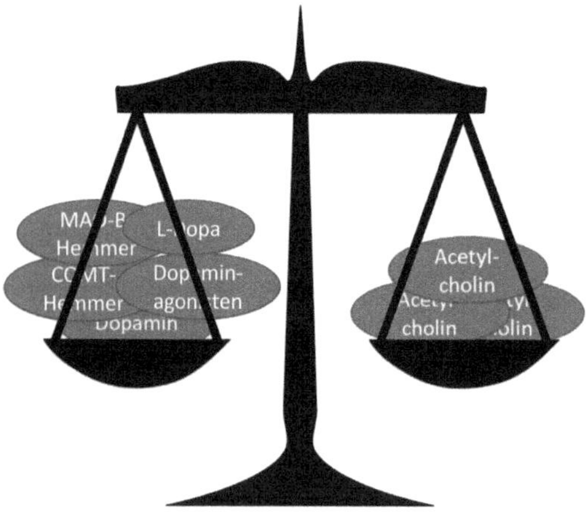

Abb. 3.2 Der relative Überschuss von Acetylcholin wird durch die Gabe von Medikamenten mit unterschiedlicher Wirkung ausgeglichen

- Anticholinergika
  Sehr wenige Patienten profitieren von Anticholinergika.
  - Sie reduzieren fast ausschließlich den Tremor.
  - Heute werden sie kaum mehr angewandt.
- NMDA-Antagonisten (Amantadin, Budipin)
  - Sie wirken antriebsaktivierend.
  - Sie reduzieren Dyskinesien.

▶ Auf das Fortschreiten der Krankheit haben die Medikamente keinen Einfluss, sodass die Symptome nach einiger Zeit wieder sichtbarer werden und sich zunehmend einschränkend auf die Selbständigkeit auswirken.

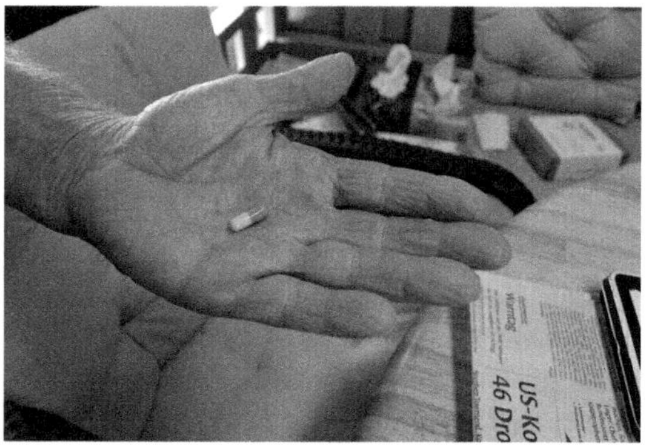

Abb. 3.3 Levodopa muss genau zu den festgelegten Zeiten eingenommen werden, um die Wirkung möglichst konstant zu halten

Wirkungsfluktuation

Im Verlauf der Erkrankung nimmt die Wirkungsfluktuation zu (siehe Abb. 3.4). Nach Einnahme der Medikamente besteht eine gute Beweglichkeit und die Mehrzahl der Symptome sind abgeschwächt oder nicht existent. Nach und nach nimmt die Wirkungsdauer der Medikamente ab. Nach zwei bis vier Stunden zeigen sich erste Wearing-Off-Symptome, d. h. Symptome wie Rigor, Bradykinese, Tremor, kognitive und psychische Einschränkungen nehmen gegen Ende der Wirkungsdauer der Medikamente zu. Kurz bevor die

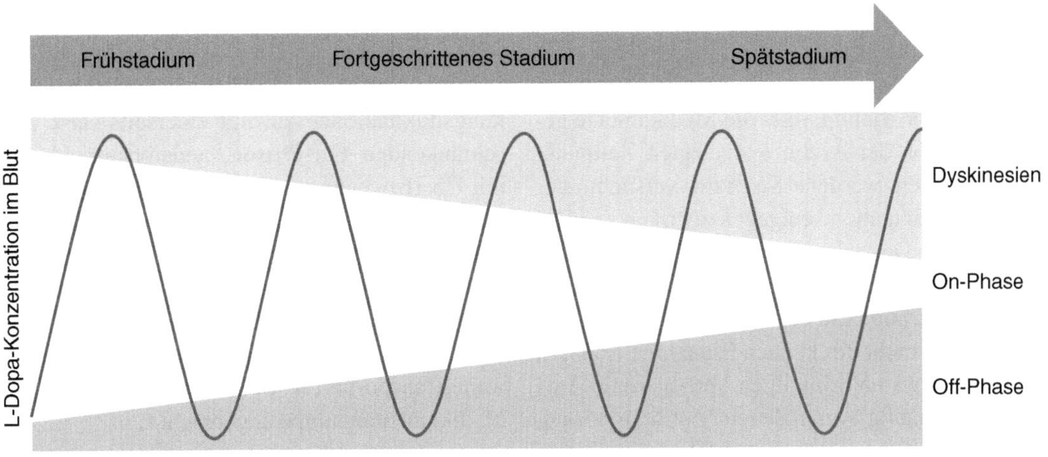

Abb. 3.4 Die Medikamentenfluktuation nimmt mit dem Fortschreiten der Erkrankung zu, sodass Phasen der Über- und Unterbeweglichkeit häufiger auftreten. (Adaptiert nach Jankovic 2005)

Symptome wieder voll ausgeprägt auftreten, sollte die nächste Medikamenteneinnahme erfolgen. Dieses Zusammenspiel der Medikamentenzusammenstellung, -dosis und des Zeitpunktes der Einnahme bedarf einer sehr feinen Abstimmung durch einen Neurologen und muss häufig mehrmals verändert werden, bis eine ausgewogene Lösung gefunden wird.

▶ Klienten müssen ihre Medikamente zu genau geplanten Zeiten einnehmen, um eine möglichst konstante Wirkung zu erzielen und Fluktuationen, mit teils starken Einschränkungen, vorzubeugen.

Im Idealfall bleibt die Beweglichkeit über den Tag durchgehend gut erhalten. Nach Jahren der Einnahme der Parkinson-Medikamente geraten die meisten Patienten jedoch gegen Ende der Medikamentenwirkung in eine sog. Off-Phase. Rigor und Bradykinese sind stark ausgeprägt, auch die psychischen und kognitiven Symptome sind verstärkt. Die Symptome haben den Betroffenen bis zur nächsten Medikamenteneinnahme im Griff. Wird die Dosis der Medikamente erhöht, um Off-Phasen zu vermeiden, kann es zu einer **Überbeweglichkeit** mit **Dyskinesien** kommen. Bewegungen sind in dem Fall zu ausladend, überschießend und weniger zielgerichtet. Die Medikamentenwirkung kann von Patient zu Patient stark variieren und verändert sich im Verlauf der Krankheit. On-Off-Symptome können medikamentengebunden oder völlig zufällig auftreten, es gibt On-Off-Phänomene, bei denen der Patient innerhalb von Sekunden zwischen und Plateau-Dyskinesien, die während der gesamten On-Phase bestehen bleiben.

▶ Dyskinesien werden vom Patienten in der Regel als weniger belastend wahrgenommen als die Off-Phase. Sie werden oftmals von Angehörigen negativer bewertet als von den Betroffenen.

Nebenwirkungen

Teilweise haben Parkinson-Medikamente erhebliche Nebenwirkungen (v. a. Dopaminagonisten), weshalb die individuelle Zusammenstellung und ihre Dosis gut mit den vorhandenen Nebenwirkungen abgewogen werden muss.

Typische Nebenwirkungen sind:

- Halluzinationen
- Störung der Impulskontrolle
- Impulskontrollstörungen bis hin zu Süchten
  - Sexsucht
  - Spielsucht
  - Internetsucht
  - Kaufsucht
  - Esssucht
  - Kleptomanie
- Verwirrtheitszustände
- Schlafstörungen

- Übelkeit
- Mundtrockenheit

Es ist sehr wichtig, dass die Medikamente genau zum von der Ärztin festgelegten Zeitpunkt eingenommen werden. So wird versucht, der Wirkungsfluktuation entgegenzuwirken, indem die nächste Dosis kurz vor dem Abklingen der davorliegenden Dosis wirkt. Die Medikamente werden im Dünndarm ins Blut aufgenommen, sie wirken also nicht direkt nach Einnahme, sondern mit einer etwa halbstündigen Verzögerung. Aufgrund der häufig vorhandenen Motilitätsstörung (eingeschränkte Bewegungsfähigkeit) des Magen-Darm-Trakts, gelangen die Medikamente nicht sofort in den Dünndarm, sondern verweilen teilweise stundenlang im Magen. Auch dies kann eine Ursache von Off-Phasen sein. Die Einnahme der Medikamente erfolgt mit einem Glas Wasser eine halbe Stunde vor oder 90 Minuten nach dem Essen.

Ernährung

Eiweißreiche Ernährung ist mit zunehmendem Alter zur Vorbeugung einer Sarkopenie (Muskelabnahme) sehr wichtig. Gleichzeitig ist die Einnahme der Medikamente mit eiweißhaltigen Lebensmitteln kontraindiziert, da dies die Wirkung von Levodopa reduziert. Das heißt, dass Fleisch und Fisch nur mit großem zeitlichem Abstand zur Medikamenteneinnahme, am besten abends, gegessen werden sollten

► Auf die bei Schluckbeschwerden häufig genutzte Methode, die Tabletten mit Joghurt zu verabreichen, sollte verzichtet werden. Stattdessen kann z. B. Apfelmus verwendet werden.

Zur Verdauungsförderung und Reduzierung von Verstopfung ist auf ballaststoffreiches Essen (Gemüse, Obst, Vollkornprodukte) und ausreichend Flüssigkeitszufuhr (ca. 2 l/Tag) zu achten. Besser als drei große Mahlzeiten am Tag sind mehrere kleine, leichte Speisen. Diese sollten in Ruhe und ohne Zeitdruck eingenommen und ausreichend gekaut werden.

3.2 Medikamentenpumpen

Im fortgeschrittenen Stadium nehmen die Wirkungsfluktuationen zu, mit einerseits stark einschränkenden Off-Phasen, andererseits Phasen mit Überbewegungen und Dyskinesien. Die Wirkungsfluktuation ist ein großer Nachteil der oralen Medikamenteneinnahme, die besonders auftritt, wenn eine Magenentleerungsstörung vorliegt und der Speisebrei mit eingenommenen Tabletten nicht vom Magen in den Dünndarm weitertransportiert wird. In diesem Fall kann eine Medikamentenpumpe angebracht sein.

Levodopa-Pumpe

Die Levodopa-Pumpe befördert das Levodopa direkt in den oberen Dünndarm, das Jejunum, wo es ohne Verzögerung aufgenommen werden kann (siehe Abb. 3.5). Dazu wird mit einem kleinen operativen Eingriff ein Stoma gelegt. Über eine Pumpe wird das Medikament, regelmäßig über den Tag verteilt, verabreicht. Dadurch ist eine durchgehende Versorgung mit L-Dopa gewährleistet und es treten keine Wirkungsschwankungen auf.

Komplikationen ergeben sich hin und wieder durch Infektionen am Stomaeingang, weshalb eine sorgfältige Hygiene eingehalten werden muss. Der Umgang mit der Pumpe und die Stomapflege kann vom Klienten oder der Angehörigen schnell erlernt werden.

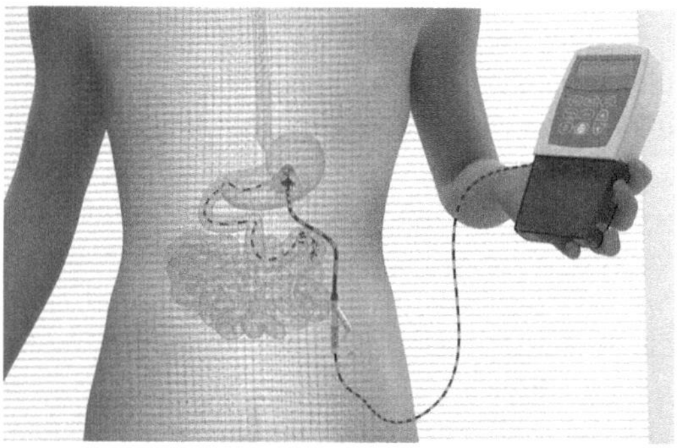

Abb. 3.5 Die Levodopa-Pumpe befördert das Medikament direkt in den oberen Dünndarm. Zum Beispiel, hier die Duodopa ® von Fa. Abbvie

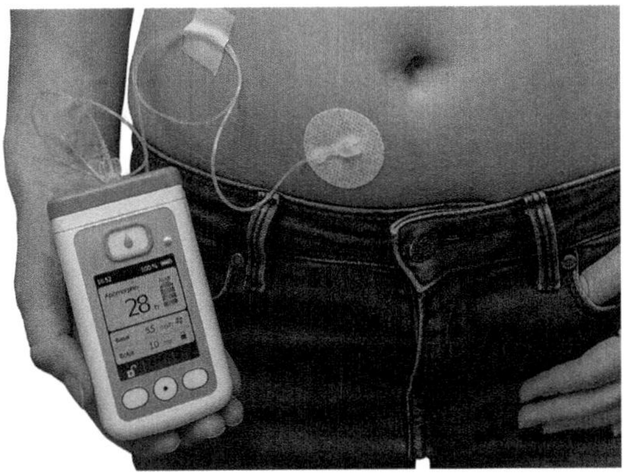

Abb. 3.6 Die Apomorphin-Pumpe spritzt das Medikament zu den programmierten Zeiten automatisch unter die Haut und beugt so Wirkungsschwankungen vor. Hier z. B. von der Fa. Licher MT GmbH

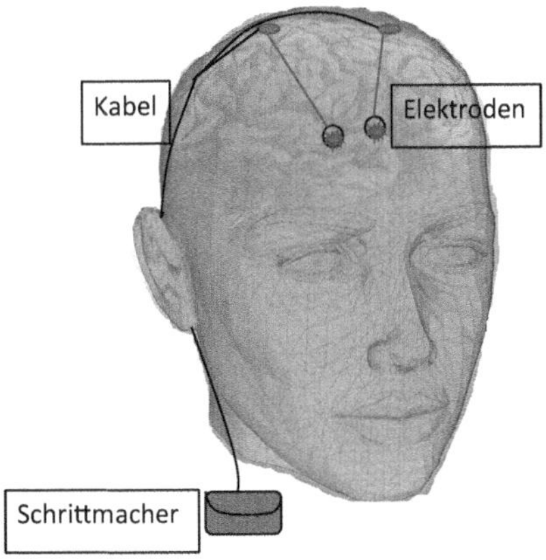

Abb. 3.7 Bei der Tiefen Hirnstimulation werden Sonden ins Gehirn eingesetzt, die über einen externen Schrittmacher elektrische Impulse zur Verbesserung vieler Parkinson-Symptome aussenden

Apomorphin-Pumpe

Apomorphin ist ein Dopaminersatz, der über eine subkutane Injektion gegeben wird (siehe Abb. 3.6). Wenn Wirkungsfluktuationen durch die Einnahme von L-Dopa zunehmen oder die pünktliche Einnahme der Tabletten nicht reibungslos funktioniert, kann die Umstellung auf eine Apomorphin-Pumpe hilfreich sein.

Über eine feine Infusionsnadel wird in vorprogrammierten Abständen automatisch die richtige Dosierung an Apomorphin unter die Haut (subkutan) gespritzt. Die Minipumpe wird um den Hals oder am Gürtel getragen. Die Handhabe kann von Klienten oder Angehörigen einfach gelernt werden. Um eine Entzündung der Einstichstelle zu vermeiden, muss die Nadel täglich versetzt und eine gründliche Hygiene eingehalten werden. Die Wirkung tritt schon 4–12 Minuten nach der Apomorphingabe ein (im Gegensatz zu mindestens 30 Minuten bei oraler Einnahme von L-Dopa).

3.3 Tiefe Hirnstimulation (THS)

Eine interessante Möglichkeit ist die tiefe Hirnstimulation (THS). Dabei werden bei einer mehrstündigen Operation am Gehirn des wachen Patienten Sonden in das Gehirn eingebracht (siehe Abb. 3.7). Über einen kleinen Apparat unter der Haut im Clavicula-Bereich, werden im Alltag konstant elektrische Impulse ins Gehirn gesandt, die die Beweglichkeit verbessern. Bradykinese und Rigor sind weniger stark ausgeprägt. Auch die Wirksamkeit bei starkem pharmakoresistentem Tremorleiden ist oftmals beträchtlich. Laut einer vielbeachteten Studie von Vitek et al. (2020) verbessern sich die Symptome im Durchschnitt für drei Stunden pro Tag.

Risiken sind Gehirnblutung beim Einsatz der Sonden, Verschlechterung der Sprache und ein Nicht-funktionieren durch Fehlplatzierung der Sonden.

Zitat

Zitat eines Parkinson-Erkrankten zum Thema THS: „Kaum einer der Docs und auch der Patienten nimmt sich genügend Zeit, die THS richtig anzupassen bzw. einzustellen. Meine Erfahrung mit den Profs ist, dass die meisten mit der Elektronik überfordert sind. Es ist eben nicht damit getan, nur die Symptome des Patienten durch einmalige Einstellung der THS zu lindern, sondern es hat jede Einstellungsänderung auch "Nebenwirkungen", die meist erst zu Hause auftreten, z. B. Süchte oder Muskelkrämpfe. Es ist eben ein Eingriff ins Gehirn, unserer Schaltzentrale, und da ganz ohne Betreuung wieder auf eigenen Beinen zu stehen … schafft nicht jeder."

Tony =(;-)° „das = sind die beiden Elektroden im Gehirn und das ° steht für den Stimulator und der lachende oder zwinkernde Smile steht für mich."

Entscheidung

Bei fortgeschrittenem M. Parkinson und manchmal schon im frühen Krankheitsverlauf bei Abnahme der Lebensqualität wird der Wunsch nach weiteren Möglichkeiten, neben der Tabletteneinnahme, größer. Die Entscheidung, ob eine THS oder eine Pumpe sinnvoll ist, sollte gut abgewogen werden. Denn die Wirksamkeit der THS ist zwar oft besser als die der Medikamentenpumpen, doch gibt es einige Faktoren, die eine Tiefe Hirnstimulation ausschließen, z. B. Demenz, Depressionen, Psychosen, Alter über 70 Jahre. Starker Tremor spricht wiederum für eine THS.

Für die Handhabe der Apomorphin- und der Levodopa-Pumpe ist das Vorhandensein von Betreuungspersonen hilfreich. Erst nach eingehender Beratung durch einen Spezialisten und evtl. Einholung einer Zweitmeinung, kann eine solch komplizierte Entscheidung gefällt werden.

Literatur und weiterführende Literatur

Biundo R, Weis L, Abbruzzese G, Calandra-Buonaura G, Cortelli P, Jori MC, Lopiano L, Marconi R, Matinella A, Morgante F, Nicoletti A, Tamburini T, Tinazzi M, Zappia M, Vorovenci RJ, Antonini A (2017) Impulse control disorders in advanced Parkinson's disease with dyskinesia: the ALTHEA study. Mov Disord 32:1557–1565. https://doi.org/10.1002/mds.27181

Buhmann C (2011) Wirkungsfluktuationen bei Morbus Parkinson. Wie Sie die kontinuierlichere Stimulation der Dopaminrezeptoren erreichen. Neurol Psychiatr 13:28–34

Deuschl G, Oertel W, Reichmann H (2016) Leitlinien für Diagnostik und Therapie in der Neurologie Idiopathisches Parkinson-Syndrom Entwicklungsstufe: S3 Kurzversion, DGN Edumat-pat-KURZLEITFADEN FUER PATIENTEN – 24-Stunden-Therapie (Version 3.0, 10/2020)

Harati A, Müller T (2013) Neuropsychological effects of deep brain stimulation for Parkinson's disease. Surg Neurol Int 4(Suppl 6):S443–S447. https://doi.org/10.4103/2152-7806.121637. PMID: 24349868; PMCID: PMC3858804

Jankovic J (2005) Motor fluctuations and dyskinesias in Parkinson's disease: clinical manifestations. Mov Disord 20(Suppl 11):S11–S16. https://doi.org/10.1002/mds.20458. PMID: 15822109

LICHER MT 03/2017 · I11_Ratgeber Apomorphin Pumpe Patient DE AT_Rev02-00 · W105

Lozano A, Dostrovsky J, Chen R, Ashby P (2002) Deep brain stimulation for Parkinson's disease: disrupting the disruption. Lancet Neurol 1(4):225–231. https://doi.org/10.1016/s1474-4422(02)00101-1. PMID: 12849455

Maricle R, Valentine R, Carter J, Nutt J (1998) Mood response to levodopa infusion in early Parkinson's disease. Neurology 50:1890–1892

Richard I, Justus A, Kurlan R (2001) Relationship between mood and motor fluctuations in Parkinson's disease. J Neuropsychiatr Clin Neurosci 13:35–41

Sturkenboom I, Thijssen M, Gons-van Elsacker J, Jansen I, Maasdam A, Schulten M, Vijver-Visser D, Steultjens E, Bloem B, Munneke M (2008) Guidelines for occupational therapy in Parkinson's disease rehabilitation. ParkinsonNet/NPF, Nijmegen/Miami

Vitek JL, Jain R, Chen L, Tröster AI, Schrock LE, House PA, Giroux ML, Hebb AO, Farris SM, Whiting DM, Leichliter TA, Ostrem JL, San Luciano M, Galifianakis N, Verhagen Metman L, Sani S, Karl JA, Siddiqui MS, Tatter SB, Ul Haq I, Machado AG, Gostkowski M, Tagliati M, Mamelak AN, Okun MS, Foote KD, Moguel-Cobos G, Ponce FA, Pahwa R, Nazzaro JM, Buetefisch CM, Gross RE, Luca CC, Jagid JR, Revuelta GJ, Takacs I, Pourfar MH, Mogilner AY, Duker AP, Mandybur GT, Rosenow JM, Cooper SE, Park MC, Khandhar SM, Sedrak M, Phibbs FT, Pilitsis JG, Uitti RJ, Starr PA (2020) Subthalamic nucleus deep brain stimulation with a multiple independent constant current-controlled device in Parkinson's disease (INTREPID): a multicentre, double-blind, randomised, sham-controlled study. Lancet Neurol 19(6):491–501. https://doi.org/10.1016/S1474-4422(20)30108-3. Epub 2020 May 26. Erratum in: Lancet Neurol. 2020 Sep;19(9):e8. PMID: 32470421

Teil II

Ergotherapeutische Grundlagen

Grundsätze der Ergotherapie 4

4.1 Betätigung

Das Hauptmerkmal der Ergotherapie ist die Betätigung. Wann immer Ergotherapeuten auf der Suche nach einer passenden Erklärung der ergotherapeutischen Arbeitsweise, ja der Essenz der therapeutischen Intervention sind – Betätigung ist das Ziel und das Werkzeug zugleich.

Betätigung, in manchen Publikationen auch Handlung genannt, ist das Tun. Dabei wird die Betätigung nicht isoliert von der Person und vom Kontext, sondern als eng mit ihnen verflochten verstanden (siehe Abb. 4.1). In diesem Buch zieht sich die Betätigungsorientierung wie ein roter Faden durch und gibt Orientierung.

Studien

Es liegen einige Studien vor, die die betätigungsorientierte Ergotherapie im Allgemeinen (Fasoli et al. 2002; Hétu und Mercier 2012; Kehoe und Rice 2016; Sackaloo et al. 2015; Wu et al. 2000; Hubbard et al. 2009; Ma et al. 1995; Law et al. 1998; Whiteford 2000; Piškur et al. 2002; Marotzki 2004) und im Besonderen für die Behandlung von M. Parkinson stützen (Murphy und Tickle-Degnen 2001; Foster et al. 2014; Sturkenboom et al. 2014).

Der Therapeut kann mit dem Wissen über die Erkenntnisse dieser Studien gegenüber sich selbst, der Klientin und dem interdisziplinären Team die Fokussierung der Therapie auf Betätigung im realen Kontext begründen. Diese handfesten Argumente, gekoppelt mit den Erfahrungswerten zahlreicher Ergotherapeuten, sollten Anlass genug sein, die Arbeitsweise auf Betätigung auszurichten.

Hürden des betätigungsorientierten Arbeitens

Immer wieder berichten Therapeuten von Hürden und Schwierigkeiten bei der Umsetzung der Betätigungsorientierung in der alltäglichen Arbeit. Einige dieser Hürden werden hier beispielhaft aufgegriffen, um erdenkliche Lösungswege aufzuzeigen.

Hürde Das Betätigungsanliegen der Klientin ist im Kliniksetting oder in der ergotherapeutischen Praxis nicht durchführbar.

Möglicher Lösungsweg Bei der simulierten Betätigung schlagen Fischer und Marterella (2019) vor, den Kontext so nah wie möglich nachzustellen. Hierbei können Fotos oder Videos des Kontexts oder der Klientin während der Betätigungsausführung hilfreich sein. In Kliniken ist es empfehlenswert, über eine möglichst umfangreiche Ausstattung an Alltagsgegenständen zu

Ergänzende Information Die elektronische Version dieses Kapitels enthält Zusatzmaterial, auf das über folgenden Link zugegriffen werden kann https://doi.org/10.1007/978-3-662-62583-5_4. Die Videos lassen sich durch Anklicken des DOI Links in der Legende einer entsprechenden Abbildung abspielen, oder indem Sie diesen Link mit der SN More Media App scannen.

A. Orellana, *Betätigungsorientierte Ergotherapie bei Morbus Parkinson*,
https://doi.org/10.1007/978-3-662-62583-5_4

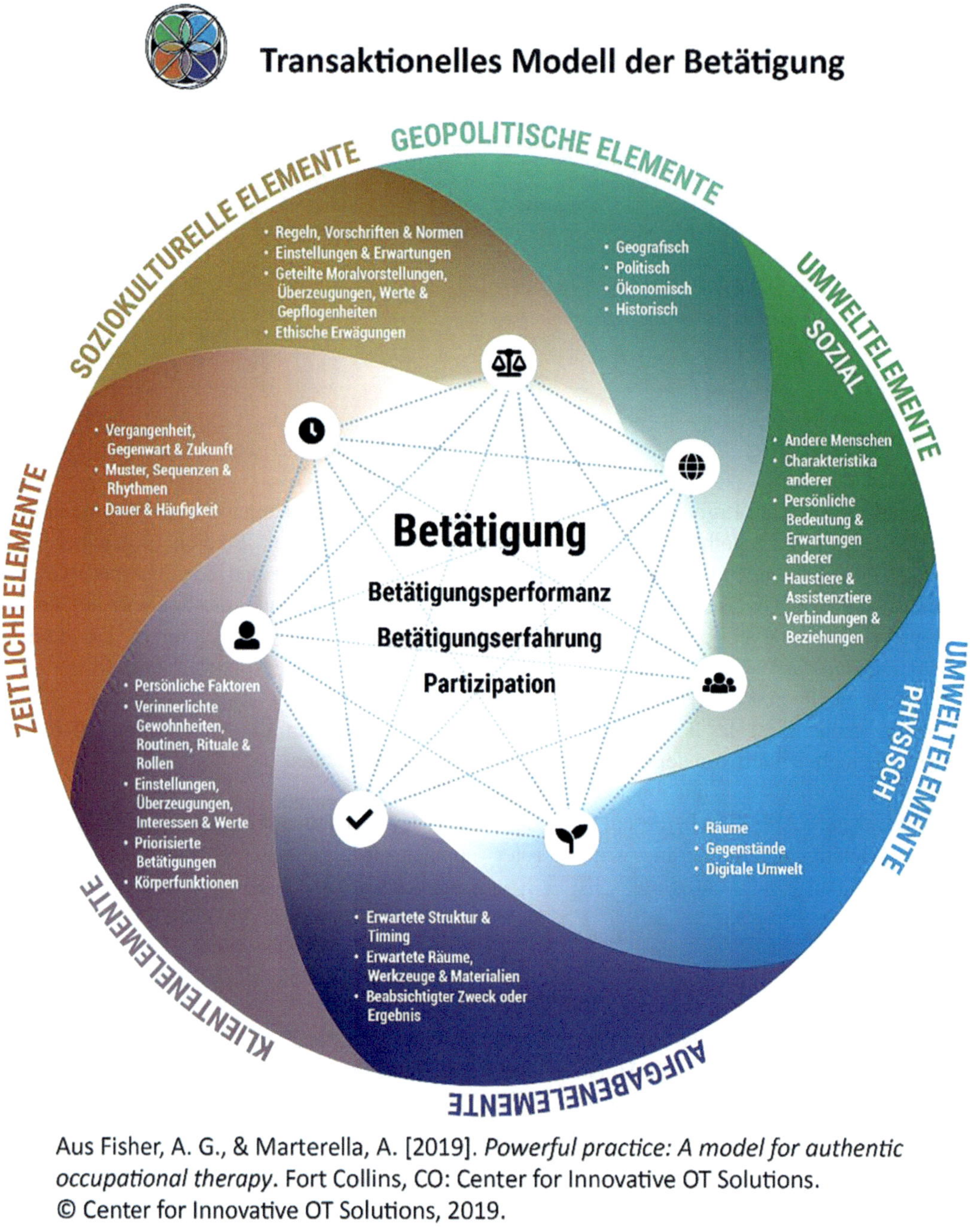

Abb. 4.1 „Transactional Model of Occupation". (Aus Fisher AG, Marterella A 2019. © Center for Innovative OT Solutions, 2019. All rights reserved)

verfügen. Obige Studien sind für die Begründung der Anschaffung gegenüber Vorgesetzten hilfreich.

Beispiel Frau K. berichtet von Schwierigkeiten beim Entnehmen der Gewürzkiste aus dem Schrank, immer wieder fallen einzelne Gewürzdosen heraus, weil sie die bilaterale Bewegung nicht gleichmäßig durchführt. Da die Gewürze in der Übungsküche der Klinik einzeln aufgestellt sind, simuliert der Therapeut die Situation. Er befüllt eine ähnlich große Kiste mit einer ähnlichen Anzahl an Gewürzdosen und platziert sie auf die geschätzte Höhe im Schrank.

Hürde Therapeut ist unsicher, wie er betätigungsorientiertes Arbeiten umsetzen soll.

Möglicher Lösungsweg Für Berufseinsteiger oder Therapeuten, die bisher funktionsorientiert gearbeitet haben, kann es hilfreich sein, sich darauf zu konzentrieren, ein von der Klientin gewähltes Ziel im Blick zu haben. Dieses Ziel sollte eine echte Betätigung aus ihrem Alltag darstellen und ihr wichtig sein. Dazu ist die Durchführung des COPM nützlich. Auch mit der Frage „In welcher Situation in Ihrem Alltag haben Sie Schwierigkeiten?" kommt man direkt zum Kern des Betätigungsproblems. Orientiert sich der Therapeut immer wieder an diesem Betätigungsziel, arbeitet er betätigungsorientiert.

Hürde Langzeitbehandlung – kein Ziel mehr

In Deutschland besteht die außergewöhnliche Gegebenheit der Langzeitverordnung von Heilmitteln bei chronischen Erkrankungen, wie Morbus Parkinson. Das ist einerseits positiv für Betroffene, weil sie uneingeschränkt therapeutische Angebote in Anspruch nehmen können. Andererseits entsteht, besonders in der Ergotherapie, nach Erreichen des Ziels ein Leerlauf, wenn kein neues Ziel gefunden wird.

Es bestehen **drei mögliche Lösungswege**:

Zum einen kann der Ergotherapeut das Ziel präventiv oder erhaltend formulieren, z. B. „Erhaltung des leserlichen Schriftbildes, um weiterhin Überweisungen selbständig ausfüllen zu können.", „Ermöglichung von sozialem Miteinander" (bei Gruppentherapie) oder „regelmäßiges Auffrischen des Geübten" (bei Dual-Task-Training). Zum anderen kann sich der Therapeut zwischenzeitlich auf körperliche oder psychische Beschwerden, wie Schmerzen oder Depressionen konzentrieren und dabei immer den Blick auf die Betätigung beibehalten. Sobald also ein Betätigungsproblem vom Therapeuten oder der Klientin erkannt wird, wird es mit in die Behandlung einbezogen.

Drittens kann die Ergotherapie abgesetzt werden, sobald das gesetzte Zeil erreicht ist, um die Therapie mit einem neuen Rezept wiederaufzunehmen, wenn die Klientin ein neues Problem findet. So bleibt die Klientin motiviert, die therapeutische Intervention kurzweilig und effektiv. Außerdem entsteht eine positive Dynamik, wenn die Therapie mit einem Erreichen des Ziels beendet wird.

Betätigung – ein verflochtener Teil des Kontexts (siehe auch Abschn. 4.3)
Aufbauend auf der Arbeit von Dewey (1989), entwickelten Forschende des Occupational Science eine transaktionale Perspektive der Betätigung. Person, Betätigung und Kontext sind untrennbar miteinander verwoben und beeinflussen sich konstant gegenseitig. Folglich führt die Veränderung des Kontexts auch zur Veränderung der Betätigungsperformanz (Art und Qualität der Durchführung der Betätigung).

▶ Die Person ist nicht die „Produzentin" der Betätigung, sondern die Betätigung ergibt sich aus dem Zusammenspiel der Person mit den unterschiedlichen Kontextfaktoren.

In der Grafik von Anne Fischer und Abbey Marterella in dem Buch „Powerful Practice" (2019) wird bildhaft dargestellt, wie alle situativen Elemente und die Betätigung aufeinander einwirken, sodass eine isolierte Betrachtung unmöglich ist siehe Abb. 4.1.

Bezieht der Therapeut alle diese Elemente in die Betrachtung einer Betätigung mit ein, so wird schnell deutlich, dass der reine Fokus auf die Klientin bei der Durchführung einer Betätigung viel zu kurzsichtig ist. Erst wenn der Blick auf das große Ganze geweitet wird und z. B. auch soziokulturelle Aspekte oder persönliche Einstellungen der Klientin berücksichtigt werden, wird eine wertfreie Beobachtung der Betätigung im Kontext möglich. Wird zum Beispiel von Seiten der Familie der Klientin erwartet, dass sie als Frau für ihren Ehemann kochen muss, liegt ein anderes soziokulturelles Element (geteilte Überzeugungen) vor, als wenn der Klient ein Mann ist und die Erwartungshaltung von Seiten der Familie ist, dass er finanziell für die Familie sorgen muss.

Doing, Being, Belonging und Becoming
Meist wird Betätigung mit einer zielgerichteten Aktivität gleichgesetzt. Wilcock und Hocking (2015) binden die vier Dimensionen Doing, Being, Belonging und Becoming in den Begriff der Betätigung ein und eröffnen so den Blickwinkel auf die passiveren Teile der Betätigung.

- Doing: entspricht der **Betätigungsperformanz**. Also die Durchführung einer Betätigung, die mit Sinnhaftigkeit gefüllt ist.
- Being: ist das Dasein sowie das Genießen und **Erleben des Moments**.
- Belonging: bedeutet die **Zugehörigkeit** zur Gemeinschaft und die soziale Interaktion.
- Becoming: ist die **Entwicklung** seiner Fähigkeiten und Kapazitäten und einer Weltanschauung.

Durch diese Sichtweise der Betätigung, in der auch Begriffe wie Genießen, Zugehörigkeit und Verständnis bedeutungsvoll sind, kann sich unser „westliches Denken" ein wenig entspannen.

► Betätigung bedeutet nicht nur tätig sein, sondern auch untätig sein.

Immer wieder begegnen den Therapeuten im Arbeitsalltag Klient*innen, für die aus Altersgründen, persönlicher Überzeugung, kultureller Herkunft oder Erkrankung das Doing weniger wichtig (geworden) ist. Anstatt in therapeutischen Aktionismus zu verfallen und die aktive Betätigung wiedererwecken zu wollen, lohnt es sich, sich die o. g. Aspekte der Betätigung zu vergegenwärtigen und ihnen Bedeutung beizumessen.

Betätigung im Alter
M. Parkinson ist eine sog. Alterskrankheit. Das Durchschnittsalter der Diagnosestellung ist etwa 60 Jahre. Dr. Katharina Röse, deutsche Professorin für Ergotherapie in Deutschland, setzte sich 2019 kritisch mit dem Umgang des Themas „Betätigung im Alter" auseinander. Sie kritisiert, dass die Mehrheit der Betätigungskonzepte das Individuum und das Aktiv-sein in den Mittelpunkt stellen. Sie fordert dazu auf, statt einer individuumszentrierten Perspektive eine kontextbezogene Perspektive einzunehmen. Gerade im Alterungsprozess verändert sich der Kontext und damit die Betätigung meist stark. Die Verantwortung nimmt ab (Kinder sind autonom, die Arbeit wird niedergelegt), oftmals steht eine Ortsveränderung an (kleine Wohnung, Heim) und enge soziale Kontakte nehmen ab (Freunde und Partner werden vermehrt krank und versterben).

Zum Thema „aktiv sein" im Alter vertritt Dr. Röse die Ansicht, dass die starke Betonung der Aktivität zu Unzufriedenheit führen kann, da eine zufriedenstellende Durchführung oftmals nicht mehr möglich ist. Aus diesem Grund ist es empfehlenswert, das **Being** und **Belonging** (siehe oben) gerade im Alter stärker zu betonen. Meist bleiben vorhandene Interessen bestehen, das aktive Ausführen (**Doing**) nimmt jedoch ab. An dessen Stelle treten Anteilnehmen an und Dasein in einer Betätigungssituation.

4.2 Klientenzentrierung

Klientenzentrierte Ergotherapie basiert auf der Grundüberzeugung, dass die Klientin fähig ist, über ihre Gesundheit zu entscheiden. Das bedeutet für Ergotherapeuten, die Klientin in jeder Phase des therapeutischen Prozesses aktiv in Entscheidungen und Umsetzung miteinzubeziehen.

Einzelklientin oder Klientengruppe
Fischer und Marterella (2019) stellen fest, dass die Klientin nicht zwingend eine einzelne Person ist. Die Klientin kann auch zwei Menschen sein z. B. Ehepartner und Patientin, Pflegekraft und Patientin, Kind und Patientin usw. Oder es sind mehrere Menschen, wie es z. B. in einer Parkinsongruppe der Fall ist, oder in einer Familie, wenn z. B die Kommunikation am Essenstisch ein Thema ist. Diese Sichtweise hilft dabei, wenn die

Entscheidung getroffen wird, wer in die Zielfindung oder die Intervention miteinbezogen werden soll.

Von der Patientin, zur Klientin

Die Klientin stand schon immer im Zentrum der Ergotherapie und doch passiert es regelmäßig, dass z. B. die Feinmotorik behandelt wird, obwohl für die Betroffene das Aufstehen aus dem Bett ein viel dringlicheres Problem ist. In der Regel kommen die Menschen als „Patientinnen" in die Ergotherapie und verlassen sie wieder als „Klientinnen". Diesen Prozess, ihre Rolle als Klientin zu finden, kann vom Ergotherapeuten aktiv unterstützt und gefördert werden. Viele Menschen mit der Parkinson-Erkrankung haben schon reichlich Therapieerfahrung und sind es dennoch gewohnt, „therapiert" zu werden. Die Einstellung: „Sie sind der Therapeut, Sie wissen, was zu tun ist.", ist die Regel.

Die klientenzentrierte Arbeitsweise ist für Therapeuten anstrengender, als eine Funktion ohne Betätigungsziel zu trainieren, da es keinen vorgefertigten Weg gibt. Denn jede Klientin, jede Situation muss individuell betrachtet werden. Und doch ist es der sinnhafteste Weg und der Weg mit der größten Wahrscheinlichkeit, nachhaltig etwas im Leben der Klientin zum Positiven zu verändern.

▶ Die Übergabe der Verantwortung vom Therapeuten an die Klientin ist von zentraler Bedeutung. Auf diese Weise macht sich die Klientin ihren Therapieprozess zu eigen und ihre intrinsische Motivation wird enorm gesteigert.

Es ist ein eindrückliches Erlebnis, wenn die Betroffene beginnt, Eigenverantwortung für ihre Therapie zu übernehmen. Schließlich kennt sich die Betroffene am besten mit ihrer individuellen Situation aus.

Zitat: „Die echten Experten für Behinderung sind die Menschen, die mit einer Behinderung leben." (Hutchinson et al. 2000)

Es entsteht ein lebendiger Austausch zwischen Therapeut und Klientin, in dem jeder seine Expertise einbringt: die Klientin über ihren Alltag und ihre Werte, der Therapeut über effektive Interventionsmöglichkeiten. Im Idealfall wird punktgenau an einer wichtigen Betätigung der Klientin mit dem passenden ergotherapeutischen Ansatz gearbeitet. Dabei ist Feingefühl notwendig, um die Klientin in ihrem eigenen Tempo mitzunehmen und eine effiziente Kooperation zu ermöglichen. Ein schrittweises Vorgehen kann helfen, einer Überforderung vorzubeugen.

Hilfreiche Sätze können dabei sein:

- Ich möchte die Therapie so individuell an Sie anpassen, wie möglich.
- Mir ist es wichtig, **Ihre** Probleme/Sichtweise/Einstellung kennenzulernen.
- Jeder Mensch ist anders und jedes Leben ist anders, deswegen möchte ich wissen, was **Ihnen** wichtig ist.
- Es gibt Studien dazu, die zeigen, dass abstraktes/funktionelles Training nicht so gut auf den Alltag übertragen wird, wie spezifisches Training der problematischen Situation.
- Überlegen Sie nochmal in Ruhe, mit welchen Situationen im Alltag Sie unzufrieden sind.
- Bitte sagen Sie mir immer, wenn Sie eigene Ideen und Vorschläge haben.
- Ich freue mich, wenn Sie auch im Laufe der Therapie Ziele oder Wünsche formulieren.

▶ Wichtige Modelle zum Weiterlesen über betätigungsorientierte und klientenzentrierte Ergotherapie sind das CMOP und OTIPM, zu denen fundierte Studien erstellt wurden.

Insgesamt lohnt sich die Mühe und Anstrengung, sich individuell mit jeder Klientin auseinanderzusetzen, anstatt ein schablonenhaftes Repertoire ablaufen zu lassen.

4.3 Kontextbezug

Der Kontext hat einen entscheidenden Einfluss auf die Betätigungsperformanz. Verändert man einen Faktor, so verändert sich auch immer die Betätigung. Dabei wird nicht nur der unmittelbare Kontext erfasst. Anne Fischer und Abbey Marterella erweitern den Blick auf alle

Kontextfaktoren, die die Betätigung beeinflussen. Sie nennen sie „situative Elemente".

Die situativen Elemente (nach Fischer und Marterella 2019) werden unterteilt in:

- Soziokulturelle Elemente
- Geopolitische Elemente
- Umweltelemente (Sozial)
- Umweltelemente (Physisch)
- Aufgabenelemente
- Klientenelemente
- Zeitliche Elemente

Mit der Erkenntnis, dass die Betätigung im verflochtenen Zusammenhang mit den situativen Elementen entsteht, verändert sich der Blick auf die Performanz und daraufhin auch der therapeutische Ansatz. So ist offensichtlich, dass eine Veränderung des Kontexts sich unmittelbar auf die Betätigung auswirkt, was im Hinblick auf die ergotherapeutische Intervention in Praxisräumen oder im Klinik-Setting Konsequenzen hat. Es gibt Evidenz dafür, dass je weiter die Intervention vom Kontext entfernt ist, desto weniger effektiv sie ist (Fasoli et al. 2002; Hétu und Mercier 2012; Kehoe und Rice 2016; Sackaloo et al. 2015; Wu et al. 2000).

In der anschaulichen Grafik (Abb. 4.1) wird dargestellt, dass es grundlegend wichtig ist, die Betätigung der Klientin als Teil eines miteinander verwobenen Gefüges aller situativen Elemente zu verstehen. In dieser Grafik wird bildhaft gezeigt, wie alle situativen Elemente und die Betätigung aufeinander einwirken, sodass eine isolierte Betrachtung unmöglich ist.

Kraus (2006) hat den Aspekt der subjektiven Wahrnehmung in ihre Definition integriert: Als Lebenswelt gilt das unhintergehbar subjektive Wirklichkeitskonstrukt eines Menschen (welches diese unter den Bedingungen ihrer Lebenslage bildet). Wenn man also über die Lebenswelt der Klientin spricht, wird, im Gegensatz zum Begriff der „Umwelt" oder des „Lebenskontexts", die **subjektive** Sichtweise des Menschen auf ihre Lebenslage betrachtet. Im Rahmen der Klientenzentrierung ist dies ein interessanter Ansatz, um die Klientin in ihrer Gesamtheit zu erkennen und hält Ergotherapeuten dazu an, auch bei der Erfassung der Kontextfaktoren die subjektive Klientinnensicht stets miteinzubeziehen.

Erst auf dieser Grundlage wird es möglich sein, das Handeln der Klientin zu verstehen. So stellt Brigitte Kohn (2019) in „Die drei Rehafelder der HoDT – eine praxisnahe Möglichkeit, um zwischen Lebenswelten zu vermitteln" die Verbindung zur „Handlungslogik" her, einem Begriff aus der HoDT. Nur wenn der Therapeut die subjektive Wirklichkeit der Klientin kennt, kann er verstehen, weshalb dieser in einer bestimmten Weise (aus seiner Sicht logisch) handelt.

Kontext: Klinik

Die Arbeit in einer Klinik ist für betätigungsorientiertes Arbeiten eine Herausforderung. Zahlreiche Hindernisse können sich einem motivierten Therapeuten in den Weg stellen. Diese sind jedoch mit ein wenig Geschick und Entschlossenheit überwindbar (s. Abb. 4.2).

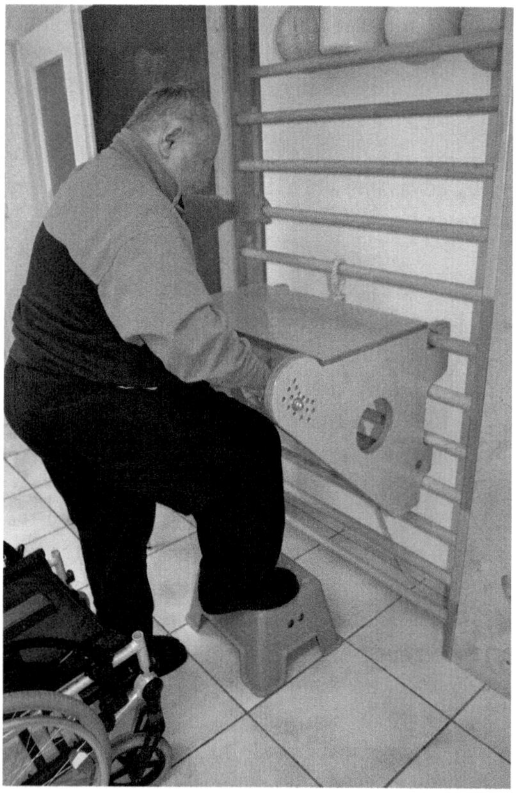

Abb. 4.2 Im Kontext der Klink ist die betätigungsorientierte Ergotherapie eine Herausforderung

Eine betätigungsorientierte Arbeitsweise ist auch im Kliniksetting umsetzbar. Welche Kontexte stehen hierfür zur Auswahl? Welche Rolle spielen Sicherheit, Zeit, Versicherung, Datenschutz, Planbarkeit, Dritte … In Tab. 4.1 sind ein paar praktische Anregungen zur Ermöglichung einer betätigungsorientierten Arbeit im Setting „Klinik". Hierzu werden die sieben Set-

Tab. 4.1 Praktische Anregungen zur Ermöglichung einer betätigungsorientierten Arbeit im Setting „Klinik"

Kontext	**Ergotherapieabteilung Einzelsetting oder Gruppe**
Beispiele	Einzelbehandlungsraum, Gruppenraum mit Behandlungsbank, Tisch,
Vorteile	• „Geschützter Bereich" • Kurzer Weg für Therapeuten • (Idealerweise) viele Materialien • Hilfsmittel zum Ausprobieren • Wenig Ablenkung • Sozialer Austausch im Gruppensetting
Nachteile	• Künstlicher Kontext • Abstrakte, funktionelle Therapie oder • Nur Simulation von Betätigung möglich • Viele Betätigungen nur teilweise oder gar nicht durchführbar
Achtung	• Informationen über Hygienevorschriften mit Hygienefachkraft der Klinik und Robert-Koch-Institut • Ausstattung der Ergotherapieabteilung mit Themenräumen (Übungsküche, Haushaltsraum, Büroraum …) und einer Vielzahl an Alltagsgegenständen (Bügeleisen, Staubsauger, Mixer, Schäler, Drucker, Ordner, Locher, Leiter, Werkzeugkasten …)
Kontext	**Patientinnenzimmer**
Beispiele	Einzelzimmer, Mehrbettzimmer
Vorteile	• Aktuelle Betätigungssituation/Lebenswelt • Körpernahe Betätigungen (Anziehen, Zähne putzen …) gut umsetzbar • Persönliche Gegenstände vor Ort • Weg für Klientin entfällt • Interdisziplinäre Zusammenarbeit möglich • Evtl. spontaner Kontakt mit Angehörigen
Nachteile	• Therapie kann von Mitpatientinnen, Pflegepersonal … unterbrochen werden • Zeitlicher Faktor (Therapeuten Weg) • Materialien und Hilfsmittel nicht vor Ort
Achtung	• Beim Mitführen von Therapiematerial auf Hygiene achten (Thema: Multiresistente Keime)
Kontext	**Station und öffentliche Bereiche der Klinik**
Beispiele	Station, Cafeteria, Kiosk, Flur, Treppe, Aufenthaltsraum, …
Vorteile	• Verschiedene Mobilitätsformen trainierbar • Simulierung von außerklinischen Betätigungen, im geschützten Rahmen • Interaktion/Kommunikation mit Menschen beobachtbar • Schrittweiser Übergang in reale Lebenswelt • Ungeplante Einflüsse nehmen zu, wie im Alltag
Nachteile	• Keine echte Betätigung in realer Lebenswelt
Kontext	**Nicht öffentliche Bereiche der Klinik**
Beispiele	Wäscherei, Personalabteilung, Anlieferung, Lager
Vorteile	• Vergrößerte Auswahl an Betätigungsmöglichkeiten • Evtl. Simulierung von Arbeitskontext möglich
Nachteile	• Erhöhter organisatorischer Aufwand • Evtl. Störung von Klinikabläufen
Achtung	• Ausdrückliche Erlaubnis von Klinikleitung einholen • Abklärung von Versicherung mit Klinikleitung • Sicherheitsvorschriften beachten (Helmpflicht, Prüfzeichen auf Geräten)
Kontext	**Außen – auf dem Klinikgelände**

(Fortsetzung)

Tab. 4.1 (Fortsetzung)

Kontext	**Ergotherapieabteilung** **Einzelsetting oder Gruppe**
Beispiele	Klinikgarten, Sitzbänke, Parkplatz
Vorteile	• Mobilität im Außenbereich trainierbar • Unebene Untergründe und Wettereinflüsse
Nachteile	• Auch nur simulierter Kontext
Kontext	**Außen – außerhalb des Klinikgeländes im öffentlichen Raum**
Beispiele	Supermarkt, Bäckerei, Straßenkreuzung, Bank, Postamt, Straßenbahn, Rolltreppe
Vorteile	• Annäherung an reale Lebenswelt • Umgang mit Erkrankung im öffentlichen Kontext (Blicke aushalten, ansprechen, um Hilfe bitten) • Erweiterte Mobilität (öffentliche Verkehrsmittel) trainierbar • Evtl. Kooperationspartner mit Fahrschule, Bäckerei …
Nachteile	• Zeitfaktor, evtl. Doppeleinheit • Unvorhersehbare Situationen möglich
Achtung	• Genaue Absprache und Dokumentation mit Ärztin und Klinikleitung, in welchem Radius möglich • Mitnahme eines Erste-Hilfe-Sets • Notfallnummer und Mobiltelefon mitführen • Datenschutz o Absprache mit Klientinnen, ob Ansprache mit oder ohne Namen o Evtl. ohne Berufskleidung, Notizblock o Diskrete Besprechung von Therapie, Abseits von Passantinnen
Kontext	**Außerhalb des Klinikgeländes an für Klientinnen relevanten Orten**
Beispiele	Haus/Wohnung der Klientin, Arbeitsplatz, gewohnter Supermarkt/Bäcker …
Vorteile	• Realer Betätigungskontext der Klientin
Nachteile	• Erhöhter organisatorischer Aufwand • Erhöhter zeitlicher Aufwand • Evtl. keine Versicherungsabdeckung
Achtung	• Abklärung mit Klinikleitung und Ärztin, inwieweit durch Versicherung abgedeckt, welche Aktivitäten möglich/nicht möglich und Dokumentation der Absprachen

tings herangezogen, die Hucke und Kuhnert (2019) unterscheiden, um eine betätigungs- und lebensweltorientierte Therapie einzuordnen.

4.4 Partizipation

Partizipation (auch Teilhabe) an einer Betätigung hat mehrere Dimensionen: persönliche Präferenz und Interesse. Was er oder sie tut, wo und mit wem; und wie viel Vergnügen und Befriedigung er oder sie dabei erfährt (Law 2002) (s. Abb. 4.3).

Um Partizipation zu messen, müssen die **Verbindungen** zwischen der Person, dem Kontext und der Betätigung betrachtet werden. Im Jahr 2001 entwickelte die WHO die ICF (Internationale Klassifikation der Funktionsfähigkeit, Behinderung und Gesundheit), darin spielt die Partizipation eine zentrale Rolle (siehe Abschn. 5.2).

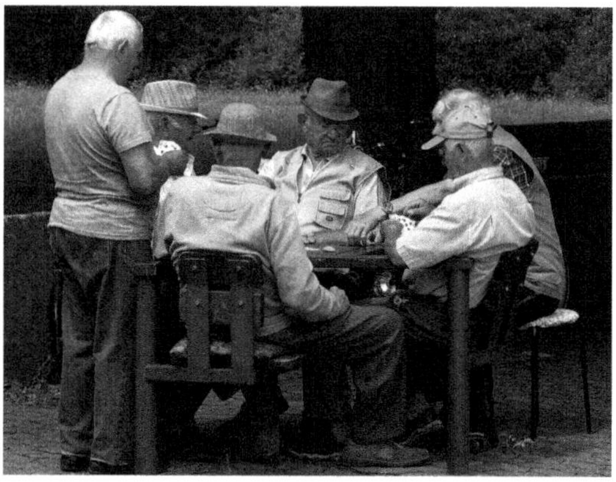

Abb. 4.3 Teilhabe; das Teilnehmen an einer bedeutungsvollen Betätigung

Bei der Entwicklung des ICF waren mehrere Ergotherapeuten involviert; dadurch hat die ergotherapeutische Sichtweise auch für die interdisziplinäre Zusammenarbeit an Bedeutung gewonnen.

- Die aktive oder passive Teilhabe an Betätigungen ist für die Lebensqualität von Parkinson-Klienten beträchtlich. Deshalb stellt die Teilhabe einen wesentlichen Arbeitsbereich der Ergotherapie dar.

In mehreren Studien wurde gezeigt, dass die Teilhabe an bedeutungsvoller Betätigung, besonders Arbeit und Freizeit, einen positiven Effekt auf Gesundheit und Wohlbefinden hat. Townsend und Polatajko (2007) erkennen, dass nicht ausschließlich Aktivität zur Partizipation führt, sondern eine Teilnahme an einer Betätigungssituation möglich ist, ohne sie aktiv durchzuführen. Das „Dabeisein" ohne Aktivität kann vor Allem im fortgeschrittenen Stadium der Parkinson-Erkrankung und im Umgang mit Apathie, Fatigue und Immobilität von Bedeutung sein und in der Ergotherapie den Blickwinkel erweitern.

4.5 Top-Down

Der Top-Down-Ansatz ist erforderlich, wenn klientenzentriert und betätigungsorientiert gearbeitet werden soll. Dies geben auch Modelle vor, die maßgeblich an der Entwicklung der aktuellen Ergotherapie beteiligt sind z. B. OTIPM, AJOT, CMOP-E.

Top-Down Vorgehen bedeutet, der Ergotherapeut:

- **erfasst** die allgemeinen Klientendaten.
- **findet heraus,** welche Betätigung der Klientin besonders wichtig ist.
- **beobachtet** diese Betätigung.
- **interpretiert,** welche Faktoren die Performanz der Betätigung beeinflussen.
- **untersucht**, nur wenn notwendig, Körperfunktionen, Kognition, Umwelt- und andere situative Elemente.

So stellt der Therapeut sicher, dass der Fokus der Intervention wirklich auf dem Anliegen der Klientin liegt. Wird hingegen damit begonnen, die Körperfunktionen zu befunden, bevor die der Klientin wichtige Betätigung herausgefunden wurde, steht automatisch die Körperfunktion im Vordergrund. Dieser Ansatz wird „Bottom-Up" genannt.

Bottom-Up Vorgehen bedeutet, der Ergotherapeut:

- **untersucht** die Körperfunktionen und/oder Kognition, Umweltfaktoren.
- **interpretiert,** welche eingeschränkten Körperfunktionen, kognitiven Einschränkungen oder Umweltfaktoren die Betätigungsperformanz beeinflussen.

Außerdem wird in diesem Fall davon ausgegangen, dass ein direkter Zusammenhang zwischen Körperfunktion und Performanz besteht, was jedoch nicht immer der Fall ist. Z. B., wenn die Klientin eine stark ausgeprägte Hypomimie zeigt (Körperfunktion), jedoch durch ihren Witz und ihre Intelligenz im Freundeskreis eine beliebte Gesprächspartnerin bleibt (Betätigung).

Zusätzlich wird beim Bottom-Up-Ansatz davon ausgegangen, dass die Betätigung sich verbessert, wenn die Körperfunktion sich verbessert. Hier belegen einige Studien, dass für den Zusammenhang limitierte Evidenz besteht. Folgende Studien entkräften den Effekt von kontextfernem funktionellem Training auf die Performanz: Díaz-Arribas et al. 2020; Mak und Hui-Chan 2008; Nieuwboer et al. 2001. Dies wäre z. B. der Fall, wenn sich die Feinmotorik, gemessen am Nine-Hole-Peg-Test, verbessert hat, die Knöpfe am Hemd jedoch noch immer nicht geschlossen werden können. Der Top-Down-Ansatz ist auch in der Übersicht des Therapieablaufs nach der „Perfect Fit"-Methode erkennbar (siehe Abb. 4.4). Die Gliederung dieses gesamten Buches und auch die Struktur innerhalb der Kapitel folgt dem Top-Down-Ansatz.

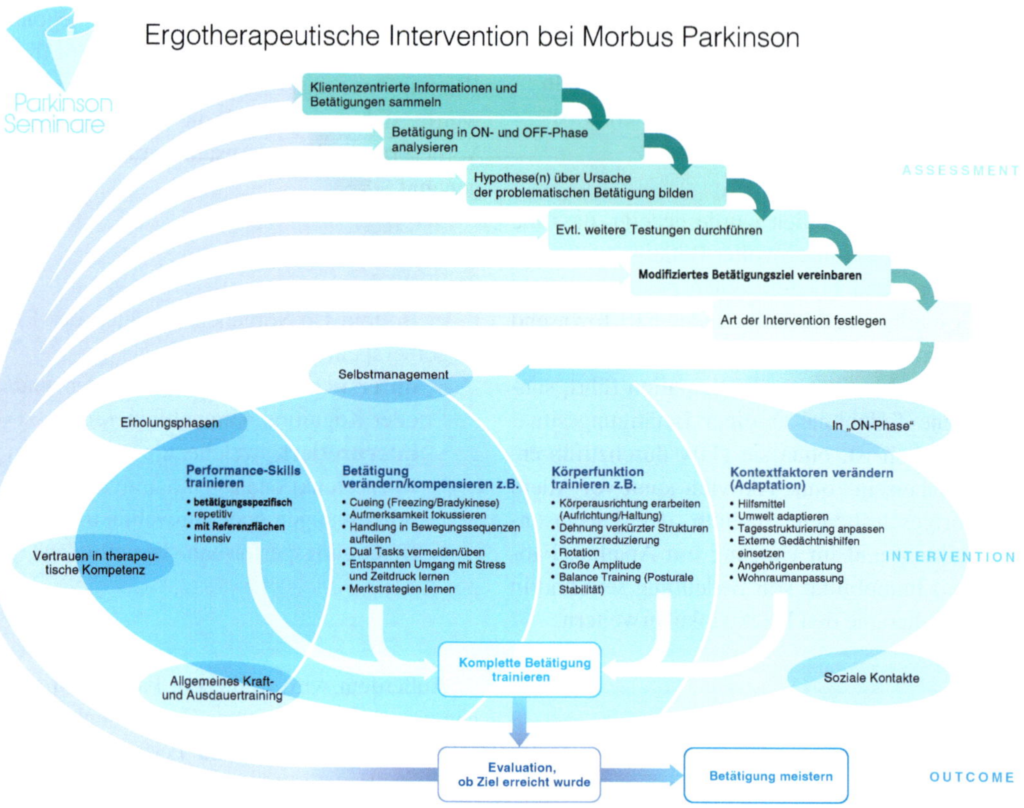

Abb. 4.4 Perfect Fit (©Martina Hoch, Amy Orellana 2020)

4.6 Flexibilität und Kreativität in der Ergotherapie

Die ergotherapeutische Intervention ist selten ein linearer Prozess, vielmehr gehören kreatives Denken, Versuch und Irrtum, professionelle Vermutung und flexibles Arbeiten zum Arbeitsalltag und sollten nicht unterschätzt werden. Denn gerade dieses flexible Denken macht aufmerksam auf notwendige Anpassung und Veränderungen im therapeutischen Prozess. Führende Ergotherapeutinnen erkennen dies:

Law et al. (1995): Eine klientenzentrierte Herangehensweise an die Praxis ist flexibel und dynamisch, mit einem Schwerpunkt auf Lernen und Problemlösung.

Robertson et al. (2015): Die Kunst der Ergotherapie betrifft die Anforderung, dass Ergotherapeuten ihre kreativen Köpfe einsetzen und sich Möglichkeiten vorstellen.

Fischer (2009): Lösungskonzepte vorzuschlagen, um sie anschließend zu evaluieren, um zu gewährleisten, dass sie effektiv sind, könnte am besten als: „die Kunst und Wissenschaft von geführtem Versuch und Irrtum“ gesehen werden.

Die in Abb. 4.4 dargestellte Übersicht des therapeutischen Prozesses zur Intervention bei M. Parkinson stellt eine Richtlinie dar, die sich in der Praxis bewährt hat. Es wird jedoch nicht dazu geraten, die Schritte strikt so abzuarbeiten. Bei Bedarf und nach kritischer Betrachtung der eigenen Arbeitsweise kann der Ergotherapeut einzelne Schritte auslassen, zusammenfassen oder auch durch eigenes Wissen ergänzen. Ein offener Austausch mit der Klientin über das therapeutische Vorgehen ist ratsam, da die Transparenz Vertrauen schafft. Die Meinung und Erfahrung der Klientin kann sehr wertvoll sein, schließlich beschäftigt sie sich täglich mit ihrer Erkrankung und ihrem Lebensalltag und ist somit eine Spezialistin für ihre Situation. Zur besseren Ansicht finden Sie die Abbildung auch online auf Springer-Link.

Literatur und weiterführende Literatur

Aragon A, Kings J (2018) Occupational therapy for people with Parkinson's, the Royal College of Occupational Therapists Specialist Section – Neurological Practice, London

Dewey J (1989) Experience and nature, 2. Aufl. Open Court, La Salle. (Original work published in 1929)

Díaz-Arribas MJ, Martín-Casas P, Cano-de-la-Cuerda R, Plaza-Manzano G (2020) Effectiveness of the Bobath concept in the treatment of stroke: a systematic review. Disabil Rehabil 42(12):1636–1649. https://doi.org/10.1080/09638288.2019.1590865. Epub 2019 Apr 24. PMID: 31017023

Dickie V, Cutchin M, Humphry R (2006) Occupation as transactional experience: a critique of individualism in occupational science. J Occup Sci 13(1):83–93. https://doi.org/10.1080/14427591.2006.9686573

Fasoli SE, Trombly CA, Tickle-Degnen L, Verfaellie MH (2002) Effect of instructions on functional reach in persons with and without cerebrovascular accident. Am J Occup Ther 56(4):380–390. https://doi.org/10.5014/ajot.56.4.380. PMID: 12125827

Fereshtehnejad S, Romenets SR, Anang JBM, Latreille V, Gagnon J, Postuma RB (2015) New clinical subtypes of Parkinson disease and their longitudinal progression: a prospective cohort comparison with other phenotypes. JAMA Neurol 72(8):863–873. https://doi.org/10.1001/jamaneurol.2015.0703

Fisher AG (2009) Occupational Therapy Intervention Process Model: A model for planning and implementing top-down, clientcentered, and occupation-based interventions. Fort Collins: Three Star Press.

Fischer A, Marterella A (2019) Powerful Practice 63–72, 207–211 CIOTS, Colorado, USA

Foster ER, Bedekar M, Tickle-Degnen L (2014) Systematic review of the effectiveness of occupational therapy-related interventions for people with Parkinson's disease. Am J Occup Ther 68(1):39–49. https://doi.org/10.5014/ajot.2014.008706. PMID: 24367954; PMCID: PMC4413458

Freysinger VJ, Alessio H, Mehdizadeh S (1993) Reexamining the morale-physical health-activity relationship: a longitudinal study of time changes and gender differences. Act Adapt Aging 17(4):25–41. https://doi.org/10.1300/J016v17n04_04

Hammell KW (2004) Dimensions of meaning in the occupations of daily life. Can J Occup Ther 71(5):296–305. https://doi.org/10.1177/000841740407100509. PMID: 15633880

Hétu S, Mercier C (2012) Using purposeful tasks to improve motor performance: does object affordance matter? Br J Occup Ther 75:367–376. https://doi.org/10.4276/030802212X13433105374314

Hubbard IJ, Parsons MW, Neilson C, Carey LM (2009) Task-specific training: evidence for and translation to clinical practice. Occup Ther Int 16(3–4):175–189. https://doi.org/10.1002/oti.275. PMID: 19504501

Hucke B, Kuhnert B (2019) Vortrag „Betätigungsorientierung umsetzen: Rahmenbedingungen und Gestaltungsmöglichkeiten im stationären und ambulanten Setting" Herbsttagung DVE des Fachausschusses Neurologie, Bochum

Hutchinson P, Pedlar A, Dunn P, Lord J, Arai S (2000) Canadian independent living centres: impact on the community. Int J Rehabil Res 23:58. https://doi.org/10.1097/00004356-200023020-00001

Kehoe R, Rice M (2016) Reality, virtual reality, and imagery: quality of movement in novice dart players. Br J Occup Ther 79. https://doi.org/10.1177/0308022615616820

Kohn B (2019) Vortrag „Die drei Rehafelder der HoDT-eine praxisnahe Möglichkeit, um zwischen Lebenswelten zu vermitteln" Herbsttagung DVE des Fachausschusses Neurologie, Bochum

Kraus B (2006) Lebenswelt und Lebensweltorientierung: eine begriffliche Revision als Angebot an eine systemischkonstruktivistische Sozialarbeitswissenschaft. Z Syst Ther Familienther 37(2):116–129. https://nbn-resolving.org/urn:nbn:de:0168-ssoar-47820-7

Law M (2002) Participation in the occupations of everyday life. Am J Occup Ther 56(6):640–649. https://doi.org/10.5014/ajot.56.6.640

Law M, Baptiste S, Mills J (1995) Client-centred practice: what does it mean and does it make a difference? Can J Occup Ther 62(5):250–257. https://doi.org/10.1177/000841749506200504. PMID: 10152881

Law M, Steinwender S, Leclair L (1998) Occupation, health and well-being. Can J Occup Ther 65(2):81–91. https://doi.org/10.1177/000841749806500204

Law M, Polatajko H, Carswell A, McColl MA, Pollock N, Baptiste S (1999) Das Kanadische Modell der Occupational Performance und das Canadian Occupational Performance Measure. In: Jerosch-Herold C, Marotzki U, Hack BM, Weber P (Hrsg) Konzeptionelle Modelle für die ergotherapeutische Praxis. Ergotherapie – Reflexion und Analyse. Springer, Berlin/Heidelberg. https://doi.org/10.1007/978-3-662-08173-0_7

Ma H, Trombly A, Robinson-Podolski C (1995) The effect of context on skill acquisition and transfer. Am J Occup Ther 53(2):138–144. https://doi.org/10.5014/ajot.53.2.138

Mak MK, Hui-Chan CW (2008) Cued task-specific training is better than exercise in improving sit-to-stand in patients with Parkinson's disease: a randomized controlled trial. Mov Disord 23:501 509. https://doi.org/10.1002/mds.21509

Marotzki U (2004) Zwischen medizinischer Diagnose und Lebensweltorientierung, Eine Studie zum professionellen Arbeiten in der Ergotherapie. Schulz-Kirchner, Idstein

Murphy S, Tickle-Degnen L (2001) The effectiveness of occupational therapy-related treatments for persons with Parkinson's disease: a meta-analytic review. Am

J Occup Ther 55(4):385–392. https://doi.org/10.5014/ajot.55.4.385

Nieuwboer A, Weerdt W, Dom R, Truyen M, Janssens L, Kamsma Y (2001) The effect of a home physiotherapy program for persons with Parkinson's disease. J Rehabil Med 33:266–272

Parkinson J (1817) An essay on the shaking palsy. J Neuropsychiatr Clin Neurosci 14(2):223–236. https://doi.org/10.1176/jnp.14.2.223. 2002 Spring; discussion 222. PMID: 11983801

Piškur B, Kinebanian A, Josephsson S (2002) Occupation and well-being: a study of some Slovenian people's experiences of engagement in occupation in relation to well-being. Scand J Occup Ther 9(2):63–70. https://doi.org/10.1080/11038120232000043

Polatajko HJ, Mandich A, Martini R (2000) Dynamic performance analysis: a framework for understanding occupational performance. Am J Occup Ther 54:65–72

Robertson D, Warrender F, Barnard S (2015) The critical occupational therapy practitioner: How to define expertise? Aust Occup Ther J 62:68–71. https://doi.org/10.1111/1440-1630.12157

Röse K (2017) Betätigung von Personen mit Demenz im Kontext Pflegeheim. Hogrefe, Göttingen

Sackaloo K, Strouse E, Rice MS (2015) Degree of preference and its influence on motor control when reaching for most preferred, neutrally preferred, and least preferred candy. OTJR (Thorofare N J) 35(2):81–88. https://doi.org/10.1177/1539449214561763. PMID: 26460470

Stadler-Grillmaier J (2007) ENOTHE-Projekt „ET-Fachterminologie" – Beitrag zur Entwicklung einer (deutschen) Fachsprache in der Ergotherapie. Ergoscience 2:100–106. https://doi.org/10.1055/s-2007-963236, Georg Thieme Verlag KG, Stuttgart/New York

Sturkenboom I, Thijssen M, Gons-van Elsacker J, Jansen I, Maasdam A, Schulten M, Vijver-Visser D, Steultjens E, Bloem B, Munneke M (2008) Guidelines for occupational therapy in Parkinson's disease rehabilitation. ParkinsonNet/NPF, Nijmegen/Miami

Sturkenboom IH, Graff MJ, Hendriks JC, Veenhuizen Y, Munneke M, Bloem BR, Nijhuis-van der Sanden MW, OTiP study group (2014) Efficacy of occupational therapy for patients with Parkinson's disease: a randomised controlled trial. Lancet Neurol 13(6):557–566. https://doi.org/10.1016/S1474-4422(14)70055-9. Epub 2014 Apr 8. Erratum in: Lancet Neurol. 2014 Jun;13(6):536. Erratum in: Lancet Neurol. 2016 Mar;15(3):241. Erratum in: Lancet Neurol. 2016 Apr;15(4):352. Erratum in: Lancet Neurol. 2016 Mar;15(3):241. PMID: 24726066

Townsend E, Polatajko H (2007) Enabling occupation II: Advancing an occupational therapy vision for health, well-being, & justice through occupation. CAOT Publishers, Ottawa

Wahl HW, Iwarsson S, Oswald F (2012) Aging well and the environment: toward an integrative model and research agenda for the future. Gerontologist 52(3):306–316. https://doi.org/10.1093/geront/gnr154. Epub 2012 Mar 14. PMID: 22419248

Weinstock-Zlotnick G, Hinojosa J (2004) Bottom-up or top-down evaluation: is one better than the other? Am J Occup Ther 58(5):594–599. https://doi.org/10.5014/ajot.58.5.594. PMID: 15481786

Whiteford G (2000) Occupational deprivation: global challenge in the new millennium. Br J Occup Ther 63:200–204. https://doi.org/10.1177/030802260006300503

Wilcock AA (1999) Reflections on doing, being and becoming*. Aust Occup Ther J 46:1–11. https://doi.org/10.1046/j.1440-1630.1999.00174.x

Wilcock AA, Hocking C (2015) An occupational perspective of health/Ann A. Wilcock, Clare Hocking SLACK Incorporated, Thorofare

Wu C, Trombly CA, Lin K, Tickle-Degnen L (2000) A kinematic study of contextual effects on reaching performance in persons with and without stroke: influences of object availability. Arch Phys Med Rehabil 81(1):95–101. https://doi.org/10.1016/s0003-9993(00)90228-4. PMID: 10638883

Teil III

Assessmentphase

Betätigungsorientierte Informationssammlung

5

Beispiel

Frau N. ist nervös. Gleich hat sie ihre erste Ergotherapie-Sitzung. Was das wohl für eine Therapie ist? Die anderen Therapeutinnen in der Klinik hat sie schon kennengerlernt – Logopäde, Physiotherapeutin und Neuropsychologin. Die waren ja alle ganz nett, aber die vielen Fragen und Tests … Wörter nachsprechen, auf einem Bein stehen, eine Uhr malen und vieles mehr. Da wird man schon etwas verunsichert. Oh, da kommt sie schon. ◀

5.1 Erste Datensammlung:

Zum Einstieg in die therapeutische Beziehung mit dem Klienten werden Daten und Hintergrundinformationen gesammelt, um sich ein umfassendes Bild des Menschen, seiner Betätigung, dem situativen Kontext und der Partizipation zu machen.

Quellen zur ersten Datenerfassung

Die Sammlung von Informationen ist kein linearer Prozess, sondern eine Mischung aus verschiedenen Quellen und Techniken. Schon vor dem Kennenlernen des Klienten beginnt die Ergotherapeutin mit der Datensammlung.

Auf der **Verordnung** der Ärztin stehen Diagnose, Nebendiagnosen und Symptome. Hier erfährt die Therapeutin, ob die M.-Parkinson-Diagnose die Haupt- oder Nebendiagnose ist, welcher M.-Parkinson-Typ besteht und welche Symptome laut Arzt im Vordergrund stehen, z. B. Tremor, Freezing. In einer ergotherapeutischen Praxis nennt der **Klient** selbst oder eine **Angehörige** häufig schon am Telefon Informationen über den Grund seiner Anmeldung, z. B. einen Sturz oder Schwierigkeiten beim Essen.

In einer Klinik können weitere Details beim **Pflegepersonal** oder aus der **Akte** erfahren werden, z. B. Umgang mit Patienten, Demenz. Bei **interdisziplinären Teamsitzungen** und in **Berichten** können die Eindrücke der angrenzenden Berufsgruppen erfahren werden, z. B. Hauptproblem aus Sicht der Physiotherapeutin.

Erstkontakt

Beim ersten Treffen mit dem Parkinson-Klienten stehen das Kennenlernen und der Aufbau einer ersten positiven Vertrauensbasis im Vordergrund. Eine tragfähige therapeutische Beziehung mit dem Klienten ist die Basis für eine effektive Therapie und wird in Abschn. 4.2 ausführlicher thematisiert. Die Therapeutin ermöglicht es dem Klienten Vertrauen zu fassen und sich zu öffnen, indem sie zugewandt, freundlich und authentisch auftritt.

Kurz-Überblick geben

Es ist eine wichtige Aufgabe der Therapeutin, beim ersten Treffen mit dem Klienten eine kurze

A. Orellana, *Betätigungsorientierte Ergotherapie bei Morbus Parkinson*,
https://doi.org/10.1007/978-3-662-62583-5_5

Erklärung zum Tätigkeitsbereich der Ergotherapie zu geben, da die meisten Menschen davon wenig Kenntnis besitzen. Hierzu kann Kap. 4 zu den Themen: Klientenzentrierung, Betätigungsorientierung und Top-Down-Ansatz hilfreich sein. Es lohnt sich, sich dazu vorab in Ruhe Gedanken gemacht zu haben, wie man in eigenen Worten die Komplexität der Ergotherapie für Laien fassbar machen kann.

▶ Folgende Punkte kann sich die Therapeutin notieren, um sich auf die Erklärung Ihrer Tätigkeit beim Erstkontakt mit einem neuen Klienten, vorzubereiten:

- persönliche Einstellung der Therapeutin zur Ergotherapie,
- Rolle der Ergotherapie in der Institution im interdisziplinären Team,
- geeignetes Beispiel, wie Intervention ablaufen kann.

Methoden zur Datenerfassung

Zur Erfassung der Daten des Klienten aus seiner eigenen Sicht, können unterschiedliche Methoden verwendet werden (siehe Tab. 5.1).

Die wichtigsten Informationen müssen nicht immer in der ersten Therapieeinheit gesammelt werden, sondern kommen oft spontan mitten in einer Intervention, wenn der Klient sich sicher fühlt. Besonders unangenehme persönliche Themen wie Inkontinenz oder Vergesslichkeit werden meist erst im Laufe der ersten Behandlungen artikuliert.

5.2 Bio-psycho-soziales Modell

Im Laufe der ersten Behandlungen erhält die Therapeutin einen umfassenden Überblick über die wichtigsten Daten des Lebenshintergrundes. Das Bio-psycho-soziale Modell, welches von der WHO im Rahmen der ICF entwickelt wurde, hat

Tab. 5.1 Methoden, die wie Werkzeuge zur Datenerfassung angewandt werden können, je nach Absicht der Therapeutin

Methode zur Datensammlung	Konzept	Kurzbeschreibung	Erfasste Daten	Art der Erfassung
Bio-psycho-soziales Modell	ICF	Auf einer übersichtlichen Seite werden die Zusammenhänge von Funktion, Aktivität, Partizipation, Kontext und personenbezogene Faktoren notiert.	Überblick über Patientendaten	Freies Interview
Betätigungsprofil	CFFP	Der Klient notiert alle Betätigungen, die er in einem Tag durchführt.	Alle bedeutungsvollen Betätigungen	Formular vom Klienten und/oder wichtigen Personen ausgefüllt
Gespräch		Im Gespräch können bisher nicht aufgenommene, auch persönliche Themen gut erfasst werden.	Nach Bedarf	Freies Gespräch
COPM	CPPF	Der Klient benennt seine Hauptprobleme bei Betätigungen, gibt die Wichtigkeit an und formuliert, mithilfe der Therapeutin 1–5 Ziele für die Therapie.	Klientenziele, Betätigungsperformanz	Halbstrukturiertes Interview
PDQ-39		Ein Kurzfragebogen, um die subjektiv eingeschätzte Lebensqualität des Klienten zu erfassen.	Lebensqualität	Fragebogen ankreuzen

sich zur Dokumentation der Datensammlung bewährt (siehe Abb. 5.1). Es ist ein international anerkanntes Gerüst zur Erfassung des gesamten Lebenshintergrundes. Die ICF hat die Absicht, die **Wechselwirkung** zwischen Gesundheitsproblem, Funktionsfähigkeit, Partizipation und Kontextfaktoren eines Menschen abzubilden, anstatt einer kausalen Sichtweise – die Krankheit führt zur Aktivitätseinschränkung und diese zur Behinderung. Die Wechselwirkung der unterschiedlichen Bereiche wird mit den Pfeilen zwischen den Komponenten dargestellt.

Dieses Umdenken in der Betrachtung des Klienten korreliert mit dem Paradigmenwechsel in der Ergotherapie zur Betätigungsorientierung und Klientenzentrierung. Die interdisziplinäre Anwendung des Bio-psycho-sozialen Modells ist in der Tat von essenzieller Bedeutung für die Rolle der Ergotherapie. Denn die ganzheitliche Sicht auf das komplexe Zusammenspiel der Komponenten, wie im Bio-psycho-sozialen Modell, ist von jeher das Spezialgebiet der Ergotherapeutinnen.

Durch die Nutzung des Bio-psycho-sozialen Models rückt der zentrale Tätigkeitsbereich der Ergotherapie, die Betätigung (im Bio-psycho-sozialen Modell **Aktivitäten** genannt) und die Teilhabe (Partizipation) in den Fokus. Der Punkt der **Teilhabe** spielt eine besondere Rolle im Bio-psycho-sozialen Modell, da die Sicherung der Teilhabe am Leben als gesamtgesellschaftliches Ziel gilt. So ist im „Übereinkommen über die Rechte von Menschen mit Behinderungen" der UN-Behindertenrechts-Konvention (2006) unter Artikel 3 nachzulesen: Allgemeine Grundsätze: „die volle und wirksame Teilhabe an der Gesellschaft und Einbeziehung in die Gesellschaft".

Und in § 4 SGB IX (2020): „Die Leistungen zur Teilhabe umfassen die notwendigen Sozialleistungen, um unabhängig von der Ursache der Behinderung (…) die persönliche Entwicklung ganzheitlich zu fördern und die Teilhabe am Leben in der Gesellschaft sowie eine möglichst selbständige und selbstbestimmte Lebensführung zu ermöglichen oder zu erleichtern."

Die Chance, die einzigartige Kompetenz der Ergotherapie zu demonstrieren, sollte wahrgenommen werden. Denn das Bio-psycho-soziale Modell erleichtert den Austausch zwischen den unterschiedlichen Berufsgruppen, da alle dasselbe Modell benutzen.

- In der Interaktion mit Ärzten kann der dynamische Prozess der Teilhabe der Klienten als Kernkompetenz der Ergotherapie kommuniziert werden.
- Bei der Zielsetzung im interdisziplinären Therapeutinnenteam kann die spezielle Interaktion von Funktion, Aktivität und Partizipation im Rahmen der Umwelt des Klienten benannt werden.
- Bei der Begründung gegenüber Krankenkassen kann die eingeschränkte Partizipation des Klienten als Begründung für die Verordnung von Ergotherapie dienen.
- Zur verständlichen Erklärung der Komplexität des Inhaltes der ergotherapeutischen Intervention kann das Bio-psycho-soziale Modell zur Veranschaulichung genutzt werden.

In der Abb. 5.1 ist der Aufbau des Modells dargestellt.

Um die Informationen abzufragen, wird ein freies Interview genutzt. Das heißt, Therapeutin und Klient führen ein teil-strukturiertes Gespräch, in dem herausgefunden wird, welche aktuellen Gesundheitsprobleme bestehen, wie diese sich auf Funktion, Aktivität und Partizipation auswirken und welche Rolle dabei Umweltfaktoren und personenbezogene Faktoren spielen. Dabei trägt die Therapeuten folgende Informationen in die zugehörigen Zellen ein:

- Gesundheitsproblem: die Diagnose und Nebendiagnosen
- Körperfunktionen und -strukturen: Körperfunktionen sind die physiologischen und psychischen Funktionen von Körpersystemen. Die Körperstrukuren sind die anatomischen Teile des Körpers. Dazu gehören z. B. mentale Funktionen, neuromuskuloskeletale Funktionen, Strukturen des Nervensystems.
- Aktivitäten: Eine Aktivität stellt die Durchführung einer Aufabe oder Handlung durch

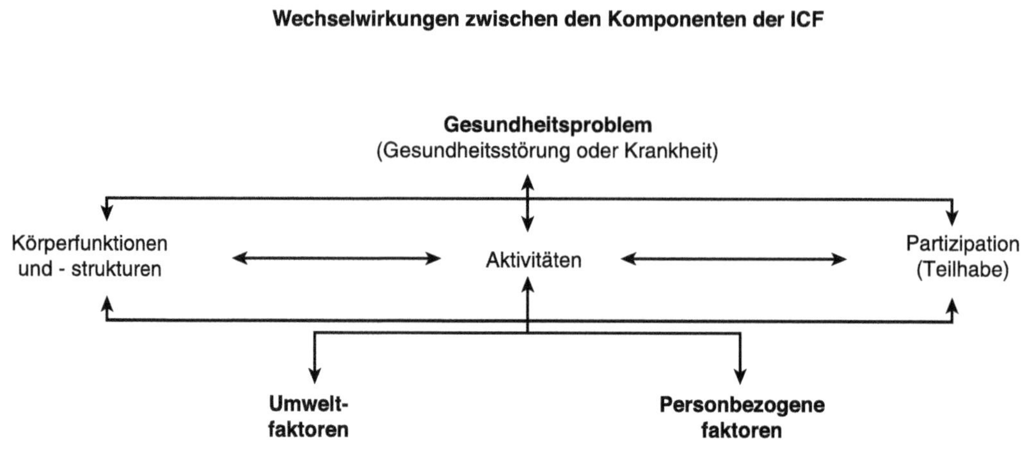

Abb. 5.1 Bio-psycho-soziales Model der ICF (2001)

Tab. 5.2 Die Zusammenhänge zwischen Körperfunktion, Aktivität und Partizipation sind auf einen Blick ersichtlich

Körperfunktion: Ruhe- und Haltetremor	⟷	**Aktivität**: Essen fällt herunter	⟷	**Partizipation**: Essen in Öffentlichkeit wird vermieden

einen Menschen in einer bestimmten Situation dar. Dazu gehören z. B. Kommunikation, Mobilität, Selbstversorgung.

- Partizipation (Teilhabe): Die Teilhabe kennzeichnet das Einbezogensein in eine Lebenssituation, z. B. Mobilität, interpersonelle Interaktionen, bedeutende Lebensbereiche (Arbeit).
- Umweltfaktoren: Umweltfaktoren bilden die materielle Umwelt (z. B. Produkte wie Medikamente und Hilfsmittel), soziale Umwelt (z. B. Unterstützung durch Familie und Vorgesetzte) und einstellungsbezogene Umwelt (z. B. Meinungen und Überzeugungen von Klient, Familie und Freunden), in der Menschen leben und ihr Dasein entfalten und die individuelles Verhalten und Handlungen beeinflussen.
- Personenbezogene Faktoren: z. B. Geschlecht, ethnische Zugehörigkeit, Alter, sozialer Hintergrund, Bildung, Beruf, Charaktereigenschaften, …

Dieses Schema erinnert die Therapeutin konstant daran, auf alle Komponenten zu achten, die einen möglichen Einfluss auf den Alltag des Betroffenen haben. Es lässt den dynamischen Prozess erkennen, den eine Behinderung mit sich bringt. Außerdem sind wechselseitige Zusammenhänge zwischen den einzelnen Komponenten auf einen Blick ersichtlich, wie im Beispiel in der Tab. 5.2 erkennbar ist.

Beim Ausfüllen des Bio-psycho-sozialen Modells können hinter den eingetragenen Stichpunkten ein Minus (-) für negative bzw. ein Plus (+) für positive Punkte notiert werden (siehe Abb. 5.2). Dies zeigt, anders als eine defizitorientierte Sichtweise, ein positiv ressourcenorientiertes Bild des Bio-psycho-sozialen Modells.

▶ Das Bio-psycho-soziale Modell kann in der Akte des Patienten als Erstes eingeheftet werden. So hat die Therapeutin immer die Übersicht vor Augen und evtl. vertretende Therapeutinnen können auf einen Blick die wichtigsten Informationen des Klienten sehen.

5.3 Betätigungsprofil

Eine gute Möglichkeit, um eine Übersicht aller Betätigungen eines Klienten zu bekommen, ist die Erstellung eines Betätigungsprofils. Hier trägt der Klient selbst, oder dessen Angehörige oder Pflegekraft alle Betätigungen in eine Tabelle

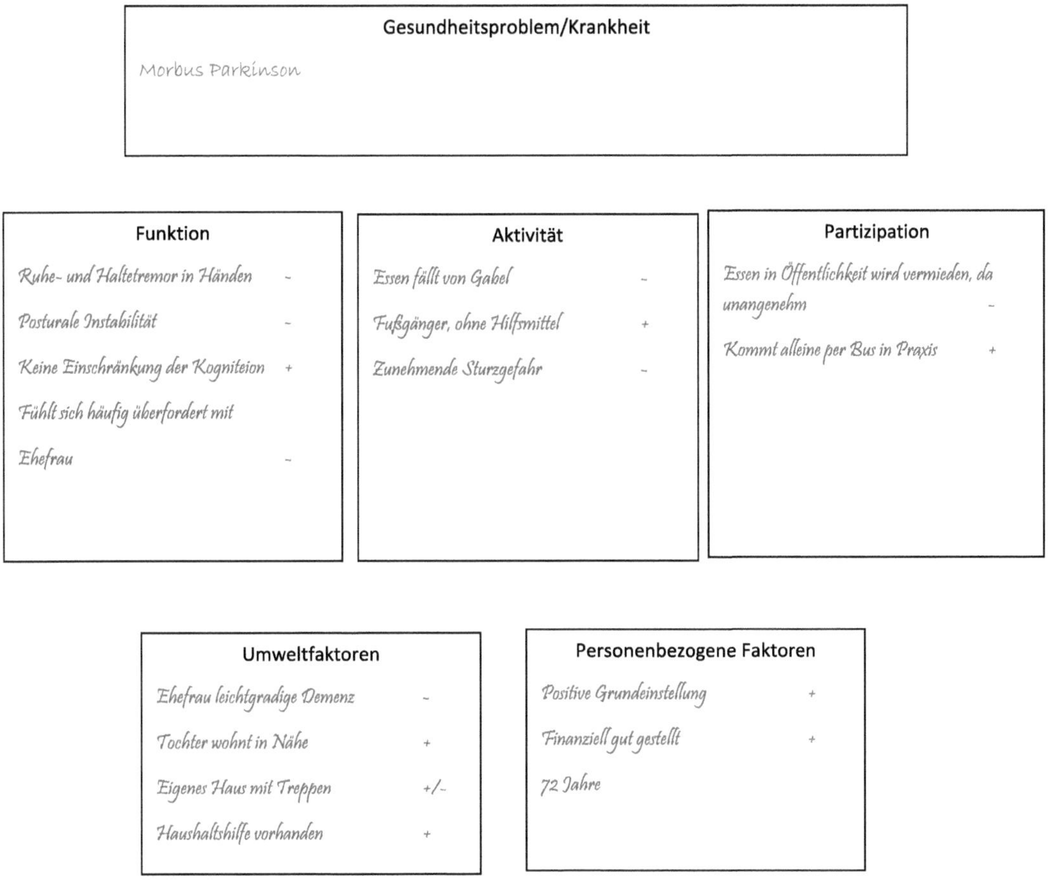

Abb. 5.2 Ausfüllbeispiel, Bio-psycho-soziales Modell

ein, die er an einem Tag ausführt und beschreibt, wie er sie durchführt, ob Hilfe benötigt wurde, welche negativen und positiven Faktoren die Betätigung beeinflussen und auftretende Symptome (z. B. Tremor, Tagesmüdigkeit, Inkontinenz). Dazu bewertet er die Performanz und die Zufriedenheit zu jeder Betätigung mit Zahlen von eins = gar nicht zufrieden, bis zehn = sehr zufrieden. Wenn die Zahlen aus kognitiven Gründen nicht eingetragen werden können, ist dies nicht notwendig. Die Beschreibung gibt meist gute Anhaltspunkte, damit die Therapeutin genauer nachfragen kann (s. Abb. 5.3).

Das Ausfüllen des Betätigungsprofils regt beim Klienten häufig eine Auseinandersetzung mit der Art von Betätigungen in seinem Alltag an. Viele Menschen machen sich beim Ausfüllen der Tabelle zum ersten Mal seit Beginn der Krankheitssymptome genauere Gedanken über Prioritätensetzung, Zufriedenheit, zeitliche Intensität, Häufigkeit und zeitliche Abfolge ihrer Betätigungen. Auch deswegen schafft es die optimale Voraussetzung, um im nächsten Schritt das COPM auszufüllen.

5.4 COPM

Das COPM (Canadian Occupational Performance Measure) ist ein validiertes, klientenzentriertes Untersuchungsinstrument des CMOP-E (Canadian Model of Occupational Performance and Engagement. Gemessen werden aus Sicht des Klienten:

- die Wichtigkeit von Betätigungen,
- die Performanz bei der Ausführung,
- die Zufriedenheit mit der Ausführung.

Betätigungsprofil

Name: Friedrich Schiller **Datum:** 11.03.2021

Ausgefüllt von: Friedrich und Erika Schiller

Uhrzeit	Tätigkeit	Beschreibung der Ausführung (Mit/ohne Hilfe, positive/negative Faktoren, auftretende Symptome)	P	Z
7:00	Aufwachen, Morgengymnastik im Bett	Zu Beginn der Übungen, Muskeln steif. Danach beweglicher.	1	1
7:20	Aufstehen, Waschen, Anziehen	Mit Hilfe (Ehefrau) bei Knöpfen und Zähneputzen, sonst selbständig, zu langsam	6	8
8:00	Frühstücken	Selbständig, Kaffee wird verschüttet, wegen Tremor	10	10
9:00	Zeitung lesen	Im Lieblingssessel, Zeitung liegt auf Knie, wegen Tremor	1	2
10:00	Fertigmachen	Jacke anziehen wackelig, Schuhe binden mit Hilfe	4	5
10:20	Fahrt zur Gymnastik	Fahrdienst	1	1
11:00	Gymnastik	V iele Übungen jetzt zu schwer, überlege aufzuhören	6	8
12:10	Rückfahrt	Fahrdienst	1	1
12:30	Mittagsschlaf	Sonst erst nach dem Essen, heute so müde, weil schlecht geschlafen	3	2
13:40	Mittagessen	Tremor besser, alles gut geklappt	1	1
14:00	Hausarbeit	Mit Ehefrau Wäsche aufhängen, mit Musik klappt zufriedenstellend	2	1
15:30	Kaffee trinken	Mit Schnabelbecher, da Tremor wieder stärker	3	5
16:30	Alleine Zuhause	Ehefrau geht einkaufen, Im Sessel Eingedöst	1	1
17:30	Essenzubereiten	Mit Ehefrau, es ist schön nützlich zu sein, etwas unsicher beim Stehen und Schneiden	4	7
19:00	Fernsehen, ins Bett gehen	Ohne Hilfe, insgesamt entspannt und müde	1	1

Abb. 5.3 Betätigungsprofil, Ausfüllbeispiel

Daraus werden bis zu fünf Betätigungsziele/ Betätigungswünsche formuliert, die der Klient selbst ausgewählt und bewertet hat. Die Therapeutin dient dem Betroffenen nur als Assistentin bei der Benennung und Einschätzung der Alltagstätigkeiten. Das Assessment wird entweder nur mit dem Parkinson-Betroffenen durchgeführt oder es wird ein Angehöriger, meist der Ehepartner, mitbefragt. Dies ist in zwei Situationen sinnvoll. Zum einen, wenn eine mittelschwere bis schwere Demenz besteht, um die Anwendung des COPM überhaupt zu ermöglichen. Zum anderen, wenn der Angehörige wesentlich in die Pflege involviert ist. In diesem Fall kommt es oft zu Konflikten im Umgang, zu fehlerhaft ausgeführter Hilfe (Transfer, Essen reichen…) und Überlastung des Angehörigen. Hierbei wird nicht nur der Patient mit Parkinson-Erkrankung als Klient gesehen, sondern die Kombination Patient – Angehörige (siehe Abschn. 1.2).

Durchführung des COPM

Zu Beginn der Erfassung wird dem Klienten kurz die Struktur des COPM gezeigt. Es werden die drei Bereiche **Selbstversorgung, Produktivität** und **Freizeit** mit knappen Unterpunkten erläutert.

Anschließend beginnt ein halbstrukturiertes Interview. Die Fragetechnik ist sehr vorsichtig. Behutsam stößt die Therapeutin die Gedanken des Klienten über seinen Tagesablauf und die darin enthaltenen Betätigungen an. Erzählt der Klient flüssig von allein, macht sich die Therapeutin Notizen und fragt nur nach, wenn Unklarheiten entstehen oder um das Problem detaillierter erfassen zu können. Fällt dem Klienten keine wichtige Tätigkeit ein, gibt die Therapeutin Stichwörter in Form von Überbegriffen vor. Zum Beispiel, „Was machen Sie in Ihrer aktiven Freizeit?“ „Haben Sie aktive Hobbies oder Interessen?“ „Gibt es da irgendwelche Probleme?“ Es wird vermieden, Beispiele zu nennen, um einer Beeinflussung entgegenzuwirken. Berichtet der Betroffene von Beeinträchtigungen auf Ebene der Körperfunktionen, werden diese auch notiert. Indem die Ergotherapeutin genau nachfragt, sollte es gelingen, die wahren Probleme bei der Betätigung herauszufinden. Zum Beispiel, „Wie wirkt sich die Steifigkeit im Körper im Alltag aus?“ oder „Wann stört Sie die Steifigkeit im Körper im Tagesablauf am meisten?“

Jede Betätigung wird vom Klienten in ihrer **Wichtigkeit** auf einer Skala von eins bis zehn eingestuft. Aus den wichtigsten Betätigungen werden **Ziele** formuliert. Hierbei benötigt der Klient meist Hilfestellung, um ein Ziel zu benennen, welches messbar und konkret ist. Zum Beispiel, anstatt: „Ich will alleine aufstehen können.“, könnte das Ziel heißen: „Aufstehen aus dem Lieblingssessel, ohne Hilfe.“ Zu jedem Ziel schätzt der Klient noch ein, wie seine **Performanz**, also die Qualität der Durchführung, ist. Dazu wird wieder die Skala von eins bis zehn genutzt. Eins = überhaupt nicht gut, zehn = besonders gut. Außerdem wird noch ein Wert für die **Zufriedenheit** mit der Performanz jeder Tätigkeit von eins bis zehn abgefragt. Diese messbaren Werte werden nach einer festgelegten Zeit (z. B. drei Monate) wieder abgefragt. So entstehen Messbarkeit und Überprüfbarkeit.

Für diese Art der Interviewgestaltung bedarf es Empathie und Geschick. Es wird empfohlen, eine Fortbildung zu diesem Thema zu besuchen, um Sicherheit in der Fragetechnik zu bekommen und eine tiefgreifende Beeinflussung des Klienten zu vermeiden. Ohne eine ausreichende Auseinandersetzung läuft man Gefahr, das COPM lediglich auszufüllen, was nicht im Sinne der Entwickler ist. Richtig angewandt ermöglicht das COPM einen ausgezeichneten Start in die therapeutische Intervention, die von Empowerment und Kooperation geprägt sein wird.

Am Ende des COPM hält die Ergotherapeutin zwischen einem und fünf Betätigungsziele oder Betätigungswünsche in der Hand, die dem Klienten wichtig sind (siehe zum Beispiel Tab. 5.3.

Die Ziele beinhalten meist eine Mischung von Betätigungen aus sehr unterschiedlichen Tätigkeitsbereichen, zum Beispiel, Mobilität, Kommunikation und Selbstversorgung. Diese Wünsche können, müssen aber nicht die endgültigen Ziele sein. Erst nach der Durchführung der Betätigungsanalyse und evtl. ergänzender Testungen bestimmen Therapeutin und Klient gemeinsam die Therapieziele (siehe Abschn. 8.1).

Tab. 5.3 Beispiel für Betätigungsziele oder -wünsche des Klienten mit von ihm angegebenen Wichtigkeit, Ausführung und Zufriedenheit mit der Ausführung (von 1 bis 10)

Problem der Betätigungsperformanz	Wichtigkeit	Ausführung	Zufriedenheit
Essen mit Messer und Gabel, ohne Essen zu verschütten (wegen Tremor)	7	3	1
Strecke von Bett zu Toilette nachts ohne Sturz laufen	5	5	4
Lauter sprechen, um am Telefon verstanden zu werden	3	4	4
Allein aus dem Bett aufstehen	3	5	3

Weitere Erfassungsmethoden von Klientenwünschen

Wenn das COPM aufgrund von eingeschränkter Kommunikation oder verminderten kognitiven Fähigkeiten nicht anwendbar ist, muss man auf andere Erfassungsmethoden zurückgreifen.

1. Befragen von nahen Angehörigen oder Pflegenden
   Dabei versucht man einfühlsam aufzudecken, welche Betätigungen wirklich für den Klienten wichtig sind. Außerdem kann so auch eine mögliche Überlastung von Angehörigen abgefragt werden. Wenn die Angehörigen nur selten oder nie zeitgleich mit der Therapeutin bei dem Betroffenen sind, kann eine Kontaktaufnahme per schriftlicher Notiz am Bettrand hilfreich sein.
2. Karten mit Aktivitäten zeigen
   Dabei werden Karten mit verschiedenen Aktivitäten gezeigt. Der Klient zeigt auf eine, die ihm wichtig ist. Hierbei können die „BIDO-G"-Karten hilfreich sein. Auf den 97 Fotokarten sind junge Erwachsene abgebildet, die unterschiedliche Alltagsaktivitäten ausführen. Dies sind Aktivitäten der verschiedenen Lebensbereiche, die in der ICF im Konzept „Aktivitäten und Partizipation" klassifiziert sind.
3. Ausprobieren und kreativ werden (s. Abb. 5.4)
   Gibt es keine Möglichkeit, vom Klienten selbst oder von Mitmenschen des Klienten Informationen über dessen Betätigungswunsch zu erfahren, muss ausprobiert werden.
   Hierbei sollte mit körpernahen Aktivitäten des täglichen Lebens begonnen werden, die der überwiegenden Mehrheit der Menschen wichtig sind, z. B:
   - Körperhygiene (Waschen, Zähne putzen, Kämmen),
   - Anziehen,
   - Essen,
   - Toilettengang,
   - Lagewechsel im Bett.

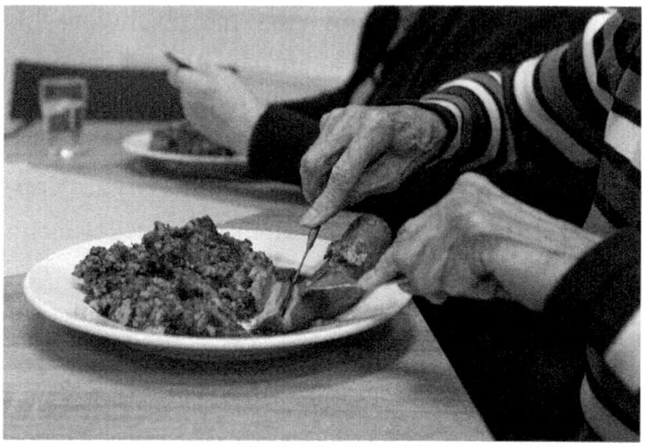

Abb. 5.4 Ausprobieren und Beobachten kann eine verbale Erfassung von Betätigungsproblemen ersetzen, wenn Klienten eine eingeschränkte Kommunikationsfähigkeit oder demenzielle Entwicklung haben

Eine weitere Art einer – dem Klienten wichtigen – Betätigung auf die Spur zu kommen ist es, persönliche Gegenstände des Klienten als Hinweis zu nutzen und in eine Aktivität einzubeziehen, z. B:

- Schminke auftragen,
- Fotobuch der Familie ansehen,
- Radio bedienen.

Von der Reaktion des Klienten auf die gemeinsame Betätigung muss die empathische Therapeutin Notiz nehmen und daraus folgern, ob sie auf dem richtigen Weg ist. Zeigt der Klient Interesse, kann die kooperative Exploration der möglichen Ausführung der Betätigung aufgenommen werden.

Beispiel

Frau N. kommt entspannt aus der ersten Ergotherapie-Stunde. Sie ist erleichtert, Tests gab es hier keine. Dafür viele Fragen. Fragen, bei denen sie wirklich in sich gehen musste. Was fällt ihr im Alltag schwer? Nicht allgemein, sondern ganz konkret. Und wie wichtig ist es ihr, in der Klinik am Laufen und am Bluse zuknöpfen zu arbeiten? Oder doch lieber am Schreiben? Es sei ganz wichtig, hat die Ergotherapeutin gesagt, dass die Ziele von ihr – der Klientin – kämen, weil nur sie ihr Leben so gut kenne. Auf dem Zimmer überlegt Frau N. nochmal, ob sie wirklich das Wichtigste erzählt hat, oder ob noch etwas fehlt. Die Ziele könne man immer anpassen, beruhigte sie die Ergotherapeutin noch beim Hinausgehen. ◀

Literatur und weiterführende Literatur

BAR, BAG BBW, Hochschule Magdeburg-Stendal (2019) Bedarfsermittlungskonzept für Leistungen zur Teilhabe am Arbeitsleben. www.bar-frankfurt.de. Zugegriffen am 02.03.2020

Bundesgesetzblatt Jahrgang 2008 Teil II Nr. 35, Artikel 3, Bonn

Bundesinstitut für Arzneimittel und Medizinpodukte (BfArM) 2020 im Auftrag des Bundesministeriums für Gesundheit (BMG) unter Beteiligung der Arbeitsgruppe ICD des Kuratoriums für Fragen der Klassifikation im Gesundheitswesen (KKG), ICD-10-GM Version 2021, Systematisches Verzeichnis, Internationale statistische Klassifikation der Krankheiten und verwandter Gesundheitsprobleme, 10. Revision, Stand: 18. September 2020, Dateiname: icd10gm2021syst_odt_20200918.pdf, Website: www.dimdi.de – Klassifikationen – Downloads – ICD-10-GM – Version 2021. Zugegriffen am 18.09.2020

Cibis W (2016) ICF-Praxisleitfaden 4, Trägerübergreifende Informationen und Anregungen für die praktische Nutzung der Internationalen Klassifikation der Funktionsfähigkeit, Behinderung und Gesundheit (ICF).Bundesarbeitsgemeinschaft für Rehabilitation (BAR) e. V, Frankfurt am Main

Law M (2002) Participation in the occupations of everyday life. Am J Occup Ther 56(6):640–649. https://doi.org/10.5014/ajot.56.6.640

Law M, Baptiste S, Mills J (1995) Client-centred practice: what does it mean and does it make a difference? Can J Occup Ther 62(5):250–257. https://doi.org/10.1177/000841749506200504. PMID: 10152881

Law M, Steinwender S, Leclair L (1998) Occupation, health and well-being. Can J Occup Ther/Revue Canadienne D'Ergothérapie 65(2):81–91. https://doi.org/10.1177/000841749806500204#

Law M, Polatajko H, Carswell A, McColl MA, Pollock N, Baptiste S (1999) Das Kanadische Modell der Occupational Performance und das Canadian Occupational Performance Measure. In: Jerosch-Herold C, Marotzki U, Hack BM, Weber P (Hrsg) Konzeptionelle Modelle für die ergotherapeutische Praxis. Ergotherapie – Reflexion und Analyse. Springer, Berlin/Heidelberg. https://doi.org/10.1007/978-3-662-08173-0_7

Sozialgesetzbuch (SGB IX), Neuntes Buch, Rehabilitation und Teilhabe von Menschen mit Behinderungen, Stand: Zuletzt geändert durch Art. 3 Abs. 6 G v. 9.10.2020 I 2075

Sturkenboom I, Thijssen M, Gons-van Elsacker J, Jansen I, Maasdam A, Schulten M, Vijver-Visser D, Steultjens E, Bloem B, Munneke M (2008) Guidelines for occupational therapy in Parkinson's disease rehabilitation. ParkinsonNet/NPF, Nijmegen/Miami

Übereinkommen über die Rechte von Menschen mit Behinderungen (Convention on the Rights of Persons with Disabilities – CRPD), Artikel 3, Menschenrechtsübereinkommen der Vereinten Nationen (2006) Generalversammlung der Vereinten Nationen

Vincon S, Romein E, Burmester S, Langsdorf S (2015) Ein roter Faden für die Therapie, Kientenzentrierte Ergotherapie in der Pädiatrie, Ergopraxis. Thieme, Stuttgart

Weinstock-Zlotnick G, Hinojosa J (2004) Bottom-up or top-down evaluation: is one better than the other? Am J Occup Ther 58(5):594–599. https://doi.org/10.5014/ajot.58.5.594. PMID: 15481786

World Health Organization & World Bank (2011) World report on disability 2011. World Health Organization. https://apps.who.int/iris/handle/10665/44575

6 Betätigungsanalyse und Hypothesenbildung

Beispiel

Herr T. hat als Betätigungswunsch „Essen ohne zu kleckern" angegeben. In den ersten Therapiestunden fällt der Therapeutin jedoch die große Unsicherheit beim Jacke anziehen auf. Auf Nachfrage gibt der Klient an, schon mal beim Jacke anziehen gestürzt zu sein. In Absprache mit Herrn T. entscheidet sie sich, die Betätigung „Jacke anziehen" genau zu beobachten, da eine erhöhte Sturzgefahr besteht und die Therapeutin einem Sturz vorbeugen möchte. ◀

Sobald der Therapeut den Betätigungswunsch der Klientin ermittelt hat, muss er die Betätigung analysieren. Die genaue Beobachtung der Klientin bei der Ausführung ihrer problematischen Betätigung ist für moderne Ergotherapeuten unumgänglich. Es ist der zentrale Inhalt des Top-Down-Ansatzes, denn nur bei der Betätigungsanalyse ist das komplexe Zusammenspiel zwischen der Betätigung und allen situativen Kontextfaktoren erkennbar.

▶ Mit der Durchführung einer Betätigungsanalyse hebt sich die Expertise der Ergotherapeuten heraus und unterscheidet sie eindeutig von allen anderen Gesundheitsberufen.

6.1 Gegenüberstellung Betätigungsanalyse – Funktionsanalyse

Bis vor zehn Jahren war es anerkannte Praxis in Deutschland, alle eingeschränkten Funktionen einer Parkinson-Klientinnen in einem ergotherapeutischen Befundbogen zu erfassen, etwa so:

Tremor ja ☐ nein ☐

Rigor ja ☐ nein ☐

Akinese:

Sprache:

Greiffunktionen:

....

Auch heute noch kann es angemessen sein, den Grad des Rigors oder das Auftreten eines Tremors zu erfassen. Die Betätigungsanalyse ist jedoch das ergotherapeutische Hauptassessment. Die Funktionen wurden aus der Annahme heraus erfasst, dass eine eingeschränkte Funktion eine eingeschränkte Performanz der Betätigung zur

A. Orellana, *Betätigungsorientierte Ergotherapie bei Morbus Parkinson*,
https://doi.org/10.1007/978-3-662-62583-5_6

Folge hat. Das kann auch zutreffen, muss jedoch nicht sein, siehe Abschn. 4.1 und 4.5. So kann z. B. eine kyphotische Haltung erkennbar sein, die im Alltag jedoch keinerlei Einschränkungen zur Folge hat. Oder ein Tremor macht der Klientin das leserliche Schreiben unmöglich, sie hat jedoch schon seit vielen Jahren alle schriftlichen Angelegenheiten per Computer erledigt. Das Schreiben mit dem Stift ist für sie also keine bedeutsame Betätigung.

6.2 Zeitpunkt der Betätigungsanalyse

Da die tageszeitliche Verfassung bei Menschen mit M. Parkinson aufgrund von Medikamentenwirkung und Fatigue schwankt, ist der gewählte Zeitpunkt der Betätigungsanalyse von grundlegender Bedeutung. Bei Betätigungen, die immer zur selben Tageszeit stattfinden, wie Mittagessen oder Transfer ins Bett, wird die Betätigung idealerweise zu der Uhrzeit beobachtet, zu der sie üblicherweise durchgeführt wird. Ist dies aus organisatorischen Gründen nicht möglich, kann ein Angehöriger gebeten werden, ein Video der Tätigkeit aufzunehmen (s. Abb. 6.1).

Bei Betätigungen, die zu wechselnden Tageszeiten stattfinden (wie Wasser trinken oder Toilettengang), ist es sinnvoll, sich zwei Mal für die Betätigungsanalyse Zeit zu nehmen: einmal in der On-Phase, wenn die Medikamentenwirkung ihren vollen Effekt hat, und einmal in der Off-Phase, wenn die Wirkung nachgelassen hat und sich die Symptome verstärkt zeigen. Dies ist nicht bei allen Klienten nötig. Im Frühstadium der Erkrankung und bei einer optimalen Medikamenteneinstellung wird meist ein Abrutschen ins Off verhindert.

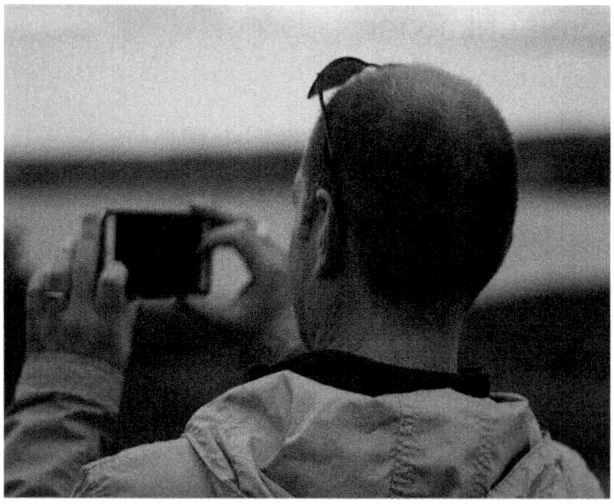

Abb. 6.1 Ein Video der Durchführung der Betätigung im gewohnten Kontext erlaubt dem Therapeuten wertvolle Einblicke

Die Fragestellung der Medikamentenwirkung kann bei der Behandlung von Menschen mit M. Parkinson ein Schlüsselfaktor beim therapeutischen Vorgehen sein (siehe Abschn. 7.8). Die Erfassung der Medikamentenwirkung im Zusammenhang mit Betätigungsperformanz ist sehr wichtig, um im Anschluss eine mögliche Ursache für die problematische Durchführung korrekt zu identifizieren. Dazu kann das Parkinson-Tagebuch im Anhang genutzt werden.

▶ Bei der Betätigungsanalyse muss immer auch die momentane Medikamentenwirkung erfasst werden, da sie erheblichen Einfluss auf die Performanz der Klientin hat.

6.3 Kontextfaktoren beim Assessment

Der situative Kontext ist unlösbar mit der Betätigung und allen anderen Kontextfaktoren verflochten. Deswegen kann eine Betätigung nicht effektiv beobachtet werden, wenn sie in einem anderen Kontext durchgeführt wird. Je weiter die Untersuchung durch den Therapeuten vom Kontext entfernt ist, desto weniger aussagekräftig ist sie. Aus diesem Grund muss der Ergotherapeut versuchen, das Assessment im reellen Kontext (z. B. im Heim der Klientin) oder so nah dran wie möglich durchzuführen. Die beste Möglichkeit dazu ist, die ergotherapeutische Intervention oder zumindest das Assessment im Hausbesuch durchzuführen.

Bei der Behandlung in einer ergotherapeutischen Praxis kann es sich lohnen, mit dem Arzt Rücksprache zu halten, wenn dieser keinen Hausbesuch verordnet hat. Nach der Erklärung, dass die Ergotherapie (oder wenigstens das Assessment) im Hausbesuch wesentlich besser auf die Klientin abgestimmt werden kann, wenn sie im Alltagskontext stattfindet, ist die Ärztin meist mit einer Änderung des Rezeptes auf „Hausbesuch“ einverstanden.

Bei einer Rehabilitation in der Klinik besteht die Möglichkeit der Betätigungsanalyse im reellen Kontext meist nicht. Vor dieser Hürde stehen Ergotherapeuten in Kliniken täglich. Sie wird auch mit Abstand am häufigsten genannt, wenn es um Schwierigkeiten bei der Umsetzung von betätigungsorientiertem Arbeiten geht. Hier einige Vorschläge, wie an das Thema des betätigungsorientierten Assessment und der Therapie in einer Klinik herangegangen werden könnte:

1. Beim Aufbau einer Ergotherapie-Abteilung eine Vielzahl von Alltagsgegenständen anschaffen und eine Therapieküche mit unterschiedlichsten Utensilien einrichten. Dies schafft von Anfang an eine Plattform, um mit Vorgesetzten und den angrenzenden Fachbereichen über die Rolle der Ergotherapie zu kommunizieren.
2. Bei einem Budget für Neuanschaffungen die Auswahl der Alltagsgegenstände erweitern. Dies kann mithilfe der ergotherapeutischen Praxismodelle gut begründet werden (siehe Kap. 2).
3. In der Klinik umschauen und erkundigen, welche vorhandenen Gegenstände es gibt, die bei Bedarf genutzt werden könnten (tiefer Sessel, Wasserkasten, Waschmaschine, Gartengeräte).
4. Angehörige bitten, entsprechende Gegenstände (oder Fotos davon) mitzubringen, um Betätigung genau nachstellen zu können.
5. Die Betätigung simulieren, also so genau wie möglich nachstellen. Dies ist bei körpernahen Alltagsaktivitäten am besten umzusetzen, da die Klientin die notwendigen Utensilien ent weder dabeihat (Haare kämmen, Zähne putzen) oder keine spezifischen benötigt (Aufstehen vom Stuhl, Essen).
6. Wenn die Betätigung sehr speziell ist und eine Nachstellung unmöglich (Autofahren, elektrische Eisenbahn bedienen), können Teilschritte nachgestellt werden (Einsteigen ins Auto, Verbindung von zwei Gleiselementen).
7. Es kann ein anderes Ziel gewählt werden, bei dem der Kontext nicht im Vordergrund steht (z. B. Treppensteigen, Kommunikation mit Unbekannten)
8. Beim Assessment des Betätigungsanliegens (siehe Abschn. 5.4) kann der Therapeut direkt nach einem Problem im **aktuellen Kontext der Klinik** fragen. Dies kann Körperhygiene, Abläufe, Tagesstrukturierung und mehr betreffen. Dies kann eine gute Möglichkeit sein, die Handlungsfähigkeit der Klientin zu ermöglichen.

6.4 Reaktive Effekte minimieren

Allein durch die Anwesenheit des Therapeuten ist die Situation verändert und das Ergebnis der Beobachtung verzerrt. Peter Atteslander stellt in diesem Zusammenhang fest, dass „jede Beobachtung im strengen Sinne teilnehmend ist“ (Atteslander 1995). Die Klientin kann sich bewusst oder unbewusst anders verhalten, weil sie jemand beobachtet. Sie kann besonders konzentriert oder auch abgelenkt sein und sie gibt sich vielleicht besondere Mühe. Auch Angehörige passen ihre Kommunikation daran an, was ihrer Meinung nach von ihnen erwartet wird. Sie zeigen sich dann mehr oder weniger geduldig und mehr oder weniger streng mit der Betroffenen. Um eine möglichst realistische Version der Betätigung beobachten zu können, ist eine genaue Besprechung zur Einführung der Betätigungsanalyse wichtig. Inhalt der Einführung sollte sein:

- Der Therapeut schafft eine freundliche, entspannte Atmosphäre.
- Er klärt, welche Betätigung beobachtet wird.
- Genauer Start und genaues Ende wird festgelegt.
- Klientin und andere anwesende Personen sollen versuchen, die Betätigung so durchzuführen wie gewöhnlich.
- Der Therapeut sollte während der Durchführung nicht angesprochen oder beachtet werden.
- Im Anschluss wird es die Möglichkeit der Besprechung geben.

- Dies ist kein Test, sondern dient lediglich der Beobachtung zur Einschätzung, woran in der Therapie gearbeitet werden kann.
- Huber (1989) spricht von einer Eingewöhnungsphase der beobachteten Personen als Mittel gegen reaktive Effekte.

6.5 Durchführung der Betätigungsanalyse

Die Durchführung der Betätigungsanalyse ist unkompliziert, wenn die Vorbereitung sorgfältig umgesetzt wurde. Der Therapeut sitzt an einem Ort, wo er der Klientin nicht im Weg ist. Er beobachtet genau die Ausführung der Betätigung und notiert sich alle Auffälligkeiten, Stärken sowie Schwächen der einzelnen Performance-Skills (Performanzfertigkeiten). Sie sind die kleinsten Einheiten, aus denen eine Betätigung zusammengesetzt ist (siehe Tab. 6.1, Abb. 6.2).

Während der Betätigungsanalyse legt der Therapeut ein besonderes Augenmerk auf die Breakdown-points – entscheidende Momente, in denen Probleme zu beobachten sind, die als Ursache für ein Nichtgelingen der Betätigung erkannt werden.

Tab. 6.1 Beispiel der einzelnen Performance-Skills einer Betätigung

Betätigung	Performance-Skills (Performanzfertigkeiten)
Anruf beantworten	In Tasche greifen
	Smartphone umfassen
	Smartphone herausziehen
	Über Display wischen
	Smartphone ans Ohr halten
	Sprechen

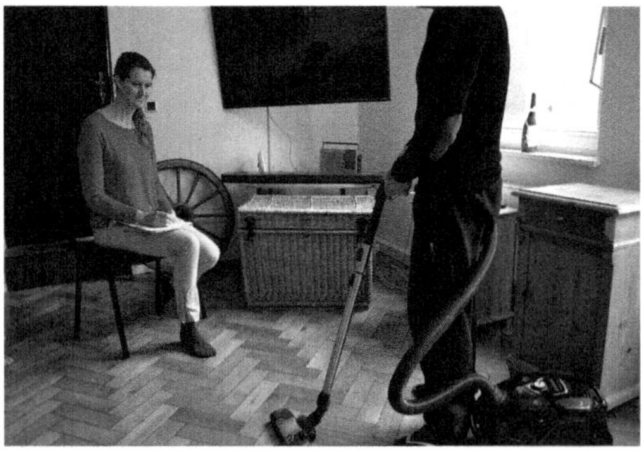

Abb. 6.2 Bei der Betätigungsanalyse beobachtet der Therapeut, ohne einzugreifen

6.6 Dokumentation

Mithilfe des Bogens zur Dokumentation der Betätigungsanalyse (siehe Anhang) lassen sich die Performance-Skills, Breakdown-Points und (hinderliche und fördernde) Kontextfaktoren der Betätigung schnell erfassen. Zusätzlich werden folgende Qualitätsfaktoren für die gesamte Durchführung der Betätigung (angelehnt an Anne Fischer) bewertet:

- Anstrengung (Grad der Anstrengung, Ungeschicklichkeit oder Ermüdung)
- Effizienz (Grad der Organisiertheit und Nutzung von Zeit, Raum oder Gegenständen)
- Sicherheit (Grad des Sicherheitsrisikos oder Verletzung der Person oder Beschädigung der Umwelt)
- Selbständigkeit (Häufigkeit der benötigten Hilfe oder verbaler Unterstützung)
- Soziale Angemessenheit (Grad der sozialen Geschicklichkeit und Reife)

6.7 Hypothesenbildung/Interpretation

Bei der Beobachtung wurde ganz bewusst darauf geachtet, nur das äußerlich Sichtbare zu dokumentieren. Dadurch wird eine vorschnelle Interpretation des Gesehenens vermieden. Mit zunehmender Erfahrung wird der Therapeut immer schneller und immer treffender Hypothesen zu den Ursachen für die problematische Betätigung entwickeln. Dabei ist eine kritische Selbstreflexion wichtig, um für falsche Hypothesen sensibel zu bleiben, und um die Therapie entsprechend anpassen zu können. So mag der Therapeut zunächst die Hypothese haben, dass das Anziehen der Klientin morgens, wegen einer eingeschränkten Kognition und daraus folgender mangelnder Strukturierung, nicht selbständig klappt. Beim Üben erkennt der Therapeut, dass die Klientin den Ablauf des Ankleidens durchaus ohne Hilfe durchführen kann. Durch die starke Verlangsamung jedoch in Zeitdruck gerät, weil der Ehemann schnell zum Frühstück möchte. Der Therapeut passt seine Hypothese an.

Bei der Hypothesenbildung weitet der Therapeut den Fokus auf alle situativen Kontextfaktoren, die auf eine Betätigung einwirken aus. Dazu kann die Abb. 4.1 in Abschn. 4.1 sehr hilfreich sein. Nach der Beobachtung der Betätigung vergegenwärtigt man sich die Gesamtheit der situativen Elemente, um nichts außer Acht zu lassen. So erhält der Ergotherapeut ein möglichst umfassendes Bild der Einflussfaktoren, die eine mögliche Ursache des Betätigungsproblems sind. Viele Therapeuten sind es gewohnt, sofort auf die Körperfunktionen zu zielen. Und bei einer chronischen Erkrankung wie M. Parkinson wird man sicherlich Einschränkungen auf der Ebene der Körperfunktionen finden. Trotzdem ist es nicht sicher, dass dies die (einzige) Ursache für ein Nichtgelingen der Aufgabe ist. Meist ist es eine Kombination von unterschiedlichen Einflüssen (s. Tab. 6.2).

Tab. 6.2 Beispiel einer Betätigungsanalyse

<table>
<tr><th colspan="3">Betätigungsanalyse Beispiel</th></tr>
<tr><td>1. Zeitpunkt</td><td colspan="2">10:45 Uhr, die gewöhnliche Therapiezeit, da die Betätigung „Jacke anziehen“ zu unterschiedlichen Uhrzeiten durchgeführt wird.</td></tr>
<tr><td>2. Kontext</td><td colspan="2">In der Ergotherapiepraxis, da die Betätigung „Jacke anziehen“ in unterschiedlichen Kontexten stattfindet.</td></tr>
<tr><td>3. Reaktive Effekte minimieren
Zur Durchführung der Betätigungsanalyse hält sich der Therapeut so gut wie möglich aus der Situation heraus.</td><td colspan="2">Dies kann dem Klienten z. B. so kommuniziert werden:
„Bitte ziehen Sie sich die Jacke so an wie immer. Tun Sie so, als wäre ich nicht da, ich bin heute nur Zuschauer. Im Anschluss besprechen wir dann meine Beobachtungen.“</td></tr>
<tr><td>4. Beobachtung
Dabei wird auf folgende Punkte geachtet:
Die Performanz der Betätigung wird genau beobachtet.
• Anstrengung
• Effizienz
• Soziale Effektivität
• Sicherheit
• Selbständigkeit
• Hypokinese
• Bradykinese
• Tremor
• Freezing</td><td colspan="2">Die Therapeutin hält sich wegen Sturzgefahr in der unmittelbaren Nähe des Klienten auf. Sie unterstützt ihn nicht bei der Handlung.
Sie macht keine Notizen, um bei Sturzgefahr zu sichern.</td></tr>
<tr><td>5. Breakdown-Points erkennen Momente in denen Probleme zu beobachten sind, die als Ursache für ein Nichtgelingen der Betätigung erkannt werden</td><td colspan="2">• Tremor ⇒ keine flüssige Handhabung der Jacke
• Gleichgewicht ⇒ Sturzgefahr</td></tr>
<tr><td>6. Dokumentation
Dabei werden Stärken genauso notiert wie Einschränkungen. Es wird darauf geachtet, zuerst nur die äußerlich beobachtbaren Teilschritte der Betätigung festzuhalten und nicht zu interpretieren.</td><td colspan="2">• Gute Beweglichkeit obere Extremität, Schürzengriff frei möglich
• Durch Tremor kann Jacke nicht sofort hinter Rücken gegriffen werden
• Kommt bei Tätigkeit aus dem Gleichgewicht, kein ausreichender Ausfallschritt zur Sturzvermeidung, Therapeutin muss sichern und halten</td></tr>
<tr><td>7. Einschätzung der Klientin erfahren</td><td>Frage: „Sind Sie zufrieden damit, wie das geklappt hat? Warum/ Warum nicht?“
„An welchem Punkt möchten Sie noch etwas verbessern?“
„Können Sie selber einschätzen, was da nicht funktioniert hat? Woran es lag?“</td><td>Antwort:
„Ich bemerke, dass ich sehr lange brauche, um die Jacke anzuziehen. Früher ging das in zwei Sekunden.“</td></tr>
<tr><td>8. Interpretation
Hypothese zur Ursache der problematischen Betätigung aufstellen</td><td colspan="2">• Stellreflexe bei axialen Bewegungen in Kombination mit Retroversion beider oberen Extremitäten eingeschränkt, hohe Sturzgefahr!
• Awareness herabgesetzt durch verminderte Propriozeption
• Keine eigenen Problemlösungsstrategien, Durchführung wie früher, Einschränkung des problemlösenden Denkens.</td></tr>
</table>

Beispiel

Herr T. zeigt gerne, wie er seine Jacke anzieht. Schnell schlüpft er mit dem rechten Arm in den Ärmel und wirft die Jacke schwungvoll hinter dem Rücken zur linken Seite. Heute sitzt die Therapeutin zur Abwechslung nicht in der Ecke und macht still Notizen in ihrem Betätigungsanalyse-Bogen. Sie steht schon bereit zum Sichern, da sie den Klienten als sehr sturzgefährdet einschätzt. Tatsächlich verliert Herr T. bei der ausholenden Bewegung das Gleichgewicht. Der rechte Arm ist schon im Ärmel „gefangen" und nicht einsatzfähig. Mit der linken Hand stützt sich Herr T. gerade noch an der Schrankwand ab, dann poltert der Körper gegen die Schrankwand, erst danach macht der Klient einen Schritt. An die Schrankwand gelehnt wurschtelt er den linken Arm in den Ärmel und zieht sie dann Stück für Stück über beide Schultern hoch. Die Knöpfe schließt er ohne Hilfe.

- „Setzen Sie sich bitte kurz, Herr T.", bittet die Therapeutin. „Ich möchte mir das kurz notieren, dann besprechen wir gemeinsam die Situation beim Jacke anziehen."
- Die Therapeutin hat sich den Performance-Skill „Jacke von rechts nach links hinter Rücken geben" als Breakdown-Point umkreist. Beim Qualitätsmerkmal „Sicherheit" steht „hoch sturzgefährdet" mit einem Ausrufezeichen!
- „So Herr T., was würden Sie sagen? Wie gut hat das mit dem Jacke anziehen geklappt? Was ist Ihnen aufgefallen?" fragt die Therapeutin.
- Herr T. antwortet: „Ich bemerke, dass ich sehr lange brauche, um die Jacke anzuziehen. Früher ging das in zwei Sekunden."

Die Therapeutin erkennt, dass die Selbsteinschätzung und die Fremdeinschätzung nicht übereinstimmen. Darin wird sie ihren Hauptfokus in der Anfangsphase der Intervention legen: Awareness für Sturzgefährdung. ◀

Literatur und weiterführende Literatur

Aragon A, Kings J (2018) Occupational therapy for people with Parkinson's, the Royal College of Occupational Therapists Specialist Section – Neurological Practice, London

Atteslander P (1995) Methoden der empirischen Sozialforschung, 2. Aufl. Sammlung Göschen de Gruyter, Berlin, S 136

Huber O (1989) Beobachtung. In: Roth E (Hrsg) Sozialwissenschaftliche Methoden, 2. Aufl. Oldenbourg, München, S 130

Law M (2002) Participation in the occupations of everyday life. Am J Occup Ther 56(6):640–649. https://doi.org/10.5014/ajot.56.6.640

Law M, Baptiste S, Mills J (1995) Client-centred practice: what does it mean and does it make a difference? Can J Occup Ther 62(5):250–257. https://doi.org/10.1177/000841749506200504. PMID: 10152881

Polatajko HJ, Mandich A, Martini R (2000) Dynamic performance analysis: a framework for understanding occupational performance. Am J Occup Ther 54:65–72

Sturkenboom I, Thijssen M, Gons-van Elsacker J, Jansen I, Maasdam A, Schulten M, Vijver-Visser D, Steultjens E, Bloem B, Munneke M (2008) Guidelines for occupational therapy in Parkinson's disease rehabilitation. ParkinsonNet/NPF, Nijmegen/Miami

Weinstock-Zlotnick G, Hinojosa J (2004) Bottom-up or top-down evaluation: is one better than the other? Am J Occup Ther 58(5):594–599. https://doi.org/10.5014/ajot.58.5.594. PMID: 15481786

7 Ergänzende Testungen

Beispiel

„Guten Morgen, Herr R.“, freundlich begrüßt die Ergotherapeutin ihren neuen Klienten. „Hallo.“, erwidert der kurz. „Heute möchte ich Sie ein wenig kennenlernen und erfahren, was Ihre persönlichen Schwierigkeiten sind, damit wir in der Therapie an den Dingen arbeiten können, die Ihnen wichtig sind.“ „Ok.“, kommt als Antwort. Auch während des COPM antwortet Herr R. zwar korrekt, aber sehr knapp auf die Fragen der Therapeutin. Zu den offenen Fragen wie „Wann im Alltag bemerken Sie Ihre Gangunsicherheit?“, gibt der Klient keine klare Antwort. In den Momenten, in denen keine Fragen gestellt werden, sitzt Herr R. scheinbar teilnahmslos auf dem Stuhl und wartet. Die Ergotherapeutin notiert: „Abklärung Demenz – Apathie“. ◀

Nach Durchführung der Betätigungsanalyse und der Hypothesenbildung ist meist schon ein sinnvoller therapeutischer Ansatz erkennbar. In einzelnen Fällen wird eine Untersuchung von zugrunde liegenden Einschränkungen auf der Körperfunktionsebene notwendig. Die nachfolgenden Tests sollen ausdrücklich **nicht** grundsätzlich angewandt werden, sondern **nur** nach einer Betätigungsanalyse erfolgen, wenn die Hypothese, durch mangelnde Kenntnis über die Einschränkungen von Körperfunktionen, nicht ausreichend gebildet werden kann. Auch dann besteht häufig die Möglichkeit, die fehlenden Informationen von angrenzenden Berufsgruppen zu erlangen, z. B. bei Physiotherapie, Logopädie, Neuropsychologie und Neurologie. Eine enge interdisziplinäre Zusammenarbeit ist für eine qualitative Behandlung des Klienten wesentlich. Dies erleichtert die Arbeit jedes Einzelnen, wirkt nach Außen stimmig und erspart dem Klienten unnötige doppelte Assessments. Zur Umsetzung des Top-Down-Ansatzes muss folgende Reihenfolge in der Ergotherapie umgesetzt werden:

1. Betätigungswunsch formulieren
2. Betätigung analysieren
3. evtl. ergänzende Testungen durchführen
4. Hypothese bilden
5. Intervention

Wie in Kap. 4 ausführlicher beschrieben, ist der Top-Down-Ansatz in Kombination mit betätigungsorientiertem Arbeiten das Kennzeichen moderner Ergotherapie und ist dessen Alleinstellungsmerkmal. In diesem Kapitel werden einzelne Tests beschrieben und Anwendungsbeispiele aufgezeigt.

▶ Eine funktionelle Testung wird in der betätigungsorientierten Ergotherapie bei Bedarf ergänzend zur Betätigungsanalyse durchgeführt, und nicht als primäre Erfassung aller Einschränkungen.

A. Orellana, *Betätigungsorientierte Ergotherapie bei Morbus Parkinson*,
https://doi.org/10.1007/978-3-662-62583-5_7

7.1 Beurteilung der Bradykinese

Eine isolierte Testung der Bradykinese kann sinnvoll sein, wenn die Medikamentenwirkung zu unterschiedlichen Tageszeiten verglichen werden soll.

Alltagsbeobachtung
Bradykinese ist das Kardinalsymptom bei der Diagnose „Morbus Parkinson", es tritt also bei jedem Klienten mit dieser Diagnose auf. Man kann Bradykinese durch Alltagsbeobachtungen erkennen.

- Hypokinese (Bewegungsamplitude ist reduziert)
- Kleinschrittiger Gang
- Mikrografie: Schriftbild ist sehr klein
- Hypomimie
- Bradykinese (Verlangsamung von Bewegungen)
- Reaktion verlangsamt, zum Beispiel Auffangen eines fallenden Gegenstandes
- Langsame Durchführung von Tätigkeiten
- Akinese (Bewegungslosigkeit)
- Freezing (plötzliche Erstarrung bei repetitiven Tätigkeiten wie Laufen, Schreiben, Zähneputzen)

Isolierte Testung
Zur isolierten Testung kann eine repetitive schnelle Wechselbewegung mit beiden Händen angeleitet werden. Dazu gehört die Diadochokinese (Drehbewegung) und das schnelle Fingertippen. Hier kann eine Hypo- und Bradykinese klar erkannt werden. In frühen Stadien kann die Bradykinese schwer zu beobachten sein, vor allem bei guter medikamentöser Einstellung. Zur Verstärkung des Symptomes kann zusätzlich zur Bewegung eine kognitive Leistung abgerufen werden. Dazu soll der Klient rückwärts zählen oder als Steigerung in Dreierschritten von 100 rückwärts zählen. Zur genauen Durchführung der Bradykinesetestung sind fachliche Videos auf YouTube zu finden, z. B. im Vortrag von Dr. D. Berg, vom Uniklinikum Tübingen.

7.2 Beurteilung des Rigors

Eine isolierte Testung des Rigors kann sinnvoll sein, wenn:

- die Therapeutin die Stärke des Rigors fühlen möchte, um die Möglichkeiten und Grenzen der therapeutischen Intervention einschätzen zu können.
- die Medikamentenwirkung zu unterschiedlichen Tageszeiten verglichen werden soll.

Isolierte Testung
Der Rigor ist ein parkinsontypisches Symptom, der bei den meisten betroffenen Menschen auftritt. Das Ausmaß des Rigors kann mit einem schnellen Test festgestellt werden. Der Klient sitzt. Die Therapeutin greift den Oberarm und den Unterarm des Patienten und sagt ihm, er soll lockerlassen. Anschließend flektiert und extendiert die Therapeutin den Ellenbogen des Betroffenen. Die Therapeutin spürt den Rigor als wächsernen Widerstand. Sollte kein Rigor festgestellt werden, kann der Patient aufgefordert werden, den anderen Arm gestreckt seitlich zu heben und zu senken (Abduktion, Adduktion), während die Therapeutin die passive Bewegung durchführt. Durch diese Ko-Innervation wird der Rigor verstärkt und sollte nun gut spürbar sein.

Das Zahnradphänomen ist möglicherweise auch feststellbar. Dies wird von der Therapeutin als ein ruckartiges Entspannen und Anspannen bei der passiven Mobilisation gespürt und durch einen zugrunde liegenden Tremor ausgelöst. Zur genauen Durchführung der Rigor-Testung sind fachliche Videos auf YouTube zu finden, z. B. im Vortrag von Dr. D. Berg, vom Uniklinikum Tübingen. Für die Therapeutin kann die Feststellung des Rigors eine Art Aha-Erlebnis sein. Die Eindrücklichkeit der Zähigkeit hilft nachzuvollziehen, gegen welche andauernden Widerstände der Klient bei jeder Bewegung kämpfen muss.

7.3 Beurteilung des Tremors

Eine isolierte Testung des Tremors kann sinnvoll sein, wenn:

- die Medikamentenwirkung zu unterschiedlichen Tageszeiten verglichen werden soll.
- aus der Betätigungsanalyse die Differenzierung des Tremor-Typs (Ruhe-, Halte- oder Aktionstremor) nicht möglich war.
- andere Einflussfaktoren auf den Tremor untersucht werden sollen (z. B. Stress, Lärm …).

Beobachtung Ruhetremor
Der parkinsonspezifische Tremor ist der Ruhetremor. Dieser kann beobachtet werden, wenn der Patient in Ruhe auf einem Stuhl sitzt. Meist tritt er in den Händen auf, aber auch in der unteren Extremität, dem Kopf und dem Oberkörper ist er zuweilen sichtbar. Sehr häufig ist das sog. **Pillendreher-Phänomen**, bei dem der Tremor in Daumen und Mittelfinger mit einer Art Pillendreher Bewegung beobachtbar ist.

Testung Aktionstremor
Auch das Auftreten von Aktionstremor oder Haltetremor ist bei M. Parkinson möglich. Zur Feststellung eines Aktionstremors wird der Patient gebeten, im Wechsel mit dem Zeigefinger auf seine Nasenspitze zu tippen und den Arm wieder auszustrecken.

Testung Haltetremor
Der Haltetremor tritt beim Halten von Gegenständen auf. Zur Untersuchung hält der Patient beide Arme ausgestreckt vor sich und hält sie dort ein paar Sekunden. Zur genauen Durchführung der Tremortestung sind fachliche Videos auf YouTube zu finden z. B. im Vortrag von Dr. D. Berg, vom Uniklinikum Tübingen.

Tremor-Dokumentation
Wichtig ist nachzufragen, ob der Tremor in bestimmten Situationen verstärkt auftritt und wann er nicht beobachtbar ist. Meist haben die Klienten schon einen Zusammenhang feststellen können. Außerdem ist es beachtenswert, dass Tremor durch Stress und Zeitdruck verstärkt wird (z. B. am Kassenautomat, wenn andere Menschen warten). Eine Verifizierung mit dem Klienten, ob dies auch bei ihm zutrifft, ist zu empfehlen. Zur genauen Abklärung kann das Parkinson-Tagebuch (siehe Abschn. 7.8 und im Anhang) vom Patienten und von Angehörigen ausgefüllt werden. So können Zusammenhänge häufig schnell aufgedeckt werden.

7.4 Beurteilung der posturalen Stabilität

Eine isolierte Testung der posturalen Stabilität kann sinnvoll sein, wenn:

- die Sturzgefahr eingeschätzt werden soll.
- die Medikamentenwirkung zu unterschiedlichen Tageszeiten verglichen werden soll.

Ein weiteres typisches Symptom bei M. Parkinson ist die herabgesetzte posturale Stabilität. Sie tritt meist später im Krankheitsverlauf auf und ist die Hauptursache von Stürzen. Da die Sturzgefahr innerhalb einer Betätigungssituation meist nur schwer mit Sicherheit zu evaluieren ist, ist eine getrennte Testung in der Ergotherapie zur Bestätigung der Vermutung empfehlenswert. Zur Einschätzung der posturalen Stabilität können zwei Testungen durchgeführt werden: der Pulsionstest und der „Timed-Up-And-Go-Test".

Pulsionstest
Der Pulsionstest ist dem UPDRS, Punkt Nr. 30, entnommen (siehe Abschn. 7.6).

Durchführung Die Therapeutin steht direkt hinter dem Patienten und zieht ihn an beiden Schultern gleichzeitig nach hinten. Die Anleitung kann wie folgt lauten: „Ich ziehe Sie gleich an den Schultern nach hinten. Versuchen Sie den Zug auszugleichen, lassen Sie sich nicht aus dem Gleichgewicht bringen. Aber keine Sorge, Sie fallen nicht um, ich halte Sie, wenn notwendig."

▶ **Cave!**
Die Therapeutin muss beim Pulsionstest darauf gefasst sein, dass der Patient keine Gleichgewichtsreaktion zeigt und muss ihn stützen, wenn dies geschieht.

Auswertung Der Pulsionstest ist **negativ**, wenn der Klient mit dem Körper und evtl. Armen den Zug ausgleicht und standhaft bleibt oder einen Ausfallschritt zur Sturzvermeidung zeigt. Der Pulsionstest ist **positiv**, wenn der Klient kleine Trippelschritte macht, die meist nicht ausreichend sind, um den Zug aufzufangen, oder aber keine Ausgleichsreaktion zeigt. In beiden Fällen muss die Therapeutin den Patienten stützen.

▶ Wenn der Pulsionstest positiv ausfällt, besteht akute Sturzgefahr! Dies sollte dem Arzt rückgemeldet und im therapeutischen Team kommuniziert werden.

Zum Pulsionstest sind fachliche Videos auf YouTube zu finden, z. B. im Vortrag von Dr. D. Berg, vom Uniklinikum Tübingen.

„Timed-Up-And-Go-Test"
Nach Podsiadlo und Richardson (1991)

Durchführung Der Klient sitzt auf einem Stuhl mit Armlehnen und lehnt sich an der Rückenlehne an. Es wird die Zeit gemessen, die der Klient von dieser Ausgangsposition benötigt, um 3 m bis zu einer Markierung auf dem Boden zu gehen, sich umzudrehen, zum Stuhl zurückzukehren und sich zu setzen. Dabei darf ein Hilfsmittel, wie ein Rollator, benutzt werden. Beim Aufstehen und Hinsetzen darf er sich auf den Armlehnen abstützen.

Auswertung
- Bis 10 Sek. – unabhängige Mobilität
- 11–20 Sek. – Mobilitätseinschränkung ohne funktionelles Defizit
- 21–29 Sek. – geringe Mobilitätseinschränkung
- Ab 30 Sek. – ausgeprägte Mobilitätseinschränkung

Zur genauen Durchführung des „Timed-Up-And-Go-Test" sind viele fachliche Videos auf YouTube zu finden.

7.5 Beurteilung der Kognition

Eine isolierte Testung der Kognition kann sinnvoll sein, wenn:

- keine Kollegin aus den angrenzenden Fachbereichen eine Testung durchgeführt hat.
- die Ergotherapeutin in der Beobachtung äußerliche Anzeichen für eine eingeschränkte kognitive Leistung (Merkfähigkeit, problemlösendes Denken) gesehen hat, sich jedoch nicht sicher ist.
- der überweisende Arzt eine ergotherapeutische Einschätzung der kognitiven Leistung eingefordert hat.
- Ärztinnen oder andere Therapeuten von einer Demenz sprechen, die Ergotherapeutin jedoch die Hypothese hat, dass die erkennbaren Einschränkungen auf die **verlangsamte Motorik** zurückzuführen sind, die Qualität der kognitiven Leistungen jedoch nicht betroffen ist.

MoCA Test (Montreal Cognitive Assessment)
In einer Cochrane-Analyse zeigte der MoCA-Test eine hohe Sensitivität, um kognitive Einschränkungen bei M. Parkinson festzustellen. Er bildet besonders Exekutivfunktionen ab, die beim IPS vordergründig eingeschränkt sind. Zusätzlich berücksichtigt er folgende kognitive Bereiche: Aufmerksamkeit und Konzentration, Gedächtnis, Sprache, visuokonstruktive Fähigkeiten, konzeptuelles Denken, Rechnen und Orientierung. Die Durchführungszeit beträgt etwa 10 Minuten.

Die Testunterlagen können auf www.mocatest.org heruntergeladen werden. Seit 2020 wird eine Zertifizierung der durchführenden Therapeutinnen verlangt.

MMST (Mini-Mental-Status-Test)
Der MMST wurde 1975 von Folstein und Kollegen entwickelt. Er ist nach dem MoCA Test der

am zweithäufigsten verwendete Test zur Erkennung von kognitiven Einschränkungen bei der Parkinson-Erkrankung. Der MMST ist im Anhang zu finden. Da eine Parkinson-Demenz mit diesem Test nicht immer angezeigt wird, empfiehlt sich zur Ergänzung der Uhrentest, siehe unten.

Auswertung
- 30 bis 28 Punkte: keine Demenz
- 27 bis 25 Punkte: leichte kognitive Beeinträchtigung
- 24 bis 18 Punkte: leichte Demenz
- 17 bis 10 Punkte: mittelschwere Demenz

Es ist zu beachten, dass die Testergebnisse sich durch **Alter**, **Bildung**, zuletzt ausgeübten **Beruf** und **kulturellen Hintergrund** beeinflussen lassen. Aus diesem Grund sollten diese Angaben bei der Testauswertung mitberücksichtigt werden.

Beobachtung im Alltag
Da der MMST milde kognitive Einschränkungen nicht misst, schlägt Dubois (2007) vor, kognitiv anspruchsvolle Betätigungen im Alltag zu beobachten oder abzufragen. Zum Beispiel können Bankgeschäfte (Überweisung), der Grad der Selbständigkeit bei der Einnahme der Medikamente, richtige Dosis und pünktliche Einnahme sowie Verhalten in sozialen Situationen auffällig sein und für eine beginnende Demenz sprechen.

Uhrentest (s. Abb. 7.1)
Ergänzend zum MMST kann der Uhrentest durchgeführt werden, da hier sowohl Exekutivfunktionen als auch räumlich-konstruktive Fähigkeiten benötigt werden.

Durchführung Der Klient wird aufgefordert, das Ziffernblatt einer Uhr in einen vorgegebenen Kreis zu zeichnen.

Anschließend soll er die Zeiger so einzeichnen, dass sie auf zehn Minuten nach elf stehen. Im Anhang ist ein Vordruck für den Uhrentest zu finden.

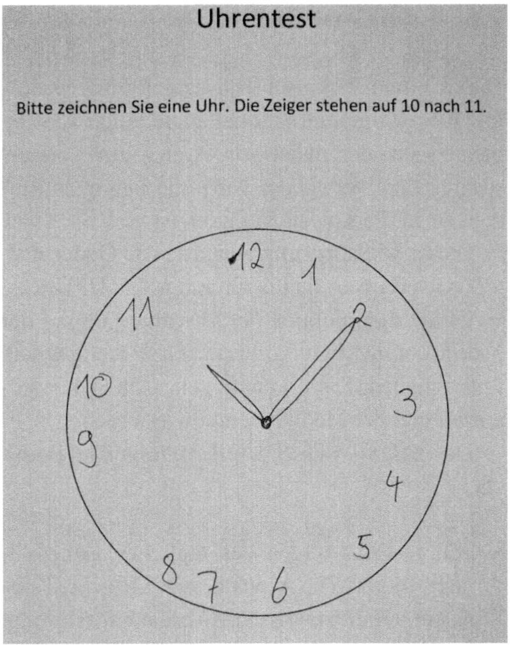

Abb. 7.1 Beispiel ausgefüllter Uhrentest, volle Punktzahl

Auswertung Der Kreis wird in vier gleich große Quadranten unterteilt, indem eine Linie durch die zwölf gezogen wird, und eine zweite Linie im rechten Winkel dazu.

Nun wird die Anzahl der Ziffern in jedem Quadranten gezählt, beginnend mit der zwölf im Uhrzeigersinn. Wenn eine Ziffer auf der Linie liegt, wird sie zum folgenden Quadranten gezählt. Drei Ziffern (egal welche) in einem Quadranten wird als korrekt gezählt (0 Punkte). Für eine fehlerhafte Anzahl der Ziffern in Quadrant 1–3 wird ein Punkt gegeben. Für eine fehlerhafte Anzahl von Ziffern im vierten Quadranten werden vier Punkte gegeben.

Bewertung:

- 0–3 Punkte – Unauffällig
- 4–7 Punkte – Auffällig (dement)

Die Zeiger (Länge, Position) bieten zusätzliche Anhaltspunkte für Auffälligkeiten der kognitiven Fähigkeiten.

7.6 MDS-UPDRS

Die „Unified Parkinsons Disease Rating Skale“, UPDRS ist ein international anerkannter Assessmentbogen, der meist von Ärzten zur Verlaufsevaluierung verwendet wird und häufig in Studien zu M. Parkinson zu finden ist.

Dieses Messinstrument wurde von Goetz et al. (2008) verbessert und heißt nun MDS-UPDRS.

Es hat die Funktion der Gesamterfassung der parkinsontypischen körperlichen Beschwerden, funktionellen Einschränkungen, Alltagskompetenzen und der Medikamentenwirkungen.

Das MDS-UPDRS Umfasst folgende Bereiche:

- Teil I: Erfahrungen des täglichen Lebens – nicht-motorische Aspekte, z. B.: Psyche, Kognition, Halluzinationen, Verdauungsstörung, Antriebsstörungen …
- Teil II: Motorische Aspekte bei Erfahrungen des täglichen Lebens, z. B.: Sprache, Speichelfluss, Essen, Ankleiden, Hobbies, Handschrift, Gehen …
- Teil III: Motorische Untersuchung, z. B.: Medikamente, Rigor, Akinese, Tremor, posturale Stabilität, Gangbild, Körperhaltung
- Teil IV: Motorische Komplikationen, z. B.: Dyskinesien, On-/Off-Phase, Fluktuation von Medikamentenwirkung

Das Assessment ist eine Kombination aus Interview mit dem Patienten und Angehörigen, sowie Beobachtung und Untersuchung. Unter www.movementdisorders.org ist ein PDF des MDS-UPDRS mit genauer Anleitung, sowie dem Assessmentbogen auf Deutsch zu finden.

7.7 Erfassung der Lebensqualität (PDQ 39)

Mit dem Parkinson Disease Questionnaire (PDQ 39) entwickelte Peto et al. (1995) einen Fragebogen, um die Lebensqualität eines Menschen mit der Parkinson-Erkrankung zu messen. Es kann ein hilfreiches Instrument in der Ergotherapie sein, um die Effektivität der Intervention messbar zu machen. Durch den Fokus auf die Emotionen und Alltagsaktivitäten erfasst dieser Fragebogen den Einfluss der ergotherapeutischen Behandlung sensibler als z. B. der UPDRS, der zu einem großen Teil die motorischen Fähigkeiten misst.

Die Lebensqualität rückte in den letzten Jahren zunehmend in den Fokus der Mediziner und ist häufiger in der Literatur und Studienmessungen zu finden. Die subjektive Wahrnehmung des Klienten wird nun in klinischen Studien auch als Effektmessung anerkannt.

Neben der Erweiterung der Evaluation medizinischer Maßnahmen um eine psychische, eine soziale (und seitens der WHO auch um eine spirituelle) Dimension, ist die Hinwendung zur subjektiven Beurteilung als das eigentlich Neue innerhalb der medizinischen Forschung anzusehen (Power et al. 1999). Diese Wahrnehmungsänderung seitens der Mediziner spiegelt sich auch in der vermehrten Nutzung des PDQ 39 wider.

▶ Ein Hauptargument der Ärzte gegen das Verschreiben von Ergotherapie ist die geringe Evidenz zur Wirksamkeit der ergotherapeutischen Intervention bei M. Parkinson, obwohl die Parkinsonleitlinien für Ärzte Ergotherapie empfehlen. Nimmt die Therapeutin nun ein Messinstrument zur Hand, welches von Ärztinnen bekannt und anerkannt ist (z. B. PDQ 39), und weist eine Verbesserung der Lebensqualität nach Abschluss der Ergotherapie damit nach, steigt das fachliche Ansehen der Ergotherapeutin und die Wahrscheinlichkeit, neue Klienten verordnet zu bekommen.

Durchführung Der PDQ 39 kann vom Klienten selbst ausgefüllt oder in einem Interview abgefragt werden. Dabei sollte keine Einflussnahme und Suggestion durch die Therapeutin erfolgen. Im Anschluss erfolgt die Auswertung zuerst der einzelnen Themenbereiche, dann des Gesamtwertes, der die Lebensqualität abbildet. Der Fragebogen umfasst acht Themenbereiche, siehe Tab. 7.1.

Der PDQ-39-Fragebogen ist online herunterzuladen.

Tab. 7.1 Themenbereiche des PDQ 39

Mobilität	• Freizeitaktivitäten • Haushaltstätigkeiten • Einkaufen • 1 km laufen • 100 m laufen • Mobilität im Haus • Mobilität außer Haus • Notwendigkeit Begleitperson • Angst zu stürzen • Ans Haus gebunden sein
Alltagsaktivitäten	• Waschen • Anziehen • Knöpfen/Schnürsenkel • Schreiben • Essen klein schneiden • Getränk halten
Emotionales Wohlbefinden	• Depression • Einsamkeit • Den Tränen nahe • Wut • Ängstlichkeit • Zukunftssorgen
Stigma	• Verheimlichung der Erkrankung • Vermeidung Essen und Trinken in Öffentlichkeit • Scham • Sorgen über Reaktionen
Soziale Unterstützung	• Nahe Beziehungen • Unterstützung durch Partner • Unterstützung durch Familie oder Freunde
Kognition	• Unerwartetes Einschlafen • Konzentration • Merkschwierigkeiten • Schlechte Träume/ Halluzinationen
Kommunikation	• Sprache • Kommunikationsprobleme • Fehlende Beachtung
Körperliches Unbehagen	• Muskelkrämpfe • Gelenkschmerzen • Hitze-/Kältegefühl

7.8 Parkinson-Tagebuch

Mit dem Parkinson-Tagebuch ist eine **Erfassung** von **Symptomen** und medikamentenbedingten **Fluktuationen** im Tagesverlauf einfach und übersichtlich durchführbar. Der Klient oder Angehörige trägt über eine Woche hinweg, in den Kalender ein, wenn bestimmte Symptome (Tremor, Schmerzen …) oder Medikamentenwirkungen (Dyskinesien, Off-Phasen) auftreten. Außerdem ist die Uhrzeit der Medikamenteneinnahme zu dokumentieren. So sind Zusammenhänge und Muster unmittelbar erkennbar. Es kann beispielsweise eine Inkonstanz der Einnahmezeit der Medikamente, medikamentenbedingte Fluktuationen oder Tagesschwankungen (z. B. bei Fatigue) festgestellt werden (siehe Abb. 7.2).

Im Anhang ist das Parkinson-Tagebuch zu finden (siehe Anhang).

7.9 Beurteilung des Wohlbefindens (Depressionen)

Mit dem Fragebogen, den die WHO (1998) entwickelt hat, kann mit nur fünf Fragen sehr präzise festgestellt werden, ob eine depressive Verstimmung vorliegt. Bei einem Punktwert unter 13, oder der Beantwortung mindestens einer Frage mit einem Punktwert von 0 oder 1, sollte die Therapeutin das Ergebnis der behandelnden Ärztin mitteilen, um eine weitere Diagnostik anzuregen. Im Anhang ist das WHO-5 zu finden (siehe Anhang).

Auswertung Punktberechnung; der Rohwert kommt durch einfaches Addieren der Antworten zustande. Der Rohwert erstreckt sich von 0 bis 25, wobei 0 geringstes Wohlbefinden/niedrigste Lebensqualität und 25 größtes Wohlbefinden, höchste Lebensqualität bezeichnen. Den Prozentwert von 0 - 100 erhält man durch Multiplikation mit 4. Der Prozentwert 0 bezeichnet das schlechteste Befinden, 100 das Beste.

7.10 Beurteilung von Fatigue

FSS (Fatigue Severity Scale)
Zur Einschätzung, ob beim Klienten eine Fatigue vorliegt, wird bei zahlreichen Krankheitsbildern die FSS eingesetzt. Dieses Assessment ist für M. Parkinson validiert und schnell durchführbar. Der FSS-Fragebogen ist im Anhang zu finden (siehe Anhang).

Parkinson Tagebuch

	Mo.	Di.	Mi.	Do.	Fr.	Sa.	So.
07:00-8:00	U	U	Levodopa, Ropinirol	U	U, Sch	U	U
08:00-09:00	Levodopa, Ropinirol	Levodopa, Ropinirol		Levodopa, Ropinirol	U, Sch	Levodopa, Ropinirol	U, St
09:00-10:00					Levodopa, Ropinirol		Levodopa, Ropinirol
10:00-11:00	Ü		Ü		Sch	Ü	
11:00-12:00	U				Sch		F
12:00-13:00	Levodopa, Ropinirol	Levodopa, Ropinirol	Levodopa, Ropinirol	Levodopa, Ropinirol	Sch	Levodopa, Ropinirol	Levodopa, Ropinirol
13:00-14:00					Levodopa, Ropinirol		
14:00-15:00							
15:00-16:00							
16:00-17:00							
17:00-18:00							
18:00-19:00	Levodopa, Ropinirol	Levodopa, Ropinirol	Levodopa, Ropinirol	Levodopa, Ropinirol	Levodopa, Ropinirol	Levodopa, Ropinirol	Levodopa, Ropinirol
19:00-20:00	F						St,U, F
20:00-21:00	F		F				St,U, F
21:00-22:00	F		F	U		U	St,U, F
22:00-23:00	F,U	U	F,U	U	U, Sch	U,Sch	St, F,U

Bitte Eintragen:

Name der eingenommenen Medikamente

U = Unterbeweglich
Ü = Überbeweglich
T = Tremor
St = Stimmung niedergeschlagen
Sch = Schmerzen
K = Konzentration, Gedächtnis eingeschränkt
F = Fatigue (sonstiges Symptom)
= (sonstiges Symptom)

Abb. 7.2 Ausfüllbeispiel des Parkinson-Tagebuchs

Auswertung Ein Mittelwert über 4 gilt als Zeichen einer erhöhten Fatigue.

Beispiel

Die Ergotherapeutin konnte ohne eine ergänzende Testung nicht feststellen, ob Herr R. eine kognitive Einschränkung hat oder eine stark ausgeprägte Apathie. Nach Abschluss des MoCA-Tests steht fest: Herr R. hat eine eingeschränkte kognitive Leistungsfähigkeit. Die Ergotherapeutin nimmt mit der Partnerin von Herr R. Kontakt auf, um gemeinsam Ziele für das tägliche Leben im familiären Kontext zu fassen. Bis zu dem Termin mit der Partnerin konzentriert sich die Therapeutin auf die körpernahen Betätigungen wie Waschen, Anziehen und Essen, um eine vermehrte selbständige Übernahme der Tätigkeiten durch den Klienten anzubahnen. ◀

Literatur und weiterführende Literatur

Burdick D, Cholerton B, Watson G, Siderowf A, Trojanowski J, Weintraub D, Ritz B, Rhodes S, Rausch R, Factor S, Wood-Siverio C, Quinn J, Chung K, Srivatsal S, Edwards K, Montine T, Zabetian C, Leverenz J (2014) People with Parkinson's disease and normal MMSE score have a broad range of cognitive performance. Mov Disord 29(10):1258–1264. https://doi.org/10.1002/mds.25924

Deuschl G, Oertel W, Reichmann H (2016) Leitlinien für Diagnostik und Therapie in der Neurologie Idiopathisches Parkinson-Syndrom Entwicklungsstufe: S3 Kurzversion, DGN

Dubois B, Burn D, Goetz C, Aarsland D, Brown RG, Broe GA, Dickson D, Duyckaerts C, Cummings J, Gauthier S, Korczyn A, Lees A, Levy R, Litvan I, Mizuno Y, McKeith IG, Olanow CW, Poewe W, Sampaio C, Tolosa E, Emre M (2007) Diagnostic procedures for Parkinson's disease dementia: recommendations from the movement disorder society task force. Mov Disord 22(16):2314–2324. https://doi.org/10.1002/mds.21844. PMID: 18098298

Goetz CG, Tilley BC, Shaftman SR, Stebbins GT, Fahn S, Martinez-Martin P, Poewe W, Sampaio C, Stern MB, Dodel R, Dubois B, Holloway R, Jankovic J, Kulisevsky J, Lang AE, Lees A, Leurgans S, LeWitt PA, Nyenhuis D, Olanow CW, Rascol O, Schrag A, Teresi JA, van Hilten JJ, LaPelle N (2008) Movement Disorder Society UPDRS Revision Task Force. Movement Disorder Society-sponsored revision of the Unified Parkinson's Disease Rating Scale (MDS-UPDRS): scale presentation and clinimetric testing results. Mov Disord 23(15):2129–2170. https://doi.org/10.1002/mds.22340. PMID: 19025984

Hagell P, Höglund A, Reimer J, Eriksson B, Knutsson I, Widner H, Cella D (2006) Measuring fatigue in Parkinson's disease: a psychometric study of two brief generic fatigue questionnaires. J Pain Symptom Manag 32(5):420–432. https://doi.org/10.1016/j.jpainsymman.2006.05.021. PMID: 17085268

Krupp L, LaRocca N, Muir-Nash J, Steinberg A (1989) The fatigue severity scale. Application to patients with multiple sclerosis and systemic lupus erythematosus. Arch Neurol 46(10):1121–1123. https://doi.org/10.1001/archneur.1989.00520460115022. PMID: 2803071

Law M, Baptiste S, Mills J (1995) Client-centred practice: what does it mean and does it make a difference? Can J Occup Ther 62(5):250–257. https://doi.org/10.1177/000841749506200504. PMID: 10152881

Macht M, Ellgring H (2018) Verhaltenstherapie bei der Parkinson-Erkrankung. Elsevier GmbH, München

Peto V, Jenkinson C, Fitzpatrick R, Greenhall R (1995) The development and validation of a short measure of functioning and well being for individuals with Parkinson's disease. Qual Life Res 4(3):241–248. https://doi.org/10.1007/BF02260863. PMID: 7613534

Podsiadlo D, Richardson S (1991) The timed „Up & Go": a test of basic functional mobility for frail elderly persons. J Am Geriatr Soc 39(2):142–148. https://doi.org/10.1111/j.1532-5415.1991.tb01616.x. PMID: 1991946

Power M, Bullinger M, Harper A, & The World Health Organization Quality of Life Group (1999). The World Health Organization WHOQOL-100: Tests of the universality of quality of life in 15 different cultural groups worldwide. Health Psychol 18(5):495–505. https://doi.org/10.1037/0278-6133.18.5.495

Skorvanek M, Goldman J, Jahanshahi M, Marras C, Rektorova I, Schmand B, van Duijn E, Goetz C, Weintraub D, Stebbins G, Martinez-Martin P (2017) Members of the MDS Rating Scales Review Committee. Global scales for cognitive screening in Parkinson's disease: critique and recommendations. Mov Disord 33(2):208–218. https://doi.org/10.1002/mds.27233.23. PMID: 29168899

Sturkenboom I, Thijssen M, Gons-van Elsacker J, Jansen I, Maasdam A, Schulten M, Vijver-Visser D, Steultjens E, Bloem B, Munneke M (2008) Guidelines for occupational therapy in Parkinson's disease rehabilitation. ParkinsonNet/NPF, Nijmegen/Miami

Tombaugh T, McIntyre N (1992) The mini-mental state examination: a comprehensive review. J Am Geriatr Soc 40:922–935. https://doi.org/10.1111/j.1532-5415.1992.tb01992.x

Watson Y, Arfken C, Birge S (1993) Clock completion: an objective screening test for dementia. J Am Geriatr Soc 41:1235–1240. https://doi.org/10.1111/j.1532-5415.1993.tb07308.x

Weinstock-Zlotnick G, Hinojosa J (2004) Bottom-up or top-down evaluation: is one better than the other? Am J Occup Ther 58(5):594–599. https://doi.org/10.5014/ajot.58.5.594. PMID: 15481786

WHO-5 (1998) Psychiatric Research Unit, WHO Collaborating Center for Mental Health, Frederiksborg General Hospital, DK-3400 Hillerød

8 Modifiziertes Betätigungsziel vereinbaren

Beispiel

Frau Sch. hat den Wunsch, wieder zu schreiben. Der Ergotherapeut erfragt, was genau sie wieder schreiben möchte, um das Ziel möglichst spezifisch erfassen zu können. Frau Sch. zieht einen Brief aus einem Stapel an Papieren. „Hier. Den habe ich von Maria bekommen, einer jungen Frau aus Weißrussland. Sie hat vor zwei Jahren hier im Heim ein Praktikum gemacht. Wir haben uns angefreundet, aber seit sie wieder in ihrer Heimat ist, habe ich sie nicht kontaktiert, weil ich nicht mehr schreiben kann.“

Der Therapeut notiert als Ziel: „Brief an Maria schreiben“. ◀

Schon zu Beginn des therapeutischen Prozesses hat der Therapeut, vielleicht mithilfe des COPM, die Klientinnenwünsche oder -ziele abgefragt und dokumentiert. Durch die zusätzliche Sammlung von Informationen über die Performanz der Betätigung, Ausprägung der Symptome, Gestaltung der Umwelt und sonstige wichtige Faktoren hat der Therapeut ein umfassendes Bild der Situation erfasst. Jetzt ist der ideale Zeitpunkt, um das von der Klientin formulierte Ziel wieder zu betrachten. In vielen Fällen kann das Klientinnenziel ohne Abänderungen übernommen werden, in anderen ist eine Modifizierung notwendig.

8.1 SMART-Ziele

Zur Orientierung dient hier die Formulierung der Ziele nach den SMART-Regeln.

S	Spezifisch
M	Messbar
A	Akzeptiert
R	Realistisch
T	Terminiert

SMART – Spezifisch

Das Ziel sollte sich nach der der Klientin wichtigen Betätigung richten und möglichst spezifisch sein. Zum Beispiel statt: „Essen verbessern.“, besser: „Suppe ohne zu kleckern essen.“ Die Formulierung des Ziels sollte für Klientin und Angehörige gut verständlich sein, also in Alltagssprache, nicht Fachsprache. Bestenfalls wird der genaue Wortlaut der Klientin übernommen. Formuliert die Klientin das Ziel funktionell oder sehr allgemein, kann der Therapeut gezielt nachfragen, z. B.: „Wann im Alltag fällt Ihnen das Feinmotorik-Problem auf?“ oder „Wann hat Ihre Müdigkeit Sie das letzte Mal davon abgehalten etwas zu tun, das Ihnen wichtig ist?“

SMART – Messbar

Um das Erreichen des Ziels überprüfen zu können, sollte es messbar sein. Dazu müssen möglichst genaue Angaben gemacht werden. Zum

A. Orellana, *Betätigungsorientierte Ergotherapie bei Morbus Parkinson*,
https://doi.org/10.1007/978-3-662-62583-5_8

Beispiel statt „verbessert laufen.", „Die Strecke vom Haus bis zum Bäcker mit Rollator, mit einer Sitzpause laufen können." Nur wenn das Ziel messbar ist, ist objektiv sicher, wann das Ziel erreicht wird. Auch für die Motivation ist es wichtig ein konkretes Ziel zu haben, auf das hingearbeitet wird. Das Erfolgserlebnis beim Erreichen des Ziels ist ein guter Punkt, um entweder die Therapie zu beenden oder um mit frischer Motivation ein neues Ziel anzugehen.

SMART – Akzeptiert

Das Ziel sollte von der Klientin akzeptiert werden. Meist ist dies ohnehin gegeben, da die Klientin nach ihren Wünschen und Zielen befragt wurde. In manchen Fällen wird jedoch ein Ziel von Ärztin, Angehörigen oder Therapeut vorgeschlagen, die etwas ändern möchten. Je nach Einsicht der Klientin wird dies von ihm unterschiedlich akzeptiert. Beispiele für diese Situationen sind:

- Sturzgefahr,
- Grad der Unterstützung durch Angehörige/ Selbständigkeit der Klientin,
- psychische Auffälligkeiten (Suchtverhalten, Unruhe),
- regelmäßige Medikamenteneinnahme,
- Gewichtszunahme,
- …

Zeigt die Klientin kein Verständnis für die Notwendigkeit des Ziels, kann ein Gespräch darüber geführt werden, welche Vorteile oder Dringlichkeit mit dem Ziel verbunden sind. Oftmals hat der Therapeut die nötigen fachlichen Argumente und Distanz zur Klientin, um ein Einlenken zu erreichen – anders als bei Angehörigen, bei denen oftmals die Beziehungsebene bei Konflikten dominiert. Sollte die Klientin jedoch nicht einsehen, weshalb das von außen bestimmte Ziel wichtig ist und keine Kooperationsbereitschaft zeigen, ist die therapeutische Intervention aussichtslos. In diesem Fall sollten Therapeut und Angehörige/Arzt abwägen, wie wichtig das Ziel ist. Bringt die Klientin sich oder andere in Gefahr, sollte z. B. nach anderen Möglichkeiten gesucht werden, um das Ziel zu erreichen (siehe Tab. 8.1). Andernfalls kann es vernachlässigt werden.

SMA*R*T – Realistisch

Ob ein Ziel realistisch ist oder nicht, ist nicht immer leicht einzuschätzen und hängt von mehreren Faktoren ab:

- der Grad der Motivation der Klientin;
- die zur Verfügung stehende Zeit;
- Vorhandensein von Demenz. Parkinson-Patientinnen, die eine demenzielle Entwicklung zeigen, haben eine erheblich geringere Chance auf Verbesserungen in anderen Bereichen;
- fördernde oder hemmende Faktoren des Kontexts (z. B. Partnerin, Wohnumgebung, finanzielle Mittel …);
- fachliche Kompetenz des Therapeuten.

Schätzt der Therapeut, nach der Betätigungsanalyse, das genannte Ziel der Klientin als unerreichbar oder nicht in der gegebenen Zeit erreich-

Tab. 8.1 Bei fehlender Problemeinsicht des Klienten, kann eine alternative Zielannäherung angestrebt werden

Problem	Alternative Zielannäherung
Sturzgefahr	• Verletzungsgefahr minimieren, z. B. durch abgerundete Kanten
Übernahme von Tätigkeiten durch Betroffene, zur Entlastung von Angehörigen	• Verminderung des Grades der Unterstützung des Angehörigen durch Einbezug von Pflegedienstleisterinnen
Psychische Auffälligkeiten (Suchtverhalten, Unruhe, Aggressionen)	• Rückzug der Angehörigen (z. B. getrenntes Schlafzimmer) • Betreuung der Betroffenen in Einrichtung (Tagespflege, Pflegeheim)
Regelmäßige Medikamenteneinnahme	• Umstellung auf Medikamentenpumpe • Tiefe Hirnstimulation • Gabe der Medikamente durch Pflegekräfte
Gewichtszunahme	• Kalorienarme Essensgabe

bar (z. B. bei einer Rehabilitation) ein, ist eine Entmutigung wie „Das können Sie nicht schaffen.“, seitens des Therapeuten ungünstig. Nichts regt die intrinsische Motivation so sehr an wie ein Ziel, das einem inneren Bedürfnis entspringt, und sei es noch so hoch gegriffen.

▶ Unrealistische Ziele bilden die Hoffnung der Klientin ab. Und die Hoffnung sollte der Therapeut der Klientin keinesfalls nehmen.

In diesem Fall kann die sog. Treppenmethode hilfreich sein. Es wird eine Treppe gezeichnet. Auf der obersten Treppenstufe steht das Ziel, welches noch außer Reichweite scheint. Gemeinsam mit der Klientin wird darüber nachgedacht, welche Fähigkeit zuerst trainiert werden muss, um dem Ziel einen Schritt näherzukommen. Auf der zweiten Stufe steht die nächste Fähigkeit, die die Klientin dem Ziel näherbringt. Siehe Abb. 8.1

Auf diese Weise wird bildlich dargestellt, welche Schritte erforderlich sind, um das große Ziel zu erreichen. Dies kann zu zwei unterschiedlichen Ergebnissen führen. Erstens: Die Klientin erkennt von allein, dass das Ziel etwas zu hoch angesetzt wurde und schließt einen Kompromiss oder sie kommt davon ab. Zweitens: Sie tut alles dafür, die jeweiligen Stufen zu erreichen, da sie ihr großes Ziel stets vor Augen hat. In beiden Fällen hat der Therapeut die Klientin ernst genommen und sie auf ihrem Weg zu ihrem persönlichen Ziel unterstützt.

SMAR*T* – Terminiert

Gleich bei der Zielformulierung sollte ein angestrebter Zeitpunkt für das Erreichen des Zieles festgelegt werden. Dies hilft dabei, realistische Ziele zu setzen und sich in dieser Zeit auf das genannte Ziel zu konzentrieren. Das Wissen um einen Zeitpunkt, bis wann das Ziel erreicht werden soll, steigert die Motivation, daran zu arbeiten.

Die Terminierung des Ziels ist nicht immer leicht einschätzbar und sollte deswegen als Richtlinie gesehen werden, nicht als feststehender Zeitpunkt. Nicht selten braucht es nur einen kleinen Input des Therapeuten, wie „Versuchen Sie die Tätigkeit mal im Sitzen.“ oder „Dieses Hilfsmittel erleichtert Ihnen das Anziehen.“, um ein Ziel innerhalb weniger Minuten zu erreichen. Andererseits kann bei degenerativen Erkrankungen das Erreichen eines Ziels sehr lange dauern oder sogar nie erreicht werden (s. Tab. 8.2 und 8.3).

8.2 Interdisziplinäre Zielfindung

Die große Bandbreite an vielfältigen Symptomen und damit einhergehenden Einschränkungen im Alltag widerspiegelnd, sind auch die Ziele einer Klientin oftmals sehr unterschiedlich. Zum Beispiel:

1. In fünf Wochen sicheres Laufen am Rollator bis zum Kiosk, ohne Stürze.

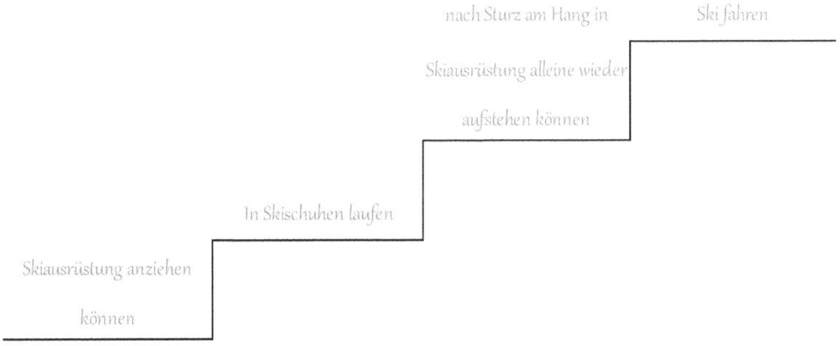

Abb. 8.1 Nicht realistische Ziele werden mit der Treppenmethode in Teilzielen Stufe für Stufe dargestellt

Tab. 8.2 Beispiel für die Formulierung von SMART-Zielen

	Terminiert	Akzeptiert	Spezifisch	Messbar
Frau K. hat	in vier Wochen	die ihr wichtigsten	Namen und Telefonnummern übersichtlich	auf ein Din A4 Blatt gesammelt.

Tab. 8.3 Beispiel für die Formulierung von SMART-Zielen. Das Ziel **r**ealistisch zu formulieren, ist eine Erinnerung für den Therapeuten und taucht nicht direkt in der Formulierung auf

	Terminiert	**A**kzeptiert+**M**essbar (durch Nachfrage)	**S**pezifisch	
Frau V. kann sich	bis zum 14. September	mit aushaltbaren	Rückenschmerzen allein ins Bett legen.	

2. In fünf Wochen leserliche Einkaufsliste schreiben.
3. Bis zum Familienfest Suppe essen, ohne sich zu verschlucken.

In der interdisziplinären Zusammenarbeit kann diese Spanne als Chance genutzt werden, indem der Ergotherapeut am Anfang der Intervention die Klientenziele im Team teilt. Es ist in ein paar Rehabilitationskliniken angewandte Praxis, dass in der ersten Teamsitzung nach Aufnahme einer neuen Klientin der Ergotherapeut die im COPM festgestellten Ziele vorträgt. Anschließend kann besprochen werden, ob es sinnvoller ist, die Ziele aufzuteilen:

z. B.
- Physiotherapie: 1. Ziel: sicheres Laufen am Rollator bis zum Kiosk, ohne Stürze
- Ergotherapie: 2. Ziel: Leserliche Einkaufsliste schreiben
- Logopädie: 3. Ziel: Essen, ohne sich zu verschlucken

Oder an das wichtigste Ziel gemeinsam herangegangen wird:

z. B.
- Physio- und Ergotherapie: 1. Ziel: sicheres Laufen am Rollator bis zum Kiosk, ohne Stürze
- Physiotherapie konzentriert sich auf:
- Kräftigung der Beine
- Schrittlänge
- Sturzprophylaxe
- Ergotherapie konzentriert sich auf:
- Dual Task beim Laufen beüben oder minimieren
- Ideale Tageszeit für die Tätigkeit ausprobieren
- Laufen in simuliertem Terraintraining

8.3 Ziele bei fortschreitender Erkrankung

Bei einer fortschreitenden Erkrankung, wie dem idiopathischen Parkinson-Syndrom, kann das Setzen von Zielen umstritten sein, da eine Verbesserung auf den ersten Blick unrealistisch erscheint und keine falschen Hoffnungen geweckt werden sollten. Andererseits sind konkrete, klientenzentrierte Ziele besonders bei einer fortschreitenden Krankheit mit einer Vielzahl an Symptomen essenziell:

- Die Klientin besinnt sich darauf, was ihr wirklich wichtig ist.
- Klientin und Therapeut fokussieren ihre Zeit und Energie auf das Ziel.
- Ziele können auch durch Veränderung der Betätigung oder Veränderung des Kontexts erreicht werden.
- Klienten erleben Selbstwirksamkeit und lernen, für ihre Bedürfnisse einzustehen.
- Durch das Setzen von Zielen werden die Erfolge sichtbar.

Trotzdem kommt es regelmäßig vor, dass die gefassten Ziele nicht erreicht werden können, weil z. B. die Symptome sich verschlechtern oder es sich als zu schwierig oder aufwändig herausstellt. Das kann für Klienten sehr belastend sein, weil durch die konstanten Rückschläge die Motivation schwindet. Auch für den Therapeuten ist der professionelle Umgang mit dem konstanten Fortschreiten der Parkinson-Erkrankung eine Herausforderung. Besonders in der Praxis, bei Langzeitpatientinnen mit Dauerverordnung, besteht die Gefahr eines „Dahinplätscherns" der Therapie ohne Ziel. Solche Phasen entstehen immer wieder. Sie sollten dazu genutzt werden, genau hinzusehen, ob noch ein Betätigungsziel besteht, oder es an der Zeit für eine Therapiepause ist.

▶ Bei Langzeitpatienten kann die Therapie frisch bleiben, indem nach Erreichen des Klientenziels eine Therapiepause eingelegt wird.

Es kann ein natürlicher Rhythmus entstehen, bei dem nach erreichtem Therapieziel eine Pause eingelegt wird, um dann, bei Auftreten eines neuen Betätigungsanliegens, die Therapie neu aufzunehmen.

Beispiel

Nach vier Wochen Schreibtraining, in denen auch die ideale Sitzhaltung beim Schreiben besprochen wurde, geeignetes Briefpapier gefunden und unterschiedliche Stifte ausprobiert wurden, schätzt der Ergotherapeut, dass Frau Sch. den Brief an Maria jetzt schreiben kann. Diese fühlt sich jedoch noch nicht bereit dazu. Sie möchte noch weiterüben, da sie ihre Schrift noch nicht ideal findet. Der Therapeut reflektiert, dass die Schrift der Klientin ungewöhnlich gleichmäßig und perfekt lesbar ist, lässt sich aber auf Wunsch der Klientin auf weitere Schreibübungen ein.

Nach weiteren vier Wochen fühlt sich Frau Sch. noch immer nicht bereit. Der Therapeut versucht ihr zu vermitteln, dass Maria sich sicherlich über den Brief freut, auch wenn Frau Sch.s Schrift nicht so perfekt ist wie früher, doch die Klientin ist nicht überzeugt. Da fällt dem Ergotherapeuten auf, er hat das Ziel nicht terminiert (T- im SMART). Er fragt Frau Sch. „Bis wann möchten Sie den Brief fertig geschrieben haben?" Sie antwortet: „In drei Wochen müsste ich das schaffen." Der Therapeut sieht auf den Kalender: „Also bis zum 7. November, ja?" „Ja." bestätigt die Klientin.

- „Gut, dann notiere ich es hier in meinen Unterlagen. Tragen Sie es doch gleich in Ihren Kalender ein, dann haben Sie eine Motivation."
- „Gute Idee," sagt Frau Sch. „dann fange ich gleich heute an, die Rose zu malen, die auf das Briefpapier soll." ◀

Literatur und weiterführende Literatur

Global Parkinson's Disease Survey (GPDS) Steering Committee (2002) Factors impacting on quality of life in Parkinson's disease: results from an international survey. Mov Disord. 17(1):60–67. https://doi.org/10.1002/mds.10010. PMID: 11835440

Law M, Baptiste S, Mills J (1995) Client-centred practice: what does it mean and does it make a difference? Can J Occup Ther 62(5):250–257. https://doi.org/10.1177/000841749506200504. PMID: 10152881

Mayor C, Roos K, Petrig A, Rossini E, Meyer S (2014) Empfehlungen zur Formulierung von ergotherapeutischen Zielen. evs-ErgotherapeutInnen Verband Schweiz, Bern. Heruntergeladen vom ErgotherapeutInnen Verband http://www.ergotherapie.chj, Zugriffsdatum 14.07.2020

Page J, Roos K, Bänziger A, Margot-Cattin I, Agustoni S, Rossini E, Meichtry M (2015) Formulating goals in occupational therapy: state of the art in Switzerland. Scandinavian Journal of Occupational Therapy. 22. https://doi.org/10.3109/11038128.2015.1049548

Radder DLM, Sturkenboom IH, van Nimwegen M, Keus SH, Bloem BR, de Vries NM (2017) Physical therapy and occupational therapy in Parkinson's disease. International Journal of Neuroscience 127(10):930–943. https://doi.org/10.1080/00207454.2016.1275617

Romein E. Klientenzentrierte Zielformulierung alle Diagnosen und Altersgruppen. http://klientenzentrierte-ergotherapie.com/Instrumente-und-Methoden-in-Ergotherapie/zielformulierung-evtl-nach-icf-alle-diagnosen-und-altersgruppen.html. Zugegriffen am 22.01.2021

Röse K (2017) Betätigung von Personen mit Demenz im Kontext Pflegeheim. Hogrefe, Göttingen

Sturkenboom I, Thijssen M, Gons-van Elsacker J, Jansen I, Maasdam A, Schulten M, Vijver-Visser D, Steultjens E, Bloem B, Munneke M (2008) Guidelines for occupational therapy in Parkinson's disease rehabilitation. ParkinsonNet/NPF, Nijmegen/Miami

Teil IV

Interventionsphase

9 Ergotherapie im Krankheitsverlauf

Je nachdem, in welchem Stadium der Parkinson-Erkrankung der Klient sich befindet, wird die ergotherapeutische Intervention individuell angepasst. Als grobe Richtlinie kann festgehalten werden, dass im Frühstadium bei jüngeren motivierten Klienten ein aktives Training von Betätigungen und Körperfunktionen sinnvoll ist. Im weiteren Verlauf verschiebt sich die Therapie in Richtung Kompensation und Adaptation. Im Endstadium der Erkrankung, wenn der Klient auf maximale Unterstützung angewiesen ist, kann eine Therapie zur Erfüllung der Grundbedürfnisse und Unterstützung von pflegenden Angehörigen adäquat sein.

► Die ergotherapeutische Intervention verändert sich teils stark im Verlauf der Parkinson-Erkrankung des Klienten, da sich auch die Symptome, innere Einstellung und persönliche Ziele des Klienten verändern.

Eine Einteilung der Krankheit in Phasen ist rein theoretisch, da M. Parkinson von Patient zu Patient unterschiedlich verläuft und auch die Kontextfaktoren nicht einheitlich sind. Dennoch ist es hilfreich, diese Einteilung vorzunehmen, um die unterschiedliche therapeutische Handhabe im Bezug zum Krankheitsverlauf darzustellen. Es wird zwischen Frühstadium, fortgeschrittenes Stadium und Spätstadium unterschieden.

9.1 Frühstadium

Beispiel

Frau F. kommt sechs Wochen nach Diagnosestellung in die Ergotherapie. Sie ist trotz ihres höheren Alters (78) im Frühstadium. Sie ist medikamentös gut eingestellt, zeigt eine leichte Bradykinese, die sich in Hypomimie, verminderter Armpendelbewegung und einer kyphotischen Haltung äußert. Außerdem berichtet sie von Schmerzen in der Brustwirbelsäule und von Niedergeschlagenheit. Außerdem fühlt sie sich nach aktiven Betätigungen, wie dem Einkaufen, müde und erschöpft. ◄

Nach der Diagnosestellung werden Menschen mit IPS medikamentös meist einige Zeit gut eingestellt. Die Symptome treten kaum noch auf und eine Fluktuation kann durch regelmäßige Medikamenteneinnahme vermieden werden. In diesem Anfangsstadium sind die Klienten meist gut beweglich, kognitiv nicht eingeschränkt und kommen im Alltag ohne große Umstellungen zurecht. Deshalb wird sie auch „Honeymoon-Phase" genannt. Eine therapeutische Intervention macht in dieser Phase Sinn, auch wenn auf den ersten

---

Ergänzende Information Die elektronische Version dieses Kapitels enthält Zusatzmaterial, auf das über folgenden Link zugegriffen werden kann https://doi.org/10.1007/978-3-662-62583-5_9. Die Videos lassen sich durch Anklicken des DOI Links in der Legende einer entsprechenden Abbildung abspielen, oder indem Sie diesen Link mit der SN More Media App scannen.

A. Orellana, *Betätigungsorientierte Ergotherapie bei Morbus Parkinson*,
https://doi.org/10.1007/978-3-662-62583-5_9

Blick oft keine gravierenden Einschränkungen zu erkennen sind.

- Coping/Krankheitsverarbeitung
  Verständlicherweise ist die Diagnose „Morbus Parkinson" ein großer Schock für die Patienten und ihre Angehörigen. Häufig hadern sie mit der Krankheit vor allem, weil sie progredient und unheilbar ist. Die Krankheitsverarbeitung benötigt Zeit und Unterstützung von allen Seiten. Konnte die Therapeutin ein vertrauensvolles Verhältnis zu dem Klienten aufbauen, kann sie durch Zuhören und Stärkung des Klienten eine Stütze sein.
  Die Frage „Wann und wie erzähle ich meinem Umfeld von der Krankheit?" ist ein komplexes Thema, welches in der Ergotherapie wiederholt besprochen werden kann und meist je nach Krankheitssymptomen und betreffender Personengruppe (nahe Angehörige, entfernte Angehörige, enge Freundinnen, Bekannte, Fremde) unterschiedlich gehandhabt wird.
  Außerdem können Klienten Themen rund um die Krankheitsverarbeitung im Rahmen einer Gruppentherapie mit Menschen in einer ähnlichen Lage besprechen (s. Abb. 9.1).
- Aufklärung
  Zwar hat jeder schon von der Krankheit „M. Parkinson" gehört und einen Betroffenen gesehen oder gekannt. Trotzdem ist erfahrungsgemäß nur geringes Wissen über die Symptome, Ursache und Prognose vorhanden. Eine Verwechslung mit MS, ALS oder Essenziellem Tremor ist nicht selten. Auch die Sorge über einhergehende Demenz, körperliche Einschränkung und frühzeitigen Tod wird häufig geäußert. Aus diesem Grund ist die Informationsvermittlung und Aufklärung ein wichtiger Teil der therapeutischen Intervention in der Frühphase.
- Aktives Training
  Im Frühstadium sind die meisten Klienten sehr motiviert, an ihren Einschränkungen zu arbeiten. Dies zeigt sich in einer großen Bereitschaft, selbstständig zu üben und auch an die Leistungsgrenze zu gehen. Das sind gute Voraussetzungen für ein aktives Training. Je höher die intrinsische Motivation, desto höher die Wiederholungszahl beim Training, desto besser auch der Outcome. Dazu sollte die Therapeutin das Wissen um den belegten positiven Effekt, den Sport und Fitness auf die nicht-motorischen Symptome und Kognition (Cusso et al. 2016), die motorischen Symptome (Alberts et al. 2001) und sogar die Krankheitsprogression (Ahlskog 2017) hat, mit dem Klienten teilen (Abb. 9.2).
- Kognition
  Da eine demenzielle Entwicklung meist erst im fortgeschrittenen Stadium eintritt, ist das Erarbeiten von Problemlösungsstrategien, gesunden Coping-Mechanismen und Strategien zum Umgang mit Symptomen z. B. Cueing (siehe Abschn. 14.1.2), Sequenzierung (siehe

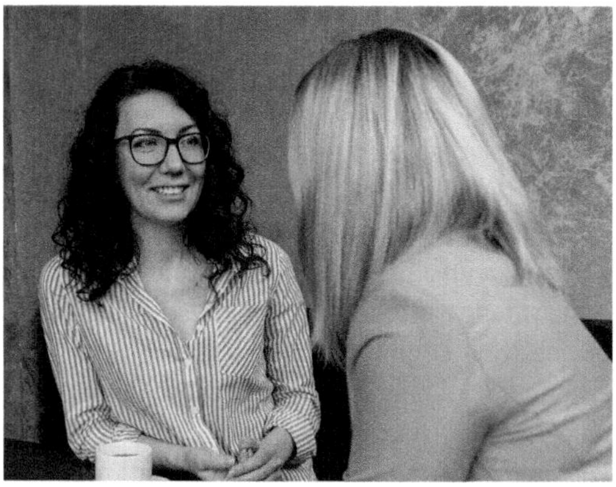

Abb. 9.1 Gespräche zur Krankheitsaufklärung und -verarbeitung sind im Frühstadium ein wichtiger Bestandteil der Ergotherapie

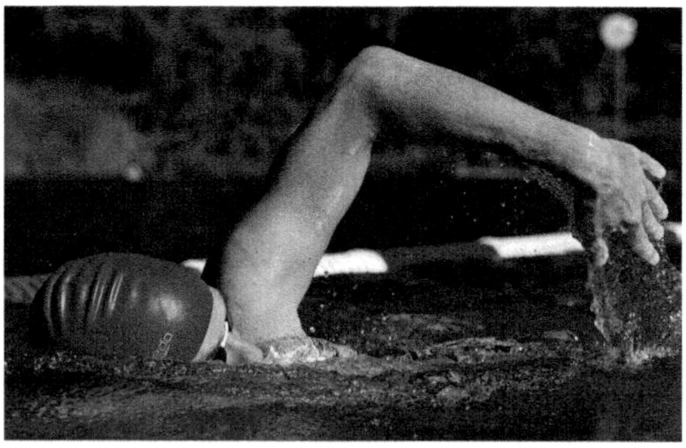

Abb. 9.2 Im Frühstadium haben Klienten oftmals eine hohe Motivation für ein aktives Training an der Leistungsgrenze, welches sich positiv auf den Krankheitsverlauf auswirkt

Abschn. 14.1.4), Vermeidung von Dual Tasks (siehe Abschn. 14.1.5) in der Frühphase noch gut möglich. Dies sollte genutzt werden, da im Laufe der Krankheit die kognitive Umstellungsfähigkeit und die Kapazität Neues zu erlernen abnimmt.

Beispiel

Frau F. hatte im COPM zwar ein motorisches Problem priorisiert, mit wachsendem Vertrauen zum Therapeuten rückten jedoch die nicht-motorischen Anliegen zunehmend in den Vordergrund. So wurden folgende Themen besprochen und bearbeitet:

- Nebenwirkungen der Medikamente (Mundtrockenheit)
- Kommunikation mit Arzt (Liste mit Fragen schreiben)
- Fragen zum Tod
- Überforderung durch vollen Terminkalender (Tagesplan ausfüllen, Prioritätenliste schreiben, unwichtiges streichen)
- Umgang mit vermehrtem Ruhebedürfnis (Einplanung von Pausen)
- Kommunikation mit Freunden, Bekannten und Unbekannten über Erkrankung (Vor- und Nachteile der Offenlegung der Erkrankung)
- Umgang mit depressiven Verstimmungen (Ruhephasen, stärkende soziale Kontakte, stärkende Aktivitäten, Reduktion der Aufgabenmenge)
- möglicher Umzug in Senioren-WG
- … ◀

9.2 Fortgeschrittenes Stadium

Beispiel

Herr J. ist ein gutgelaunter Mensch. Es fallen ihm viele mögliche Bereiche in seinem Leben ein, an denen er arbeiten könnte. Das Schreiben, sein Büro neu ordnen, „schöner Essen“, lauter sprechen. Hauptsächlich kommt er aber in die Reha wegen seiner häufigen Stürze. Mit Rollator lässt er sich in der Öffentlichkeit nicht sehen, aber er weiß, dass es nicht so weiter gehen kann. Entweder er wird wieder stabiler oder er muss ins Heim. ◀

Im fortgeschrittenen Stadium nehmen die motorischen und nicht-motorischen Symptome auch während der On-Phase zu. Die Fluktuation der Medikamentenwirkung nimmt zu, sodass Hyperkinesien (Überbeweglichkeit) und akinetische Zustände (Unbeweglichkeit) vermehrt auftreten. Die Arbeitsfähigkeit ist meist nicht mehr gegeben und auch im Alltag zeigen sich immer mehr Probleme. Es besteht eine größere Abhängigkeit von äußerlicher Hilfe durch Angehörige oder Pflegepersonen. Die therapeutische Intervention verlagert sich in dieser Phase. Es entsteht vermehrt Bedarf für kompensatorische Methoden oder adaptive Mittel.

- Coping/Krankheitsverarbeitung
  Die Auseinandersetzung mit der Krankheit ist nun nichts Neues mehr, findet bei einer progredienten Erkrankung jedoch stetig statt, da immer neue oder veränderte Symptome auftreten. Als klientenzentrierte Therapeutinnen sind Ergotherapeutinnen einzigartig dazu ausgebildet, die Krankheitsverarbeitung und die Auswirkung auf den Alltag zu unterstützen. Themen wie die zunehmende Hilfebedürftigkeit, verminderte Mobilität, äußeres Erscheinungsbild und eine Vielzahl an individuellen, persönlichen Anliegen können aufkommen.
- Sturzprävention
  Stürze stellen einen gravierenden Meilenstein bei M. Parkinson dar. Nach einem Sturz ist die Wahrscheinlichkeit, innerhalb der folgenden drei Monate erneut zu stürzen, erhöht.
  Aus diesem Grund ist eine Sturzprophylaxe mit Gleichgewichts- und Pulsionstraining (siehe Abschn. 14.1.2) frühzeitig indiziert. Zusätzlich sollte die Ergotherapeutin eine Wohnraumberatung durchführen um Stolperfallen zu identifizieren (siehe Abschn. 15.2).
- Kompensation und Adaptation
  Mit der Verschlechterung der Symptome, evtl. vermindertem Antrieb und einer demenziellen Entwicklung nimmt die Effektivität der aktivierenden Therapie langsam ab. An dessen

Stelle treten das Einüben von Kompensationsmethoden (Cueing, Entspannungstechniken, Merkstrategien … siehe Kap. 14) und der Einsatz von Adaptionen (Hilfsmittel, Wohnraumanpassung, Veränderung der Umwelt siehe Kap. 15).

- Angehörigenberatung
  Im fortgeschrittenen Stadium übernehmen Partnerinnen oder andere Angehörige zunehmend Aufgaben bei der Haushaltsführung, unterstützen den Betroffenen bei der Mobilität und führen pflegerische Tätigkeiten aus. Ergotherapeutinnen können in dieser Phase Tipps und Tricks bei der Handhabung vermitteln (z. B. Zeitdruck minimieren, Drehen im Bett, Kommunikation).
  Ein weiterer wichtiger Aspekt ist, dass viele Angehörige im Spätstadium in eine Überlastung geraten. Um dem vorzubeugen, ist eine frühzeitige Begleitung und Aufklärung der pflegenden Angehörigen wichtig (z. B. professionelle Unterstützung durch ambulante Pflege, Selbsthilfegruppen, Stressmanagement). Mehr Informationen dazu sind in Abschn. 15.1 zu finden).

Beispiel

Sobald Herr J. in der Reha ankommt, bekommt er einen Rollator. Naserümpfend nimmt er ihn entgegen. „Damit sehe ich so alt aus.", bemerkt er. Doch sobald er sieht, dass hier fast alle damit herumlaufen, nimmt er ihn doch mit zum Essensraum. In der Physiotherapie ist das Ziel schnell klar: Sturzprävention. In der Logopädie will er an einer lauteren Stimme arbeiten. In der Ergotherapie nennt er zunächst das Schreiben als wichtigstes Ziel, bis ihm die Ergotherapeutin versichert, dass Sturzprävention auch für die Ergo ein wichtiges Tätigkeitsfeld ist. Zusammen begeben sie sich auf Ursachenforschung. Wann genau treten die Stürze auf? In welchem Raum? Zu welcher Uhrzeit? Hat es etwas mit Müdigkeit oder Ablenkung zu tun? Welche Hilfsmittel könnten noch hilfreich sein? Herr J. ist überrascht, wie alltagsnah dieses Thema sein kann. ◀

9.3 Spätstadium

Beispiel

Frau V. kommt schon seit vielen Jahren zur Ergotherapie in die Praxis. Immer, wenn es wieder eine Verschlechterung gibt oder sie mit einer Situation zu Hause nicht zurechtkommt, holt sie sich ein Rezept. Mittlerweile holt der Ehemann die Rezepte. Frau V. sitzt meist im Rollstuhl und ist bei der Selbstversorgung auf die Pflege und Hilfe ihres Mannes angewiesen. An der Tagesstrukturierung und Planung nimmt die Klientin nicht mehr aktiv teil, es ist für sie kognitiv nicht mehr möglich. ◀

Folgende Meilensteine kennzeichnen den Beginn des Spätstadiums.

- Regelmäßige Stürze
- Visuelle Halluzinationen
- Demenz
- Aufnahme ins Pflegeheim notwendig

Nach dem Auftreten dieser Meilensteine spricht man von einem exponentiellen Verlauf. Das heißt für die Praxis: Wenn die Meilensteine zu beobachten sind, ist mit einem rapiden Abbau des Klienten zu rechnen. Vom Auftreten der Meilensteine bis zum Tod vergehen im Durchschnitt etwa fünf Jahre. Welches Bild sich genau im Spätstadium zeigt, ist bei dieser diversen Erkrankung sehr unterschiedlich. So können motorische Symptome wie Dysphagie und Bettlägerigkeit dominieren oder aber nicht-motorische Symptome, wie Demenz, Psychosen und Depression.

Die Spätphase beim M. Parkinson wird über die starke Abhängigkeit von einer Pflegeperson zur Verrichtung der Aktivitäten des täglichen Lebens, bis hin zur Bettlägerigkeit, definiert. Jedoch tritt nur bei 5 % der Parkinson-Betroffenen eine Bettlägerigkeit oder Abhängigkeit vom Rollstuhl ein. Im Spätstadium ist nicht mit funktionellen Verbesserungen zu rechnen. Vielmehr geht es um vier wichtige Aspekte, erstens die Verbesserung der Lebensqualität, zweitens die Erfüllung der Grundbedürfnisse, drittens die Vermeidung von Sekundärschäden (Prophylaxe von Kontrakturen,

Pneumonie, Thrombose, Dekubitus und Stürze) und viertens die Ermöglichung von (passiver) Teilhabe.

Verbesserung der Lebensqualität

Im Verlauf der Erkrankung nimmt die subjektiv erlebte Lebensqualität der Klienten stark ab. Durch die große Abhängigkeit von anderen Personen, depressive Verstimmung, große Immobilität und zum Teil starke Schmerzen, empfinden viele Klienten kaum noch Lebensfreude. In der Ergotherapie aktivierte, oftmals kleine Veränderungen können eine große Wirkung auf die erlebte Lebensqualität der Klienten haben. Hierzu ein paar praktische Anregungen:

- Verständliche Erklärung der Krankheit, Symptome und Wirkung der Medikamente,
- Begrüßung mit Händedruck oder fester Berührung an Schulter,
- direktes Ansprechen des Klienten,
- gemeinsames Lesen eines aufheiternden Gedichtes des Lieblingsautors,
- Trinken des Nachmittagskaffees auf der Terrasse, statt im Aufenthaltsraum des Pflegeheims,
- gemeinsames Ausprobieren der elektrischen Eisenbahn (früheres Hobby),
- selbständiges Gesicht waschen, bei sonstiger vollkommener Abhängigkeit von Pflegeperson,
- Anregung der Mithilfe des Klienten beim Kochen, z. B. Gurke schneiden, Karotte schälen,
- Lagerung mit Blick zum Fenster,
- Fotomobile über Bett, mit Bildern von Familie,
- Fotoalbum gemeinsam betrachten (s. Abb. 9.3),
- Handmassage, auch von Angehörigen durchführbar.

Erfüllung der Grundbedürfnisse

Ausgehend von der **Maslowschen Bedürfnispyramide** (Maslow 1943) haben Menschen folgende Bedürfnisse (nach Wichtigkeit sortiert):

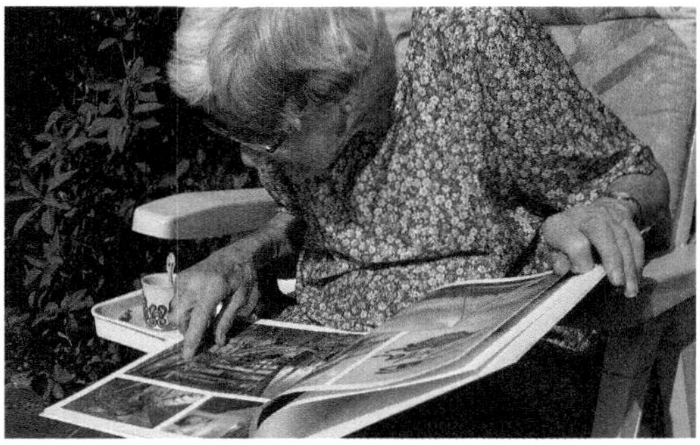

Abb. 9.3 Einfache Betätigungen, wie gemeinsames ansehen eines Fotoalbums, können in der Spätphase der Erkrankung die Lebensqualität merklich verbessern

- Körperliche Grundbedürfnisse: Atmung; Wärme; Trinken; Essen; Schlaf (Ruhe und Entspannung),
- Sicherheit: Unterkunft/Wohnung; Gesundheit; Schutz vor Gefahren; Ordnung (Gesetze, Rituale),
- Soziale Beziehungen: Freundeskreis; Partnerschaft; Liebe; Nächstenliebe; Sexualität; Fürsorge; Kommunikation.

Eine Grundannahme der **Ergotherapie** ist, dass es ein menschliches Bedürfnis ist, tätig zu sein und an Betätigungen teilzuhaben. Die therapeutische Interventionsbeispiele in Tab. 9.1 sind von den o. g. Bedürfnissen abgeleitet.

Vermeidung von Sekundärschäden

Durch die Zunahme der Immobilität und Verstärkung der Symptome im fortgeschrittenen Stadium, treten gehäuft Sekundärschäden auf. Dazu gehören Kontrakturen, Pneumonie, Thrombose, Dekubitus und Sturzfolgen (Frakturen, Fallangst). Für bettlägerige Klienten besteht eine stark erhöhte Gefahr, einen oder mehrere der genannten Sekundärschäden zu entwickeln. Aus diesem Grund hat die regelmäßige Mobilisation aus dem Bett oberste Priorität (Abb. 9.7).

▶ Im Fall einer Bettlägerigkeit des Klienten kann eine Langzeitbehandlung in der

Tab. 9.1 Therapeutische Interventionsbeispiele

	Bedürfnis	Beispiele
Körperliche Grundbedürfnisse	Atmung	• Aufsetzen an Bettkante oder in Stuhl • Mobilisierung • Atemübungen (Abb. 9.4) • Atemanregende Massage • Frischluftversorgung (Fenster öffnen, raus gehen)
	Wärme	• Angepasste Raumtemperatur • Nicht zu warm, wegen möglicher gestörter Temperaturregulation
	Trinken	• Dem Klienten angenehme Getränke anbieten (Tee, Saft …) • Trinkmenge besprechen (Kognition – Inkontinenz)
	Essen	• Liste mit gut schluckbarem Essen machen • Proteine wichtig im Alter (Sarkopenie Vorbeugung) • Proteine nicht mit Medikamenteneinnahme essen
	Schlaf (Ruhe, Entspannung)	• Im Tagesplan fest einplanen • Wichtigkeit von Schlaf und Ruhe für Aktivität und Energie vermitteln
Sicherheit	Unterkunft/ Wohnung	• Wohnung/Haus durch Hilfsmittel und Wohnraumberatung sicher machen (s. Abb. 9.5) • Umzug in Heim planen (Liste mit Gegenständen die mitgenommen werden, Heime recherchieren)
	Gesundheit	• Besprechen von Einfluss von Aktivität, Sozialkontakten und Ernährung auf psychische und körperliche Gesundheit • Fokussierung auf Ressourcen und positive Aspekte des Lebens
	Schutz vor Gefahren	• Sturzgefahr durch Gleichgewichtsübungen, Vermeidung von Stolperfallen in der Wohnung und Hilfsmittelversorgung reduzieren
	Ordnung (Gesetze, Rituale)	• Therapie klar strukturieren • Ziele setzen und Intervention transparent darauf abstimmen • Das Leben durch Kalender und Tages-/Wochenplan strukturieren • Teilhabe an Familienritualen wieder ermöglichen (gemeinsames Essen, Feiern …)
Soziale Beziehungen	Freundeskreis	• Reflektieren, wer wirkliche Freundinnen sind • Mit diesen Menschen regelmäßigen Kontakt anstreben • Um Hilfe bitten
	Partnerschaft	• Bewusst werden, dass Rollenveränderung unumgänglich ist (Hilfsbedürftiger – Helfender) • Dysbalance vermeiden, durch Hilfe holen von außen • Partnerschaft aktiv leben durch bewusste gemeinsame Aktivitäten (s. Abb. 9.6)
	Liebe	• Lernen, Liebe auf unterschiedliche Arten zu zeigen (Worte, Brief, Nachricht, Geschenk, Aufmerksamkeit) • Nähe zur Familie suchen
	Nächstenliebe	• Trotz eigener Erkrankung Unterstützung an andere weitergeben (z. B. über Selbsthilfegruppen, in Familie) • Freundlicher Umgang mit allen Menschen (Nachbarn, Therapeutinnen, Partner)
	Sexualität	• Therapeutin sollte kommunizieren, dass Sexualität auch ein Thema in der Ergotherapie sein kann • Probleme erfragen, Umgehens weisen und Sex-Hilfsmittel besprechen

(Fortsetzung)

Tab. 9.1 (Fortsetzung)

	Bedürfnis	Beispiele
	Fürsorge	• Im Rahmen der eigenen Möglichkeiten fürsorgliche Tätigkeiten für Partnerin und Familie übernehmen (Tee kochen, Rückenmassage anbieten) • Evtl. Haustier aufnehmen • Garten/Pflanzen pflegen
	Kommunikation	• Unterschiedliche Kommunikationswege ausprobieren • Rollenspiele zur Verbesserung der Kommunikation • Logopädie anregen, wenn notwendig
Tätig sein	Selbstversorgung	• Übernahme basaler körperlicher Versorgung (Gesicht waschen, Hände eincremen) • Transfer im Bett (Drehung) • Miteinbeziehen in Regelung persönlicher Angelegenheiten (Fragen nach Essenswünschen)
	Produktivität	• Besuch alter Arbeitsstelle • Kontakt mit ehemaligen Arbeitskolleginnen aufrechterhalten • Übernahme kleiner Haushaltstätigkeiten (Wäsche falten, Pflanzen gießen)
	Freizeit	• Neue Hobbys suchen (Fotografieren, Musik hören) • Alte Hobbys adaptieren (Hörbuch statt lesen, Schach zusehen statt spielen) • Aktive Freizeit anpassen (Reisen für Menschen mit Behinderung)

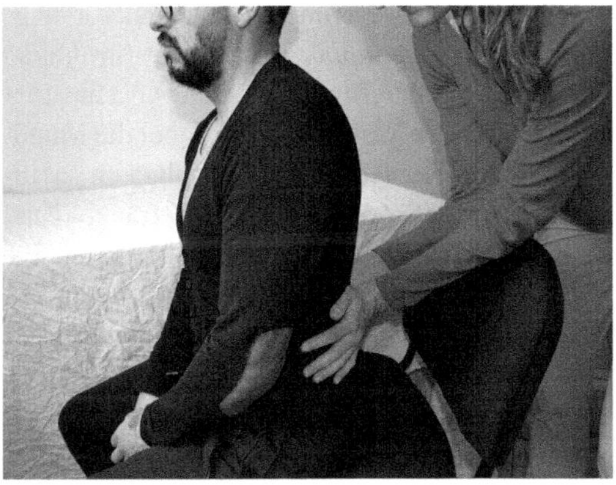

Abb. 9.4 Atemübungen fördern die tiefe Atmung und beugen einer Pneumonie vor. Um eine Zwerchfellatmung anzuleiten, wird der Klient dazu aufgefordert bei der **Einatmung** gegen die, am unteren Rücken platzierten, Hände der Therapeutin zu atmen. Alternativ kann der Klient seine eigenen Hände auf den Bauch legen und dagegen atmen

Ergotherapie sinnvoll sein, um eine regelmäßige Mobilisation zu gewährleisten und Sekundärschäden vorzubeugen.

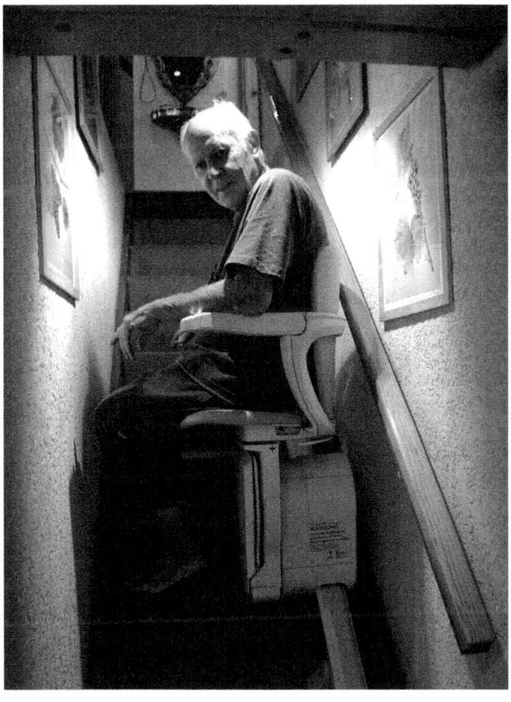

Abb. 9.5 Durch eine Wohnraumanpassung kann das selbständige Leben im eigenen Heim ermöglicht werden

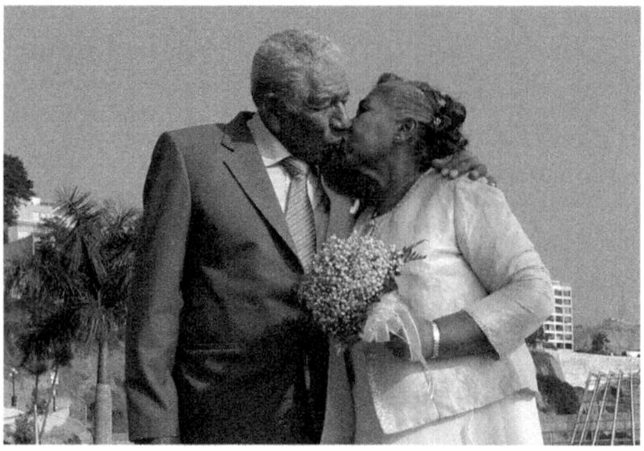

Abb. 9.6 In der Ergotherapie können Anregungen für eine Verwirklichung von Fürsorge und Partnerschaft gegeben werden. So kann dieses menschliche Grundbedürfnis auch in der Spätphase der Erkrankung erfüllt werden

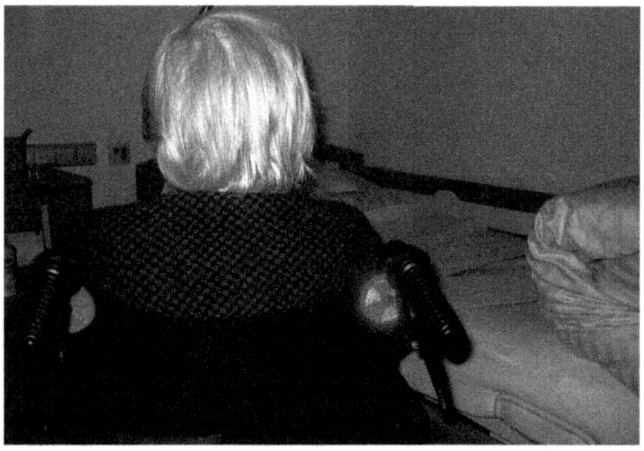

Abb. 9.7 Tägliche Mobilisierung aus dem Bett ist im Spätstadium wichtig zur Pneumonieprophylaxe, Dekubitusprophylaxe, Kontrakturenprophylaxe und Thromboseprophylaxe

Kontrakturenprophylaxe

Durch den zunehmenden Rigor und die vermehrte Hypokinese können Muskeln verkürzen und längerfristig Kontrakturen entstehen. Typische Bereiche sind die Flektoren der Hände, die ventrale Seite des Halses und Oberkörpers, Hüftbeuger und Fußflektoren.

Je nach betroffenem Körperbereich wird das Stehen, der Transfer, der Einsatz der Hände oder die Aufrichtung behindert. Schon frühzeitig im Krankheitsverlauf ist es sinnvoll, durch regelmäßige körperliche Aktivität und Sport Muskelverkürzungen vorzubeugen, denn bestehende Kontrakturen sind kaum wieder rückgängig zu machen. Aktive Mobilisation kann durch passive Mobilisation und Dehnen sowie Lagerung im Bett unterstützt werden.

Pneumonie Prophylaxe

Eine Pneumonie gehört zu den häufigsten Todesursachen beim IPS. Sie kann durch Schluckstörungen und mangelnde Mobilisation hervorgerufen werden. Zur Vorbeugung muss genau beobachtet werden, ob eine Schluckstörung vorliegt. Häufiges Verschlucken oder Rasselgeräusche beim Atmen sind Zeichen, dass das Schlucken nicht physiologisch abläuft. Eine Untersuchung bei einer Hals-Nasen-Ohren-Ärztin ist ratsam.

> **Cave!**
> Wenn nach dem Trinken Rasselgeräuschen beim Atmen zu hören sind könnte eine unerkannte Schluckstörung vorliegen, was zu einer Pneumonie führen kann.

Für eine Verbesserung des Schluckvorgangs beim Trinken, kann das Trinken mit Strohhalm oder einem Trinklernbecher (siehe Abschn. 15.3 Hilfsmittel) von Vorteil sein, da dabei die Mundspannung höher ist, was das Schlucken fazilitiert. Auch das Andicken von Getränken und Suppen ist eine Möglichkeit. Eine regelmäßige Mobilisation in den Sitz ist notwendig, um den Abtransport von in die Lunge eingetretener Flüssigkeit zu ermöglichen. Zusätzlich können atemstimulierende Maßnahmen hilfreich sein. Wenn noch keine logopädische Intervention erfolgt, sollte die Ergotherapeutin dies veranlassen.

Thromboseprophylaxe

Der wichtigste Faktor zur Vorbeugung einer Thrombose ist die Mobilisation. Der Klient sollte regelmäßiges Aufstehen in den Tagesablauf integrieren. Außerdem sind Eigenübungen zur Aktivierung der Muskelpumpe im Bett oder im Sitz sinnvoll. Dabei unterstützt die Muskelbewegung die Venen dabei, das Blut zurückzutransportieren (siehe Abb. 9.8, Video 9.8). Auch das Tragen von Thrombosestrümpfen gehört zur Thromboseprophylaxe.

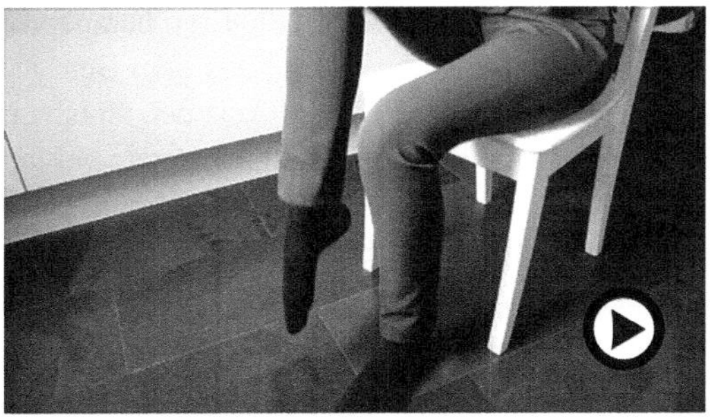

Abb. 9.8 mit Video 9.8 Zur Thromboseprophylaxe können Übungen zur Aktivierung der Muskelpumpe durchgeführt werden (▶ https://doi.org/10.1007/000-2x5)

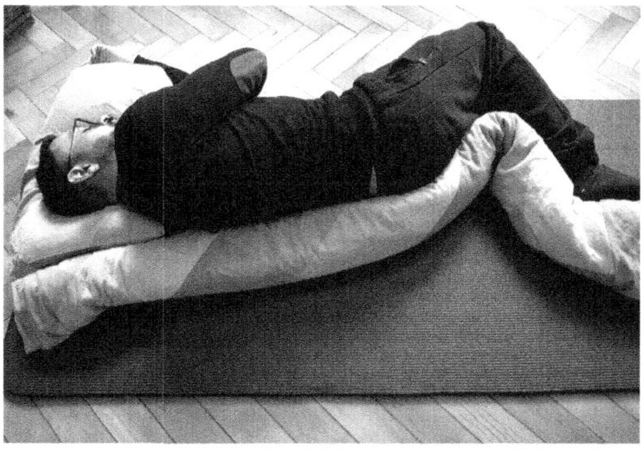

Abb. 9.9 Bei immobilen Klienten kann eine dynamische Lagerung ihn dabei unterstützen, Mikrobewegungen im Bett zu machen, um einem Dekubitus vorzubeugen. Eine längs zusammengerollte Bettdecke gibt etwas Unterstützung im Rücken um eine Seitdrehung zu ermöglichen, ohne Bewegungseinschränkend zu wirken

Dekubitusprophylaxe

Im fortgeschrittenen Stadium fällt es Klienten zunehmend schwer, sich im Bett zu drehen, wodurch die Dekubitus-Gefahr zunimmt. Das unbewusste nächtliche Drehen bei Gesunden fehlt bei Menschen mit M. Parkinson. Selbst wenn sie nachts wach werden, ist es ihnen oftmals nicht möglich, sich ohne Hilfe umzudrehen. Die Ermöglichung der selbständigen Drehung im Bett hat dabei oberste Priorität. Das kann durch Training der Rotation im Liegen mit Handlungshilfen geschehen (z. B. Beine anstellen). Zusätzlich kann der Einsatz von Hilfsmitteln notwendig sein (z. B. Bettgriff, Schlaufenband am Bettrand). Ist die aktive Drehung nicht mehr möglich, wird eine dynamische Lagerung notwendig, d. h. eine Unterstützung im Rücken (z. B. zusammengerollte Bettdecke), um die Seitlage zu ermöglichen. Dabei sollte überflüssiges Lagerungsmaterial vermieden werden, damit der Klient noch mit Mikrobewegungen eine bequeme Schlafposition finden kann und dadurch selbständig zur Dekubitusprophylaxe beitragen kann (s. Abb. 9.9).

Auf die Lagerung des Kopfes muss bei Menschen mit der Parkinson Erkrankung besonders geachtet werden. Durch den Rigor kann das „Kopfkissenphänomen" entstehen. Die ventrale Halsmuskulatur ist sehr fest und kann nicht entspannt werden. Wird der Kopf nicht unterlagert (meist mit zwei Kissen) hängt der Kopf in der Luft (s. Abb. 9.10). Auch eine regelmäßige Mobilisation aus dem Bett in den Sitz und Stand trägt zur Dekubitusprophylaxe bei.

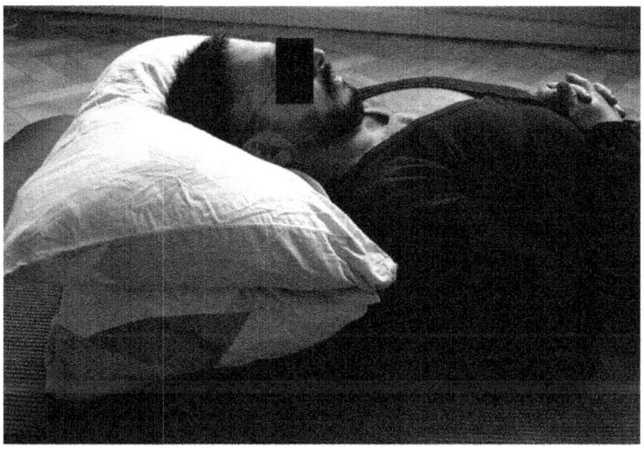

Abb. 9.10 Bei starkem Halsrigor muss der Kopf gut unterlagert werden (zwei Kissen), sonst kann der Klient ihn nicht ablegen und er hängt in der Luft

Sturzprophylaxe

Zur Vermeidung von Stürzen im Spätstadium ist eine durchdachte Hilfsmittelversorgung erforderlich. Meist wird ein Rollator notwendig. Die Versorgung mit einem Rollstuhl ist bei täglichen Stürzen oder Immobilität angemessen. Auch das Üben von sicheren Transfers z. B. Bett Rollstuhl, Rollstuhl-Toilette und Rollstuhl-Auto, evtl. mit Anleitung eines Angehörigen, kann eine wichtige Sturzprophylaxe darstellen. Weitere Aspekte zur Sturzvermeidung siehe Abschn. 14.4.3.

Unterstützung von pflegenden Angehörigen

Angehörige von Menschen mit M. Parkinson im Spätstadium begleiten den Betroffenen in der Regel schon viele Jahre. Sie geraten immer mehr in die Rolle des Pflegenden und fühlen sich häufig überfordert, ohne eine Möglichkeit der Entlastung erkennen zu können. Hier fällt der Ergotherapeutin die Aufgabe zu, der Angehörigen neue Wege aufzuzeigen und sie, wenn erwünscht, dabei zu begleiten. Dazu gehört z. B. Organisation von ambulanter Pflege, Aufnahme in Seniorenheim recherchieren, Hilfsmittelberatung zur Entlastung (Pflegebett, Toilettenstuhl, elektrischer Sessel mit Aufstehhilfe), Wohnraumberatung (evtl. Badumbau, rollstuhlgerechte Wohnung). Für weitere Informationen zur Angehörigenberatung (siehe Abschn. 15.1).

Passive Teilhabe ermöglichen

Der Idee von Wilcock (1999) folgend, gehört zur Betätigung nicht nur das Tun (Doing), sondern auch das Sein (Being), Zugehörigkeit (Belonging) und Entwicklung (Becoming). Demnach kann auch das „Dabeisein" bei der Betätigung anderer Menschen ein wertvolles Geschehen sein, welches die Lebensqualität steigert. Besonders Betroffene im Spätstadium, denen oftmals wenig Handlungsmöglichkeiten gegeben sind, sind meist dafür dankbar, das Gefühl der Zugehörigkeit erleben zu können. Z. B. Teilnehmen am Gottesdienst, beim Literaturkreis zuhören, Fußballspiele besuchen. Für weitere Informationen zu Teilhabe (Partizipation) siehe Abschn. 4.4.

► Das „Dabeisein" ohne Aktivität kann mit Blick auf die Parkinson-Erkrankung im fortgeschrittenen Stadium und im Umgang mit Apathie, Fatigue und Immobilität von Bedeutung sein und in der ergotherapeutischen Intervention neue Handlungsmöglichkeiten eröffnen .

Beispiel

Obwohl Frau V. keine körperlichen oder kognitiven Verbesserungen mehr erzielt, finden sich doch immer wieder kleine Ziele, die relevant sind. So ist ihr das Kartenschreiben an Weihnachten ein wichtiges Anliegen, weshalb sie es gerne mit der Ergotherapeutin gemeinsam macht. Außerdem hat die Ergotherapeutin schon den Transfer ins und aus dem Bett geübt. Sie haben die Wichtigkeit der täglichen Mobilisation besprochen und dafür einen Plan geschrieben (Motomed, Stehübungen, Dehnungsübungen). Außerdem wurde die Handhabung bei der Pflege und Unterstützung seiner Frau schon häufig mit dem Ehemann durchgesprochen und ausprobiert. Und immer wieder ist die Therapie ein Ort des Wohlfühlens und der Erholung, an dem Probleme ausgesprochen werden können, aber auch gelacht wird (Tee trinken, Entspannungsmassage, Gespräche). ◄

Literatur und weiterführende Literatur

Ahlskog JE (2017) Aerobic Exercise: Evidence for a Direct Brain Effect to Slow Parkinson Disease Progression, PhD, MD. Mayo Clinic Proceedings 93:3; 360–372

Alberts JL, Linder SM, Penko AL, Lowe MJ, Phillips M (2001) It is not about the bike, it is about the pedaling: forced exercise and Parkinson's disease. Exerc Sport Sci Rev 39(4):177–86. https://doi.org/10.1097/JES.0b013e31822cc71a. PMID: 21799425. https://doi.org/10.1016/j.mayocp.2017.12.015

Cusso ME, Donald KJ, Khoo TK (2016) The impact of physical activity on non-motor symptoms in Parkinson's disease: a systematic review. Front Med (Lausanne) 3:35

Deuschl G, Oertel W, Reichmann H (2016) Leitlinien für Diagnostik und Therapie in der Neurologie Idiopathisches Parkinson-Syndrom Entwicklungsstufe: S3 Kurzversion, DGN

Global Parkinson's Disease Survey (GPDS) Steering Committee (2002) Factors impacting on quality of life in Parkinson's disease: results from an international survey. Mov Disord 17:60–67. https://doi.org/10.1002/mds.10010

Gravell R, Duncan GW, Khoo TK, Burn DJ, Sayer AA, Barker RA, Lawson RA, Yarnall AJ (2018) Multimorbidity predicts quality of life but not motor severity in early Parkinson's disease. J Parkinsons Dis 8(4):511–515. https://doi.org/10.3233/JPD-181428. PMID: 30248064

Hoehn MM, Yahr MD (1967) Parkinsonism: onset, progression, and mortality. Neurology 50(2):318. and 16 pages following. PMID: 9484345. https://doi.org/10.1212/wnl.50.2.318

Laupheimer M, Härtel S, Schmidt S, Bös K Exercise training –/INS; effects of MOTOmed® exercise on typical motor dysfunction in Parkinson's disease. J Neurol Sci 333:e123

Law M (2002) Participation in the occupations of everyday life. Am J Occup Ther 56(6):640–649. https://doi.org/10.5014/ajot.56.6.640

Law M, Baptiste S, Mills J (1995) Client-centred practice: what does it mean and does it make a difference? Can J Occup Ther 62(5):250–257. https://doi.org/10.1177/000841749506200504. PMID: 10152881

Law M, Steinwender S, Leclair L (1998) Occupation, health and well-being. Can J Occu Ther 65(2):81–91. https://doi.org/10.1177/000841749806500204

Maslow AH (1943) A theory of human motivation. Psychol Rev 50(4):370–396. https://doi.org/10.1037/h0054346

Radder DLM, Sturkenboom IH, van Nimwegen M, Keus SH, Bloem BR, de Vries NM (2017) Physical therapy and occupational therapy in Parkinson's disease. Int J Neurosci 127(10):930–943. https://doi.org/10.1080/00207454.2016.1275617

Röse K (2017) Betätigung von Personen mit Demenz im Kontext Pflegeheim. Hogrefe, Göttingen

Sacheli MA, Murray DK, Vafai N, Cherkasova MV, Dinelle K, Shahinfard E, Neilson N, McKenzie J, Schulzer M, Appel-Cresswell S, McKeown MJ, Sossi V, Jon Stoessl A (2018) Habitual exercisers versus sedentary subjects with Parkinson's disease: multimodal PET and fMRI study. Mov Disord 33(12):1945–1950. https://doi.org/10.1002/mds.27498. PMID: 30376184

Sturkenboom I, Thijssen M, Gons-van Elsacker J, Jansen I, Maasdam A, Schulten M, Vijver-Visser D, Steultjens E, Bloem B, Munneke M (2008) Guidelines for occupational therapy in Parkinson's disease rehabilitation. ParkinsonNet/NPF, Nijmegen/Miami

Uhrbrand A, Stenager E, Pedersen MS, Dalgas U (2015) Parkinson's disease and intensive exercise therapy – a systematic review and meta-analysis of randomized controlled trials. J Neurol Sci 353(1–2):9–19. https://doi.org/10.1016/j.jns.2015.04.004.Epup. PMID: 25936252

Varanese S, Birnbaum Z, Rossi R, Di Rocco A (2011) Treatment of advanced Parkinson's disease. Parkinsons Dis 2010:480260. https://doi.org/10.4061/2010/480260. PMID: 21331376; PMCID: PMC3038575

Wilcock AA (1999) Reflections on doing, being and becoming*. Australian Occupational Therapy Journal 46:1–11. https://doi.org/10.1046/j.1440-1630.1999.00174.x

10 Positive Einflussfaktoren auf Therapie

Eine ergotherapeutische Intervention richtet sich nach dem Ziel, das für die Klientin wichtig ist. Zusätzlich existieren einige Einflussfaktoren, die jede therapeutische Intervention bei Morbus Parkinson positiv beeinflussen. Das sind: das Selbstmanagement der Klientin, das Vertrauen in die therapeutische Kompetenz, allgemeines Kraft-/ und Ausdauertraining, „On-Phase" während der Therapie, regelmäßige Erholungsphasen. In „Perfect Fit" siehe Abb. 4.4 sind die positiven Einflussfaktoren in den kleinen Ovalen um das große Oval der Interventionen abgebildet. Diese Faktoren sollten im Idealfall gegeben sein, um eine optimale Therapie zu ermöglichen. Natürlich ist das selten die Realität. Ein paar der Einflussfaktoren sind oftmals nicht gegeben oder sind sogar als negative Faktoren präsent. Zum Beispiel, dass die Klientin nicht nur keine regelmäßigen Erholungsphasen einrichtet, sondern, dass sie sogar konstant über ihre körperlichen Grenzen geht und dadurch völlige Erschöpfung erreicht.

► Bestenfalls sollten die positiven Einflussfaktoren vorhanden sein, um die therapeutische Wirksamkeit zu unterstützen. Deswegen ist es sinnvoll fehlende Einflussfaktoren im Rahmen der ergotherapeutischen Intervention zu fördern.

Die positiven Einflussfaktoren wirken wie ein Beförderer für die ergotherapeutische Intervention für Menschen mit Parkinson. Wenn vorhanden, können sie die individualisierte Therapie verstärken und zur vollen Entfaltung bringen. Die positiven Einflussfaktoren wirken unterstützend auf die therapeutische Intervention. Zum Beispiel hat die Klientin Vertrauen in die therapeutische Kompetenz – wird sie für die Therapie empfänglich sein. Im gesamten Verlauf der Therapie sollte der Therapeut die Einflussfaktoren im Blick haben. Wenn ihm auffällt, dass ein Punkt fehlt oder ungenügend ausgeprägt ist, kann er es in die Therapie mitaufnehmen, obwohl es nicht ausdrücklich als Ziel genannt wurde.

10.1 Selbstmanagement

Beispiel

Frau M. verlässt die Praxis etwas verwirrt. Die Therapeutin hat sie gefragt, was **sie** verbessern möchte. „Das muss doch die Therapeutin wissen, nicht ich," erzählt sie ihrem Mann. „Sie weiß doch was Parkinson ist und was man da macht." „Vielleicht möchte sie ja deine Sicht wissen, schließlich ist es ja dein Leben" überlegt der Ehemann. ◄

Da Parkinson eine chronische Erkrankung ist, mit der der Patient sein Leben lang leben muss, ist eine innere Akzeptanz und ein aktiver Umgang mit der Erkrankung sowohl für das Coping als auch für eine effektive Therapie notwendig.

A. Orellana, *Betätigungsorientierte Ergotherapie bei Morbus Parkinson*,
https://doi.org/10.1007/978-3-662-62583-5_10

Klientinnen mit einem guten Selbstmanagement wirken in ihrem Auftreten gefestigt und zielgerichtet. Sie haben gelernt, ein akzeptierendes Verhältnis zu ihrer Krankheit aufzubauen und Veränderungen als Herausforderung zu sehen, die sie engagiert angehen.

Kurz nach Diagnosestellung überwältigt der Schock viele Klientinnen. Je nach Persönlichkeit der Klientinnen können sie in Untätigkeit verfallen. Sätze wie: „Es bringt doch eh alles nichts!" oder „Die Therapeuten/Ärztinnen wissen am besten, was zu tun ist," werden geäußert. Ergotherapeuten können Klientinnen in dem Prozess zum Erlernen eines guten Selbstmanagements unterstützen.

▶ Ein gutes Selbstmanagement der Klientin führt zu selbständiger Zielsetzung, Eigeninitiative bei der Umsetzung der Ziele und Problemlösungsverhalten. Dadurch fühlen sich Klienten beim Umgang mit ihrer Erkrankung fähig, was sich positiv auf die Lebensqualität auswirkt.

Kessler und Liddy untersuchten (2017) ergotherapeutische Programme zur Förderung des Selbstmanagements bei Menschen mit Parkinson. Sie stellten fest, dass Selbstmanagement-Programme, die in die Rehabilitation eingebettet sind, vielversprechend sind. Dabei sollten Zielsetzung, Problemlösung, Inklusion von Pflegenden und unterstützende Freunde in das Programm eingeschlossen werden.

Wann indiziert?
„Selbstmanagement" wird selten von Klientinnen als konkretes Ziel formuliert. Der Therapeut kann das Thema aufgreifen, wenn er erkennt, dass die Klientin sich weitgehend passiv verhält und Problemlösungsstrategien nicht oder kaum anwendet.

Es gibt bei Menschen mit Morbus Parkinson zwei Hauptgründe für die eingeschränkte Umsetzung von Problemlösungsstrategien. Zum einen, wenn die exekutiven Funktionen der Klientin herabgesetzt sind, also die kognitive Flexibilität, die Inhibition und das Arbeitsgedächtnis nicht problemlos funktionieren. Zum anderen, wenn die Diagnose kürzlich gestellt wurde oder die Klientin (auch nach längerer Erkrankung) Auffälligkeiten im Coping zeigt. Hinweise dafür können sein:

- Niedergeschlagenheit/depressive Verstimmung,
- passive Einstellung,
- keine eigenen Ziele oder Wünsche für Therapie,
- keine Durchführung von Eigenübungen.

Setting Ein Selbstmanagement-Training ist besonders gut geeignet als **Gruppentherapie**, da die Klientinnen sich gegenseitig unterstützen und Informationen austauschen. Besonders der Erfahrungsaustausch wird von Teilnehmerinnen meist als große Bereicherung gewertet. Natürlich kann das Thema bei Bedarf auch in die **Einzeltherapie** eingewoben werden. So bietet sich zum Einstieg der Therapieeinheit meist eine passende Gelegenheit, um über Erlebtes und den Umgang mit der Erkrankung zu sprechen und gegebenenfalls hilfreiche Tipps zu geben. Die Vermittlung von Strategien im Umgang mit der Krankheit ist in solch „kleinen Häppchen" oft für die Klientin leichter annehmbar und auch die Umsetzung im Alltag ist leichter realisierbar.

Werden Angehörige als erweiterte Klientinnen in die Therapie einbezogen, ist das Thema Selbstmanagement besonders wichtig. Die Reaktionen auf eine chronische Erkrankung können weit auseinander gehen. Verdrängung, Vermeidung von Informationen, Rückzug oder auch Aktionismus, aktives Suchen von Informationen und sozialem Austausch, sind Beispiele für mögliche Arten der Verarbeitung. Im Rahmen der Ergotherapie ist es möglich, Arten der Verarbeitung gemeinsam zu reflektieren.

Umsetzung
Der Ergotherapeut kann zur Strukturierung des Selbstmanagements der Klientin den Bogen „Selbstreflexion" verwenden (Siehe Anhang und Abb. 10.2). Darin füllt die Klientin, allein oder mit Angehörigen oder Therapeut zusammen, die

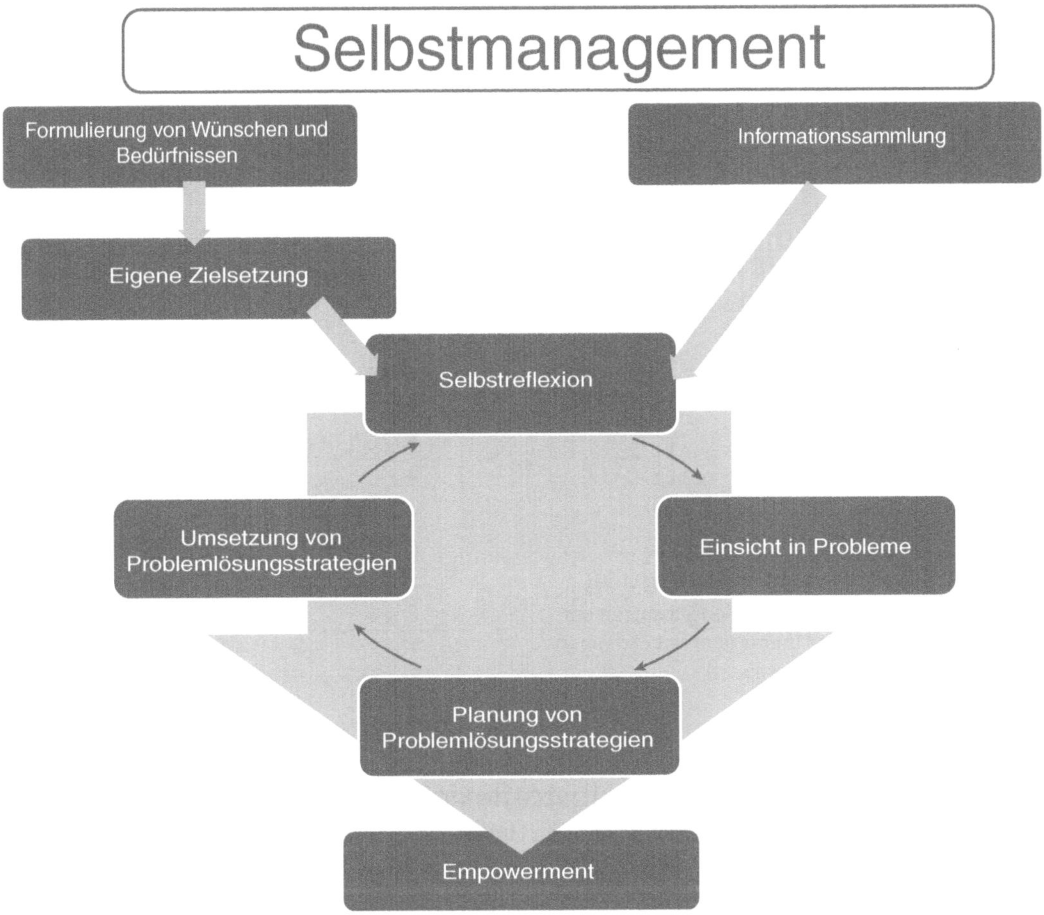

Abb. 10.1 Prozess des Selbstmanagement

vorgegebenen Schritte aus. Es macht Sinn, den Bogen nicht auf ein Mal auszufüllen, sondern von Therapieeinheit zu Therapieeinheit, um den Veränderungsprozess damit zu begleiten. Die genaue Art und Weise des Einsatzes des Bogens ist der therapeutischen Einschätzung des behandelnden Ergotherapeuten überlassen.

In der Abb. 10.1 ist der Prozess des Selbstmanagements dargestellt: Zuerst benennt die Klientin eine konkrete, problematische Situation. Dann formuliert die Klientin ihre Wünsche und Bedürfnisse und drückt sie als Ziele aus. Nach einer Informationssammlung, wie diese Ziele erreicht werden können, reflektiert sie über ihre momentane Umgangsweise mit dem vorhandenen Problem und welche Gefühle, Gedanken und Reaktionen sie in der Situation hat. Durch die Reflexion und das schriftliche Festhalten, erlangt sie eine Einsicht in problemhafte Umgangsweisen. Durch die Einsicht kann sie, evtl. mithilfe des Therapeuten, eine Problemlösungsstrategie entwickeln. Bei der nächsten Gelegenheit setzt sie die Problemlösungsstrategie um. Daraufhin reflektiert sie, ob sie mit den veränderten Gefühlen, Gedanken und/oder Reaktionen ihr Ziel erreicht. Wenn nein, geht sie in die Selbstreflexion und beginnt den Kreislauf nochmals. Wenn ja, führt der Prozess zu Empowerment und positivem Selbstmanagement.

Menschen mit einem funktionierenden Selbstmanagement durchlaufen diesen Prozess meist auf einer unbewussten Ebene. In der Regel hat jedoch jeder einzelne Situationen, in denen das Selbstmanagement defekt ist und der Prozess

Selbstreflexion

Situation: Schreibtisch ist mit Papieren überladen und unübersichtlich

Tragen Sie eine konkrete Situation ein, die Sie belastet.

Wünsche und Bedürfnisse

Machen Sie ein Brainstorming zu Ihren eigenen persönlichen Wünschen und Bedürfnissen, zur obigen Situation.

Mehr Platz auf dem Schreibtisch
Ordnung
Mehr Platz und Ordnung im Kopf
Weniger Papierkram und Verantwortung

Eigene Ziele

Formulieren Sie Ziele, um Ihre Wünsche zu erfüllen

- Nur einen Papierstoß auf Schreibtisch
- Wieder Zeit zum Buch lesen haben
-
-
-

Informationssammlung

Tragen Sie hier ein, welche Quellen Sie nutzen um Informationen über das Thema (s.o) zu bekommen. (Websites, Broschüren, Therapeut)

Quellen	Gelesen
Mit Therapeut sprechen	
Online Erkundigen wegen Bürohilfe	

Selbstreflexion

Machen Sie sich Gedanken zur obigen Situation. Wann tritt die Situation ein? Wie fühlen Sie sich dabei? Was denken Sie dabei? Wie reagieren Sie darauf?

Gefühle	Gedanken	Reaktion
1. Konstanter Druck durch unerledigte Büroarbeit Gefühl der Wertlosigkeit und Ineffizienz 2. Schwierig Aufgabe an Sohn abzugeben, möchte ihn nicht belasten	1. Warum kriegst du das nicht auf die Reihe? 2. Der Arme, hat schon so viel zu tun.	1. Vermeidung Ablenkung durch Fernsehen 2. Spreche Sohn nicht an

Problemlösungsstrategien/Alternative Umgangsweise

Welche Strategien können Sie anwenden, um die Situation zu verbessern.

1. Statt Vermeidung, Sohn ansprechen, ob er mir ein Mal die Woche hilft die Papiere zu sortieren. (Abgeben)
2. Sohn ansprechen und sofort die Option einer Bürokraft als Alternative ansprechen. Er soll ehrlich sagen, ob er Zeit hat und wählen

Nach der Umsetzung der Problemlösungsstrategien, gehen Sie nochmals zur „Selbstreflexion" zurück und schreiben mit anderer Farbe ein, welche Gefühle, Gedanken und Reaktionen Sie jetzt haben und passen Sie die Problemlösungsstrategien gegebenenfalls an.

Abb. 10.2 Ausgefülltes Beispiel für die Anwendung des Selbstreflexionsbogens. Mit momentaner Umgangsweise (1.) und Umgangsweise nach erster Reflexion (2.)

stockt. In diesem Fall kann eine fachliche Begleitung des Therapeuten hilfreich sein.

Problematische Situation Wählen Um den Prozess des Selbstmanagement zielgerichtet führen zu können, ist die Wahl einer konkreten problematischen Situation notwendig. Dies kann eine Konfliktsituation, eine Situation der Überforderung, ein Gefühl des „Nicht-Weiterkommens" oder der Ziellosigkeit und viele andere sein.

Formulierung von Wünschen und Bedürfnissen In einer stark hierarchischen Einstellung im Gesundheitsbereich, in dem Ärzte als allwissend und Patientinnen als Leidende gesehen werden, ist der Gedanke, dass „Patientinnen" zu „Klientinnen" werden und ihre eigenen Wünsche und Ziele aussprechen, häufig nicht leicht zu akzeptieren. Auch den Klientinnen selbst fällt es oft schwer, aus der Rolle des passiven Opfers herauszuwachsen. Sätze wie „Sie wissen es doch am besten!", oder „Es soll halt besser werden," werden gerne von Klientinnen erwidert, wenn sich der Therapeut nach ihren Bedürfnissen erkundigt. Viele Klientinnen sind positiv überrascht, dass sie ironischerweise noch nie als Spezialistinnen für ihre eigenen Bedürfnisse gesehen wurden und direkt danach gefragt wurden.

Sobald die Klientin erkennt, dass es in der Ergotherapie genau darum geht und alle Ergotherapeuten es als selbstverständliche Grundlage für eine gelingende Intervention sehen, kann eine klientenzentrierte Kommunikation auf Augenhöhe stattfinden. In der Arbeitspraxis hat sich gezeigt, dass die meisten Klientinnen sehr dadurch gestärkt werden, wenn sie als Expertinnen für ihr eigenes Leben dazu aufgefordert werden, Wünsche auszuformulieren, sodass sie beginnen, auch anderen Therapeuten, Ärzten und Angehörigen gegenüber für ihre eigenen Bedürfnisse einzustehen. Durch das konkrete Auseinandersetzen mit dem Thema innerhalb der Ergotherapie finden sie die richtigen Worte auch außerhalb.

Eigene Zielsetzung Sobald die Klientin ihre eigenen Problempunkte herausgefunden hat, gelingt der folgende Schritt meist ohne weiteres Zutun – ein Ziel wird formuliert. Gelingt es also der Klientin mithilfe des Ergotherapeuten, die innere Haltung zu verändern und ein aktives Selbstmanagement zu entwickeln, ist es ihr von da an möglich, ohne Hilfe bedeutungsvolle Betätigungen und daraus folgende Ziele zu formulieren. Es zählt wohl zu den erfüllendsten Momenten als Ergotherapeut, wenn die Klientin aus Eigeninitiative ein Ziel in die Therapie mitbringt, welches der Therapeut nicht in Erwägung gezogen hätte.

Zusätzlich zum Gespräch mit der Klientin dient das COPM als validiertes Assessment dazu, Klientinnen in einem halb strukturierten Interview zu unterstützen, die eigenen Bedürfnisse und Ziele zu erkennen und auszuformulieren (siehe Abschn. 5.4). Außerdem sollten die Ziele nach den SMART-Regeln formuliert werden (siehe Tab. 10.1 und Abschn. 8.1)

Beispiel

Folgendes Ziel wurde von Frau T. als wichtigstes ausgesucht (A): In den kommenden drei Wochen (T) selbständig mit einem Wochenkalender (R) & (S) umgehen, um die regelmäßigen Termine ohne Hilfe (M) wahrnehmen zu können. ◀

Informationssammlung In einer (2002) von der „Global Parkinson's Disease Survey (GPDS) Steering Committee" durchgeführten Studie über Lebensqualität wurden Faktoren ermittelt, die

Tab. 10.1 Ziele sollten nach den SMART-Regeln formuliert werden

S	-	Spezifisch	Eine spezifische Betätigung oder Situation
M	-	Messbar	Mit messbaren Angaben, zur Überprüfung. Zum Beispiel Menge, Zeit, Häufigkeit, Distanz
A	-	Akzeptiert	Von der Klientin akzeptiert, also ein ihr wichtiges Ziel
R	-	Realistisch	Ein nach Einschätzung des Therapeuten realistisches Ziel, welches in der festgelegten Zeit (siehe terminiert) erreichbar ist
T	-	Terminiert	Zur Überprüfbarkeit, konkreter Zeitpunkt, bis wann Ziel erreicht werden soll

eine Auswirkung auf die subjektiv empfundene Lebensqualität bei Parkinson haben. Nach dem positiven Test auf Depressionen war an zweiter Stelle der Umfang der Information über die Erkrankung bei Diagnosestellung der wichtigste Indikator für den Grad der empfundenen Lebensqualität.

Um die Krankheit selbstbestimmt angehen zu können, ist es notwendig, Informationen über neuronale Zusammenhänge, Symptome, Verlauf, Medikamente und Perspektiven der Erkrankung zu haben. Die Beschaffung von Informationen ist auf vielfältige Weise möglich. Dabei kann der Ergotherapeut unterstützen. Folgende Quellen können hilfreich sein (s. Abb. 10.3):

- Selbsthilfegruppen
- Websites (siehe Tab. 10.2)
- Broschüren
- Zeitschriften
- Bücher
- Ratgeber
- Artikel
- Nachfragen bei Therapeuten und Arzt

Eine Auseinandersetzung mit o. g. Medien ist therapieunterstützend. Sie können sowohl innerhalb der Therapie, gemeinsam mit dem Therapeuten, als auch in Eigenarbeit zu Hause oder auf dem Patientenzimmer durchgesehen und reflektiert werden. In einer randomisierten, kontrollierten Studie von Grosset und Grosset (2005) konnte eindeutig ein signifikanter Einfluss medizinischer Aufklärung auf Patientenverhalten, hier in Form der Medikamenteneinnahmepünktlichkeit, nachgewiesen werden.

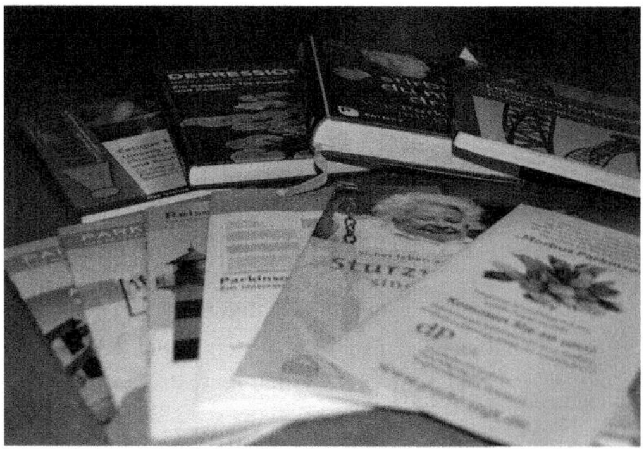

Abb. 10.3 Eine Vielzahl an unterschiedlichen Druckmedien sind zum Thema Parkinson oder spezifische Symptome erhältlich

Bei der Aufklärung über die Krankheit sollte eine psychische oder kognitive Überforderung der Klientin vermieden werden. Auch das Recht auf Nichtwissen muss beachtet werden. Erkennt der Therapeut Anzeichen dafür, dass die Klientin neues Wissen über die Parkinson-Erkrankung nicht wünscht – wie ablenkendes Verhalten oder stark emotionale Reaktionen – ist ein vorsichtiger Umgang mit dem Thema ratsam. Vielleicht ist ein späterer Zeitpunkt passender oder eine andere Art der Aufklärung ist für diese Person einfacher zu verarbeiten. Eine Unterteilung in kleinere Portionen macht den Inhalt der Informationen für die Klientin besser fassbar. Optimalerweise macht der Therapeut in diesem Fall das Angebot, Informationen mit der Klientin zu recherchieren und wartet dann darauf, dass sie auf ihn zukommt.

Die meisten Klientinnen durchlaufen im Krankheitsverlauf Phasen unterschiedlicher Intensität und Arten des Auseinandersetzens mit ihrer Krankheit. Nach einer besonders intensiven Zeit des Umgangs mit der Erkrankung, z. B. wäh-

Tab. 10.2 Übersicht über Websites für Betroffene

https://www.parkins-on-line.de/	PARKINSonLINE ev., Parkinson-Selbsthilfegruppe im Internet
https://www.parkinson-vereinigung.de/	Deutsche Parkinson Vereinigung eV.
https://www.nakos.de/	Nationale Kontakt- und Informationsstelle zur Anregung und Unterstützung von Selbsthilfegruppen
https://www.parkinson-gesellschaft.de/	Deutsche Gesellschaft für Parkinson und Bewegungsstörungen
https://www.jung-und-parkinson.de/	Jung & Parkinson die Selbsthilfe eV.
https://www.jupa-dpv.de/startseite/	JuPa – zu jung für Parkinson? Die Informationsseite für jung erkrankte Menschen
www.teamdopamin.de	Eine große Sammlung parkinsonrelevanter Themen von Betroffenen und Angehörigen verfasst.

rend einer Rehabilitation, kann eine Zeit des „einfach vor sich hin lebens“ folgen. An die Stelle der Trauer nach der Diagnosestellung tritt nicht selten ein flapsiger oder sogar ironischer Ton. All diese Formen sind natürlich und sollten vom Therapeuten respektiert werden. Die Aufgabe des Therapeuten ist es also, der Klientin **Informationsquellen aufzuzeigen**, relevante **Informationen zu portionieren**, sie verständlich zu **erklären** und gegebenenfalls **ruhen zu lassen**, wenn eine Überforderung droht.

Selbstreflexion Eine Reflexion der eigenen Einstellungen und Handlungen ist notwendig, um ein gesundes Selbstmanagement entwickeln zu können. Nur, wenn sich die Klientin bewusst darüber ist, wie sie mit der Krankheit, den Symptomen und den damit zusammenhängenden Situationen umgeht, können Schlüsse daraus gezogen werden, ob das Verhalten gewinnbringend ist, oder ob eine Verhaltensänderung hilfreich wäre. Im Gespräch mit dem Therapeuten oder anderen Klientinnen kann sich die Klientin achtsam fragen, welche

- Gefühle,
- Gedanken,
- Reaktionen

sie in bestimmten Situationen hatte und diese schriftlich festhalten. Dazu kann der Selbstreflexionsbogen (siehe Anhang) genutzt werden. Alternativ ist die Übersicht in Tab. 10.3 hilfreich, um die Unterschiede von Gefühlen, Gedanken und Reaktionen und die Zusammenhänge miteinander herauszuarbeiten. Anschließend formuliert die Klientin, mit welchen alternativen Gedanken und Reaktionen sie bei einem Wiederauftreten der Situation zur Problemlösung beitragen könnte.

Problemlösungsstrategien
Oftmals stößt die kritische Auseinandersetzung mit Gefühlen, Gedanken und Reaktionen in schwierigen Situationen einen Veränderungsprozess an, der keiner weiteren Unterstützung durch den Therapeuten bedarf. Ist dies nicht der Fall, kann der Therapeut durch Nachfragen in den darauffolgenden Therapieeinheiten oder durch die kooperative Erarbeitung von Problemlösungsstrategien die Klientin langsam zu mehr Selbstmanagement hinführen.

Dieser Prozess enthält einen Kreislauf, der von der Selbstreflexion zur Einsicht in Probleme führt; durch diese Einsicht wird gemeinsam ein Plan zur Problemlösung entwickelt, den die Klientin anschließend umsetzt. Die Umsetzung

Tab 10.3 Kurzer Selbstreflexionsbogen

Machen Sie sich Gedanken zur obigen Situation. Wann tritt die Situation ein? Wie fühlen Sie sich dabei? Was denken Sie dabei? Wie reagieren Sie darauf?

Wann: ______________________________

Gefühle	Gedanken	Reaktion	alternative Gedanken und Reaktionen

wird wiederum reflektiert, womit der Kreislauf geschlossen ist und die Klientin zu Empowerment gelangt.

Beispiel

Nach mehreren Monaten bei der Ergotherapie, kommt Frau M. in die Praxis: „Frau W. wir müssen ein neues Ziel vorne anstellen! Unser Sohn heiratet bald und ich möchte unbedingt auf seiner Hochzeit tanzen. Wegen meiner Fallangst bin ich aber sehr nervös. Können Sie mir damit helfen?“ ◀

10.2 Vertrauen in therapeutische Kompetenz

Beispiel

Herr H. ist nervös. Fast hätte er wieder die Therapie vergessen. Letzte Woche kam er aus Nervosität eine Stunde zu früh. Hat er auch an alles gedacht? Hausschlüssel, die Ergotherapie-Mappe, das Handy. Er kommt pünktlich, muss aber noch auf Toilette. Herr H. entschuldigt sich ausgiebig. ◀

Die Grundlage für die therapeutische Intervention ist das Vertrauen der Klientin in die therapeutische Kompetenz. Zahlreiche Autoren benennen die Wichtigkeit der therapeutischen Beziehung für ein erfolgreiches Outcome der Therapie. Auch die Klientinnen sehen es als sehr wichtig an, mit dem Therapeuten eine gute Beziehung zu haben.

▶ Eine achtsame Reflexion des Therapeuten zu seiner Kommunikationsweise, zum eigenen Auftreten und dem äußeren Erscheinungsbild und bei Bedarf einer Anpassung dieser, können das Vertrauen der Klientin in den Therapeuten fördern.

Das Gefühl des Vertrauens entsteht einerseits durch unbestimmbare zwischenmenschliche Prozesse, andererseits können eindeutige Faktoren genannt werden, die förderlich sind:

- Einfühlsame Kommunikation
  Die Art und Weise, wie der Therapeut mit der Klientin spricht, welche Mimik und Gestik er verwendet und wie gut er seinem Gegenüber zuhört, ist ausschlaggebend dafür, ob der Therapeut als einfühlsam und kompetent wahrgenommen wird.
- Wahrnehmen der Klientin und ihrer Wünsche und Werte
  Bei einer solch schweren Erkrankung wie dem Morbus Parkinson mit seinen vielgestaltigen Symptomen, ist es als Therapeut manchmal nicht leicht, über das äußerliche Erscheinungsbild hinwegzusehen und den Menschen zu erkennen. Durch bewusstes Zuhören und Nachfragen erfährt der Therapeut, was der Klientin wichtig ist und Letztere fühlt sich wahrgenommen.
- Fachliche Kompetenz
  Durch Berufserfahrung und Auseinandersetzung mit der Krankheit (z. B. Fachliteratur, fachlicher Austausch mit Kolleginnen, Fortbildung …) wächst die fachliche Kompetenz des Therapeuten.
  Eine wichtige Voraussetzung für die Therapie ist, sich als Therapeut das Fachwissen anzueignen, um der Klientin das Wissen anschließend vereinfacht zu vermitteln. Auf diese Weise entsteht eine Transparenz, die für das Vertrauensverhältnis förderlich ist.
  Auch Berufsanfängerinnen können aufgrund ihrer soliden Ausbildung oder ihres Studiums, plus angelesenem Fachwissen, welches speziell auf die Situation der Klientin passt, selbstsicher auftreten und der Klientin ihre Fachkompetenz zeigen.
- Äußerliches Erscheinungsbild
  Der erste Eindruck der Klientin vom Therapeuten ist meist oberflächlich. Das äußere Erscheinungsbild des Therapeuten wird wahrgenommen und beeinflusst unbewusst das Vertrauen in die therapeutische Kompetenz. Folgende Aspekte sollten vom Therapeuten selbstkritisch beachtet werden:
  - Gepflegtes Äußeres,
  - Art der Arbeitskleidung (sportlich, elegant, einheitliche Arbeitskleidung),

  - Namensschild,
  - Haltung, Gestik, Mimik (aufrecht, freundlich).

  Auch das Erscheinungsbild der Praxis oder Ergotherapie-Abteilung hat einen Einfluss auf das Vertrauen in die therapeutische Kompetenz.

  Hier können folgende Punkte beachtet werden:
  - Sauberkeit,
  - Ordnung,
  - neue, moderne Therapiemittel,
  - ansprechende Dekoration/Bebilderung.
- Umgang mit antriebsarmen amimischen Klientinnen

  Durch die Bradykinese wird die Bewegungsamplitude und -geschwindigkeit immer geringer. Da auch die Mimik, Gestik und Sprachlautstärke reduziert sind, ist die Übertragung auf die gesamte Therapiesituation inklusive des Therapeuten häufig beobachtbar. Da Menschen ihr Gegenüber unbewusst spiegeln, wirkt die verminderte Motorik der Patientin „ansteckend" auf das Gegenüber.

  Dem sollte der Therapeut aktiv entgegenwirken:
  - Bewusst lebendiges Auftreten des Therapeuten,
  - bewusst ausdrucksstarke Mimik verwenden,
  - bewusste Steuerung der Sprachmelodie und Lautstärke,
  - „lockere" Atmosphäre kreieren durch „Plaudern" und „Witzeln",
  - angenehmes Ambiente durch frische Blumen, hellen Raum, freundliche Mitarbeiter.
- Es lohnt sich, als Therapeut seine eigene Wirkung zu reflektieren und gegebenenfalls anzupassen, ohne verkrampft zu versuchen fröhlich zu sein. Vielmehr wird allein mit der bewussten Entscheidung, lebendig und ausdrucksstark aufzutreten, die innerliche Einstellung auch nach außen sichtbar und wirkt dabei nicht zwanghaft, sondern natürlich.
- Diskreter Umgang mit persönlichen Daten der Klientin,
- Pünktlichkeit,
- Humor und angenehme Atmosphäre.

In Anbetracht der gravierenden Einschränkungen durch die Erkrankung und die undurchsichtige Prognose, ist es verständlich, dass sowohl den Klientinnen und Angehörigen als auch den Therapeuten hin und wieder eine betrübte Stimmung überkommt. Ein warmer Tee im richtigen Moment und Humor auch in schwierigen Augenblicken können die Lage erträglicher machen und die Bindung zwischen Klientin und Therapeut festigen.

Beispiel

„Herr H., setzen Sie sich erst einmal! Wir haben keinen Stress." Beruhigt ihn die Therapeutin. Sie macht ihm einen Tee, fragt ihn nach seiner Woche und hört in Ruhe zu." Nach 10 Minuten atmet Herr H. wieder ruhig und lächelt. Die Therapeutin macht einen Vorschlag: „Ich habe mir für heute etwas überlegt, das Sie Ihrem Ziel, wieder ordentlicher zu Essen, ein Stück näherbringt. Sind Sie bereit?" ◀

10.3 Allgemeines Kraft- und Ausdauertraining

Beispiel

„Früher habe ich mich doch so gerne bewegt," äußert Frau I. gegenüber ihrer Schwester. „Seit ich nicht mehr schwimmen kann, geht mein Sport gegen Null." Wovon sie ihrer Schwester nicht erzählt, ist die Mattigkeit, die sie innen spürt, die große Leere und das Gefühl von „wozu auch, es hilft doch eh nichts." ◀

In einem systematischen Review von Brienesse und Emerson (2013) wurde festgestellt, dass Krafttraining sich positiv auf die Kraft, Mobilität und andere funktionelle Tätigkeiten aus wirkt.

Ausdauertraining hat einen umfassenden positiven Einfluss. Cusso et al. (2016) wiesen verbesserte nicht-motorischen Symptome (z. B. Depression, Apathie, Verdauung) und Kognition nach. Ahlskog (2017) konnte nachweisen, dass Ausdauertraining sich positiv auf die motorischen Symptome (z. B. Bradykinese, Koordination, Posturale Stabilität) auswirkt und Alberts et al. (2001) gehen sogar davon aus, dass die Krankheitsprogression verlangsamt wird. Es ist zum Abschluss dieser Veröffentlichung noch nicht abschließend geklärt, ob Fitnesstraining den progredienten Verlauf der Krankheit definitiv verlangsamen kann, es wird aber zunehmend davon ausgegangen.

Kraft- und Ausdauertraining gehören nicht zum primären Arbeitsfeld von Ergotherapeuten, trotzdem ist das Wissen über den positiven Effekt auf den Verlauf der Erkrankung von großer Bedeutung.

Petzinger et al. beschreiben in ihrem Artikel (2013) dass auch in einem von Parkinson betroffenen Gehirn, mit Dopaminmangel und eingeschränkten Abläufen, Veränderungen auf neuronaler Ebene möglich sind. Studien belegen, dass eine kortikostriatale Plastizität mit vermehrter Dopaminausschüttung durch körperliches Training angeregt wird.

Petzinger et al. beschreiben, dass die Kombination aus Fitnesstraining und dem Üben einer Betätigung zu Veränderungen im Gehirn führt. Einerseits wird die Synapsenstärke erhöht, durch vermehrte Ausschüttung von Neurotransmittern, einer größeren Rezeptorendichte und Dendritenbildung. Andererseits verbessert sich die gesamte Gehirngesundheit, durch verbesserte trophische Faktoren (Wachstumsfaktoren), vermehrte Durchblutung, gestärktes Immunsystem, vermehrte Neurogenese (Neubildung von Nervenzellen) und verbesserten Stoffwechsel.

Durch die erhöhte Synapsenstärke und verbesserte Gehirngesundheit ist die Verschaltung zwischen den Gehirnabschnitten verstärkt. Daraus resultiert eine verbesserte Performanz in der Motorik, Kognition und Stimmung/Motivation (s. Abb. 10.4).

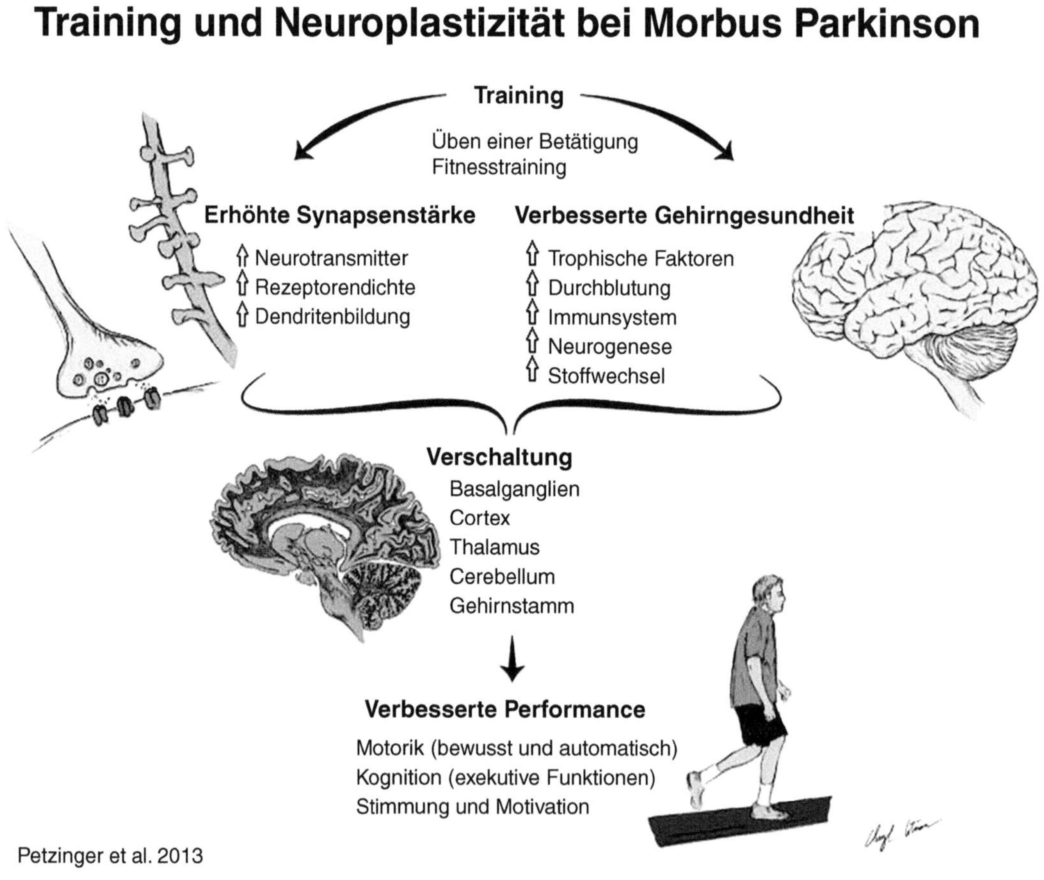

Abb. 10.4 Eigene Darstellung. (In Anlehnung an Petzinger et al. 2013)

Ergotherapeutische Möglichkeiten für Kraft- und Ausdauertraining **Aufklärung der Klientin** Durch die Informierung der Klientin über das Potential des Gehirns, sich trotz der Erkrankung positiv zu verändern, befähigt der Therapeut sie zum Selbstmanagement. Zur Aufklärung dienen Informationsflyer, YouTube, Videos, Übungsbücher ...

▶ Das Fitnesstraining aller Art sich positiv auf zahlreiche Parkinson-Symptome auswirkt, ist unumstritten und sollte deshalb in jeder multimodalen Therapie seinen Platz haben.

Übung innerhalb der Therapie Abwechselnd mit der Übung der Betätigung, der Besprechung von Tagesstrukturierung oder Entspannungsübungen können auch innerhalb der ergotherapeutischen Intervention ein Fitnesstraining oder Kraftübungen durchgeführt werden. In welchem Umfang dies stattfindet, muss der Therapeut abwägen. Zwischen „kurz durchsprechen und zeigen" bis zu „momentan ist es meine Hauptintervention" ist alles möglich, solange es ergotherapeutisch begründbar ist.

Beispiel: Frau T. ist schon seit acht Monaten in ergotherapeutischer Behandlung. Es wurden in der Ergotherapie schon einige Ziele erreicht:

- Selbständig baden (Badewannenbrett verordnet und Nutzung geübt)
- Umgang mit Fatigue (Tagesstrukturierung, Pausen einplanen, delegieren)
- Leserlichen Einkaufszettel schreiben (liniertes Papier, Cueing)

Durch das komplexe Symptombild von Frau T. treten regelmäßig Situationen im Alltag auf, die im Rahmen des Selbstmanagements von Frau T. und ihrem Ehemann als Probleme definiert werden und als Ziel in die Ergotherapie gebracht werden. Dazu gehören z. B. Ziele zu folgenden Themen: Sturzprävention, Kommunikation am Telefon, äußerliches Erscheinungsbild, Anleitung der Angehörigen bei Sicherung der Betroffenen.

Der Therapeut hat sich dazu entschieden, ein Fitnessprogramm in die therapeutische Intervention einfließen zu lassen. Dies ermöglicht drei Dinge: Erstens wirkt sich das Ausdauertraining, wie oben beschrieben, positiv auf die Gehirngesundheit und damit auch auf Gleichgewicht, kognitive Flexibilität, Wachheit ... aus. Zweitens bilden die Fitnessübungen eine Struktur für die Therapie. Der Therapeut kommt regelmäßig zum Hausbesuch in die Familie, geht eine Runde mit der Klientin walken und ist präsent, wenn die Klientin Probleme oder Fragen zu weiteren Themen hat. Der Therapeut erkennt oft auf einen Blick, wenn es eine Veränderung gegeben hat, wie z. B ein verbundener Arm wegen eines Sturzes. Drittens kann die Klientin durch das regelmäßige Üben sicher mit den Walkingstöcken umgehen und schließt sich hin und wieder einer Nachbarin beim Spaziergang an.

Eigentraining außerhalb der Therapie Erklärt der Therapeut der Klientin den Zusammenhang zwischen regelmäßigem, intensivem Fitnesstraining und Verbesserung der zerebralen Leistungsfähigkeit, kann es ideal als Ergänzung der Therapie durchgeführt werden. Innerhalb der Ergotherapie können folgende Anstöße gegeben werden:

- Vorschlag von möglichen sportlichen Aktivitäten (siehe Tab. 10.4)
- Gemeinsames Initiieren des Trainings, z. B. in Therapie walken, Hometrainer aus Keller holen ...
- Recherche über Gruppen z. B. Sportverein, Fitnessstudio, Laufgruppen
- Hilfen wie Fitness-Apps und Schrittzähler vorstellen
- Trainingspartner engagieren (Freunde, Familie, Nachbarn)

Zur „Kontrolle" kann der Ergotherapeut einen Trainingsplan erstellen, welchen er wöchentlich kontrolliert. Dies kann die Disziplin erhöhen und schafft eine gute Möglichkeit, Fragen zum Trai-

Tab. 10.4 Sportarten, bei denen eine Evidenz für einen positiven Effekt auf den Körper, das Wohlbefinden und den Alltag von Menschen mit M. Parkinson besteht

Sportart	Positiver Effekt auf
Tanzen (v. a. Tango, aber auch andere Standardtänze)	Gleichgewicht, Ausdauerleistung, Krankheitsprogression, Freezing, Gehfähigkeit bei Dual-Task-Bedingungen, Lebensqualität
Tai-Chi	Gleichgewicht, reduzierte Sturzhäufigkeit, Schrittlänge
Nordic Walken	Unklare Studienlage, evtl. Gehfähigkeit, Gleichgewicht, Lebensqualität
Yoga	Posturale Stabilität, Sturzgefahr, Gehfähigkeit, Bradykinese, Rigor, Lebensqualität, Ängste, Depression
Boxen	kleine Studie, Gleichgewicht, Gehfähigkeit, ADLs, Lebensqualität
Fahrradfahren	Gehfähigkeit, Gleichgewicht
Motomed ®	Gehfähigkeit, Gleichgewicht, Fein- und Handmotorik

ning zu besprechen. Für weitere Informationen zu Eigenübungen siehe Kap. 17.

Wenn zusätzlich zur Ergotherapie eine physiotherapeutische Behandlung stattfindet, ist eine Abstimmung mit den Kollegen notwendig, um Überschneidungen zu vermeiden und einen optimalen Behandlungsplan zu erhalten. Wenn die Physiotherapie das intensive Fitnesstraining abdeckt, kann sich die Ergotherapie ganz auf die vielfältigen weiteren Aufgabenbereiche konzentrieren.

▶ Parkinson-Betroffene haben häufig über die Jahre eine Vielzahl an Eigenübungs- und Trainingsprogrammen von unterschiedlichen Therapeuten bekommen, sodass ein Überfluss an Erwartungen paralysierend wirkt. In diesem Fall ist die Fokussierung auf ein bis zwei Ziele in enger Abstimmung mit angrenzenden Berufsgruppen sinnvoll.

Übertrag in den Alltag Während einer Rehabilitation oder eines Klinikaufenthalts sind Klientinnen meist motiviert, wesentlich häufiger und intensiver zu trainieren, um merkliche Fortschritte zu erzielen. Dies sollten die Therapeuten entschieden nutzen, in dem sie ein zielgerichtetes intensives Therapiepaket schnüren, welches sich präzise nach den Bedürfnissen der Klientin richtet und sie maximal fördert. Dazu gehört ein Fitnesstraining am oberen Leistungslimit. Meist wird dies hauptsächlich von der Physiotherapieabteilung übernommen. Um das Momentum der erreichten Verbesserungen zu nutzen, ist eine Fortsetzung des Trainings nach Entlassung aus der Klinik sinnvoll. Diese Aufgabe der Alltagsübertragung kann der Ergotherapeut übernehmen. Dazu sind die Punkte unter „Eigentraining außerhalb der Therapie" (s. o.) anwendbar.

Umfang des Fitnesstrainings In Anlehnung an die Empfehlung der WHO in den „Richtlinien zu körperlicher Aktivität und Bewegungsmangel" sollen Menschen mit chronischen Erkrankungen mindestens 2,5 Std./Woche mit erhöhtem Puls trainieren. Dies ist eine handfeste Richtlinie, die auf mehreren Studien über allgemeine Gesundheit basiert. Wichtig ist bei der Festlegung einer Trainingszeit für Klientinnen, sich immer nach dem Grad der Fitness und den Vorerfahrungen der Klientinnen zu richten. Eine Überforderung hat den negativen Effekt, dass die Betroffene gar nicht dazu motiviert ist, die Übungen durchzuführen. Es ist zu empfehlen, mit weniger Übungszeit zu beginnen und diese langsam zu steigern.

Art des Fitnesstrainings Zunächst ist das Wichtigste, dass die sportliche Aktivität, die die Klientin regelmäßig als Fitnesstraining durchführt, ihr Freude bereitet. Denn nur dann wird die Klientin genug Motivation und Disziplin aufbringen, um es intensiv, regelmäßig und dauerhaft durchzuführen. Aus diesem Grund sollte der Therapeut zuerst von gegebenen Interessen oder früher ausgeführten Sportarten ausgehen und anregen, diese wieder intensiver aufzunehmen. Zeigt die Klientin kein Interesse mehr oder ist es evtl. zu gefährlich (z. B. Reiten, Schwimmen) oder nicht mehr durchführbar (z. B. Tennis, Skifahren), sollte der Therapeut neue sportliche Betätigungsfelder vorschlagen und wenn möglich ausprobieren lassen. Dabei sind aktive, rhythmische

Sportarten passiven, statischen Sportarten vorzuziehen (s. Abb. 10.5 und 10.6). In Tab. 10.4 werden einige Sportarten vorgestellt, zu denen es wissenschaftliche Untersuchungen gibt, und welche positiven Effekte sich jeweils zeigten.

Intensität Der Schlüsselfaktor beim Fitness- oder Ausdauertraining ist eine moderate oder hohe Intensität der Durchführung. Die Klientin muss also dazu motiviert werden, am oberen Leistungslimit zu trainieren, sodass die Herzfrequenz sich erhöht. Nur so sind Verbesserungen der Symptome erreichbar. Ist eine hohe Intensität aus Gründen des mangelnden Antriebs, Sicherheitsbedenken oder kognitiven Einschränkungen nicht umsetzbar, ist auch ein Training mit moderater bis niedriger Intensität akzeptierbar. Diese Art des Trainings unterstützt die Statuserhaltung.

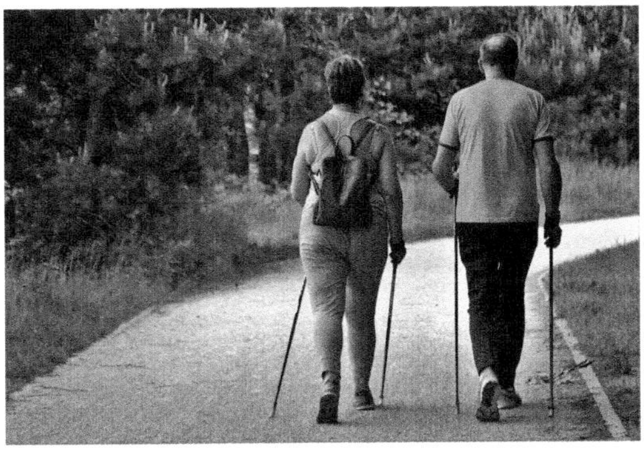

Abb. 10.5 Nordic Walken ist für Menschen mit M. Parkinson eine gute Möglichkeit, wöchentlich 2,5 Stunden Fitnesstraining nachzukommen

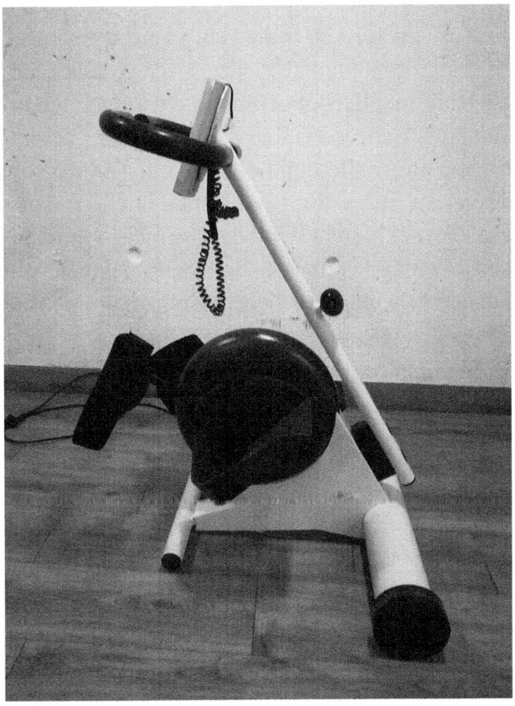

Abb. 10.6 Motomed ® ist eine gute Möglichkeit regelmäßig zu trainieren

In Untersuchungen mit motorunterstütztem Heimtrainer (Motomed ®) und Tandemrad führten Patienten ein sog. „forced training" (gezwungenes Training) durch, bei dem die Geschwindigkeit über der lag, die die Klientin selbst durchführen würde. Die Patientin lässt sich nicht passiv führen, sondern macht die Bewegung aktiv mit. Es zeigten sich nicht nur Verbesserungen in der Gehfähigkeit, sondern auch in der Finger- und Handmotorik. Dies bekräftigt die Hypothese, dass „forced training" zentralmotorische Steuerungsprozesse beeinflusst. Auf nicht-motorische Symptome scheint „forced training" keinen Einfluss zu haben.

Schon länger bekannt ist der Fakt, dass Fahrradfahren Menschen mit M. Parkinson auch im späteren Stadium der Erkrankung häufig noch möglich ist. In einer Studie von Storzer et al. (2017) wurden bei Betroffenen mit implantierten Dioden zur tiefen Hirnstimulation die Gehirnströme gemessen, während sie Fahrrad fuhren. Dabei wurde festgestellt, dass subthalamic beta power (13–35 Hz) beim Fahrradfahren unterdrückt wird. Die beta power ist bei Menschen mit Parkinson in der Regel pathologisch erhöht. Eine Störfrequenz von 18 Hz, die beim Freezing normalerweise auftritt, wird, wie in der Untersuchung festgestellt wurde, noch mehr unterdrückt und könnte neue Richtungen für therapeutische Interventionen aufweisen (s. Abb. 10.7).

Gedanken zu ergotherapeutischer Behandlung vs. Fitnesstraining Wenn es wissenschaftlich belegt ist, dass Fitnesstraining, Krafttraining und Fahrradfahren die Motorik im **gesamten** Körper verbessern, auch die Hand- und Feinmotorik – braucht es dann überhaupt noch Ergotherapie?

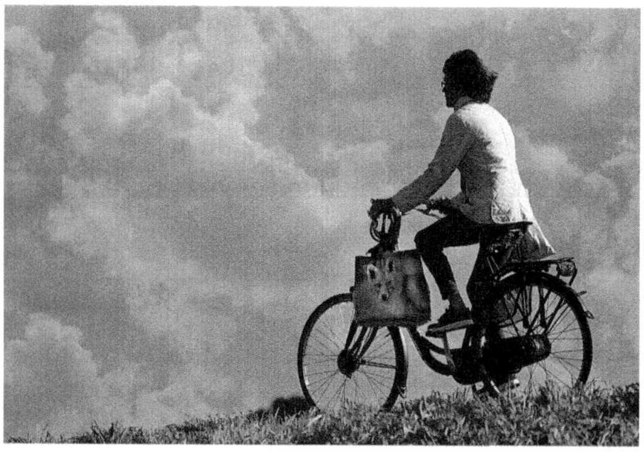

Abb. 10.7 Fahrradfahren ist auch im fortgeschrittenen Krankheitsverlauf oftmals noch möglich und hat laut Studien einen unterdrückenden Effekt auf neuronale Störfrequenzen, die Freezing auslösen

Jeder Ergotherapeut kommt wohl hin und wieder an diesen Punkt des Zweifelns an der Effektivität der ergotherapeutischen Intervention. Bedenkt man die genaue Bedeutung der Verbesserung der Gehfähigkeit, des Gleichgewichts und der Feinmotorik im Kontext einer multidimensionalen Erkrankung wie dem Parkinson-Syndrom, erkennt man die Lücken, die entstehen, wenn man nur die motorischen Symptome betrachtet. Um eine wirkliche Verbesserung zu erzielen, müssen zusätzlich zur Verbesserung der motorischen Symptome auch die damit verwobenen nicht-motorischen Symptome beachtet werden, und es ist entscheidend, inwieweit sich beides auf die Betätigung und die Teilhabe der Klientin in ihrer spezifischen Situation auswirkt. Nur dann machen motorische Verbesserungen auch Sinn, weil die Klientin die Veränderung auch in ihrem täglichen Leben bemerkt. Passend dazu wird in Kap. 4 näher auf die Themen Betätigungsorientierung (Abschn. 4.1) Klientenzentrierung (Abschn. 4.2) und die Bedeutung des Kontexts (Abschn. 4.3) eingegangen.

Die WHO definiert im Rahmen des ICF (2001), dass die Betätigung der Klientin und damit zusammenhängende Partizipation am gesellschaftlichen Leben eine zentrale Rolle in der Rehabilitation spielen. Da auch Ärztinnen mit dem ICF arbeiten, rückt dieser Gedanke immer mehr in den Fokus des Bewusstseins aller im Gesundheitsbereich arbeitenden Menschen. Mit diesem Ansatz arbeiten die Ergotherapeuten schon immer und ganz selbstverständlich. Deshalb sollten alle Ergotherapeuten ihre Position zum Thema Klientenzentrierung und Betätigung entschlossen einnehmen und auch uneingeschränkt vertreten.

Zu intensiv? In keiner Studie über Fitnesstraining wurden negative Auswirkungen von intensivem Training auf Symptome und Krankheitsverlauf der Parkinson-Erkrankung gefunden. Trotzdem sollte der Therapeut mit gewisser Vorsicht vorgehen. Es gilt zu bedenken, dass Parkinson eine Alterskrankheit ist; 75 % der Menschen über 70 Jahre haben eine Multimorbidität mit zwei oder mehr gleichzeitig auftretenden chronischen, physischen oder mentalen Beschwerden. Die Zahl der Parkinson-Erkrankten mit Komorbiditäten differiert nicht von denen mit anderen Krankheitsbildern. Die Wahrscheinlichkeit, dass die Klientin zusätzlich eine koronare Herzkrankheit, Osteoporose, Zustand nach Apoplex oder eine weitere gesundheitliche Einschränkung hat, ist hoch und nicht immer ist intensives Fitnesstraining damit vereinbar.

Zusätzlich ist zu bedenken, dass die Diagnose M. Parkinson hin und wieder falsch gestellt wird. Es kann möglicherweise auch ein zerebraler Insult Auslöser für die Parkinson-ähnlichen Symptome sein. In diesem Fall wäre ein Training am oberen Leistungslimit evtl. kontraindiziert. Wenn ein Zweifel besteht, wird dazu geraten, ein intensives Training vorher mit dem behandelnden Arzt abzusprechen und eine obere Grenze für Puls und Blutdruck während der Übung festzulegen.

Beispiel

Ein paar Wochen später ruft Frau I. ihre Schwester an: „Ich habe dir doch von meinem Wunsch erzählt, mehr Sport zu machen. Meine Ergotherapeutin hat mir geraten, mir einen Sportpartner zu suchen, damit ich dranbleibe. Könnte ich zwei Mal die Woche mit dir laufen, wenn du mit Ricky Gassi gehst? Wir haben das mit den Walkingstöcken ausprobiert, das macht richtig Spaß und ich komme ganz schön in Schwung.“ ◀

10.4 In On-Phase

Beispiel

Als der Therapeut ins Patientenzimmer kommt, sitzt Herr Qu. bewegungslos an der Bettkante. Auf dem Weg zur Ergotherapie-Abteilung heben sich Herrn Qu`s Füße kaum vom Boden ab und er kommt bei jeder äußeren Ablenkung ins Freezing. Sie gehen ein paar Schritte – eine Tür geht auf – Herr Qu. steht. Sie gehen wieder ein paar Schritte – die Farbe des Bodens ändert sich – Herr. Qu. steht … Als sie im Behandlungsraum ankommen, braucht Herr Qu. eine kleine Pause. Der Therapeut sieht auf die Uhr, das Schreibtraining wird heute wieder nicht möglich sein. ◀

In den ersten Jahren nach der Parkinson-Diagnose ist der Patient medikamentös meist gut eingestellt. Der Grad der Fluktuationen ist so niedrig, dass der Patient immer im On bleibt. Die Medikamenteneinnahme wird so koordiniert, dass der L-Dopa-Spiegel nie unter ein Level rutscht, in dem Off-Symptome wie Freezing-Episoden und starke Bradykinese auftreten. Damit ist eine gute Beweglichkeit mit geringen Einschränkungen durch Bradykinese durchgehend gegeben.

Nach durchschnittlich 5–6 Jahren entstehen größere Fluktuationen, gegen Ende der Einnahmezeit des Medikaments beginnt das sog. Wearing-off: Rigor und Bradykinese sowie nicht-motorische Symptome wie Ängste und Apathie nehmen zu. Aber auch in die entgegengesetzte Richtung können Veränderungen in Form von Überbeweglichkeit beobachtet werden. Diese sog. Peak-dose-Dyskinesien treten kurz nach Einnahme des L-Dopa auf. Das heißt, der Patient erlebt zunehmend sowohl Überbeweglichkeit (Dyskinesien) als auch Unterbeweglichkeit (Off-Symptomatik). Die Zeit, in der die Medikamentenwirkung und damit die Beweglichkeit ideal ist, wird „On-Phase" genannt. Diese wird im Krankheitsverlauf immer kürzer, der Intervall der Medikamentengabe wird verkürzt, um den Fluktuationen bestmöglich entgegenzuwirken. Für weitere Informationen zur Medikamentenfluktuation siehe Abschn. 3.1. In der Abb. 3.2 unter Abschn. 3.1 ist die Medikamentenfluktuation anschaulich dargestellt.

Die Lernfähigkeit des Gehirns ist in der On-Phase am größten. Dopamin, das „Belohnungshormon", spielt eine wichtige Rolle beim Erlernen oder Umlernen. Deswegen ist es eine große Hilfe, wenn beim Trainieren einer Betätigung oder Körperfunktion, aber auch beim Anwenden neuer Hilfsmittel oder neuer Strategien der Patient im On ist. Das L-Dopa versetzt das Gehirn in einen lernfähigen Status, und das in der Therapie geübte Verhalten kann sich besser im Gehirn verankern.

▶ Wenn möglich sollte die Therapie in der On-Phase durchgeführt werden, da dann eine bestmögliche Versorgung des Gehirns mit Dopamin besteht und damit die beste Voraussetzung für „lernen" gegeben ist.

Bei den meisten Parkinson-Klientinnen in frühen Krankheitsstadien, die sich die meiste Zeit des Tages im On befinden, ist die Therapiezeit meist noch frei wählbar. Nur früh morgens, bevor die Medikamente eingenommen wurden, lässt sich eine Off-Phase beobachten.

Bei Klientinnen im fortgeschrittenen oder Spätstadium kann der Therapeut durch ein Gespräch mit Klientin, Angehörigen, Arzt oder Pflegekraft herausfinden, wann die beste Tageszeit für die Therapie ist. Nicht immer lässt sich die On-Phase genau vorherbestimmen. Einflussfaktoren wie Tagesverfassung, Abweichung der Einnahmezeit der Medikamente oder Verdauungsstörungen verändern die Wirkung der Medikamente und erschweren, besonders im fortgeschrittenen Stadium der Erkrankung, die Therapieplanung.

In der Klinik kommt erschwerend hinzu, dass Klientinnen häufig zur Medikamenteneinstellung aufgenommen wurden. Sie sind dann für einen Großteil des Aufenthaltes nicht gut eingestellt und befinden sich oftmals über Stunden oder Tage im Off-Zustand. In diesem Fall nutzt der Therapeut seine Flexibilität und erarbeitet Strategien für den Umgang mit Off-Phasen, macht eine Entspannungstherapie oder übt mit Angehörigen das Handling der bewegungslosen Betroffenen. Für weitere Ideen siehe Abschn. 14.19.

Hin und wieder kann eine Intervention in der Off-Phase auch therapeutisch gewünscht und geplant sein. In dieser Einheit können z. B. die Strategien, die vorher bei guter Beweglichkeit gefestigt wurden, jetzt auf die eingeschränkte Tageszeit übertragen werden.

Beispiel

Der Therapeut hat die Therapiezeit um eine Stunde nach hinten verlegen lassen. Herr Qu. tritt dynamisch durch die Tür zum Behandlungszimmer. „Wird heute geschrieben?" fragt er, seinen Schreibfüller schwingend. ◀

10.5 Erholungsphasen

Beispiel

Frustriert wirft Herr L. sein Handtuch in die Umkleidekabine. Heute hat er nur 800 Meter geschafft, nicht einmal die Hälfte seines früheren Schwimmpensums. Er ist enttäuscht, er hat die Artikel gelesen. Bei Parkinson ist körperliche Fitness das A und O. Die Beweglichkeit bleibt so länger gut, die Stimmung ist besser und die Schlafstörungen sind weniger stark ausgeprägt. Und jetzt? Er schafft einfach immer weniger. ◀

▶ Erholungsphasen sollten ein fester Bestandteil im Tagesablauf jedes Parkinson-Klientinnen sein.

Überforderung Durch das langsame Fortschreiten der Erkrankung führen viele Klientinnen ihren Alltag weiter wie bisher und geraten zunehmend in eine Überforderung.

Fatigue gehört mit einer Prävalenz von 37 %-65 % zu den schwerwiegendsten Symptomen bei der Parkinson-Erkrankung und beeinflusst die Lebensqualität stark. 56 % der Betroffenen geben Fatigue unter den ersten drei am stärksten behindernden Symptomen der Erkrankung an. Weitere Informationen zum Umgang mit Fatigue sind in Abschn. 14.11 zu finden. Nicht nur die Klientinnen, bei denen eine Fatigue diagnostiziert wurde, sollten auf Erholungsphasen achten. Zu wissen, wann es Zeit ist, die Ansprüche an sich selbst herunterzusetzen und allgemein zu entschleunigen, fällt vielen Klientinnen schwer. Jüngere Klientinnen stehen evtl. noch im Berufsleben und haben eine Familie zu versorgen und das Gefühl „irgendwie weitermachen zu müssen". Ältere Betroffene haben oft ihr ganzes Leben lang „geschafft und gemacht", sie fühlen sich unproduktiv, und es fällt ihnen schwer, auch Mal nichts zu tun.

Aufklärung und Akzeptanz Eine Aufklärung über das Fatigue-Syndrom und eine Spiegelung o. g. Einstellungen kann eine hilfreiche Einleitung für ein Gespräch darüber sein. Hierbei kann der Bogen zur Selbstreflexion hilfreich sein (siehe Anhang).

Viele Klientinnen benötigen eine Art „Erlaubnis" des Therapeuten, Pause zu machen. Mit der Erklärung, dass eine Erholungsphase bei Parkinson notwendig ist, um wieder Kräfte zu sammeln und tatkräftig seinen Alltag oder die Übungen anzugehen, wächst die Akzeptanz der Klientin. Hat die Klientin verstanden und akzeptiert, dass Erholungsphasen ein wichtiger Teil des Alltags sind, um die Aktivitätsphasen zu ermöglichen, geht man in die konkrete Planung über.

Planung der Erholung

- Zeitpunkt

Durch das Ausfüllen eines Wochenplans (siehe Anhang) entsteht eine übersichtliche Aufstellung, wann die kräftezehrenden Aktivitäten stattfinden, wo natürliche Pausen entstehen (z. B. Mittagspause), und wo etwas umorganisiert werden sollte, um eine Erholungspause zu ermöglichen (z. B. vor oder nach einer kräftezehrenden Aktivität).

- Art der Erholung

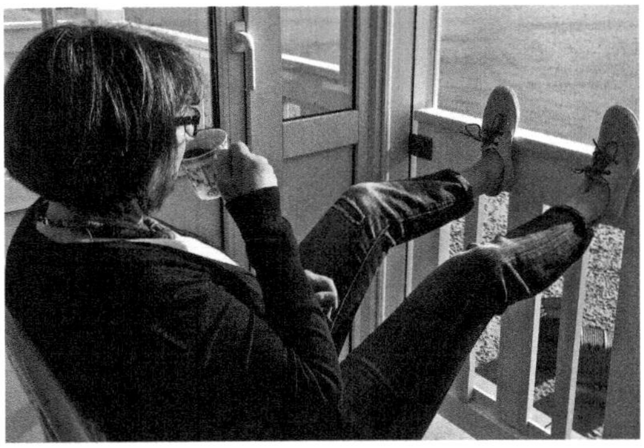

Abb. 10.8 Ruhige Erholungsphasen sind für Menschen mit Parkinson wichtig, um mit frischer Energie in den Alltag oder ins Training zu starten

Es bestehen viele Möglichkeiten, eine Erholungspause durchzuführen (s. Abb. 10.8). Je nach Situation und persönlicher Vorliebe sollte besprochen und experimentiert werden, mit welcher Art der Pause die Klientin am meisten Erholung findet. Beispiele sind:

- Schlaf
- Kurzschlaf
- Meditation
- Beine hochlegen
- Ruhige Musik hören
- Warmgetränk
- In der Natur ruhen

Was für gesunde Menschen erholsam sein kann – spazieren gehen, Gartenarbeit oder stricken – mag für Parkinson-Erkrankte zwar auch eine angenehme, ruhige Aktivität sein, kann jedoch nicht als Erholung gelten. Dazu muss man sich das Krankheitsbild nochmal ins Gedächtnis rufen. Alle Bewegungen, die vor der Erkrankung automatisiert waren und mit minimaler neuronaler Aktivität abgerufen wurden, müssen nun bewusst durchgeführt werden und benötigen wesentlich mehr Gehirnkapazität. Dies muss den Klientinnen und vor allem auch pflegenden Angehörigen und Pflegekräften vermittelt werden, um die Möglichkeit einer **wirklichen** Erholung zu schaffen. Die Klienten sollen wirklich nichts tun, während sie sich ausruhen.

- Ort der Erholung

Wo ist ein passender Ort, um eine Pause zu machen? Um alle möglichen Hindernisse zu beseitigen, wird mit der Klientin der genaue Ort für eine Erholungsphase besprochen. Dabei sollte beachtet werden, dass

- Ruhe herrscht,
- keine Störung auftritt,
- es bequem ist,
- die Klientin selbständig die gewünschte Position einnehmen kann.

Beispiel

Als Herr L. seiner Ergotherapeutin vom Abfall seiner sportlichen Leistungen erzählt, hört sie ihm gut zu. Sie weiß, dass es ihm persönlich sehr wichtig ist, sportlich zu sein. Herr L. ist fit. Er schwimmt drei Mal die Woche und geht zusätzlich ins Fitnessstudio. Der Therapeut erzählt Herrn L. von den Untersuchungen, die sagen, dass Erholungspausen auf die Ausprägung der Symptome auch einen großen Einfluss haben, und dass es darauf ankommt, eine gesunde Balance von Fitness und Erholung zu finden. Zusammen erarbeiten sie einen Fitness- und Erholungsplan, nach dem er sich fortan richtet. ◀

10.6 Soziale Kontakte

Beispiel

Herr V. blättert in seinem Adressbuch. Die Menschen darin, früher gute Bekannte und Freunde, sind nur noch Namen. Weit entfernte Erinnerungen. Wie ist es nur dazu gekommen, dass keiner ihm mehr nahesteht, überlegt Herr V. Ein paar Freunde haben sich gleich nach der Diagnose verflüchtigt. Ihnen war es wahrscheinlich zu viel. Sie waren unsicher, wie sie mit ihm umgehen sollten, oder hatten einfach keine Lust mit ihm in der Öffentlichkeit Blicke auf sich zu ziehen. Aber was war mit Eymen passiert? Und Irma und Jakob? Er wusste es nicht mehr. Über die Jahre hatten die Aktivitäten abgenommen, bei denen er aktiv mitmachen konnte und die Ausreden der Freunde haben zugenommen. Schon bitter. Er schlägt das Büchlein wieder zu, es macht ihn sentimental darin zu blättern. ◀

Winter et al. untersuchten in einer Studie (2010) den Zusammenhang von Lebensqualität und Anzahl der Mitglieder im Haushalt bei 100 Menschen mit M. Parkinson. Dabei stellten sie fest, dass die Lebensqualität höher war, je mehr soziale Unterstützung (Haushaltsmitglieder) sie hatten. Und Holt-Lunstad et al. wiesen (2010) in einer vielbeachteten Studie die positive Auswirkung von sozialen Interaktionen auf die Lebenserwartung nach. Basierend auf diesem Wissen ist es sinnvoll, sich in der Ergotherapie mit dem Thema sozialer Interaktion zu befassen (s. Abb. 10.9).

Stellt der Therapeut bei der Sammlung der Informationen über die Klientin fest, dass wenige oder keine sozialen Kontakte vorhanden sind, kann das in die therapeutische Intervention mit einfließen.

- Gruppenbehandlung
  Eine gute Möglichkeit, soziale Interaktion zu ermöglichen, sind Gruppenbehandlungen. Hier kann in lockerer Runde, mit Spaß und Verständnis, mit anderen Betroffenen ein Austausch stattfinden. Oftmals entstehen wertvolle Bekanntschaften, hin und wieder sogar neue Freundschaften.
- Vorstellung von Gruppen
  In der Nähe der Klientin sind meist verschiedene Gruppenangebote zu finden. Diese vorhandenen Gruppen sind ideale Orte, um Gleichgesinnte zu treffen. Oftmals braucht es nur den Vorschlag des Therapeuten oder ein gemeinsames Ansehen der Website oder eines Flyers der in Frage kommenden Gruppen. Es ist aber auch möglich, die Klientin beim ersten Mal zu einer neuen Gruppenaktivität zu begleiten, um die Hemmschwelle zu verringern.
  Mögliche Gruppen sind:
  - Selbsthilfegruppen,
  - Seniorengruppen (Tanzen, Singen, Ausflüge, Gymnastik …),
  - Kirchengruppen,
  - Chor,
  - Vereine (Sport, Musik),
  - Volkshochschulangebote (Sprache lernen, kreative Angebote …),
  - uvm.
- Kommunikation fördern
  Bei der Kommunikation von Parkinson-Betroffenen mit Mitmenschen entstehen häufig Missverständnisse. Dies kann daran liegen, dass die nonverbalen Kommunikationswege des Erkrankten erheblich reduziert sind. Mimik und Gestik sind verringert. Aber auch die verbale Kommunikation kann unter dem Morbus Parkinson leiden. Die Stimme ist leiser und schlecht verständlich, Antworten kommen häufig verzögert und sehr kurzgehalten. All diese Punkte können der Klientin in der Ergotherapie gespiegelt werden. Gemeinsam mit der Klientin sollte der Therapeut Alternativen suchen (Schriftweg, gemeinsame Erlebnisse), eine lebendige Kommunikation trainieren und in Rollenspielen erproben.
- Alte Kontakte auffrischen
  Durch die Krankheit verlieren sich manche engen Bindungen zu Freunden oder Familie. Oftmals sind sich frühere Kontakte nicht sicher, wie sie mit dem Menschen mit Parkinson umgehen sollen. Oder die Kommunika-

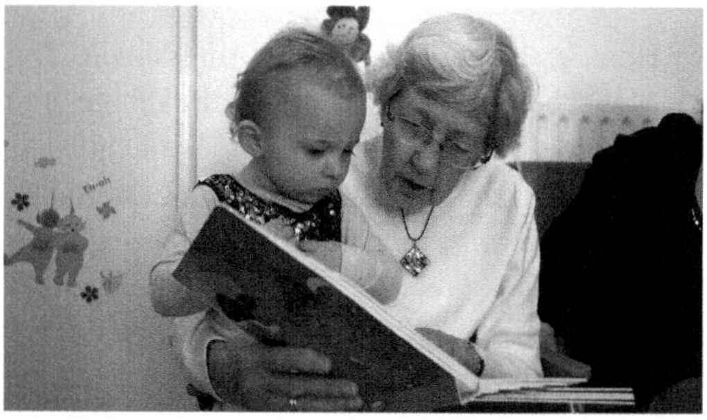

Abb. 10.9 Soziale Kontakte erhöhen die Lebensqualität erheblich und lenken die Aufmerksamkeit auf die wertvollen Bereiche des Lebens

tion hat durch die mangelnde Initiative der Betroffenen nachgelassen.
Wenn die Klientin es wünscht, kann der Therapeut diese alten Kontakte einladen, mit zur Therapie dazu zu kommen, um mögliche Verhaltensweisen oder Interaktionsideen zusammen zu besprechen. Dazu gehören Kommunikationsregeln (z. B. Zeit lassen, Nachfragen, Erinnern lauter zu sprechen), aber auch praktische Vorschläge, wie die Klientin unterstützt werden kann und welche Aktivitäten und Ausflugsmöglichkeiten weiterhin beiden möglich sind.

- Kontaktaufnahme
  Durch die Abnahme der Kommunikationsfähigkeit und des Antriebes fällt es vielen Menschen mit Parkinson schwer, den Kontakt mit Freundinnen und Familie zu halten. Die Kommunikation kann in der Ergotherapie angebahnt werden. Dazu können Briefe, Karten oder Geschenke (z. B. zum Geburtstag oder Feiertagen) dienen, die in der Ergotherapie gestaltet, geschrieben und versandt werden. Einladung von Familie oder Freunden zu einfachen Aktivitäten (z. B. Kaffee trinken, Kartenspielen). Auch alle anderen Formen der Kommunikation sind möglich, je nach Präferenz der Klientin, z. B. E-Mails, Telefonate, Nachrichten mit dem Smartphone, Videonachrichten oder -anrufe mit dem Smartphone und die persönliche Verabredung.

Beispiel

Herr V. swiped über sein Handy. „Wer nutzt heute noch Adressbücher?" denkt er. Seine Ergotherapeutin hat ihm gesagt, dass es wichtig ist, mit seinen Freunden aktiven Kontakt zu halten. „Wen rufe ich heute an?" Er sieht seine Kontaktliste durch – so viele neue Namen, die netten Menschen gehören. Herr V. hat gelernt, seine Erkrankung bei den neuen Freunden vom Dartclub und dem Singkreis schnell zu thematisieren. So entstehen keine unangenehmen Situationen – sie wissen gleich, was los ist, und dass es wirklich komplett still sein muss, wenn er auf die Dartscheibe zielt, weil sonst Gefahr besteht, dass er jemanden am Fuß trifft. ◀

Literatur und weiterführende Literatur

Ahlskog JE (2017) Aerobic exercise: evidence for a direct brain effect to slow Parkinson disease progression, PhD, MD. Mayo Clin Proc 93(3):P360–P372

Alberts JL, Linder SM, Penko AL, Lowe MJ, Phillips M (2001) It is not about the bike, it is about the pedaling: forced exercise and Parkinson's disease. Exerc Sport Sci Rev 39(4):177–186. https://doi.org/10.1097/JES.0b013e31822cc71a, https://doi.org/10.1016/j.mayocp.2017.12.015. PMID: 21799425

Aragon A, Kings J (2018) Occupational therapy for people with Parkinson's, the Royal College of Occupational Therapists Specialist Section – Neurological Practice, London

Bergmann MF, Chlond MA, Schnoor H (2016) Evaluation eines psychosozialen Trainings für Parkinson-Betroffene: Eine randomisierte kontrollierte Studie zur Untersuchung der Effekte auf die gesundheitsbezogene Lebensqualität und die Krankheitsverarbeitung sowie weitere Parameter. Philipps-Universität Marburg

Bombieri F, Schena F, Pellegrini B, Barone P, Tinazzi M, Erro R (2017) Walking on four limbs: a systematic review of nordic walking in Parkinson disease. Parkinsonism Relat Disord 38:8–12. https://doi.org/10.1016/j.parkreldis.02.004. Epub 2017 Feb 6. PMID: 28202374

Brienesse LA, Emerson MN (2013) Effects of resistance training for people with Parkinson's disease: a systematic review. J Am Med Dir Assoc 14(4):236–241. https://doi.org/10.1016/j.jamda.2012.11.012. Epub. PMID: 23318666

Combs SA, Diehl MD, Staples WH, Conn L, Davis K, Lewis N, Schaneman K (2011) Boxing training for patients with Parkinson disease: a case series. Phys Ther 91(1):132–142. https://doi.org/10.2522/ptj.20100142. Epub 2010 Nov 18. PMID: 21088118

Cusso ME, Donald KJ, Khoo TK (2016) The impact of physical activity on non-motor symptoms in Parkinson's disease: a systematic review. Front Med (Lausanne) 3:35

de Dreu MJ, van der Wilk AS, Poppe E, Kwakkel G, van Wegen EE (2012) Rehabilitation, exercise therapy and music in patients with Parkinson's disease: a meta-analysis of the effects of music-based movement therapy on walking ability, balance and quality of life. Parkinsonism Relat Disord 18(Suppl 1):S114–S119. https://doi.org/10.1016/S1353-8020(11)70036-0. PMID: 22166406

Farley B, Fox CN, Ramig L, McFarland D (2008) Intensive amplitude-specific therapeutic approaches for Parkinson's disease: toward a neuroplasticity-principled rehabilitation model. Topics Geriatr Rehab 24:99–114

Foster ER, Bedekar M, Tickle-Degnen L (2014) Systematic review of the effectiveness of occupational therapy-related interventions for people with Parkinson's disease. Am J Occup Ther 68(1):39–49. https://doi.

org/10.5014/ajot.2014.008706. PMID: 24367954; PMCID: PMC4413458

Global Parkinson's Disease Survey (GPDS) Steering Committee (2002) Factors impacting on quality of life in Parkinson's disease: results from an international survey. Mov Disord 17:60–67. https://doi.org/10.1002/mds.10010

Grosset KA, Grosset DG (2005) Patient-perceived involvement and satisfaction in Parkinson's disease: Effect on therapy decisions and quality of life. Mov Disord 20:616–619. https://doi.org/10.1002/mds.20393

Hackney ME, Earhart GM (2009) Effects of dance on movement control in Parkinson's disease: a comparison of Argentine tango and American ballroom. J Rehabil Med 41(6):475–481. https://doi.org/10.2340/16501977-0362. PMID: 19479161; PMCID: PMC2688709

Holt-Lunstad J, Smith TB, Layton JB (2010) Social relationships and mortality risk: a meta-analytic review. PLoS Med 7(7):e1000316. https://doi.org/10.1371/journal.pmed.1000316. PMID: 20668659; PMCID: PMC2910600

Jankovic J (2005) Motor fluctuations and dyskinesias in Parkinson's disease: clinical manifestations. Mov Disord 20(Suppl 11):S11–S16. https://doi.org/10.1002/mds.20458. PMID: 15822109

Kessler D, Liddy C (2017) Self-management support programs for persons with Parkinson's disease: an integrative review. Patient Educ Couns 100(10):1787–1795. https://doi.org/10.1016/j.pec.2017.04.011.Epub. PMID: 28465112

Kohl M (2017) Mehr Sein als Schein? Wie Therapeuten Placebo-Effekte steuern können, Unternehmen Praxis, Kiel

Kwok JYY, Kwan JCY, Auyeung M, Mok VCT, Lau CKY, Choi KC, Chan HYL (2019) Effects of mindfulness yoga vs stretching and resistance training exercises on anxiety and depression for people with parkinson disease: a randomized clinical trial. JAMA Neurol 76(7):755–763. https://doi.org/10.1001/jamaneurol.2019.0534. PMID: 30958514; PMCID: PMC6583059

Law M, Baptiste S, Mills J (1995) Client-centred practice: what does it mean and does it make a difference? Can J Occup Ther 62(5):250–257. https://doi.org/10.1177/000841749506200504. PMID: 10152881

Law M, Polatajko H, Carswell A, McColl MA, Pollock N, Baptiste S (1999) Das Kanadische Modell der Occupational Performance und das Canadian Occupational Performance Measure. In: Jerosch-Herold C, Marotzki U, Hack BM, Weber P (Hrsg) Konzeptionelle Modelle für die ergotherapeutische Praxis. Ergotherapie – Reflexion und Analyse. Springer, Berlin/Heidelberg. https://doi.org/10.1007/978-3-662-08173-0_7

Li F, Harmer P, Fitzgerald K, Eckstrom E, Stock R, Galver J, Maddalozzo G, Batya SS (2012) Tai chi and postural stability in patients with Parkinson's disease. N Engl J Med 366(6):511–519. https://doi.org/10.1056/NEJMoa1107911. PMID: 22316445; PMCID: PMC3285459

Ni M, Mooney K, Signorile JF (2016) Controlled pilot study of the effects of power yoga in Parkinson's disease. Complement Ther Med 25:126–131. https://doi.org/10.1016/j.ctim.2016.01.007. Epub 2016 Feb 10. PMID: 27062960

Palmadottir G (2006) Client-therapist relationships: experiences of occupational therapy clients in rehabilitation. Br J Occup Ther 69:394–401. https://doi.org/10.1177/030802260606900902

Petzinger GM, Fisher BE, McEwen S, Beeler JA, Walsh JP, Jakowec MW (2013) Exercise-enhanced neuroplasticity targeting motor and cognitive circuitry in Parkinson's disease. Lancet Neurol 12(7):716–726. https://doi.org/10.1016/S1474-4422(13)70123-6. PMID: 23769598; PMCID: PMC3690528

Power M, Bullinger M, Harper A, The World Health Organization Quality of Life Group (1999) The World Health Organization WHOQOL-100: tests of the universality of quality of life in 15 different cultural groups worldwide. Health Psychol 18(5):495–505. https://doi.org/10.1037/0278-6133.18.5.495

Radder DLM, Sturkenboom IH, van Nimwegen M, Keus SH, Bloem BR, de Vries NM (2017) Physical therapy and occupational therapy in Parkinson's disease. Int J Neurosci 127(10):930–943. https://doi.org/10.1080/00207454.2016.1275617

Reynolds GO, Otto MW, Ellis TD, Cronin-Golomb A (2016) The therapeutic potential of exercise to improve mood, cognition, and sleep in Parkinson's disease. Mov Disord (1):23–38. https://doi.org/10.1002/mds.26484. Epub 2015 Dec 30. PMID: 26715466; PMCID: PMC4724300

Sacheli MA, Murray DK, Vafai N, Cherkasova MV, Dinelle K, Shahinfard E, Neilson N, McKenzie J, Schulzer M, Appel-Cresswell S, McKeown MJ, Sossi V, Jon Stoessl A (2018) Habitual exercisers versus sedentary subjects with Parkinson's disease: Multimodal PET and fMRI study. Mov Disord 33(12):1945–1950. https://doi.org/10.1002/mds.27498. PMID: 30376184

Sacheli MA, Neva JL, Lakhani B, Murray DK, Vafai N, Shahinfard E, English C, McCormick S, Dinelle K, Neilson N, McKenzie J, Schulzer M, McKenzie DC, Appel-Cresswell S, McKeown MJ, Boyd LA, Sossi V, Stoessl AJ (2019) Exercise increases caudate dopamine release and ventral striatal activation in Parkinson's disease. Mov Disord 34(12):1891–1900. https://doi.org/10.1002/mds.27865. Epub. PMID: 31584222

Storzer L, Butz M, Hirschmann J, Abbasi O, Gratkowski M, Saupe D, Vesper J, Dalal SS, Schnitzler A (2017) Bicycling suppresses abnormal beta synchrony in the Parkinsonian basal ganglia. Ann Neurol 82(4):592–601. https://doi.org/10.1002/ana.25047. Epub 2017 Oct 10. PMID: 28892573

Sturkenboom I, Thijssen M, Gons-van Elsacker J, Jansen I, Maasdam A, Schulten M, Vijver-Visser D, Steultjens E, Bloem B, Munneke M (2008) Guidelines for occupational therapy in Parkinson's disease rehabilitation. ParkinsonNet/NPF, Nijmegen/Miami

Tenison E, Smink A, Redwood S, Darweesh S, Cottle H, van Halteren A, Haak P, Hamlin R, Ypinga J, Bloem B,

Ben-Shlomo Y, Munneke M, Henderson E (2020) Proactive and integrated management and empowerment in Parkinson's disease: designing a new model of care. Parkinson's Dis:1–11. https://doi.org/10.1155/2020/8673087

Uhrbrand A, Stenager E, Pedersen MS, Dalgas U (2015) Parkinson's disease and intensive exercise therapy – a systematic review and meta-analysis of randomized controlled trials. J Neurol Sci 353(1-2):9–19. https://doi.org/10.1016/j.jns.2015.04.004. Epup. PMID: 25936252

Van Puymbroeck M, Walter AA, Hawkins BL, Sharp JL, Woschkolup K, Urrea-Mendoza E, Revilla F, Adams EV, Schmid AA (2018) Functional improvements in Parkinson's disease following a randomized trial of yoga. Evid Based Complement Alternat Med 3:8516351. https://doi.org/10.1155/2018/8516351. Erratum in: Evid Based Complement Alternat Med. 6;2018:4523743. PMID: 29967649; PMCID: PMC6009016.

WHO guidelines on physical activity and sedentary behaviour (2020) World Health Organization, Geneva; Licence: CC BY-NC-SA 3.0 IGO

Winter Y, von Campenhausen S, Gasser J, Seppi K, Reese JP, Pfeiffer KP, Bötzel K, Oertel WH, Dodel R, Poewe W (2010) Social and clinical determinants of quality of life in Parkinson's disease in Austria: a cohort study. J Neurol 257(4):638–645. https://doi.org/10.1007/s00415-009-5389-7. Epub 2009 Nov 28. PMID: 19946784

World Health Organization (2001) International classification of functioning, disability and health: ICF. World Health Organization. https://apps.who.int/iris/handle/10665/42407

11 Interventionsarten

Nach der Interpretation der Betätigungsanalyse und gegebenenfalls der Durchführung weiterer Testungen, findet die Entscheidungsfindung der Ergotherapeutin für eine Intervention statt. Obwohl in der schematischen Übersicht „Perfect fit" in Abb. 4.4 die einzelnen Interventionen im großen Oval in vier Spalten aufgeteilt sind, ist es in der praktischen Arbeit weder gängig noch sinnvoll, eine Interventionsart isoliert durchzuführen. Vielmehr wählt die Therapeutin aus jedem Bereich die Punkte aus, die für die spezielle Situation des Klienten geeignet sind.

▶ Die Trennung der Interventionsarten im „Perfect fit" (siehe Abb. 4.4) bildet nicht die Realität ab, da die Therapeutin sie in der therapeutischen Praxis selten getrennt nutzt, sondern beliebig kombiniert. Es dient vielmehr der Entscheidungsfindung.

Für ein besseres Verständnis der unterschiedlichen therapeutischen Möglichkeiten werden hier die fünf Interventionsarten getrennt beschrieben. Jede Therapeutin kann so im Therapieprozess reflektieren, welche Intervention sie nutzt und warum. Dies kann vor allem hilfreich sein, wenn Therapeutin und Klient das Gefühl haben, nicht weiterzukommen, oder dass dieser Weg nicht zum gefassten Ziel führt. Die fünf Interventionsarten sind:

1. Performance-Skills (Performanzfertigkeiten) trainieren
2. Betätigung verändern
3. Betätigungsspezifische Körperfunktionen trainieren
4. Kontextfaktoren verändern – Adaptation
5. Komplette Betätigung trainieren

11.1 Performance-Skills (Performanzfertigkeiten) trainieren

(siehe Abb. 4.4 Spalte 1)

Betrachtet man eine Betätigung, lässt sie sich in Einzelschritte zerlegen. Ein Performance-Skill ist die kleinste mögliche Bewegungseinheit innerhalb einer Betätigung. Die Betätigung „Aufstehen" kann beispielsweise in folgende Performance-Skills unterteilt werden:

1. An Stuhlkante rutschen
2. Füße unter Stuhl positionieren
3. Hände auf Armlehnen stützen
4. Gewicht nach vorne verlagern
5. Aufstehen

Bei der Betätigungsanalyse stellt die Therapeutin gegebenenfalls fest, dass eins oder mehrere dieser einzelnen Performance-Skills innerhalb der gezeigten Betätigung eingeschränkt sind und die erfolgreiche Durchführung behindert oder scheitern lässt. In diesem Fall spricht man von einem Breakdown-Point. Die Therapeutin

A. Orellana, *Betätigungsorientierte Ergotherapie bei Morbus Parkinson*,
https://doi.org/10.1007/978-3-662-62583-5_11

erkennt z. B., dass der Klient beim Aufstehen das Gewicht nicht ausreichend nach vorne verlagert, und dadurch eine Falltendenz nach hinten besteht. In diesem Fall macht es Sinn, für die Betätigung des Aufstehens die im „Perfect fit" (Abb. 4.4) erste Spalte „Performance-Skill trainieren" zu wählen und gezielt an der Gewichtsverlagerung zu arbeiten (für eine ausführliche Beschreibung des Training der Performance-Skills siehe Kap. 13).

11.2 Betätigung verändern

(siehe Abb. 4.4, 2. Spalte)

Häufig erkennt die Therapeutin bei der Betätigungsanalyse, dass der Klient etwas an der Betätigung verändern muss, damit er diese erfolgreich durchführen kann. Es gibt eine Vielzahl an Möglichkeiten, eine Betätigung zu verändern, um zum Ziel zu gelangen. Hier wird mit Evidenzbasierter Praxis (EBP) vorgegangen. Die Therapeutin weiß aus der Fachliteratur, welche möglichen Interventionsarten es gibt, oder liest es sich für diese spezifische Problemstellung an.

Wenn der Klient z. B. beim Aufstehen ins Freezing kommt, kann die Therapeutin mit ihm verschiedenartige Cues ausprobieren. Sie kann versuchen, ob ein lautes „Hoch" die Bewegung des Aufstehens kraftvoll initiiert. Oder vielleicht funktioniert es besser, wenn sich der Klient auf die Oberschenkel klatscht, um das Aufstehen zu starten. Es kann jedoch sein, dass Cues keine wesentliche Verbesserung des Aufstehens bewirken. In dem Fall exploriert die Therapeutin weiter. Ist es evtl. hilfreich, wenn der Klient die Arme beim Aufstehen schwungvoll nach vorne bringt? In Kap. 14 sind viele Interventionsmöglichkeiten beschrieben, bei denen die Betätigung verändert wird. Dort sind sie den jeweils vordergründigen Symptomen zugeordnet.

11.3 Betätigungsspezifische Körperfunktionen trainieren

(siehe Abb. 4.4 Spalte 3)

Möglicherweise ist die Ursache für die gescheiterte Durchführung einer Betätigung in einer eingeschränkten Körperfunktion zu finden. Dann geht die Therapeutin davon aus, dass die Betätigung nur verbessert werden kann, wenn die Funktion verbessert wird.

Definition nach Stadler-Grillmaier (2007), Funktion: – Zugrunde liegende physische, psychische und kognitive Komponenten, die Betätigungs-/Handlungs-/Beschäftigungsperformanz ermöglichen.

Beobachtet die Therapeutin beim Aufstehen des Klienten aus dem Stuhl z. B., dass die Beine zittern und der Klient auf halbem Weg zum Aufstehen wieder in den Stuhl zurückfällt, könnte eine Kraftminderung in den Beinen vorliegen. In diesem Fall kann die Ergotherapeutin der Physiotherapie seine Beobachtung schildern, damit die Beinkraft an Geräten trainiert werden kann. Auch in der Ergotherapie sind kräftigende Übungen im Stehen sinnvoll. Außerdem kann das Aufstehen wiederholt sehr langsam durchgeführt werden, was zu einer Kräftigung der Beine führt. So arbeitet die Therapeutin an der Körperfunktion und bindet sie gleichzeitig in die Betätigung mit ein, was einen Übertrag in den Alltag fördert. In Kap. 14 sind unter den jeweiligen Symptomen unter Anderem funktionelle Übungen zu finden.

11.4 Kontextfaktoren verändern – Adaptation

(siehe Abb. 4.4 Spalte 4)

Die vierte Möglichkeit, ergotherapeutisch zu intervenieren, ist, Kontextfaktoren zu verändern. Besonders im fortgeschrittenen Verlauf der Parkinson-Erkrankung wird diese Interventionsart vermehrt genutzt, da sie die Durchführung der Betätigung gewährleistet und Partizipation ermöglicht, auch wenn durch Training oder Veränderung der Betätigung sich keine Verbesserung erzielen lässt.

Insbesondere bei einer degenerativen Erkrankung, die von körperlichem Abbau und sozialem Rückzug geprägt ist, ist es wichtig, die Optionen der Adaptation auszuschöpfen. Dazu muss die

Therapeutin die genauen Kontextfaktoren kennen und in ihre Therapieplanung einbeziehen. Zugleich sollte die Therapeutin eine große Auswahl an Mitteln kennen, um die Kontextfaktoren zu verändern. Dazu zählen die Beratung der Angehörigen, das in Betracht ziehen von Hilfsmitteln sowie die Wohnraumberatung. Um dem Klienten das Aufstehen aus dem Stuhl zu ermöglichen, ist z. B. ein Austausch des Stuhles denkbar. Ein Stuhl, der nicht wegrutscht, sondern stabil steht, und außerdem eine erhöhte Sitzfläche bietet, erleichtert das Aufstehen enorm. Oder die Angehörige muss angeleitet werden, wie er dem Betroffenen beim Aufstehen die beste Unterstützung geben kann. Z. B. nicht unter der Achsel nach oben ziehen, sondern dafür sorgen, dass die Füße unter, nicht vor, dem Körper stehen. Der Angehörige sollte zur Sicherung vor dem Betroffenen stehen. Auch ein Haltegriff an der Wand neben dem Stuhl ist eine mögliche Adaptation der Umwelt, die zielführend sein kann. Für Mehr zum Thema Kontextfaktoren verändern/Adaptation siehe Kap. 15.

11.5 Komplette Betätigung trainieren

(siehe Abb. 4.4 unten im Oval)

Im Anschluss an die vier Interventionsformen „Performance-Skill trainieren", „Betätigung verändern", „Körperfunktionen trainieren" oder „Kontextfaktoren verändern", muss der Transfer in den Alltag geschehen, indem die Betätigung als Ganzes trainiert wird. So ist die Verbindung der therapeutischen Intervention zum gewählten Betätigungsziel für den Klienten transparent. Er erkennt, dass durch das repetitive Training einer Bewegungseinheit, das Verändern von Kleinigkeiten im Handlungsablauf, das Training von abstrakten Körperfunktionen oder die Adaptation der Umwelt, die komplette Betätigung am Ende besser gelingt. Gleichzeitig können Therapeutin und Klient überprüfen, ob der Klient seinem Ziel näherkommt, oder ob evtl. ein weiteres Instrument eingesetzt werden muss bzw. etwas an der Interventionsart verändert werden sollte. Mehr Informationen zum Thema „Komplette Betätigung trainieren" ist in Kap. 16 zu finden.

> Der therapeutische Prozess ist ein konstantes Reflektieren und Anpassen.

Dem dynamischen Prozess ist immer das bedeutungsvolle Betätigungsziel übergeordnet, welches von der Therapeutin und vom Klienten fortwährend im Blick behalten wird. So führt der Klient das Aufstehen vom Stuhl am Ende der Therapiestunde ohne Anleitung oder Hilfestellung der Therapeutin nochmals durch. Der Klient erhält die Chance, das Geübte oder Veränderte in der Betätigung einzusetzen. Bei Bedarf können weitere notwendige Veränderungen besprochen werden, wie einen Angehörigen zur Sicherung neben sich stehen zu haben.

Literatur und weiterführende Literatur

Aragon A, Kings J (2018) Occupational therapy for people with Parkinson's, the Royal College of Occupational Therapists Specialist Section – Neurological Practice, London

Foster ER, Bedekar M, Tickle-Degnen L (2014) Systematic review of the effectiveness of occupational therapy-related interventions for people with Parkinson's disease. Am J Occup Ther 68(1):39–49. https://doi.org/10.5014/ajot.2014.008706. PMID: 24367954; PMCID: PMC4413458

Law M (2002) Participation in the occupations of everyday life. Am J Occup Ther 56(6):640–649. https://doi.org/10.5014/ajot.56.6.640

Law M, Baptiste S, Mills J (1995) Client-centred practice: what does it mean and does it make a difference? Can J Occup Ther 62(5):250–257. https://doi.org/10.1177/000841749506200504. PMID: 10152881.

Law M, Steinwender S, Leclair L (1998) Occupation, health and well-being. Can J Occup Ther 65(2):81–91. https://doi.org/10.1177/000841749806500204

Murphy S, Tickle-Degnen L (2001) The effectiveness of occupational therapy–related treatments for persons with Parkinson's disease: a meta-analytic review. Am J Occup Ther 55(4):385–392. https://doi.org/10.5014/ajot.55.4.385

Radder DLM, Sturkenboom IH, van Nimwegen M, Keus SH, Bloem BR, de Vries NM (2017) Physical therapy and occupational therapy in Parkinson's disease. Int J Neurosci 127(10):930–943. https://doi.org/10.1080/00207454.2016.1275617

Stadler-Grillmaier J (2007) ENOTHE-Projekt „ET-Fachterminologie" – Beitrag zur Entwicklung einer (deutschen) Fachsprache in der Ergotherapie. Ergoscience 2:100–106. https://doi.org/10.1055/s-2007-963236, Georg Thieme KG, Stuttgart/New York

Sturkenboom I, Thijssen M, Gons-van Elsacker J, Jansen I, Maasdam A, Schulten M, Vijver-Visser D, Steultjens E, Bloem B, Munneke M (2008) Guidelines for occupational therapy in Parkinson's disease rehabilitation. ParkinsonNet/NPF, Nijmegen/Miami

12 Entscheidung für Intervention

Beispiel

Die Tasse rutscht, wie in Zeitlupe, seitlich vom Teller herunter und fällt krachend zu Boden. Herr N. beschimpft sich selber: „Wie kann man nur so blöd sein!", er greift wütend den Teller und zerschmettert ihn auch am Boden. Später am Nachmittag kommt er in die Küche. Der Kühlschrank steht auf. Herr N. schlägt sich selber auf den Oberschenkel „Schon wieder! Immer lässt du den Kühlschrank auf! Du A … loch!" Ein paar Tage später will Herr N. sich sein Insulin spritzen. Aber wo ist die Spritze? Gerade war sie noch da. Hektisch sucht er auf dem Tisch, unter den Papieren, im Regal und auf dem Boden. Verschwunden. „Das kann doch nicht wahr sein" murmelt er, „du Idiot!". Als oberstes Ziel sagt Herr N. der Therapeutin: „Wieder besser mit mir selber umgehen." ◀

Welche Interventionsmethoden in welcher Kombination und Reihenfolge umgesetzt werden, fällt in die Expertise des Therapeuten und kann nicht pauschal festgelegt werden. Die flexible und individuelle Kombination verschiedener Interventionen macht sogar die einzigartige ergotherapeutische Wirkungsweise aus und sollte ausdrücklich das Mittel der Wahl sein. Für eine verbesserte Anschaulichkeit und zur Strukturierung der ergotherapeutischen Arbeit, wird die Interventionsmöglichkeiten in fünf Bereiche unterteilt:

1. Performance-Skills trainieren
2. Betätigung verändern/kompensieren
3. Körperfunktionen trainieren
4. Kontext verändern/adaptieren
5. Komplette Betätigung trainieren

(siehe „Perfect fit" Abb. 4.4)

Um die adäquate Interventionsart für die Klientin festzulegen, sollten folgenden Punkte beachtet werden:

1. Krankheitsphase
2. Kognitive Kompetenzen der Klientin
3. Prognostische Einschätzung des Therapeuten
4. Grad der Motivation
5. Zeitaufwand
6. Wunsch der Klientin
7. Wunsch betroffener Dritter (Angehörige, Pflege)

12.1 Krankheitsphase

In frühen Krankheitsphasen der Parkinson-Erkrankung ist die zerebrale Flexibilität meist noch nicht eingeschränkt. Trophische Faktoren, die Durchblutung des Gehirns, das Immunsystem, die Neurogenese und der Stoffwechsel sind weitgehend funktionsfähig und tragen zu einer gesunden Gehirnstruktur bei, sodass der Abbau der dopaminergen Zellen durch Restrukturierung im Gehirn teilweise kompensiert werden kann. Diese

A. Orellana, *Betätigungsorientierte Ergotherapie bei Morbus Parkinson*,
https://doi.org/10.1007/978-3-662-62583-5_12

Tatsache trägt maßgeblich zur Entscheidungsfindung der Intervention bei, denn eine trainierende Therapie hat wesentlich größere Erfolgschancen bei einem Gehirn, in dem Neuroplastizität und damit das Lernen noch gut möglich ist.

Auch die Motivation einer Klientin, die sich in einem frühen Stadium ihrer Krankheit befindet, ist meist wesentlich größer. Verständlicherweise sinkt die Bereitschaft vieler Klientinnen, nach zahlreichen Rehabilitationsmaßnahmen, therapeutischen Behandlungen und medizinischen Interventionen, bei der aktuellen Therapie wieder alles zu geben. Es kann eine sog. Therapiemüdigkeit eintreten. Dies ist ein natürlicher Prozess und sollte vom Therapeuten wertfrei als solcher gesehen werden. Folglich führt eine frühe Krankheitsphase häufig zu einer eher aktiven Therapie (1. Betätigung trainieren oder 3. Körperfunktionen trainieren) eine spätere Krankheitsphase eher zu einer aktiven Therapie mit weniger Intensität (2. Betätigung verändern/kompensieren) oder passiveren Therapie (4. Kontext verändern/adaptieren).

12.2 Kognitive Kompetenzen der Klientinnen

Von Patientin zu Patientin variiert die Ausprägung der Demenz stark – von keiner Einschränkung bis zu schwersten kognitiven Beeinträchtigungen. Bei einer demenziellen Entwicklung wird von einer geringen Retention von neu gelernten Verhaltensweisen ausgegangen. Das heißt, dass das Beüben einer Betätigung selten zu einer Verbesserung der Betätigung führen wird, da im Prozess des Erlernens, der Abspeicherung und des Abrufs mit Einschränkungen gerechnet werden muss. Wenn der Therapeut unsicher ist, wie gut die Lernfähigkeit der Klientin noch ist, wird dazu geraten, eine Probeeinheit durchzuführen. In dieser kann durch repetitive, aktive Durchführung (nicht durch Erklären) der Betätigung das prozedurale Lernen aktiviert werden und der Therapeut bekommt ein Gefühl dafür, ob es eine zielführende Interventionsmöglichkeit ist. Ansonsten ist eine kompensatorisch-adaptive Therapie (2. und 4.) am sinnvollsten.

12.3 Prognostische Einschätzung des Therapeuten

Eine Prognose zur Wirkungsfähigkeit der Therapie ist für Therapeuten ein schwieriger, aber notwendiger Teil der Arbeit. Mit zunehmender Berufserfahrung nimmt die Genauigkeit der Einschätzung zu. Bei Nachfragen seitens Patientinnen und Angehörigen nach der Prognose, z. B. „Kann das wieder besser werden?" oder „Bringt das überhaupt noch etwas?", muss der Therapeut sorgfältig abwägen, wie er seine Antwort formuliert, um weder falsche Hoffnungen zu wecken noch die Motivation zu dämpfen. Für die Therapie eine klare prognostische Einschätzung zu treffen ist dagegen notwendig, um einen therapeutischen Leitfaden zu haben, die therapeutischen Mittel zu begründen und beides der Klientin und angrenzenden Berufsgruppen klar zu kommunizieren. In diese therapeutische Prognose fließen verschiedene Argumente:

- Krankheitsphase
- Demenzielle Entwicklung
- Einschätzung des Arztes
- Literatur und Studien zum Thema
- Bisherige Erfahrung des Therapeuten
- Motivation und Disziplin der Klientin

Nach Abwägung der o. g. Punkte fasst der Therapeut seine Erkenntnisse zusammen, um eine Entscheidung für eine der fünf Interventionsmöglichkeiten zu treffen.

12.4 Grad der Motivation

Herabgesetzte Motivation
Eine fehlende oder herabgesetzte Motivation der Klientin, sich aktiv an der Therapie zu beteiligen, kann eine Vielzahl an Gründen haben.

- Fatigue
- Depressive Verstimmung
- Zweifel am Outcome („Das bringt doch eh alles nichts")
- Mangelndes Verständnis oder Vergessen

- Therapeutischer Ansatz richtet sich nicht nach dem Ziel der Klientin
- Fehlen einer therapeutischen Beziehung
- Generelle Zufriedenheit mit aktueller Situation

Die Frage, inwieweit der Therapeut versuchen sollte, die Motivation der Klientin zu erhöhen, hängt mit den oben aufgelisteten Ursachen für den mangelnden Antrieb zusammen und sollte sensibel gehandhabt werden. Fakt ist: Mit einem Menschen ohne Motivation kann keine effektive Therapie durchgeführt werden, da ein Negativkreislauf entsteht (siehe Abb. 12.1).

▶ Die intrinsische Motivation der Klientin ist eine Grundbedingung für eine erfolgreiche Therapie.

Um einen Negativkreislauf zu vermeiden, muss der Therapeut die Ursache des Motivationsmangels ermitteln. Da jede Therapiesituation individuell zu betrachten ist, können hier nur Denkanstöße gegeben werden. Lösungen für mangelnde Motivation müssen immer klienten- und kontextspezifisch gefunden werden (siehe Tab. 12.1).

Hoher Grad der Motivation

Besonders in frühen Krankheitsphasen oder nach einer medikamentösen Veränderung oder Tiefen

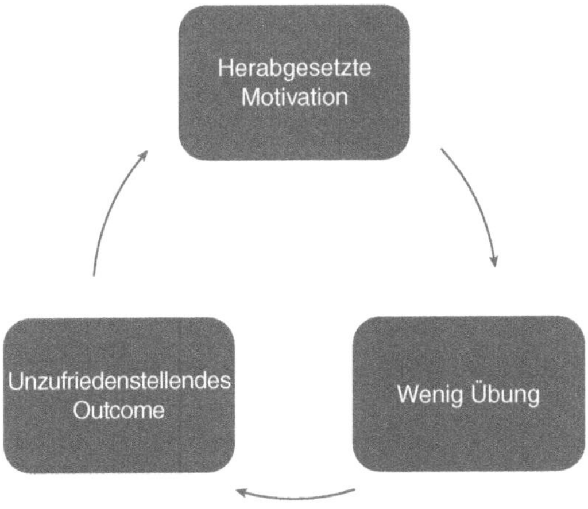

Abb. 12.1 Negativkreislauf der herabgesetzten Motivation

Tab. 12.1 Gedankenansätze zur Lösungsfindung bei herabgesetzter intrinsischer Motivation der Klientin

Ursache für herabgesetzte Motivation	Lösungsvorschlag
Fatigue	• Umstellung der Medikamente • Zeitliche Veränderung der Medikamenteneinnahme • Zeitliche Umstellung der Therapie • Veränderung der Tagesstrukturierung (siehe Abschn. 14.8.3) • Passive Teilhabe ermöglichen • In Abschn. 14.11 ist eine ausführliche Beschreibung der Intervention bei Fatigue zu finden.
Depressive Verstimmung	• Umstellung der Medikamente • Siehe Abschn. 14.10, Depressionen und Ängste • Passive Teilhabe ermöglichen
Zweifel am Outcome („Das bringt doch eh alles nichts.“)	• Abgabe der Verantwortung an Klientin • Auseinandersetzung mit Gründen für die Zweifel • Erklärung, warum Ergotherapie sinnvoll und wissenschaftliche Studienlage • Absetzen der Therapie, evtl. Wiederaufnahme bei Meinungsänderung
Mangelndes Verständnis oder Vergessen	• Erklärung, warum Ergotherapie sinnvoll und wissenschaftliche Studienlage • Bezug zum Klientenziel herstellen, • „Einfach beginnen“. Durch das **Tun** positiven Effekt erfahren • Ziele visualisieren mit Bildern und Schlagwörtern
Therapeutischer Ansatz richtet sich nicht nach dem Ziel der Klientin	• Zurück zur klientenzentrierten Zielfindung siehe Kap. 5 und 8
Fehlen einer therapeutischen Beziehung	• An therapeutischer Beziehung arbeiten (siehe Abschn. 10.2 positive Einflussfaktoren: Vertrauen in therapeutische Kompetenz) • Therapeutenwechsel
Generelle Zufriedenheit mit aktueller Situation, kein Leidensdruck	• Zurück zur Zielfindung siehe Kap. 5 und 8 • Bei Überlastung von Angehörigen, Fokus auf Angehörige richten • Akzeptanz und Absetzen der Ergotherapie

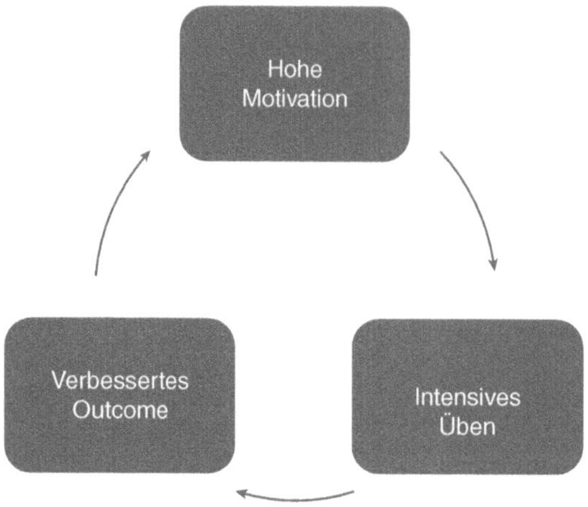

Abb. 12.2 Positiver Motivationskreislauf

Hirnstimulation haben Klientinnen häufig einen hohen Grad an Motivation. Die Plastizität des Gehirns und damit das Erlernen von Neuem ist eng mit den Emotionen verbunden. Je freudiger und inspirierter der Mensch an eine Aufgabe herangeht, desto mehr Synapsen werden gebildet und desto mehr Neurotransmitter werden ausgeschüttet. Mit diesen Klientinnen ist ein aktives Üben der Betätigung oder einzelner Körperfunktionen bedeutend effektiver als bei herabgesetzter Motivation. So kann sich ein positiver Kreislauf entwickeln (siehe Abb. 12.2).

Zusammenfassend kann festgestellt werden, dass ein hoher Grad an Motivation für **übende** Therapieformen spricht (1. Betätigung trainieren, 3. Körperfunktionen trainieren). Bei einem niedrigen Grad an Motivation sollte zunächst die Ursache identifiziert werden, um sich in Zusammenarbeit mit der Klientin damit auseinanderzusetzen. Wenn die Motivation niedrig bleibt, werden **aktive** Therapieformen **mit weniger Intensität** (2. Betätigung verändern/kompensieren) oder eher **passive, kompensatorische** Therapien bevorzugt (4. Kontextfaktoren verändern/adaptieren).

12.5 Zeitaufwand

Je nach Setting und Dringlichkeit kann der Zeitfaktor für die erste Entscheidung, welche Therapieform einzuleiten ist, ausschlaggebend sein.

- **Aktuelle Situation:** Ist der von der Klientin genannte Betätigungswunsch an den aktuellen Kontext gebunden, wird meist nach einer schnellen Lösung gesucht, also eine Veränderung der Kontextfaktoren.
  - **Beispiel:** Die Klientin ist in der Klinik durch die schnelle Abfolge von Therapien gestresst, weil sie nicht zu spät kommen möchte.
  - **Therapeutische Entscheidung:** Veränderung der Kontextfaktoren – Die Abfolge der Therapieeinheiten wird, nach Absprache im Team, umstrukturiert.
- **Zeitlimit:** Muss das Ziel zu einem bestimmten Zeitpunkt erreicht werden, wird eine kurzfristige therapeutische Intervention gewählt.
  - **Beispiel:** Klientin hat in wenigen Tagen einen Banktermin und hat Sorge, wichtige Fragen zu vergessen.
  - **Therapeutische Entscheidung:** Veränderung der Kontextfaktoren – Therapeut und Klientin denken gemeinsam über Fragen nach und schreiben eine Liste als Gedächtnisstütze.
- **Längerfristige Veränderung gewünscht:** Eine ähnliche Situation tritt regelmäßig auf und soll auf längere Sicht verbessert werden.
  - **Beispiel:** Die Klientin möchte generell bei behördlichen Terminen besser vorbereitet sein.
  - **Therapeutische Entscheidung:** Betätigung verändern – Strategien zur Verbesserung der Strukturierung und Merkhilfen selbst erstellen (Kalenderführung, Notizzettel …)
  - **Oder therapeutische Entscheidung:** Betätigung trainieren – im Rollenspiel werden verschiedene Termine durchgespielt und anschließend besprochen.

12.6 Wunsch der Klientin

Bei einer klientenzentrierten Arbeitsweise wird im Verlauf der kompletten Therapie eine kooperative Beziehung zur Klientin beibehalten. Wenn der Ergotherapeut die Klientin als „Spezialisten für ihre Situation“ anerkennt, muss auch die Entscheidungsfindung, welche Interventionsart angewandt wird, mit ihr zusammen erfolgen. Sobald der Therapeut die anderen Faktoren abgeklärt hat, macht er für die Klientin seine Herangehensweise transparent und erfragt deren Sichtweise. Eine offene Neugier hilft dem Therapeuten dabei, die Einstellungen und Wünsche der Klientin wirklich zu verstehen und ernst zu nehmen. Nicht selten überraschen die Klientinnen mit ihrem Witz, ihrer präzisen Einsicht und mit kreativen Ideen, die gewinnbringend auf die Therapie einwirken.

▶ Durch die Erfragung der Wünsche, erfährt die Klientin eine Wertschätzung seitens des Therapeuten und ist sicherlich bereit, sich verstärkt aktiv zu involvieren und motiviert mitzuarbeiten.

Beispiele für Fragen an die Klientin können sein:

- „Ich habe mir seit der letzten Therapie Gedanken zu den Möglichkeiten gemacht, um gemeinsam an Ihrem Ziel zu arbeiten. Aber zuerst würde mich interessieren, was Sie für Ideen haben."
- „Mir ist Ihre Sicherheit beim Laufen wichtig. Können Sie sich vorstellen, einen Rollator auszuprobieren?"
- „Sie sagten ja, das Essen ist Ihnen wichtig. Haben Sie zu Hause schon verschiedene Möglichkeiten ausprobiert?"
- „Ich denke, Sie können mit täglichem intensiven Üben Ihre Handschrift wieder leserlich machen. Sind Sie dazu motiviert? Oder sollen wir uns lieber mit anderen Möglichkeiten befassen, wie der Nutzung eines Computers?"

12.7 Wunsch betroffener Dritter

Wenn der Begriff „Klientin" weiter gefasst wird und – statt nur den Patientinnen – auch die nahen Angehörigen oder Pflegekräfte mit einem Betätigungsanliegen umfasst, werden deren Wünsche und Meinungen natürlich auch in die Therapie einbezogen. Durch das tägliche Zusammensein oft über Jahre erfasst der Angehörige oder Pflegende das Leben der Parkinson-Betroffenen sehr detailliert. So können sie wertvolle Einsichten zur Therapie beisteuern, die der Therapeut durch seine „Außensicht" nicht erkennen kann, z. B. ob die Eigenübungen wirklich durchgeführt werden, womit die Betroffene ihren Alltag füllt, ob sich eine demenzielle Entwicklung im Alltag bemerkbar macht, wie stark die Belastung für den Angehörigen ist …

Bei der Befragung von Dritten muss immer mit Bedacht vorgegangen werden und aufmerksam zwischen eigenen Interessen und Interessen im Sinne der Patientin unterschieden werden. Auch auf problematische Dynamiken zwischen Pflegenden und Patientin oder komplizierte Abhängigkeitsbeziehungen sollte der Therapeut achten und entsprechend den Fokus immer bei der Klientin lassen.

Beispiel

Um das Ziel von Herrn N. greifbarer zu machen und es konkret auf den Alltag zu beziehen, erfragt die Therapeutin, wann genau er sich in der Woche danach schlecht behandelt hat. Herr N. berichtet von dem Vorfall mit dem Kühlschrank. Da gedankliche Prozesse eine Körperfunktion darstellen, hat die Therapeutin die Hypothese, dass ein Umdenken stattfinden kann, damit Herr N. sich trotz des offen gelassenen Kühlschranks nicht mehr selbst beschimpft (prognostische Einschätzung der Therapeutin). Außerdem ist Herr N. sehr offen dafür, sich selbst zu reflektieren (Motivation).

Die Therapeutin entscheidet sich deshalb für die Interventionsart **Körperfunktion trainieren**. Gemeinsam erarbeiten sie eine liebevollere Kommunikation mit sich selbst, wenn er nächstes Mal den Kühlschrank offenlässt. Diese eine Situation im Leben von Herrn N. ist nun entschärft, aber es gibt noch mehr.

Herr N. berichtet von der Situation mit der Tasse, die zu Boden fiel, und wie er in seiner Wut den Teller hinterherschmiss. Der Therapeutin fällt auf, dass das Tragen des Tellers und der Tasse zur Küche für Herrn N., der mit Bradykinese am Stock geht (Krankheitsphase), zu schwierig ist und auch durch Training nicht wesentlich verbessert werden kann (prognostische Einschätzung der Therapeutin). Sie entscheidet sich für die Interventionsart **Kontextfaktoren verändern.** In Zukunft nutzt Herr N. einen Servierwagen, um Geschirr zwischen Küche und Esstisch zu transportieren.

Im dritten Beispiel, das Herr N. nennt, geht es um die Situation mit der verlorenen Spritze. Zunächst hat die Therapeutin die Hypothese, dass durch eine bessere Ordnung und Struktur die Spritze nicht verloren gehen würde (**Kontextfaktoren verändern**). Auf Nachfrage erkennt sie jedoch, dass Herr N. eine klare Struktur hat und über seinen Diabetes genau Buch führt, er jedoch durch seine beginnende Parkinson-Demenz (kognitive Kompetenzen des Klienten) hin und wieder durcheinanderkommt. Außerdem möchte Herr N. die Struktur nicht ändern, da er gut damit zurechtkommt (Wunsch des Klienten). Also entscheidet sich die Therapeutin für die **Veränderung der Betätigung**. Die Therapeutin zeigt Herrn N. eine Atemübung, die er anwenden kann, wenn er spürt, dass sein Stresspegel steigt. Sie besprechen, dass er sich in Situationen, in denen er sich aufregt, zuerst hinsetzen und durchatmen soll, um dann in Ruhe weiterhandeln zu können – z. B. zu überlegen, wo er die Spritze das letzte Mal hatte. ◀

Literatur und weiterführende Literatur

Fischer A, Marterella A (2019) Powerful Practice. CIOTS, Fort Collins, S 63–72, 207–211

Foster ER, Bedekar M, Tickle-Degnen L (2014) Systematic review of the effectiveness of occupational therapy-related interventions for people with Parkinson's disease. Am J Occup Ther 68(1):39–49. https://doi.org/10.5014/ajot.2014.008706. PMID: 24367954; PMCID: PMC4413458

Law M (2002) Participation in the occupations of everyday life. Am J Occup Ther 56(6):640–649. https://doi.org/10.5014/ajot.56.6.640

Law M, Baptiste S, Mills J (1995) Client-centred practice: what does it mean and does it make a difference? Can J Occup Ther 62(5):250–257. https://doi.org/10.1177/000841749506200504. PMID: 10152881.

Law M, Steinwender S, Leclair L (1998) Occupation, health and well-being. Can J Occup Ther 65(2):81–91. https://doi.org/10.1177/000841749806500204

Radder DLM, Sturkenboom IH, van Nimwegen M, Keus SH, Bloem BR, de Vries NM (2017) Physical therapy and occupational therapy in Parkinson's disease. Int J Neurosci 127(10):930–943. https://doi.org/10.1080/00207454.2016.1275617

Robertson D, Warrender F, Barnard S (2015) The critical occupational therapy practitioner: how to define expertise? Aust Occup Ther J 62:68–71. https://doi.org/10.1111/1440-1630.12157

Sturkenboom I, Thijssen M, Gons-van Elsacker J, Jansen I, Maasdam A, Schulten M, Vijver-Visser D, Steultjens E, Bloem B, Munneke M (2008) Guidelines for occupational therapy in Parkinson's disease rehabilitation. ParkinsonNet/NPF, Nijmegen/Miami

Tenison E, Smink A, Redwood S, Darweesh S, Cottle H, van Halteren A, Haak P, Hamlin R, Ypinga J, Bloem B, Ben-Shlomo Y, Munneke M, Henderson E (2020) Proactive and integrated management and empowerment in Parkinson's disease: designing a new model of care. Parkinson's Dis:1–11. https://doi.org/10.1155/2020/8673087

13 Performance-Skills (Performanzfertigkeiten) trainieren

(siehe Abb. 4.4 Spalte 1)

Beispiel

Frau F., 79 Jahre, alleinlebend und mit einem aktiven Sozialleben, trägt häufig und leidenschaftlich Kleider. Nun kommt sie seit kurzem nicht mehr ganz an die Kleiderstange ihres Kleiderschranks heran und möchte nicht jedes Mal auf eine Trittleiter steigen. Deshalb sammeln sich die feinen Kleider nun auf der Sessellehne in ihrem Schlafzimmer. ◄

Ein Performance-Skill (Performanzfertigkeit) ist die kleinste mögliche Bewegungseinheit innerhalb einer Betätigung. Am Beispiel „trinken" können folgende Performance-Skills erkannt werden:

1. Blick zum Glas wenden
2. Hand zielgerichtet zum Glas bewegen
3. Hand öffnen
4. Glas greifen
5. Hand mit Glas zum Mund führen
6. Glas kippen und trinken
7. Schlucken
8. Hand mit Glas wieder auf Tisch stellen
9. Hand öffnen
10. Arm und Hand wieder in Ruheposition ablegen

Hat die Therapeutin ein problematisches Performance-Skill identifiziert, spricht man vom Break-Down-Point. Es muss nicht zwingend die komplette Betätigung geübt werden, um eine zufriedenstellende Ausführung zu erreichen. Es kann genügen, nur am Break-Down-Point zu üben. Sobald dieser gelingt und wieder in die gesamte Betätigung integriert wird, sollte auch sie gelingen. Es werden vier Komponenten definiert, die im Training eines Performance-Skills bei Menschen mit M. Parkinson enthalten sein müssen:

1. betätigungsspezifisch
2. repetitiv
3. intensiv
4. mit Referenzflächen

13.1 Betätigungsspezifisch

Einige Studien belegen, dass abstraktes Üben einer Bewegung nicht die beste Möglichkeit ist, um Alltagshandlungen zu verbessern (siehe Abschn. 4.1). Somit ist das Üben mit sog. Therapiemitteln, wie Stangen, Bällen, Ringen und Knete, nicht sinnvoll und sollte höchstens ergänzend eingesetzt werden. Vielmehr muss die Therapiesituation genau – oder so genau wie möglich – der Betätigung im Alltag des Klienten gleichen.

Ergänzende Information Die elektronische Version dieses Kapitels enthält Zusatzmaterial, auf das über folgenden Link zugegriffen werden kann https://doi.org/10.1007/978-3-662-62583-5_13. Die Videos lassen sich durch Anklicken des DOI Links in der Legende einer entsprechenden Abbildung abspielen, oder indem Sie diesen Link mit der SN More Media App scannen.

A. Orellana, *Betätigungsorientierte Ergotherapie bei Morbus Parkinson*,
https://doi.org/10.1007/978-3-662-62583-5_13

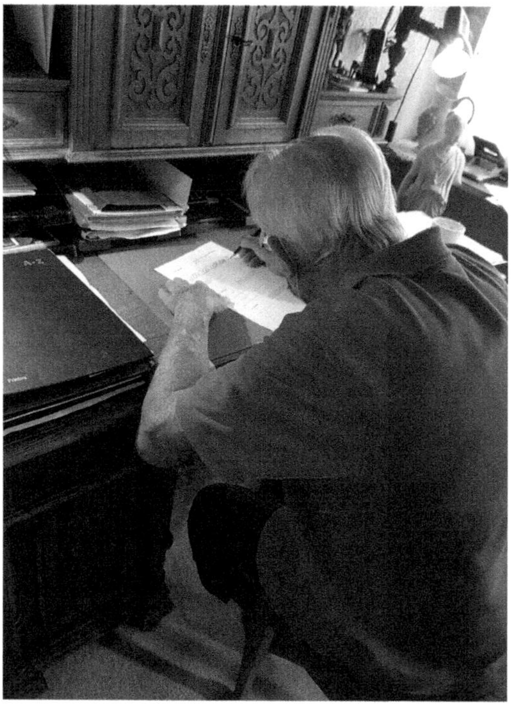

Abb. 13.1 Betätigungsspezifisch – der Klient übt das Schreiben in seinem gewohnten Kontext „Büro“

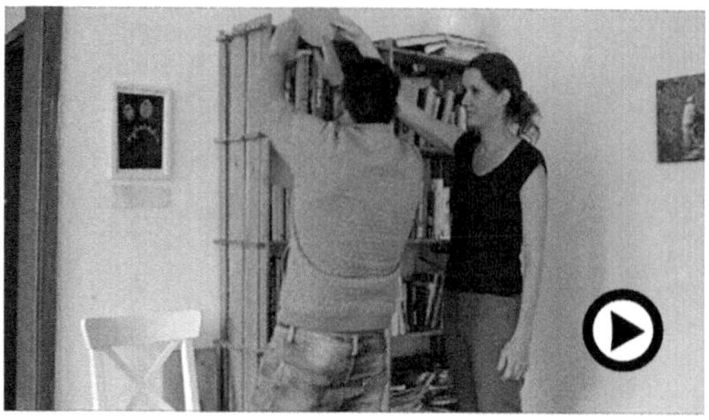

Abb. 13.2 Betätigung: Korb auf Regal abstellen. Performance-Skill: Aufrichten mit Anheben des Korbes über Kopf – repetitiv, intensiv und mit Referenzflächen. Zunächst simplifiziert, ohne Korb … (▶ https://doi.org/10.1007/000-2x8)

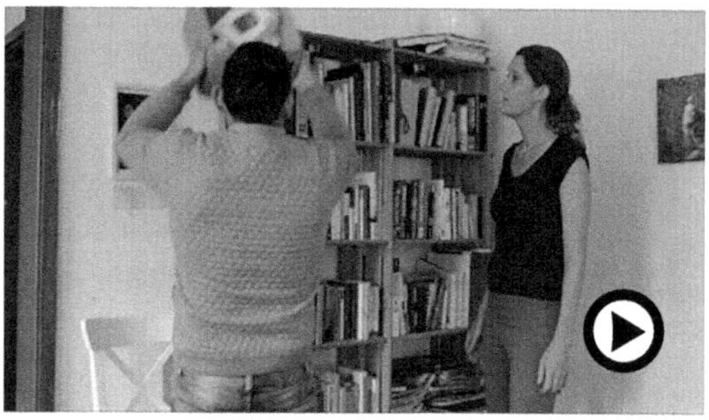

Abb. 13.3 … dann Performance-Skill mit Korb (▶ https://doi.org/10.1007/000-2x7)

Es wird also im selben Kontext mit den Materialien, Werkzeugen und Personen geübt, die auch sonst gegeben sind (s. Abb. 13.1).

Um das intensive Üben zu ermöglichen, kann es hilfreich sein, die Betätigung während des Trainings zu vereinfachen und den Break-Down-Point isoliert zu üben. Der Break-Down-Point ist der Moment, an dem die Betätigung scheitert oder eingeschränkt durchführbar ist (siehe Kap. 6).

Beispiele:

- **Betätigung:** Korb auf Regal stellen
  - **Break-Down-Point:** Aufrichtung beim nach oben Strecken
  - Vereinfachung: Um die Schnelligkeit der Bewegung zu ermöglichen, wird das Platzieren des Korbes zunächst nicht mit geübt. Der Klient übt nur die schnelle Bewegung der Aufrichtung samt Streckung der Arme mit dem gefüllten Korb (siehe Video 13.2 in Abb. 13.2 und Video 13.3 in Abb. 13.3).
- **Betätigung:** Aufstehen aus dem Bett ohne Hilfe
  - **Break-Down-Point:**
    1. Drehen im Bett
    2. Stresssteigerung durch Ehepartnerin
  - **Vereinfachung:** Die Betätigung „Aufstehen aus dem Bett“ wird im Alltag mit der Ehefrau zur Sicherung durchgeführt. In der Therapie trennt die Ergotherapeutin die beiden Break-Down-Points voneinander, um sich zuerst auf die motorische Komponente konzentrieren zu können. Später wird er eine intensive Angehörigenberatung durchführen, um das Vorgehen der Ehefrau in der Situation zu besprechen und zu trainieren. So wird die Partnerin gebeten, zunächst beim Training nicht anwesend zu sein.
- **Betätigung:** Löffeln der Suppe am Familientisch

- **Break-Down-Point:** Suppe wird durch Tremor vom Löffel verschüttet
- **Vereinfachung:** Die Therapeutin übt mit dem Klienten zunächst mit leerem Löffel die Bewegungsabfolge mit viel Unterstützungsfläche. Das heißt, der Ellenbogen wird aufgestützt und der rechte Arm wird mit der linken Hand stabilisiert. Sobald dieser Bewegungsablauf durch das Training routiniert ist, wird die Komponente der Suppe dazu genommen. Auch wird das Essen am Familientisch zunächst zurückgestellt, um die Ablenkungsfaktoren zu reduzieren. Nach dem schrittweisen Einüben der Betätigung ist das gemeinsame Essen am Tisch jedoch entscheidend. Denn nur, wenn diese erhöhte Anforderung vom Klienten bewältigt werden kann, ist das Ziel erreicht.

▶ Die Betätigung wird zwar **simplifiziert**, jedoch **nicht abstrahiert**.

Das abstrakte Üben als Ersatz oder als Vorbereitung für die tatsächliche Tätigkeit des Klienten, wurde lange in der ergotherapeutischen Ausbildung gelehrt und findet dementsprechend Anwendung in zahlreichen Institutionen. Es gibt jedoch wissenschaftliche Studien, die zeigen, dass kein Übertrag auf andere Tätigkeitsfelder stattfindet. Wenn der therapeutische Inhalt also „Knetübungen" ist, dann ist der Klient im Anschluss vielleicht der Meister der Knete – meistert jedoch nicht den Umgang mit Messer und Gabel. Andere Studien zeigen klar auf, dass das Trainieren einer konkreten Betätigung zu einer Verbesserung dieser Betätigung führt (siehe Kap. 4).

13.2 Repetitiv

Die zweite Komponente beim Training eines Performance-Skills ist die Repetition. Das Ziel beim Trainieren einer Betätigung ist die Veränderung des Verhaltens. Um dies zu erreichen, muss „Lernen" erfolgen. Lernen wird von Myers (2008) und Atkinson et al. (2000) als „durch Erfahrung entstandene, relativ überdauernde Verhaltensänderung" definiert. Auf neuronaler Ebene lässt sich „Lernen" als Strukturveränderung im Gehirn erkennen. Es entstehen neue neuronale Vernetzungen. Dazu gehören vor allem die Synapsenbildung, aber auch eine vermehrte Ausschüttung von Neurotransmittern und Neurogenese (die Bildung neuer Nervenzellen). Je mehr synaptische Verknüpfungen entstehen und sich durch Wiederholung festigen, desto besser kann das Erlernte in bereits bekanntes Verhalten integriert werden.

▶ Die Wiederholung (Repetition) ist beim Lernen ein ausschlaggebender Faktor. Durch Repetition werden die neuronalen Verbindungen verstärkt, wohingegen nicht genutzte Verbindungen verblassen.

Erfahrungsgemäß muss eine hohe Zahl an Wiederholungen hintereinander, ohne falsche Durchführung, erfolgen, um motorisches Lernen zu manifestieren. Wie häufig genau wiederholt werden muss, um eine Verhaltensänderung zu erreichen, hängt von mehreren Faktoren ab:

- Alter des Menschen
- Gehirngesundheit
- Aufmerksamkeit während des Trainings
- Motivation des Menschen
- Emotionale Einbindung/persönliche Wichtigkeit
- Medikamentenwirkung (z. B. L-Dopa bei M. Parkinson)

In der Fachliteratur werden unterschiedliche Angaben zu notwendigen Wiederholungszahlen gemacht. Die Zahlen liegen jedoch immer weit über denen, die die Klienten erfahrungsgemäß im Rahmen der Ergotherapie schaffen. Um einen Richtwert zu haben, wird von einer Repetitionszahl von 900 ausgegangen. Es sind also 900 richtige Wiederholungen einer Handlung hintereinander notwendig. Diese 900 Mal werden in kleine Übungsportionen aufgeteilt.

Mindestens 900 Wiederholungen in drei Wochen!

= 60× pro Tag, fünf Mal pro Woche

= 3 × 20 Mal pro Tag

Besser häufiger und kurz als einmal lange trainieren.

Erklärt die Therapeutin dem Klienten die Wichtigkeit der Repetition für ein erfolgreiches Outcome der Therapie, ist die Wahrscheinlichkeit höher, dass er dies auch in Eigenübungen zu Hause umsetzt. Die Angabe einer festen Anzahl der Wiederholungen motiviert zusätzlich, anstatt zu sagen „Üben Sie so häufig, wie es geht." Besonders junge Klienten oder Klienten, die musikalisch oder sportlich auf hohem Niveau geübt haben, zeigen ein großes Maß an Disziplin. Das repetitive Üben ist ihnen schon bekannt und vor allem die Erfahrung, dass die Repetition Erfolg ermöglicht.

▶ Eine Form der Motivation, um die 60 Wiederholungen pro Tag zu schaffen, kann ein Trainingskalender sein, in dem der Klient selbst das Training dokumentiert. Dazu werden für jeden Tag, an dem das Training 3 × 20 Mal durchgeführt wurde, ein Häkchen oder ein Smiley in den Kalender eingetragen.

Apps, z. B. „therapio", können den Klienten bei der Dokumentation unterstützen. Fitness-Armbänder werden meist als Schrittzähler genutzt. Da die Schritte jedoch anhand von Armschwungbewegungen gezählt werden, lassen sie sich, je nach Übung, auch zum Messen der Anzahl der Repetitionen nutzen.

13.3 Intensiv

Die dritte Komponente des Trainings eines Performance-Skills ist die Intensität. Dieses Attribut wird von Therapeutinnen oft unterschätzt, wird jedoch von einer zunehmenden Anzahl von Studien über motorische Therapien für M. Parkinson gestützt (Ebersbach et al. 2010; Uhrbrand et al. 2015; Farley et al. 2008. Um das Wort „intensiv" zu definieren, unterteilt man es in weitere Merkmale:

- aufmerksam,
- rhythmisch,
- mit großer Amplitude,
- mit Motivation.

Liest man sich die obigen Begriffe nochmal durch, fällt auf, dass sie das genaue Gegenteil der Merkmale der Parkinson-Erkrankung sind, die sich langsam, in sich gekehrt, arrhythmisch, reduziert und antriebsarm zeigt. Es wird also den Parkinson-Symptomen durch eine Umkehr ins Gegenteil entgegengewirkt.

Aufmerksam

Damit die Intensität des Trainings des Performance-Skills nicht nachlässt, muss der Klient mit seiner Aufmerksamkeit stets auf die Tätigkeit fokussiert sein. Folgende Faktoren können die Aufmerksamkeit positiv beeinflussen:

- Der Klient muss den Ablauf des Trainings verstehen.
- Es sollten keine ablenkenden Einflüsse (Angehörige, Fernseher, Mobiltelefon) einwirken.
- Eine allgemein gute Vigilanz des Klienten (Tageszeit, Ausgeruhtsein) unterstützt positiv.
- Ein äußerliches „Wecken" der Aufmerksamkeit durch Signalwörter wirkt unterstützend.

Rhythmisch

Rhythmus wird bei der Parkinson-Therapie schon lange eingesetzt. So sind die Musik- und Tanztherapie bewährte Therapiemethoden. Klienten berichten von einer „Leichtigkeit" und „Lockerheit", die sie schon lange nicht mehr erlebt haben. Auch wissenschaftlich lassen sich verbesserte Schrittlänge und verbesserte Beweglichkeit nachweisen (Hackney und Earhart 2009). Um einen rhythmischen Übungsablauf zu erstellen ist, wie oben beschrieben, eine Reduktion auf einen Performance-Skill und ein klarer Anfangs- und Endpunkt der zu übenden Bewegung notwendig. Bei langen, komplexeren Bewegungsabläufen ist ein rhythmisches Üben nicht möglich. Der Rhythmus kann verbal angeleitet werden

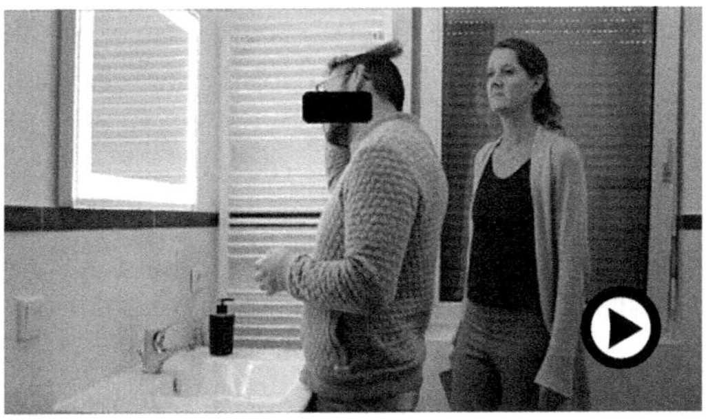

Abb. 13.4 Betätigung Haare bürsten. Break-Down-Point: Klient perseveriert, bürstet nicht am Hinterkopf (▶ https://doi.org/10.1007/000-2x6)

(siehe Video in Abb. 13.4) durch Klatschen, durch Klopfen vorgegeben bzw. mit Musik unterstützt werden oder die Therapeutin macht die Übung parallel mit. Die letzte Option animiert den Klienten sicherlich am meisten mit Energie weiter zu üben.

Mit großer Amplitude

Die Amplitude der Motorik nimmt im Verlauf der Krankheit immer weiter ab. Um diese Gegebenheit auszugleichen, werden die Performance-Skills mit bewusst großen, ausholenden Bewegungen trainiert. Dies erscheint den Klienten oftmals übertrieben. Durch ihre veränderte Wahrnehmung empfinden sie die Bewegung als übermäßig ausholend. Ermöglicht die Ergotherapeutin mit einem Spiegel oder einer Videoaufnahme einen visuellen Abgleich, stellen Klienten fest, dass die Bewegung im Normbereich liegt, wenn sie sich übermäßig groß anfühlt. Diese falsche Wahrnehmung kann durch wiederholtes Trainieren sowie verbale und visuelle Rückmeldung korrigiert werden.

▶ Um eine vergrößerte Amplitude zu erreichen können auch Bilder unterstützend sein.

- Gestikulieren – wie ein Dirigent
- Mimik – wie ein Clown
- Gehen – wie ein Soldat/König

Mit Motivation

Den Grundstein für die Eigenmotivation des Klienten hat die Therapeutin schon in der Assessmentphase gelegt, als sie mit dem Klienten zusammen ein Betätigungsziel erarbeitete, das diesem wichtig ist. Durch die bei der Parkinson-Erkrankung häufig auftretenden, abgeflachten Emotionen und depressiven Verstimmungen ist die Motivation, aktiv zu trainieren, häufig herabgesetzt. Es kann sogar dazu führen, dass ein neues Ziel oder eine andere (passivere) Therapiemethode gewählt werden müssen, um ein positives Outcome zu erzielen. Bevor dieser Weg eingeschlagen wird, sollte die Therapeutin ermitteln, ob die Motivation des Klienten extern angeregt werden kann. Dafür kann die Therapeutin folgende Methoden anwenden:

- Klient an Ziel erinnern
- Visualisierung des Ziels durch ein Bild
- Gedankliche Vorstellung, das Ziel schon erreicht zu haben
- Verbal motivierende Stichwörter (gut, weiter, super …)
- Messung des Erfolgs nach jeder Runde, um Verbesserung anzuzeigen
- Geleistete Wiederholungen der Übung dokumentieren (Motivationsplan)

Manche Klienten profitieren davon, wenn die Therapeutin motivierende kleine Cue-Wörter (Signalworte) nutzt. Da diese Art des Trainings wie „Antreiben“ oder „Drill“ wirken kann, ist eine vorherige Erklärung gegenüber dem Klienten und anderen Anwesenden unverzichtbar, um Unannehmlichkeiten vorzubeugen. Außerdem sollte auf eine äußerst freundliche Stimmlage und Mimik geachtet werden. Die beste Wortwahl beim Anspornen muss jede Therapeutin für sich herausfinden, damit es für sie und den Klienten animierend und natürlich ist. Im Video zu Abb. 13.2 ist ein Beispiel zu den Signalwörtern zu hören.

Es ist sinnvoll, die Nutzung von Signalwörtern intermittierend einzusetzen, das heißt, Pausen zu machen und die Signalwörter später wieder einzusetzen. So wird dem Umstand vorgebeugt, dass die Signalwörter Teil der Hintergrundgeräusche werden und nicht mehr bewusst wahrgenommen werden. Auf manche Klienten wirkt es ablenkend oder irritierend, wenn die Therapeutin Signalwörter nutzt. In diesem Fall kann es sinnvoll sein, nur zu Beginn der Übung ein Signalwort zu nutzen (z. B. „Und los!"). Obwohl die Intensität für das motorische Lernen wichtig ist, muss die Therapeutin darauf achten, dass der Klient nicht zu intensiv übt. In den europäischen Leitlinien für Physiotherapie (Keus et al. 2014) werden folgende Punkte genannt, bei denen das Training beendet werden sollte, und mit einem Arzt Rücksprache gehalten werden soll.

- Übelkeit
- Gefühl der Enge oder Schmerzen in der Brust, die länger als einige Minuten andauern
- Ungewöhnlich starke Atemlosigkeit, wie etwa mehr als 40 Atemzüge pro Minute
- Schwere Fatigue oder Dyspnoe
- Schwindel oder Benommenheit
- Das Gefühl, dass das Herz zusätzliche Schläge macht oder Schläge auslässt
- Schmerzen
- Kalter Schweiß

13.4 Mit Referenzflächen

Referenzflächen geben dem Klienten bei jeder erfolgreich durchgeführten Bewegung ein sensorisches, visuelles und auditives Feedback. Die Eigenwahrnehmung der Körperhaltung und der Motorik ist mit vermehrter Rigidität reduziert. Dies zeigt sich in der Verringerung der Amplitude der Bewegungen und ist auf eine Verarbeitungsstörung von propriozeptiven Reizen in den Basalganglien zurückzuführen. Bei repetitiven Bewegungen, z. B. Armschwung, Haare bürsten oder Schreiben, ist bei den ersten Ausführungen noch eine Amplitude im Normbereich zu beobachten, diese nimmt mit jeder Wiederholung etwas ab.

Die therapeutische Wirksamkeit der externen Fokussierung der Aufmerksamkeit wurde in einigen Studien belegt. Fordert man Menschen mit posturaler Instabilität und Ängsten auf, sich auf den Untergrund zu konzentrieren (nicht auf die Füße oder darauf geradezustehen) nimmt die posturale Stabilität zu und die Angst ab (Jazaeri et al. 2018). Auch auf das motorische Lernen bei Parkinson-Betroffenen hat die externe Fokussierung der Aufmerksamkeit eine positive Wirkung. So konnten Kakar et al. (2013) zeigen, dass die Aufforderung, beim Erlernen des Dartspielens sich auf den Dart, die Scheibe und den Flug des Darts zu fokussieren – anstatt auf die Handhaltung und Bewegung des Armes –, zu einer größeren Treffsicherheit führte.

Die Notwendigkeit der visuellen Kontrolle zur genauen Durchführung zielgerichteter Bewegungen mit der oberen Extremität wurde mehrfach bestätigt (Torres et al. 2011; Majsak et al. 1998; Adamovich et al. 2001)

Um die externe Fokussierung und visuelle Kontrolle der Bewegung zu unterstützen, werden Referenzflächen eingesetzt. Eine Referenzfläche sollte folgende Eigenschaften aufweisen:

- Idealgröße zwischen 15 cm und 25 cm Durchmesser: Laut einer Studie von Fernandez et al. (2018) besteht bei Parkinson-Kranken (wie auch bei gesunden Personen) eine gegenläufige Abhängigkeit von Schnelligkeit und Genauigkeit einer zielgerichteten Bewegung, das sog. speed-accuracy trade-off (Geschwindigkeit-Genauigkeit Abtausch). So wirkt sich eine kleine Referenzfläche negativ auf die Schnelligkeit der Bewegung aus.
- Klar visuell abgegrenzt, z. B. Farbkreis oder bestimmter Gegenstand (Schublade, Toaster …)
- Klarer sensorischer Reiz bei Berührung (fester Untergrund, nicht weich)
- Klarer auditiver Reiz bei Berührung (fester Untergrund, nicht weich)

Durch das klare visuelle Ziel und die klare sensorische und auditive Rückmeldung bei Berührung, kann der Klient selbständig kontrollieren, ob die Bewegung eine ausreichend große Amplitude hatte, und so seine eingeschränkte propriozeptive Eigenwahrnehmung kompensieren. Der Klient sollte dazu aufgefordert werden, jede Bewegung visuell zu verfolgen, da dies nachgewiesenermaßen die Zielgenauigkeit verbessert.

▶ Referenzflächen bieten dem Klienten klare visuelle, auditive und/oder sensorische Rückmeldung, dass die Bewegung mit ausreichender Amplitude durchgeführt wurde. Damit wird die Einschränkung der Propriozeption kompensiert.

Auch gesunde Menschen nutzen Referenzflächen im Alltag, ohne sich dessen bewusst zu sein. Es ist die sensorische, auditive und/oder visuelle Rückmeldung des Objektes, dass die Betätigung erfolgreich war, z. B.:

- Schließen der Tür: das Klacken des Türschlosses und der Widerstand des Türrahmens
- Haare kämmen: der Wegfall des Widerstandes der Bürste in den Haaren, sobald die Haare durchgekämmt sind, evtl. visuelle Kontrolle
- Aufhängen eines Bildes: die Gewichtabnahme durch den Nagel
- Licht geht an, wenn Lichtschalter betätigt wurde

Für das Training mit Parkinson-Klienten nutzen wir die vorhandenen Referenzflächen, machen sie dem Klienten bewusst und fügen zur Verstärkung der Rückmeldung bei Bedarf weitere hinzu, z. B.:

- **Haare kämmen**: Therapeutin hält ein Buch in den Nacken, um auditive und stärkere sensorische Rückmeldung zu erhalten, sobald die Haare durchgekämmt sind (siehe Video 13.5 in Abb. 13.5).
- **Aufrichtung**: Da gesunde Menschen die Rückmeldung nur aus den Propriozeptoren im Körper erhalten, Hinzunahme der Wand als sensorische Rückmeldung am Rücken (siehe Video 13.6 Abb. 13.6).
- **Schreiben**: Verstärkung der Linien, um visuelle Rückmeldung zu intensivieren (siehe Abb. 13.7).

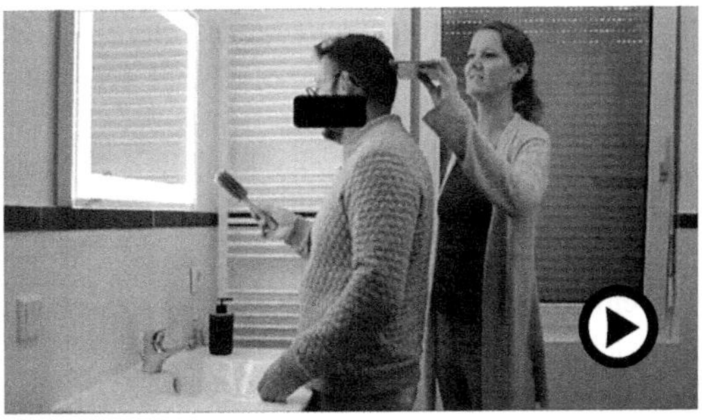

Abb. 13.5 Betätigung: Haare bürsten. Performance-Skill: Hinterkopf bürsten. Referenzfläche (Buch) (▶ https://doi.org/10.1007/000-2x9)

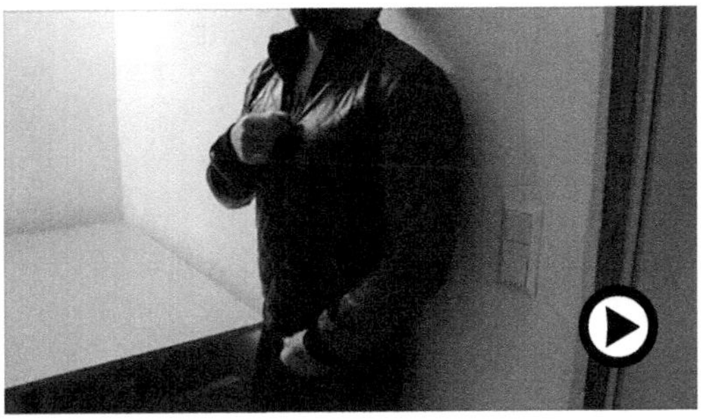

Abb. 13.6 Aufrichtung mit der Wand als Referenzfläche (▶ https://doi.org/10.1007/000-2xa)

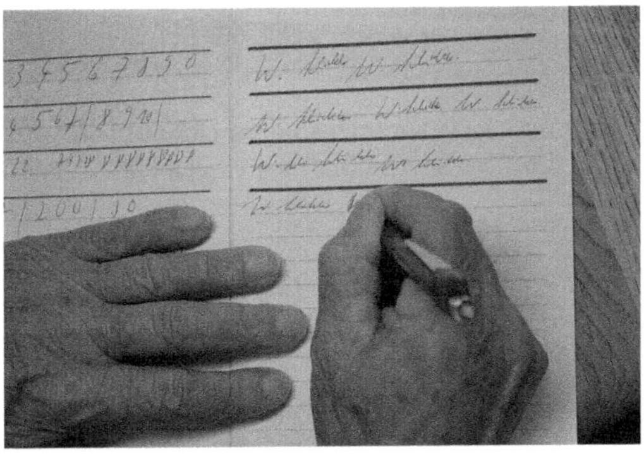

Abb. 13.7 Nachgezogene Linien als Referenzflächen beim Schreiben um Mikrografie vorzubeugen

Übertrag in den Alltag

Das Ziel des Trainings ist der Übertrag in die alltägliche Betätigung. Dazu gibt es drei mögliche Fälle:

1. Wenn die Referenzfläche ein schon im Alltag vorhandener Gegenstand ist, findet der Übertrag ohne Hindernisse statt.
2. Wenn die Referenzfläche künstlich für das Training eingefügt wurde, kann die Therapeutin mit dem Klienten besprechen, die Referenzfläche auch im Alltag zu verwenden (siehe Abb. 13.8, 13.9 und 13.10)
   oder
3. Die Referenzfläche wurde künstlich für das Training eingefügt, soll oder muss aber nicht im Alltag verwendet werden. In diesem Fall muss diese künstliche Komponente des Trainings stufenweise zurückgenommen werden, bis sie nicht mehr benötigt wird.

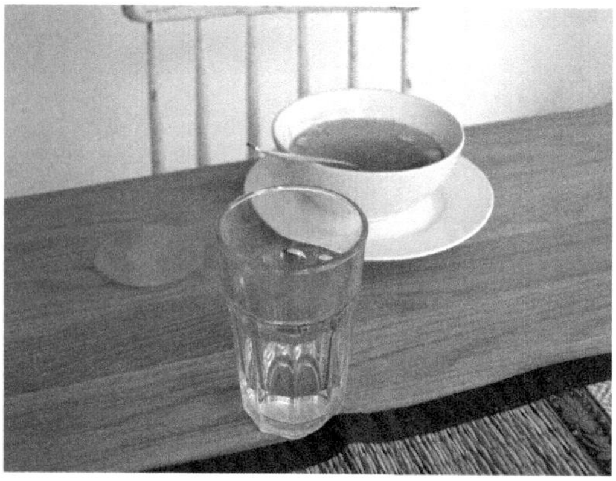

Abb. 13.8 Der Referenzkreis erinnert Klienten im Alltag daran, den Tisch als Unterstützung für den Ellenbogen zu nutzen

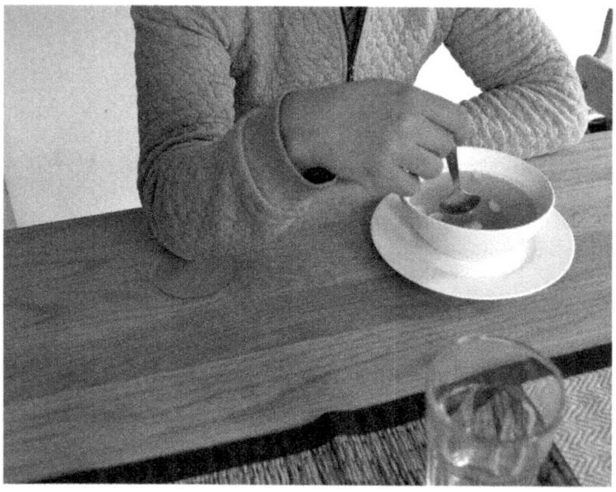

Abb. 13.9 Durch Aufstützen des Ellenbogens wird der Tremor verringert

Bei einer konstanten Nutzung einer Referenzfläche verlässt sich der Klient immer auf die externe Kontrolle der Bewegung. Das therapeutische Ziel ist es aber, dass er seine Körperwahrnehmung neu anpasst und sich verstärkt darauf verlassen kann. Eine Studie zeigt, dass sich ein Verhältnis von „mit Referenzfläche" zu „ohne Referenzfläche" von 6 zu 1 positiv auf den Lernprozess auswirkt. Im Trainingsprozess wird also nach sechs Durchführungen die Referenzfläche einmal entfernt und schon für die achte Wiederholung wieder eingesetzt.

▶ Als Referenzfläche kann ein farbiger, laminierter Kreis mit Kitt (z. B. Patafix) oder aus Antirutschfolie am Zielpunkt angebracht werden, damit der Klient eine externe Kontrolle hat, die visuell klar erkennbar ist. Diese Referenzfläche lässt sich innerhalb eines Trainingsablaufs mehrmals entfernen und wieder anbringen (s. Abb. 13.11 und 13.12).

Beispiel

Frau F. trägt ihr Lieblingskleid, es schwingt bei jedem Schritt um ihre Beine. Sie sieht daran herunter. Auf dem schönen blauen Stoff ist keine Falte zu erkennen. Sie freut sich darüber, dass die Ergotherapeutin ihr Ziel so ernst genommen hat. „Kleider auf die Kleiderstange hängen können". Zusammen hatten sie nochmal ausprobiert, ob sie nicht doch auf eine

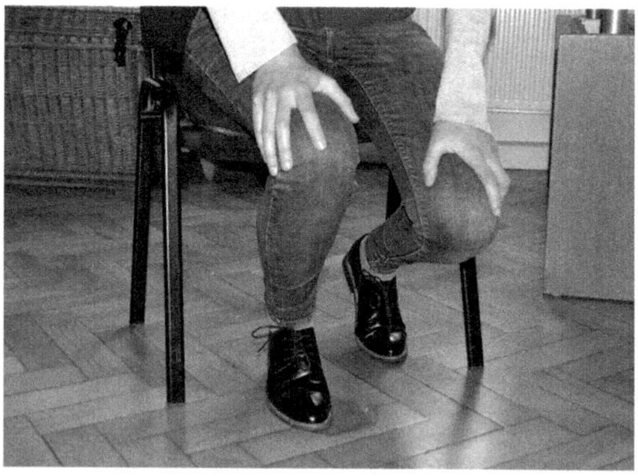

Abb. 13.10 Referenzkreis aus Antirutschfolie im Alltag als Positionierungshilfe und Cueing beim Aufstehen

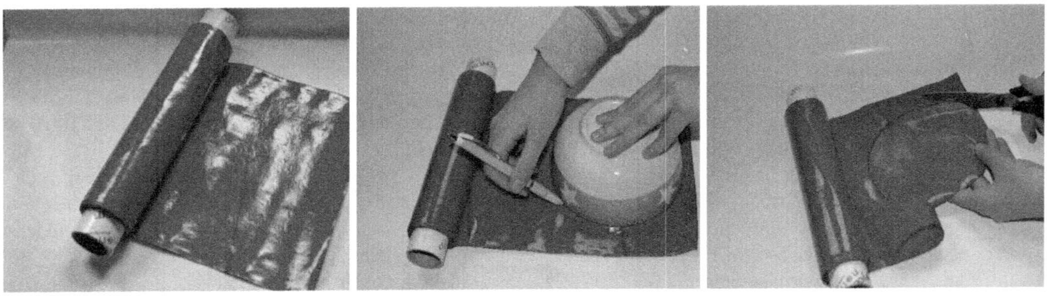

Abb. 13.11 Herstellung von Referenzkreisen aus Antirutschfolie

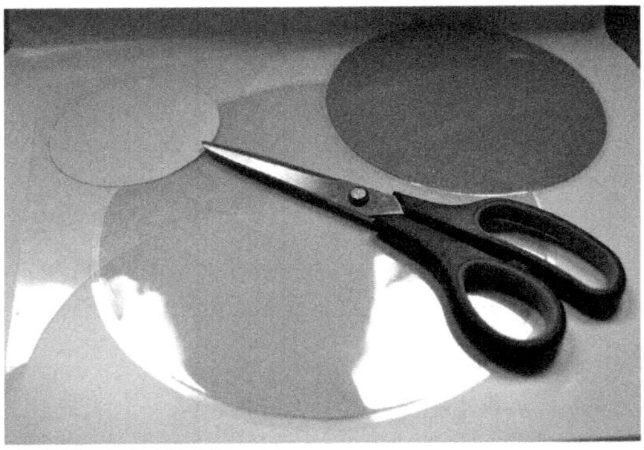

Abb. 13.12 Herstellung von Referenzkreisen aus laminiertem Papier

Trittleiter steigen könnte. Das war aber wirklich zu wackelig. Da hat die Therapeutin ihr im Spiegel ihren Rundrücken von der Seite gezeigt und dass sie 10 cm weiter hochkommt, wenn sie sich vom Rücken aus streckt. Das haben sie zusammen geübt: bücken – strecken, bücken – strecken, erst ohne Kleid zur Stange hoch, dann mit dem leeren Bügel und dann mit dem Kleid, immer wieder, bis es in Fleisch und Blut übergegangen ist. Jetzt hängen die Kleider wieder, anstatt über der Stuhllehne Falten zu sammeln. ◀

Literatur und weiterführende Literatur

Adamovich SV, Berkinblit MB, Hening W, Sage J, Poizner H (2001) The interaction of visual and proprioceptive inputs in pointing to actual and remembered targets in Parkinson's disease. Neuroscience 104(4):1027–1041. https://doi.org/10.1016/s0306-4522(01)00099-9. PMID: 11457588

Aman JE, Elangovan N, Yeh IL, Konczak J (2014) The effectiveness of proprioceptive training for improving motor function: a systematic review. Front Hum Neurosci 8:1075. https://doi.org/10.3389/fnhum.01075. PMID: 25674059; PMCID: PMC4309156

Atkinson R, Derry S, Renkl A, Wortham D (2000) Learning from examples: instructional principles from the worked examples research. Rev Educ Res 70:181. https://doi.org/10.3102/00346543070002181

Ebersbach G, Ebersbach A, Edler D, Kaufhold O, Kusch M, Kupsch A, Wissel J (2010) Comparing exercise in Parkinson's disease – the Berlin LSVT®BIG study. Mov Disord 25(12):1902–1908. https://doi.org/10.1002/mds.23212. Erratum in: Mov Disord.;25(14):2478. PMID: 20669294

Farley B, Fox CN, Ramig L, McFarland D (2008) Intensive amplitude-specific therapeutic approaches for Parkinson's disease: toward a neuroplasticity-principled rehabilitation model. Topics Geriatr Rehab 24:99–114

Fasoli SE, Trombly CA, Tickle-Degnen L, Verfaellie MH (2002) Effect of instructions on functional reach in persons with and without cerebrovascular accident. Am J Occup Ther 56(4):380–390. https://doi.org/10.5014/ajot.56.4.380. PMID: 12125827

Fernandez L, Huys R, Issartel J, Azulay JP, Eusebio A (2018) Movement speed-accuracy trade-off in Parkinson's disease. Front Neurol 9:897. https://doi.org/10.3389/fneur.2018.00897. PMID: 30405521; PMCID: PMC6208126

Foster ER, Bedekar M, Tickle-Degnen L (2014) Systematic review of the effectiveness of occupational therapy-related interventions for people with Parkinson's disease. Am J Occup Ther 68(1):39–49. https://doi.org/10.5014/ajot.2014.008706. PMID: 24367954; PMCID: PMC4413458

Hackney ME, Earhart GM (2009) Effects of dance on movement control in Parkinson's disease: a comparison of Argentine tango and American ballroom. J Rehabil Med 41(6):475–481. https://doi.org/10.2340/16501977-0362. PMID: 19479161; PMCID: PMC2688709

Hétu S, Mercier C (2012) Using purposeful tasks to improve motor performance: does object affordance matter? Br J Occup Ther 75:367–376. https://doi.org/10.4276/030802212X13433105374314

Hubbard IJ, Parsons MW, Neilson C, Carey LM (2009) Task-specific training: evidence for and translation to clinical practice. Occup Ther Int 16(3–4):175–189. https://doi.org/10.1002/oti.275. PMID: 19504501

Jazaeri SZ, Azad A, Mehdizadeh H, Habibi SA, Mandehgary Najafabadi M, Saberi ZS, Rahimzadegan H, Moradi S, Behzadipour S, Parnianpour M, Taghizadeh G, Khalaf K (2018) The effects of anxiety and external attentional focus on postural control in patients with Parkinson's disease. PLoS One 13(2):e0192168. https://doi.org/10.1371/journal.pone.0192168. PMID: 29390029; PMCID: PMC5794142

Kakar C, Zia N, Sehgal S, Kushwaha S (2013) Effect of external and internal focus of attention on acquisition, retention, and transfer phase of motor learning in Parkinson's disease. Hong Kong Physiother J 31:88–94. https://doi.org/10.1016/j.hkpj.2013.02.001

Kehoe R, Rice M (2016) Reality, virtual reality, and imagery: quality of movement in novice dart players. Br J Occup Ther 79. https://doi.org/10.1177/0308022615616820

Keus SHJ, Munneke M, Graziano M, et al (2014) Europäische Physiotherapie Leitlinie beim idiopathischen Parkinson-Syndrom.; KNGF/ParkinsonNet, die Niederlande; https://www.parkinsonnet.info/euguideline

Klockgether T, Dichgans J (1994) Visual control of arm movement in Parkinson's disease. Mov Disord 9:48–56. https://doi.org/10.1002/mds.870090108

Law M (2002) Participation in the occupations of everyday life. Am J Occup Ther 56(6):640–649. https://doi.org/10.5014/ajot.56.6.640

Law M, Steinwender S, Leclair L (1998) Occupation, health and well-being. Can J Occup Ther 65(2):81–91. https://doi.org/10.1177/000841749806500204

Majsak MJ, Kaminski T, Gentile AM, Flanagan JR (1998) The reaching movements of patients with Parkinson's disease under self-determined maximal speed and visually cued conditions. Brain 121(Pt 4):755–766. https://doi.org/10.1093/brain/121.4.755. PMID: 9577399

Myers KA (2008) Using learning reconsidered to reinvent disability education. About Campus 13:2–9. https://doi.org/10.1002/abc.246

Redgrave P, Rodriguez M, Smith Y, Rodriguez-Oroz MC, Lehericy S, Bergman H, Agid Y, DeLong M, Obeso JA (2010) Goal-directed and habitual control in the basal ganglia: implications for Parkinson's disease. Nat Rev Neurosci 11(11):760–772. https://doi.org/10.1038/nrn2915

Sackaloo K, Strouse E, Rice MS (2015) Degree of preference and its influence on motor control when reaching for most preferred, neutrally preferred, and least preferred candy. OTJR (Thorofare N J) 35(2):81–88. https://doi.org/10.1177/1539449214561763. PMID: 26460470

Sturkenboom I, Thijssen M, Gons-van Elsacker J, Jansen I, Maasdam A, Schulten M, Vijver-Visser D, Steultjens E, Bloem B, Munneke M (2008) Guidelines for occupational therapy in Parkinson's disease rehabilitation. ParkinsonNet/NPF, Nijmegen/Miami

Torres EB, Heilman KM, Poizner H (2011) Impaired endogenously evoked automated reaching in Parkinson's disease. J Neurosci 31(49):17848–17863. https://doi.org/10.1523/JNEUROSCI.1150-11.2011. PMID: 22159100; PMCID: PMC3294266

Uhrbrand A, Stenager E, Pedersen MS, Dalgas U (2015) Parkinson's disease and intensive exercise therapy – a systematic review and meta-analysis of randomized controlled trials. J Neurol Sci 353(1–2):9–19. https://doi.org/10.1016/j.jns.2015.04.004.Epup. PMID: 25936252

Williams AJ, Peterson DS, Ionno M, Pickett KA, Earhart GM (2013) Upper extremity freezing and dyscoordination in Parkinson's disease: effects of amplitude and cadence manipulations. Parkinsons Dis 2013:595378. https://doi.org/10.1155/2013/595378. Epub. PMID: 24027652; PMCID: PMC3763266

Wulf G, Landers M, Lewthwaite R, Töllner T (2009) External focus instructions reduce postural instability in individuals with Parkinson disease. Phys Ther 89(2):162–168. https://doi.org/10.2522/ptj.20080045. Epub 2008 Dec 12. PMID: 19074619

14 Betätigungsorientierte Therapieansätze für parkinsonspezifische Themen

Dieses umfangreiche Kapitel ist nach Symptomen gegliedert. Hier finden sich hauptsächlich die Interventionsarten „Betätigung verändern" (siehe Abb. 4.4 Spalte 2) und „Betätigungsspezifische Körperfunktionen trainieren" (siehe Abb. 4.4 Spalte 3) wieder, doch auch Aspekte des Trainings der Betätigung und Veränderung von Kontextfaktoren (siehe Abb. 4.4 Spalte 1 und 4) fließen in die symptomspezifischen therapeutischen Ansätze ein.

14.1 Bradykinese

14.1.1 Symptombeschreibung

Die Bradykinese wirkt sich verlangsamend auf die gesamte Motorik aus. Bewegungen werden mit einer geringen Amplitude und teilweise stark verlangsamt durchgeführt. In vielen Publikationen wird die Akinese als Synonym für Bradykinese genutzt. Dies ist nicht ganz korrekt und in englischsprachigen Veröffentlichungen nicht vorzufinden.

- **Akinese** = A-kinese = keine Bewegung
- **Bradykinese** = Brady-kinese = verlangsamte Bewegung
- **Hypokinese** = Hypo-kinese = Unterbewegung (weniger ausladend)

Alle drei o. g. Probleme können bei Menschen mit M. Parkinson auftreten. Dabei ist die Willkürmotorik des gesamten Körpers betroffen.

Fragt man die Betroffene, welche Symptome sie wahrnimmt, wird manchmal Schwäche benannt. Meist liegt jedoch bei der Messung keine Kraftminderung vor, sondern die Bradykinese wird von der Klientin als solche interpretiert. Eines der ersten Auffälligkeiten ist oftmals der **reduzierte Armschwung** beim Gehen, zunächst einseitig, später beidseitig. Später kommen **Hypomimie**, im Deutschen auch **Maskengesicht** genannt, mit einem ausdrucksarmen bis starren Gesicht, manchmal einem offenen Mund und seltenem Lidschlag hinzu. Durch die **Amplitudenabnahme** der Motorik werden Bewegungen kleiner ausgeführt, z. B. beim Klatschen und Winken, sowie die Gestik beim Sprechen.

Für die Durchführung von Betätigungen wird mehr Zeit benötigt als vor der Erkrankung. Dies fällt vor allem bei täglichen Verrichtungen auf, wie Anziehen, Duschen oder Spülmaschine ausräumen. **Feinmotorische Tätigkeiten**, wie das Binden einer Schleife oder die Manipulation von Geldmünzen, sind stark verlangsamt und zunehmend eingeschränkt. Typischerweise kommt es zu einer **Mikrografie**. Die Schrift ist beim Anset-

Ergänzende Information Die elektronische Version dieses Kapitels enthält Zusatzmaterial, auf das über folgenden Link zugegriffen werden kann https://doi.org/10.1007/978-3-662-62583-5_14. Die Videos lassen sich durch Anklicken des DOI Links in der Legende einer entsprechenden Abbildung abspielen, oder indem Sie diesen Link mit der SN More Media App scannen.

A. Orellana, *Betätigungsorientierte Ergotherapie bei Morbus Parkinson*,
https://doi.org/10.1007/978-3-662-62583-5_14

zen zum Schreiben noch groß und flüssig. Die Schriftgröße nimmt im Verlauf jedoch stetig ab, rutscht häufig unter die Linie und wird immer weniger lesbar. In manchen Fällen endet das letzte Wort in einem Strich. Und selbst die Klientin kann das Geschriebene nicht mehr entziffern. Auch die **Grobmotorik** ist betroffen. So ist der Transfer ins Bett und aus dem Bett sowie das Aufstehen ein häufiges Problem.

Die **Stimme** wird oft **leiser** und monoton (**Hypophonie**) und es kann eine Dysarthrie auftreten, sodass die Klientin teilweise nicht gut verstanden werden kann. Es kann zu **Speichelfluss** kommen, der nicht auf vermehrte Speichelproduktion zurückzuführen ist, sondern auf die reduzierte Schluckhäufigkeit.

Der **Gang** wird **kleinschrittiger** bis hin zu **Trippelschritten**, die Füße werden kaum vom Boden abgehoben. Bei allen Aktivitäten kann eine Zunahme der Brady- und Hypokinese bei repetitiven Tätigkeiten, wie Haare bürsten oder Tisch abwischen, beobachtet werden. Das äußere Erscheinungsbild der Parkinson-Erkrankung wird stark von der Bradykinese geprägt. Klientinnen erscheinen oftmals antriebsarm und niedergeschlagen, was jedoch irreführend sein kann.

► Hinter dem unbewegten Äußeren verbirgt sich häufig ein vollkommen gegensätzlicher Charakter. Aber Witz, Interesse und Freude können durch die Bradykinese nur stark reduziert nach außen kommuniziert werden.

Freezing

Vor allem im späteren Verlauf der Erkrankung kann es zu Freezing-Episoden kommen. In diesen fühlt sich die Betroffene wie festgefroren. Es tritt eine plötzliche Unfähigkeit ein, eine Bewegung zu initiieren oder fortzuführen. Besonders häufig ist dies beim Laufen zu beobachten („freezing of gait"), aber auch in der oberen Extremität und beim Sprechen. Durch die Propulsion (Neigung zum Vorwärtsfallen) entsteht ein Ungleichgewicht. Dieser Gleichgewichtsverlust kann nicht, wie bei Gesunden, abgefangen werden, da Ausgleichsbewegungen im Oberkörper und

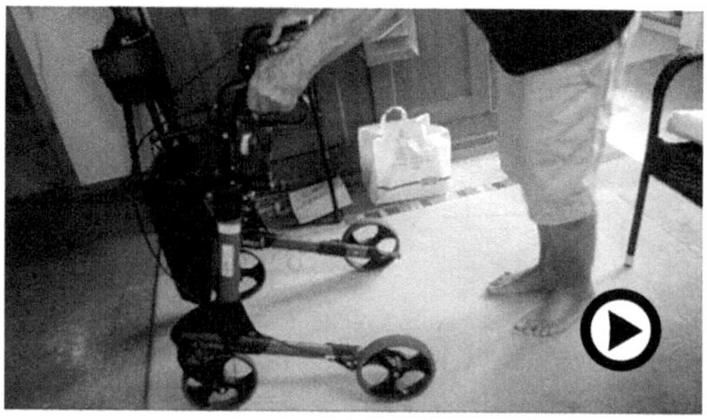

Abb. 14.1 Freezing und Trembling-In-Place beim Loslaufen, Ausgelöst durch Dual-Task (sprechen mit der Therapeutin) (► https://doi.org/10.1007/000-2y4)

Schutzschritte ebenfalls nicht initiiert werden können. Es kommt zum Kniezittern („Trembling-In-Place" oder „Knee-Trembling") oder zu Trippelschritten auf der Stelle (Festination) oder mit minimalem Weggewinn (Jacobs et al. 2009). Die Sturzgefahr nimmt zu.

Meist treten Freezing-Episoden während Off-Phasen ein, wenn die Dopaminsättigung im synaptischen Spalt der Nervenfasern reduziert ist, jedoch ist ein Auftreten in der On-Phase auch möglich (s. Video 14.1, Abb. 14.1).

Auslösend für eine Freezing-Episode können äußerliche Faktoren sein, die die Aufmerksamkeit minimal vom Laufen ablenken, z. B.:

- Geräusch (auch Ansprechen),
- enger Durchgang (z. B. Türrahmen),
- Wechsel des Bodenbelags,
- Bewegung im Blickfeld (z. B. vorbeifahrendes Auto).

Auch innere Faktoren können ein Freezing provozieren:

- Stress,
- Angst,
- Schlafmangel,
- Dual-Tasks (z. B. Sprechen beim Laufen),
- Richtungswechsel beim Laufen.

Meist hält eine solche Blockade wenige Sekunden an und wird von der Klientin selbst oder durch einen äußeren Reiz aufgelöst.

▶ **Cave!** Beim Laufen stellt das Freezing eine erhöhte Sturzgefahr dar, da der Oberkörper die Vorwärtsbewegung durchführt, wobei es zu einer Dysbalance kommt. Der notwendige Schutzschritt zur Sturzvermeidung tritt nicht ein und es kommt zum Sturz.

14.1.2 Cueing

Beispiel

Herr C. steht an der Fußgängerampel und wartet nervös auf das grüne Männchen. Feierabendverkehr – er weiß, er muss schnell sein, keiner will auf einen alten Mann warten, der noch bei rot mitten auf der Kreuzung schlurft. Sobald die Ampel umspringt, geht ein Ruck durch seinen Körper, aber es kommt kein Schritt. Zweiter Versuch – er ist wie festgefroren. Beim dritten Versuch schafft er es, die Straße zu kreuzen. Mitten auf der Fahrbahn ändert sich die Beschaffenheit des Asphalts, Herr C. nimmt dies wahr und steht plötzlich wieder still, mitten auf der Kreuzung. ◀

Arten von Cues Zur Vermeidung von Freezing, und auch um der Amplitudenminderung entgegenzuwirken, existiert eine sehr gut erforschte, auch in der Praxis etablierte Methode: das Cueing. „Cue" ist das englische Wort für „Hinweisreiz". Da der Impulsreiz nicht aus dem Gehirn kommt, wird er von außen als „Cue" gegeben und die Hemmung der Motorik wird überwunden.

Man unterscheidet zwischen Initiierungs-Cue und regelmäßigen Cues. Der Initiierungs-Cue wird eingesetzt, wenn eine Bewegung nicht begonnen werden kann, wie beim Aufstehen, Loslaufen oder Greifen der Tasse. Repetitive Cues helfen bei der Weiterführung einer repetitiven Bewegung wie Laufen, Treppe steigen, Brot schneiden oder Kämmen. Zunächst gilt es festzustellen, welche Art der Cues zur Klientin passen. Es gibt folgende Cues:

1. Visuelle,
2. auditive,
3. taktile/propriozeptive,
4. kognitive.

Visuelle Cues
Als visuelles Cue kann alles genutzt werden, was sich gerade am jeweiligen Aufenthaltsort findet: siehe Tab. 14.1, oder es können an wichtigen Punkten visuelle Cues angebracht oder mitgenommen werden, siehe Tab. 14.2.

Auditive Cues
Auditive Cues können von der Patientin selbst oder von einem Begleiter oder Hilfsmittel produziert werden (siehe Tab. 14.3).

Tab. 14.1 Schon vorhandene Gegebenheiten können als visuelle Cues genutzt werden

Unregelmäßigkeit im Gehweg	Initiierungs-Cues
Licht/Schatten	
Kaugummi am Boden	
Schwelle	
Spalten zwischen Gehwegplatten	Repetitive Cues
Linien an Bordsteinkante	
Treppenstufen	

Tab. 14.2 Visuelle Cues können an wichtigen Orten angebracht werden

Bohnen/Steinchen in Tasche zum Werfen und darüber Steigen	Initiierungs-Cues
Einen Gegenstand den Weg entlang kicken	
Fuß des Begleiters, zum Übersteigen	
Anti-Freezing Stock (siehe Abschn. 15.3)	
Laserstock (siehe Abschn. 15.3)	
Laserschuhe (siehe Abschn. 15.3)	Repetitive Cues
Gegen Stock treten	
Tapelinien am Boden, an engen Stellen	
Tapekreuz am Boden, für Drehung (siehe Abb. 14.2, Video 14.3 zu Abb. 14.3)	
einer Person beim Gehen zusehen	
Linien beim Schreiben (siehe Abschn. 14.20 Schreibtraining)	

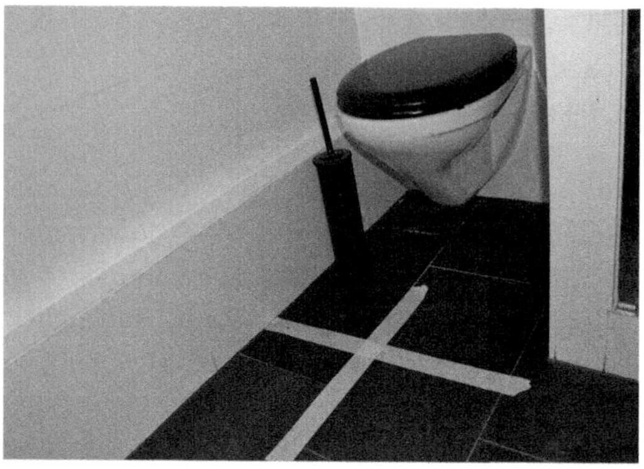

Abb. 14.2 Kreuz vor Toilette, als Cue für die Drehung

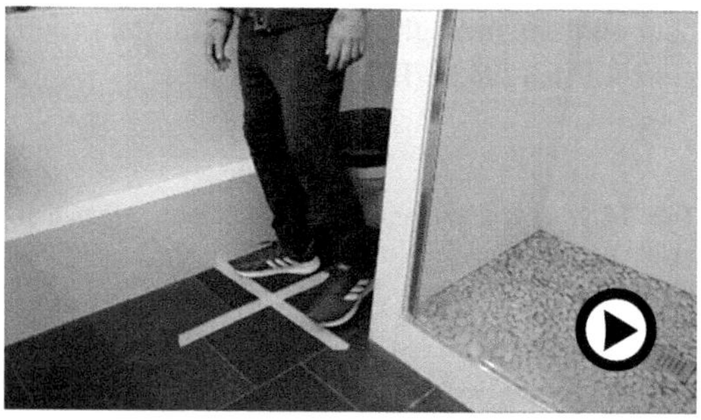

Abb. 14.3 Anwendung des Kreuzes zur Drehung vor Toilette (▶ https://doi.org/10.1007/000-2xc)

Tab. 14.3 Beispiele für auditive Cues

„Los", „Ja" oder anderes verbales Signal (siehe Video 14.4 zu Abb. 14.4)	Initiierungs-Cues
Klatschen	
Auf Schritte hören	Repetitive Cues
Auf Takt der Walkingstöcke hören	
Metronom, auch als App	
Zählen	
Singen	
Auf Ticken der Uhr hören	

Taktile/propriozeptive Cues

Auch taktile und propriozeptive Cues können von der Patientin selbst oder von einer Begleiterin oder einem Hilfsmittel produziert werden (siehe Tab. 14.4).

Kognitive (interne) Cues

Die eleganteste Lösung, da sie vollkommen intern abläuft, ist die Nutzung von kognitiven Cues.

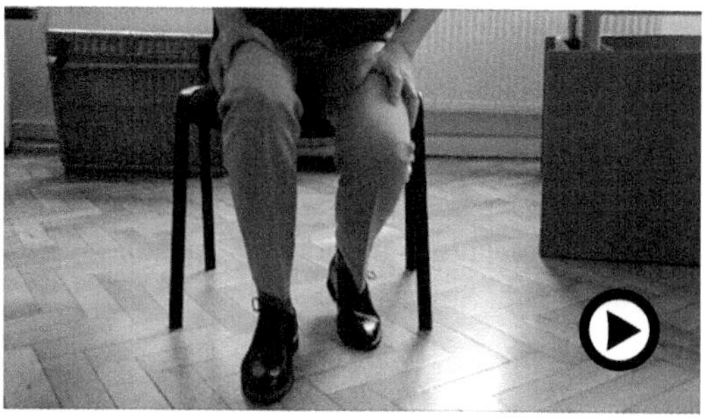

Abb. 14.4 Auditives Cue: „Hoch" beim Aufstehen (▶ https://doi.org/10.1007/000-2xd)

Tab. 14.4 Beispiele für taktile und propriozeptive Cues

Auf Schulter, Schenkel klopfen beim Aufstehen (siehe Video 14.5 zu Abb. 14.5)	Initiierungs-Cues
Gewicht hin und her verlagern zum Anlaufen	
stampfen	Repetitive Cues
Vibration in Mobiltelefon als App (MoveApp)	
Gewichte an Füßen	
Band an Rollator befestigen, mit Schritten dagegen treten (siehe Abb. 14.6 und Video 14.7 zu Abb. 14.7)	
Ball an Schnur, beim Laufen dagegentreten (siehe Abb. 14.8 und Video 14.9 zu Abb. 14.9)	

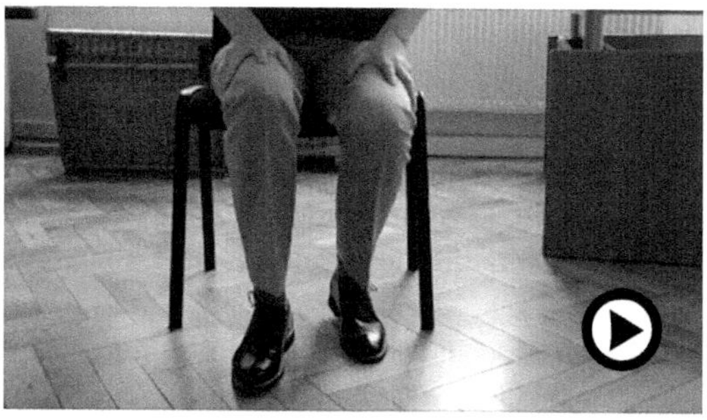

Abb. 14.5 Taktiles Cue: auf Schenkel klatschen, zum Aufstehen (▶ https://doi.org/10.1007/000-2xe)

Diese internen Cues sind in Untersuchungen als effektiver als externe Cues bestätigt worden (singen gegenüber Musik hören). Dabei nutzt die Patientin ihre Fantasie, um sich den passenden Cue vorzustellen, anstatt dass er von außen kommt. So werden die bei gesunden Menschen

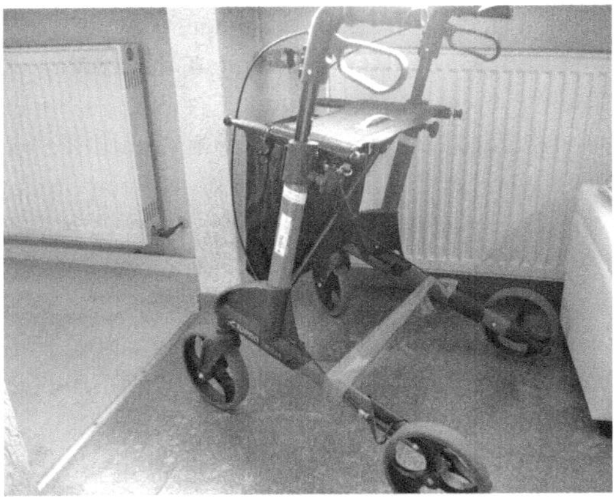

Abb. 14.6 Band an Rollator für große Schritte

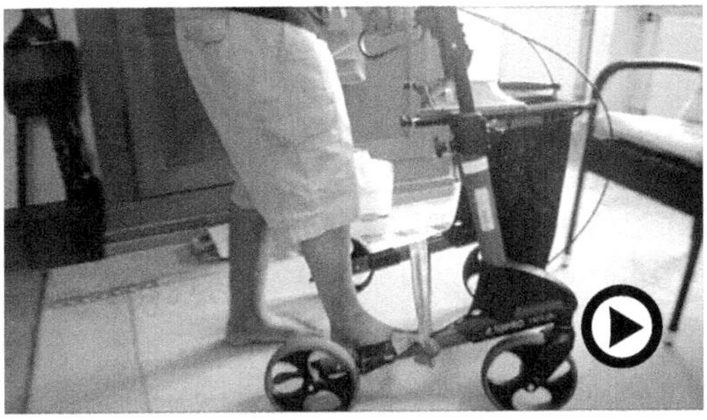

Abb. 14.7 Taktiles Cueing, Band an Rollator für große Schritte (▶ https://doi.org/10.1007/000-2xf)

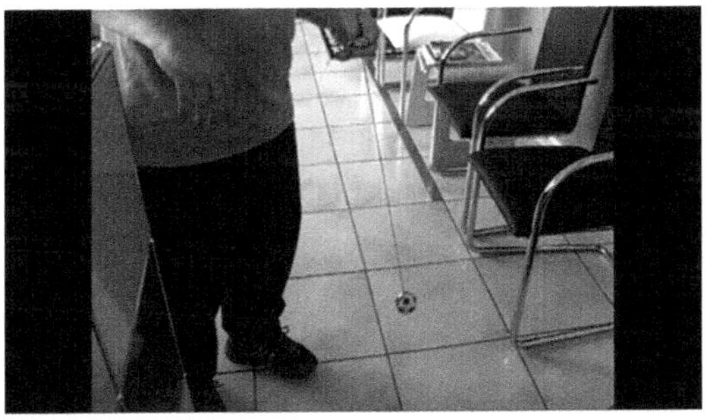

Abb. 14.8 Taktiles Cueing: Ball an Band um dagegen zu treten

ablaufenden Prozesse der Bewegungsinitiierung in den Basalganglien umgangen und auf die Cortexebene verlagert. Alle oben gelisteten visuellen, auditiven und taktil/propriozeptiven Cues können

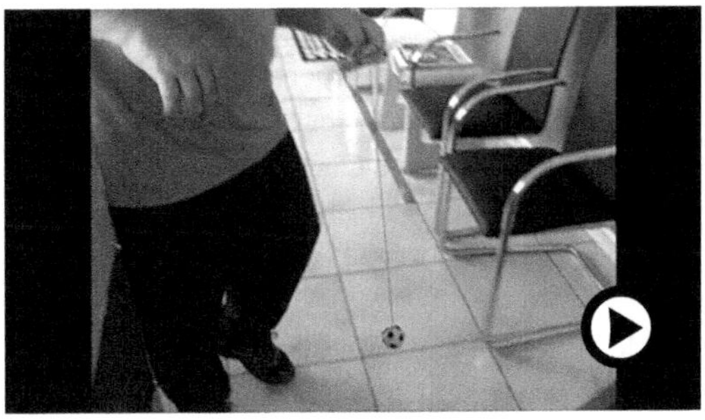

Abb. 14.9 taktiles Cueing: Ball an Band um dagegen zu treten (▶ https://doi.org/10.1007/000-2xg)

Tab. 14.5 Beispiele für kognitive Cues

Einen großen Stein visualisieren	Initiierungs-Cues
„Ja“ oder anderes Start-Wort lautlos vorsagen	
Das Antippen an Schulter von Partner vorstellen	
Ein Lied lautlos singen	Repetitive Cues
Lautlos zählen	

mit ein wenig Übung als kognitive Cues fungieren. Als besonders erfolgreich haben sich in der Praxis die kognitive Cues in Tab. 14.5 erwiesen.

Anwendung der Cues Um den passenden Cue für die Klientin zu finden, sollten verschiedene Hinweisreize aus den o. g. sensorischen Bereichen ausprobiert werden. In dieser therapeutischen Intervention dürfen Klientin, Angehörige und Therapeut uneingeschränkt kreativ sein und eigene Ideen einbringen.

> Wichtig ist, dass die Cues kurz und eindeutig sind, Therapeut und Angehörige sollten auf ablenkende, einleitende Sätze und Berührungen verzichten. Statt: „So jetzt bitte aufstehen.“ Besser: „Los!“. Statt am Arm tätscheln, besser einen kurzen Klaps auf die Schulter.

Cueing und Demenz
Bei der Auswahl des Cues sollte eine mögliche demenzielle Entwicklung beachtet werden.

- Einschränkung der Merkfähigkeit -> externe Cues durch die Begleitperson,
- leichte Herabsetzung der Merkfähigkeit -> externe oder kognitive Cues,
- keine kognitive Einschränkung -> kognitive Cues.

Meist stellt sich schnell ein geeignetes Cue heraus. Mit diesem können nun alle relevanten Situationen aus dem Alltag geübt werden, in denen Freezing auftritt. Nachdem ein Cue genug geübt wurde, kann es sinnvoll sein, ihn in einen kognitiven Cue zu „verwandeln", um ihn in sozialen Situationen unauffällig einsetzen zu können. Wichtig ist, dass die Klientin selbständig oder ggf. mit Unterstützung eines Angehörigen an den Einsatz des Cues denkt und ihn auch richtig anwendet. Da Freezing meist in Stresssituationen auftritt, scheitert die erfolgreiche Anwendung häufig an diesem Punkt. Zum Umgang mit Stress sind in Abschn. 14.8 weitere Hilfestellung zu finden.

Nachdem ein Cue eine Weile gebraucht wurde, kann es passieren, dass er an Potenz verliert. Man geht davon aus, dass der bekannte Cue im Gehirn in den automatisierten Bewegungsablauf integriert wird, was die Effektivität erheblich abschwächt, da die automatisierten Bewegungsabläufe die häufigsten Freezing-Situationen hervorrufen. Aus diesem Grund ist eine Änderung des Cues oftmals notwendig. Sobald die Klientin und Angehörige das Prinzip des Cueings verstanden haben, werden sie meist selbst kreativ und erfinden eigene Cues, die zu ihnen passen.

Studienlage

In einer Studie von Dr. Nieuwboer et al. (2007) war der positive Effekt des Cueings auf das Freezing, die Gehgeschwindigkeit und die Balance während des Einsatzes signifikant. Nach sechs Wochen wurde eine beträchtliche Abnahme der positiven Auswirkung festgestellt. Daraus lässt sich folgern, dass Cues fortlaufend angewandt und abgewandelt werden müssen. Eine regelmäßige Auffrischung des Trainings in der Ergotherapie ist sinnvoll.

Der Einsatz von Cues für die obere Extremität wurde bisher nur in kleinen Studien untersucht. Es lässt sich die Tendenz erkennen, dass sie wirksam sind. Ma et al. (2011) zeigten, dass auditives Cueing beim Reichen und Greifen zu einer schnelleren, kräftigeren Bewegung führt, die jedoch weniger flüssig ist. In einer anderen Studie war die Bewegung zusätzlich flüssiger, es bedarf also noch weiterer Untersuchungen, um zu einheitlichen Ergebnissen zu kommen.

Etabliert und mehrfach untersucht ist der Einsatz von Linien beim Schreiben. Wobei die obere und untere Linie als Cues dienen, um eine Mikrografie zu vermeiden. Eine Reihe weiterer Studien belegen, dass visuelle Cues die eingeschränkte propriozeptive Wahrnehmung kompensieren und bei einer Vielzahl von Bewegungen eine effektive Motorik ermöglichen. Dazu gehören zielgerichtetes Ausstrecken des Armes, Greifen, koordinierte Arm- und Rumpfbewegung, wiederholte Armbewegungen und Laufen. (Adamovich et al. 2001; Muratori et al. 2008; Majsak et al. 1998; Klockgether und Dichgans 1994; Harrison et al. 2018; Nackaerts et al. 2015)

Beispiel

Als Herr C. mitten auf der Kreuzung ins Freezing kommt, fällt ihm die Ergotherapie ein. Er atmet einmal tief aus und wieder ein, stellt sich vor, es läge ein dicker Ast vor ihm auf dem Boden, macht beherzt einen großen Schritt darüber und erreicht die gegenüberliegende Seite gerade, als die ruhelosen Autofahrer ihre Motoren hochfahren. ◀

14.1.3 Aufmerksamkeit fokussieren

Beispiel

Herr P. bemerkt, dass er immer dann ins Stocken gerät, wenn sein Smartphone in seiner Hosentasche klingelt oder piept. Diese kleine Ablenkung, gekoppelt mit dem Impuls, das Smartphone aus der Tasche zu ziehen, behindert ihn nun immer wieder im Alltag. Inmitten einer Betätigung, wie dem Essen, Anziehen oder Laufen, meldet sich sein Telefon und Herr P. kommt zum Stillstand. Erst nach mehreren Sekunden schafft er es, aus dem Freezing wieder herauszukommen, und nach weiteren Sekunden kann er die erhaltene Nachricht ansehen oder den Anruf beantworten (meist zu spät). Herr P. fühlt sich dadurch sehr eingeschränkt und es ist ihm peinlich, wenn es in sozialen Situationen geschieht. ◄

Bei der Ausführung von automatisierten Bewegungen wird im gesunden Gehirn ein Kreislauf von den Basalganglien zum motorischen Kortex in Gang gesetzt. Dieser Kreislauf ist im Parkinson-Gehirn durch das fehlende Dopamin unterbrochen. Deswegen muss die Betroffene die Bewegungsabläufe, die früher automatisiert abliefen, zunehmend bewusst steuern. Der Vorteil einer automatisierten Bewegung ist, dass sie quasi unbeachtet neben einer anderen Bewegung durchgeführt werden kann. Da die betroffene Parkinson-Klientin ihre volle Aufmerksamkeit für die (früher automatische) Bewegung benötigt, kann keine zweite Bewegung durchgeführt werden und die Klientin stockt. Im schlimmsten Fall kommt es (aus ungeklärten Gründen) zum Freezing.

Therapeutische Intervention

Häufig kommt es in einer durchgeführten Betätigung immer in einem bestimmten Moment zum Freezing oder zu einem Zusammenbruch des Handlungsablaufs. In dem Fall kann durch die Fokussierung der Aufmerksamkeit auf diesen Moment die Problematik behoben werden.

Training der Aufmerksamkeitsfokussierung (s. Video 14.10 zu Abb. 14.10)

- **Informierung**: Zunächst ist es wichtig, der Klientin die gestörten Abläufe im Gehirn zu erklären. Das erlangte Verständnis gibt der Klientin die Gelegenheit, sich mit ihrer Erkrankung auseinanderzusetzen und ermöglicht die Offenheit für eine therapeutische Intervention.
- **Definierung des problematischen Moments**: Durch die Betätigungsanalyse erkennt und definiert der Therapeut den genauen Moment, in dem es zum Stocken der Handlung kommt.

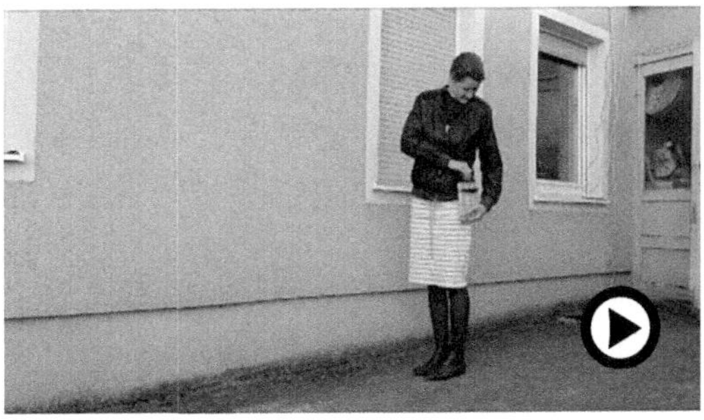

Abb. 14.10 Fokussierung der Aufmerksamkeit. Mobil Telefon klingelt, stehen bleiben, visuelle Kontrolle, kompletter Fokus auf Handlung (▶ https://doi.org/10.1007/000-2xh)

Eine Videoaufzeichnung kann zur Unterstützung gemacht werden. So kann gemeinsam mit der Klientin von außen die Betätigung analysiert werden.

- **Unterbrechung anderer Handlungen**: Die Klientin sollte parallellaufende Handlungen kurz unterbrechen, damit sie die Aufmerksamkeit voll auf den problematischen Moment fokussieren kann. Dies kann sie verbal durch ein laut ausgesprochenes oder gedachtes „**Stopp**!" unterstützen.
- **Kompletter Fokus**: Die Klientin wird angeleitet, die Aufmerksamkeit komplett zu fokussieren. Das bedeutet die uneingeschränkte gedankliche Konzentration auf die Aktivität in dem Moment.
- **Visuelle Kontrolle**: In dem Moment der fokussierten Aufmerksamkeit wird die aktive Hand visuell fixiert, da dies den Fokus nochmal verstärkt.
- **Verbalisierung**: Eine laut ausgesprochene oder gedankliche Verbalisierung zur Unterstützung der Initiierung der Motorik mag ergänzt werden, z. B. Ha!, Ja!, Los!
- **Üben in der Therapie**: Innerhalb der therapeutischen Intervention wird die Betätigung, mithilfe der oben beschriebenen Methode, wiederholt durchgeführt. Der Therapeut erinnert an die wichtigen Punkte oder führt die Betätigung parallel durch, damit die Klientin durch Nachahmung lernt.
- **Übertrag in den Alltag**: Damit die Fokussierung der Aufmerksamkeit auch im Alltag umgesetzt wird, können Erinnerungen helfen z. B.

- Zettel
- Angehörige
- Eigenübungen zu Hause

Beispiel

Der Therapeut **informiert** Herrn P., dass automatisierte Bewegungen durch den Dopaminmangel nicht mehr flüssig abgerufen werden können. Alle Bewegungen, die man schon hunderte Male gemacht hat und ohne nachzudenken ausführt, wie z. B. die Brille auf der Nase nach oben zu schieben oder das Telefon aus der Tasche zu ziehen, sind automatisiert. Er erklärt ihm, dass es wahrscheinlich auch in Zukunft länger als früher dauern wird, dass er aber durch die Methode der „Fokussierung der Aufmerksamkeit" erreichen kann, dass die Bewegung und der Ablauf flüssiger werden.

Zunächst entscheiden Therapeut und Herr P., die Einstellungen des Smartphones zu ändern, sodass es bei Nachrichten nicht mehr klingelt, sondern nur bei Anrufen. Dann besprechen sie die Handlung „Anruf beantworten" in Kombination mit einer konkreten Situation – dem Laufen auf dem Gehweg –, da dies häufig vorkommt und Herrn P. am stärksten belastet. Durch die Videoanalyse der Betätigung sehen Therapeut und Herr P., dass er während des Laufens versucht, das Smartphone aus der Tasche zu ziehen, und dabei sowohl das Laufen als auch die Tätigkeit der Hände ins Freezing geraten. Sie besprechen, dass er zuerst stehen bleiben soll, wenn das Smartphone klingelt. Damit wird das Laufen **unterbrochen**.

Während der Klient das Smartphone aus der Tasche zieht, soll er sich **komplett** darauf **fokussieren** und die Hand **visuell** fixieren. Er kann ein leises „So" **aussprechen**, um die Bewegung zu initiieren. Diese Sequenz wird sowohl **innerhalb der Therapie**, ohne Ablenkung, als auch als **Eigenübung** zu Hause trainiert. Sobald Herr P. die Abfolge verinnerlicht hat, wird die Handlung auch in der Öffentlichkeit geübt. Da es nicht immer vorhersehbar ist, wann das Telefon klingelt, ist von Herrn P. viel Selbstdisziplin bei der Umsetzung der erarbeiteten Methode im **Alltag** gefragt.

Nach fünf Wochen des Trainings gelingt es Herrn P. in den meisten Situationen, die „Fokussierung der Aufmerksamkeit" umzusetzen. Er berichtet, dass er zwar nicht schneller geworden ist, durch die Methode jedoch nach außen hin nicht so ungeschickt aussieht und sich auch sicherer fühlt. ◄

14.1.4 Aufteilung in Sequenzen

Beispiel

Herr P. eilt in Richtung Toilette. Er weiß, es muss schnell gehen – die lästige Dranginkontinenz. An der Tür angekommen, versucht er mit der rechten Hand elegant den Rollator weiterzuschieben, um gleichzeitig mit Links die Tür zu öffnen. Es gibt ein Durcheinander, die Tür hängt am Rollator, der Ärmel am Türgriff. Herr P. stockt, zerrt und schiebt, bis er endlich wieder freikommt. Rückwärts geht er in Richtung Toilette, zieht den Rollator hinterher und kommt nun nicht mehr an die Tür, um sie zu schließen. Wieder stockt, zerrt und zieht er, bis der Rollator neben ihm steht und der Griff zur Türklinke gelingt. Er schließt schnell die Tür. Nun klappt er den Toilettendeckel hoch, blickt jedoch gleichzeitig auf seinen Hosenknopf, der als nächstes dran ist. Und nochmal stockt er, blickt zum Deckel, klappt ihn nach oben und schafft es gerade noch rechtzeitig, die Hose zu öffnen, herunterzuziehen und sich auf die Klobrille zu setzen. „Das muss doch auch anders gehen," mutmaßt er. ◄

Bei komplexen Betätigungen können Menschen mit M. Parkinson in ein Stocken oder Freezing geraten. Dies passiert, meist entweder, wenn versucht wird, zwei Bewegungen zur gleichen Zeit durchzuführen, oder die darauffolgende Bewegung bereits mental geplant wird, während die vorherige Bewegung noch nicht abgeschlossen ist. In beiden Fällen wird teilweise auf automatisierte Bewegungsabläufe zurückgegriffen, die durch den Dopaminmangel im Parkinson-Gehirn nicht flüssig ausführbar sind – es kommt zum Stocken. Die genauen pathophysiologischen Abläufe beim Freezing sind nicht bekannt.

▶ Eine Umstellung oder Vereinfachung der Betätigung ist vielen Parkinson-Klientinnen nicht möglich, da sie meist auch eine Einschränkung der exekutiven Funktionen haben. D. h., kognitive Flexibilität und Problemlösungsstrategien sind eingeschränkt. Die Klientin benötigt dazu therapeutische Unterstützung.

Vor allem bei komplexen Betätigungen ist die Aufteilung in Sequenzen eine wirkungsvolle Methode, um Handlungsabläufe flüssig und erfolgreich zu meistern. Es gibt hierzu zwei Studien. Sie belegen einen positiven Effekt auf die Initiierung und das Anhalten des Laufens, das Drehen während des Laufens, das Drehen im Bett und das Aus- und Einsteigen vom und ins Bett sowie das Hinsetzen und Aufstehen (Kamsma et al. 1995) und (Nieuwboer et al. 2001).

Im Zusammenhang mit Demenz ist die **Sequenzierung**, auch **Chaining** genannt, ein bewährtes Mittel bei komplexen Betätigungen, wie Kaffeekochen oder Wäschewaschen. Wozu es leider keine Studien bei M. Parkinson gibt, ist die Wirksamkeit von Sequenzierung auf manuelle Tätigkeiten. Aus der praktischen Erfahrung heraus scheint es jedoch in vielen Fällen effektiv zu sein.

In ihrer Studie zielten Kamsma und Kollegen (1995) darauf ab, eine komplexe Betätigung, die in der normalen Ausführung schnell, mit zeitgleichen und teils automatisierten Bewegungen durchgeführt wird, mit neuen Strategien für Menschen mit der Parkinson-Erkrankung zu vereinfachen. Es war ihnen wichtig, die einzelnen Bewegungen voneinander zu entkoppeln und mit hoher Aufmerksamkeit ausführen zu lassen. Folgende Punkte wurden als Voraussetzung für die Strategien für komplexe Bewegungssequenzen definiert:

1. Sie müssen **schrittweise strukturiert** sein, jeder Schritt umfasst eine einzige, einfache Bewegung oder eine einfache Kombination von Bewegungen.
2. Diese Schritte werden als Sequenz, **in logischer Abfolge**, aneinandergereiht. Wenn die Sequenz komplett durchgeführt wurde, muss es zum gewünschten Ergebnis führen.
3. **Jeder Schritt** muss **isoliert** ausgeführt werden können und in eine stabile Halteposition münden. Von dieser ausgehend muss der folgende Schritt initiiert werden können, sodass eine Überlagerung und eine daraus folgende Komplikation und zeitliche Beschränkung vermieden wird.
4. Bei der Durchführung der Schritte muss die Klientin die maximale Möglichkeit zur **bewusst kontrollierten** Durchführung haben – wenn möglich mit taktiler, visueller oder auditiver Kontrolle.
5. Wegen der Komplexität von axialen Bewegungen und der Schwierigkeit einer bewusst kontrollierten Durchführung ist es wichtig, **Rotationsbewegungen einzuschränken**.

▶ Eine Fotosequenz, die am Ort der Ausführung aufgehängt wird, erinnert die Klientin an die schrittweise Durchführung.

Zusätzlich sind kurze Signalwörter sinnvoll. Sie können mit dem Handlungsschritt laut gesprochen werden, um die Bewegung einzuleiten.

Beispiel

Es wurden zunächst zwei Veränderungen der Umwelt für die Betätigung von Herrn P. besprochen. Erstens wird der Toilettendeckel nach dem Toilettengang nicht zugeklappt, damit der Handlungsablauf beim nächsten Toilettengang einen Schritt weniger beinhaltet und somit schneller durchführbar ist. Zweitens trägt der Klient entweder Hosen mit Gummibund oder verwendet einen speziellen Hosenknopf mit elastischem Gummi- oder Silikonband an Hosen mit Knopf. Dadurch wird das hektische Öffnen des Knopfes vermieden und die Betätigung läuft schneller. Nach drei Monaten des Übens hat sich die Sequenzierung für den Toilettengang von Herrn P. bewährt (siehe Tab. 14.6.

Tab. 14.6 Beispiel für Sequenzierung des Toilettengangs

	Beschreibung	Verbalisierung
1.	Zügiges Laufen an Toilettentür vorbei, Rollator an besprochener Stelle abstellen	An Tür vorbei – Stopp
2.	Rollator feststellen	Bremsen fest – Stopp
3.	Rollator loslassen und zur Tür drehen (Rollator bleibt draußen stehen)	Loslassen und drehen – Stopp
4.	Tür öffnen, mit links	Tür auf – Stopp
5.	Eintreten, dabei an Türrahmen mit rechter Hand festhalten	Rein laufen – Stopp
6.	Im Uhrzeigersinn drehen	Rechts drehen – Stopp
7.	Links festhalten, rechts schließt die Tür	Tür zu – Stopp
8.	Rechts und links an Haltegriffen festhalten, einen Schritt rückwärts zu Toilette	Festhalten, zurück – Stopp
9.	Hose und Unterhose herunter ziehen	Hose runterziehen – Stopp
10.	Setzen	Setzen

Die gemessene Zeit für die Tätigkeit ist ein paar Sekunden kürzer. Und durch den klaren Ablauf ist Herr P. weniger gestresst, was sich positiv auf die Dranginkontinenz auswirkt. Zusätzlich ist die Sturzgefahr gering. ◀

14.1.5 Dual-Tasks

Beispiel

Frau Z. hat Nachmittagsbesuch von ihrer Nachbarin. Den Kaffee hat sie vor ihrem Eintreffen schon zubereitet, Kekse und Tablett liegen bereit. Sie freut sich auf das gemütliche Treffen mit ihrer Bekannten. Vorsichtig trägt sie alles auf dem Tablett ins Wohnzimmer. „Du wirst nicht glauben, was der Kater gestern Nacht gemacht hat …“, beginnt die Nachbarin. Frau Z. kommt zu der Engstelle zwischen Sofa und Ablage und gerät ins Stocken. Als sie versucht, sich durch die Engstelle zu manövrieren, gerät das Tablett in Schräglage, das Milchkännchen kippt um. Schnell eilt die Freundin zur Hilfe und nimmt Frau Z. das Tablett ab. Enttäuscht läuft Frau Z. in die Küche zurück, um einen Lappen zu holen. Der Vorfall ist ihr sehr unangenehm, die Freude gedämpft. ◀

Dual-Task-Aufgaben, also Aufgaben, bei denen zwei (oder mehr) Tätigkeiten gleichzeitig durchgeführt werden, fallen Parkinson-Betroffenen (bei fortschreitender Erkankung zunehmend) schwer. Dies liegt daran, dass bei einer Dual-Task-Aufgabe eine Tätigkeit automatisiert weiterlaufen muss, während die andere Tätigkeit mehr Aufmerksamkeit benötigt. Durch die gestörten Abläufe im Limbischen System, die durch den Dopaminmangel ausgelöst wurden, übernimmt der Kortex im Parkinson-Gehirn auch die Steuerung von früher automatisierten Tätigkeiten. Soll das Gehirn sich nun bewusst auf zwei parallel laufende Tätigkeiten konzentrieren, kann es zu einer Überlastung kommen. Eine oder mehr Tätigkeiten brechen zusammen, der Fluss ist gestört und die Klientin kann die Betätigung oftmals nicht oder nur zum Teil erfolgreich beenden.

Typische Dual-Tasks, die bei M. Parkinson eingeschränkt sind:

- Schlucken und Sprechen (z. B. in sozialen Situationen Essen)
- Laufen und Zuhören (z. B. Spaziergang mit Partnerin)
- Transfer und Anweisungen befolgen (z. B. Transfer aus Bett mit Pflegeperson)
- Schreiben und Nachdenken, wie der Satz weitergeht (z. B. beim Briefeschreiben)
- Autofahren
- Laufen und Mobiltelefon beantworten
- Laufen und Schlüssel aus der Jackentasche holen
- …

Es gibt zwei mögliche Verfahrensweisen für Dual-Task-Aufgaben bei M. Parkinson. Entweder die Dual-Tasks werden vermieden oder sie werden geübt. Sobald der Klientin und – ganz wichtig – auch dem Angehörigen der Zusammenhang zwischen Dual-Tasks und Problemen beim Ablauf (z. B. Freezing) erklärt wird, erkennen sie es häufig als Ursache für viele problematische Betätigungen im Alltag. Anschließend können sie gemeinsam mit dem Therapeuten daran arbeiten, Dual-Tasks im Alltag weitgehend zu vermeiden. Bezogen auf o. g. Beispiele, sind in Tab. 14.7 ein paar Lösungsvorschläge.

Tab. 14.7 Beispiele für die Vermeidung von Dual-Task-Aufgaben

Dual-Task (s. Abb. 14.11)	Lösungsidee
Schlucken und Sprechen	Am Esstisch bewusst erst schlucken, dann Sprechen
Laufen und Zuhören	Mit Spazierpartner besprechen, dass während des Laufens nicht gesprochen wird, sondern in der Pause auf der Parkbank
Transfer und Anweisung	Anweisungen von Pflegeperson müssen kurz sein und nur **vor** den Handlungsschritten oder in Handlungspausen gegeben werden
Schreiben und Nachdenken	Beim Schreiben zuerst überlegen, welcher Satz (oder Satzteil) geschrieben wird, dann durchführen, anschließend wieder Pause zum Nachdenken
Autofahren	Bei deutlichen Dual-Task-Schwierigkeiten sollte das Autofahren aufgegeben werden
Laufen und Mobiltelefon beantworten	Beim Klingeln des Telefons stehen bleiben, antworten, nach dem Auflegen weiterlaufen
Laufen und Schlüssel aus der Tasche holen	Schlüssel erst direkt vor der Tür, nach dem Stehenbleiben, herausholen.

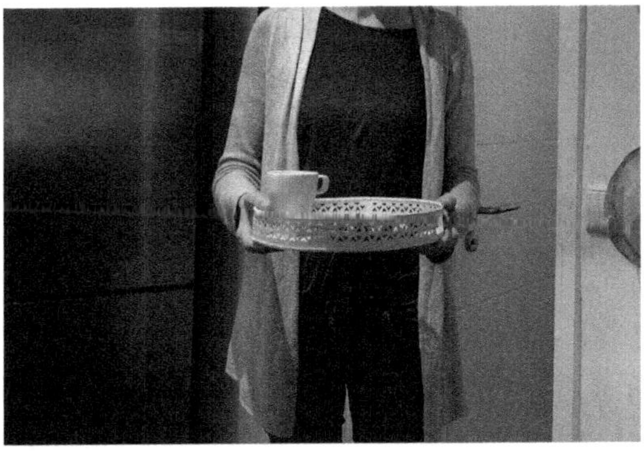

Abb. 14.11 Typisches Dual-Task: Tablett tragen und laufen

Bei einigen Dual-Tasks ist eine Vermeidung nicht möglich oder die Klientin wünscht sich, es weiterhin zusammen durchzuführen. In diesem Fall ist auch eine Beübung von Dual-Tasks möglich (Canning 2005; Strouwen et al. 2017). Demnach ist das Trainieren von Dual-Tasks möglich. Folgendes Vorgehen wird empfohlen:

1. **Aufgabenspezifisch**: Das abstrakte Üben von Dual-Tasks wird nicht empfohlen. Nach einem Dual-Task-Training in einem Hindernisparcours mit spontan zugeworfenen Bällen kann nicht erwartet werden, dass im Anschluss das Einpacken der Einkäufe und gleichzeitiges Hören des Kaufbetrags verbessert möglich ist. Vielmehr muss die spezifische Situation entweder reell oder simuliert trainiert werden. Z. B.: Klientin packt Dinge in eine Tasche und versucht, vom Therapeuten gesagte Geldbeträge zu hören und sich zu merken.
2. **Tätigkeiten einzeln oder zusammen trainieren**: Strouwen et al. (2017) verglichen, ob es beim Dual-Task-Training besser ist, die einzelnen Tätigkeiten einzeln nacheinander oder zusammen zu üben. Im Ergebnis stellten sie fest, dass beide Methoden gleich wirksam sind. Es liegt also im Ermessen des Therapeuten zu entscheiden, welche Art des Trainings in dem spezifischen Fall vorzuziehen ist.
3. **Eigenübung**: Je häufiger das Dual-Task-Training wiederholt wird, desto flüssiger wird der Ablauf der Betätigung. Ein Eigentraining auf dem Klientinnenzimmer oder zu Hause ist also eine große Unterstützung der Therapie. Oftmals sind Angehörige gerne bereit, die Eigenübungen zu begleiten.
4. **Regelmäßige Auffrischung**: Wie bei allen Arten von Training mit Menschen mit der Parkinson-Erkrankung, nimmt der Effekt des Trainings mit der Zeit ab. Es wird also vorgeschlagen, alle 3–5 Wochen die Trainingssequenz zu wiederholen.

Beispiel

Einen Monat später hat Frau Z. wieder Besuch von Ihrer Nachbarin. Sie freut sich, ist aber auch nervös. „Ich möchte dir kurz etwas erklären," beginnt sie. „Der Parkinson wirkt sich ja auf sehr unterschiedliche Art und Weise aus. Bei mir ist es zum Beispiel so: Wenn ich zwei Sachen gleichzeitig tue – also Dinge, die ich früher automatisch gemacht habe –, dann hänge ich. Das liegt am Dopaminmangel im Gehirn."

- „Ich helfe dir gerne."
- „Ich möchte den Kaffee gerne selber rüber tragen, schließlich bist du mein Gast. Ich habe das geübt in der Ergotherapie. Nur um eins möchte ich dich bitten. – Ich kann nicht gleichzeitig das Tablett tragen und dir zuhören. Lass uns also erst wieder sprechen, wenn ich sitze."
- „Oh, natürlich. Jetzt verstehe ich es auch."

Die nächsten Besuche verlaufen reibungslos. Nach einem Jahr fühlt sich Frau Z. weniger sicher und trotz Dual-Task-Trainings stockt sie häufig beim Tablett tragen. Sie entscheidet sich, nach Beratung der Ergotherapeutin, einen Servierwagen zu kaufen. ◀

14.1.6 Große Amplitude

Beispiel

Hr. K. ist häufig bedrückt und von sich selbst enttäuscht. Die Ärztin hat eine Depression diagnostiziert, was Herr K. anzweifelt und ihn noch mehr ins Grübeln bringt. Seine ganze Körperhaltung ist zusammengesunken, der Kopf nach unten gebeugt, die Schultern fallen nach vorne, sein Rücken ist gekrümmt. Er verbringt viel Zeit sitzend auf seinem Stuhl. In den letzten Monaten haben sich seine Aktivitäten aufgrund der Beschränkungen der Corona-Pandemie zusehends reduziert. Es ist Herrn K. bewusst, dass Bewegung wichtig ist, aber diese kostet ihn große Überwindung. Die gezeigten Schwungübungen empfindet er als langweilig. ◀

Die bei Menschen mit M. Parkinson typische Hypokinese ist meist bei jeder Betätigung sichtbar. Das Bewegungsausmaß ist reduziert, obwohl in den muskuloskelettalen Strukturen primär keine Schädigung vorliegt. Die Motorik wirkt gedrosselt und ist auch beim Armschwung, der Mimik und Gestik deutlich sichtbar. Der Ursprung der reduzierten Amplitude liegt in der veränderten Körperwahrnehmung. Die Propriozeption ist deutlich reduziert. Die propriozeptive Wahrnehmung fungiert als „innerer Kalibrator" im Gehirn der Klientin, gibt Rückmeldung über die durchgeführte Bewegung. Da dies bei Menschen mit Morbus Parkinson fehlerhaft ist, kommt es zu einer Hypokinese.

Zum Erreichen einer vergrößerten Amplitude muss die Motorik neu kalibriert werden. Dies geschieht bestenfalls durch ein intensives, repetitives, aufmerksames Training der Betätigung oder einer Performanzfertigkeit (Performance-Skill), siehe Kap. 13. Zur **Unterstützung** der betätigungsspezifischen Therapie ist ein abstraktes Training von ausladenden Bewegungen sinnvoll, um die allgemeine Beweglichkeit zu erhalten. Auch diese sollte folgende Komponenten aufweisen:

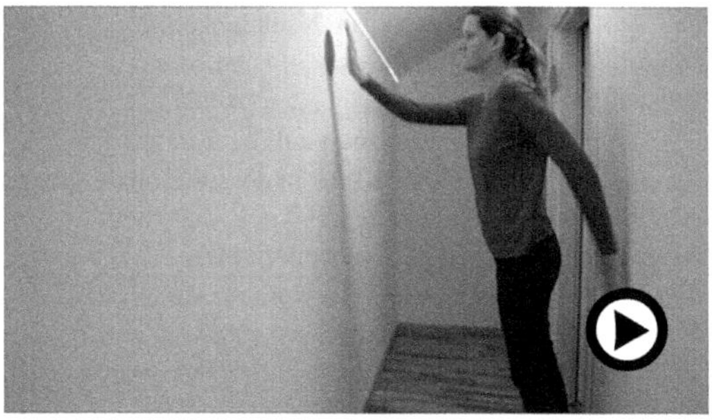

Abb. 14.12 Armschwung mit Referenzflächen (▶ https://doi.org/10.1007/000-2xj)

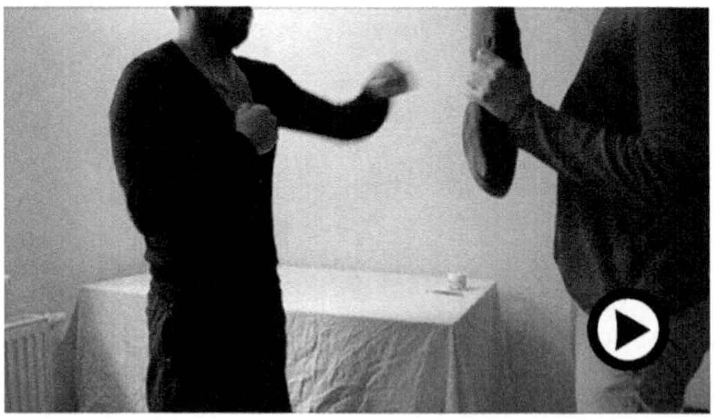

Abb. 14.13 Boxen (▶ https://doi.org/10.1007/000-2xk)

- repetitiv
- intensiv
- aufmerksam
- mit Referenzflächen (s. Video 14.12, Abb. 14.12, Video 14.13, Abb. 14.13)

Amplitudentraining in der Betätigung

Neben dem abstrakten Amplitudentraining kann das Bewegungsausmaß konkret für eine Betätigung trainiert werden. Der Therapeut identifiziert zunächst den Moment in dem die Betätigung scheitert, den sog. Break-Down-Point. Dazu sollte eine Betätigungsanalyse durchgeführt werden (siehe Kap. 6). Dann trainiert die Klientin genau diesen Break-Down-Point repetitiv, intensiv und mit Referenzflächen. Diese Vorgehensweise wird in Kap. 13 ausführlich erarbeitet. Dafür sollten Referenzflächen eingesetzt werden. Am besten werden vorhandene Flächen als Referenzflächen festgelegt, die bei der Bewegungsdurchführung erreicht werden müssen.

Beispiele sind beim Tischabwischen die Tischkante und beim Brilleputzen der Brillenrahmen (siehe Video 14.14, Abb. 14.14 und Video 14.15, Abb. 14.15). Wenn keine natürlichen Referenzflächen vorliegen, können „künstliche" Flächen zu Trainingszwecken eingesetzt werden. Als hilfreich haben sich laminierte Kreise aus buntem Papier erwiesen, die an der Stelle platziert werden, die beim Amplitudentraining erreicht werden soll (siehe Abb. 14.16).

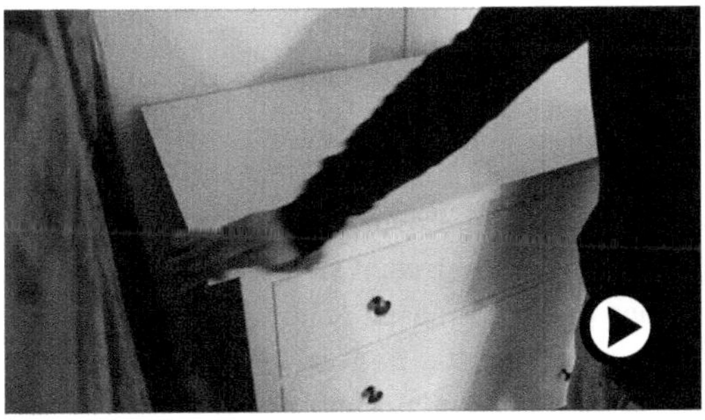

Abb. 14.14 Oberfläche abwischen. Der Klient wischt bewusst von einer Kante zur Anderen, um Hypokinese zu vermeiden (▶ https://doi.org/10.1007/000-2xm)

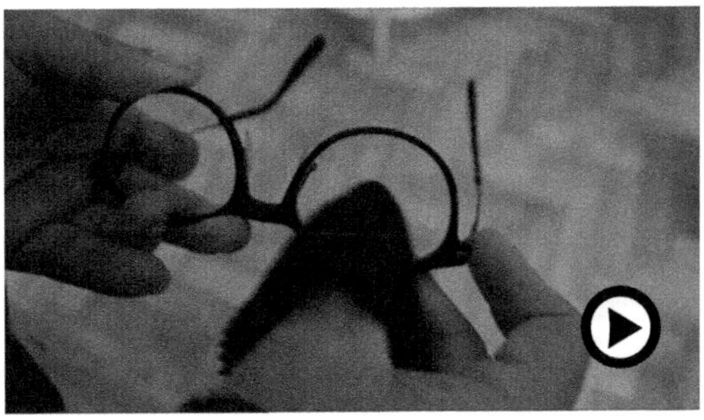

Abb. 14.15 Brille Putzen. Der Klient wird angeleitet von Rand zu Rand zu putzen, um Hypokinese zu vermeiden (▶ https://doi.org/10.1007/000-2xn)

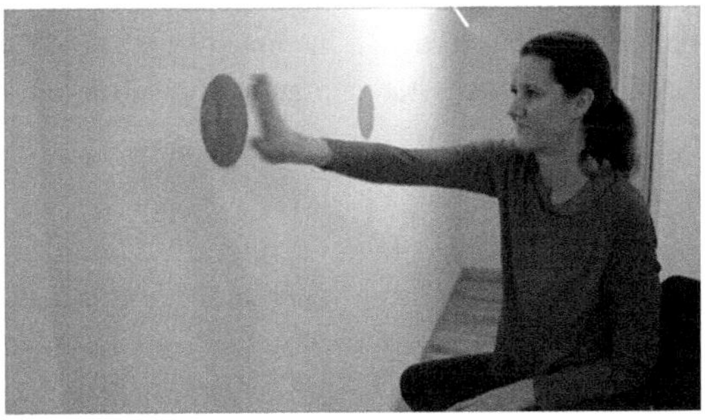

Abb. 14.16 Farbige Referenzkreise unterstützen die Klientin darin, beim Training die große Amplitude beizubehalten

BIG-Therapie

Das LSVT-BIG-Programm wurde aus dem „Lee Silverman Voice Treatment" (LSVT-LOUD) weiterentwickelt, bei dem es um die Sprechlautstärke geht. Bei der BIG-Therapie ist das Ziel eine möglichst große Bewegungsamplitude zu erreichen. Dazu werden bestimmte Bewegungsabfolgen eingeübt, die verschiedene Komponenten vereinen: maximale Amplitude, Rotation, Cueing, Stimme, aktive Dehnung und Rhythmus. Zusätzlich entwickelt der Therapeut individuell gestaltete funktionelle Komponenten, die sich nach den Schwierigkeiten des Klienten richten.

Das Training ist sehr intensiv mit einer hohen Übungshäufigkeit. Es besteht aus 16 Übungseinheiten, aufgeteilt in vier Sitzungen pro Woche für vier Wochen. Jede Übungseinheit dauert eine

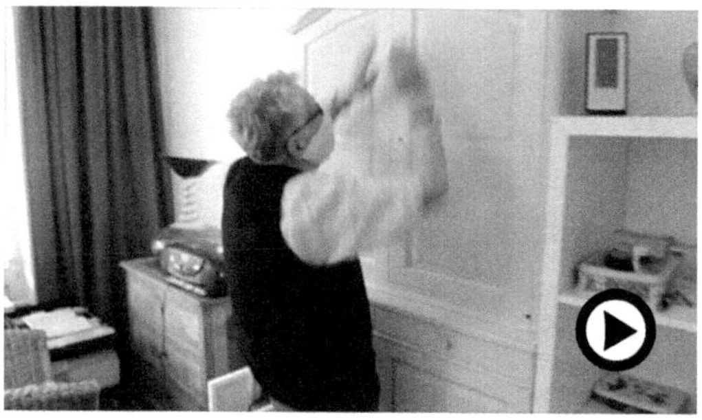

Abb. 14.17 Musik kann bei Amplitudentraining Rhythmus unterstützen und generell stimmungsaufhellend wirken (▶ https://doi.org/10.1007/000-2xp)

Stunde. Zusätzlich sollen tägliche Eigenübungen durchgeführt werden. In mehreren Studien konnte die Effektivität nachgewiesen werden.

Beispiel

Einer Eingebung folgend setzt die Therapeutin bei der nächsten Therapieeinheit Musik während den Übungen ein. „Mozart ist mein Leben," sagt Herr K. mit Tränen in den Augen, dann setzt er mit einem Lächeln schwungvoll und rhythmisch zu seinen Übungen an (s. Video 14.17, Abb. 14.17). ◀

14.2 Rigor

14.2.1 Symptombeschreibung

Der Rigor ist ein erhöhter Grundtonus der Muskulatur und tritt bei M. Parkinson im gesamten Körper auf, dabei ist er in den Flexoren stärker ausgeprägt als in den Extensoren. Die Betroffenen haben das Gefühl, sich konstant gegen eine bremsende Festigkeit zu bewegen. Beim passiven Mobilisieren einer Extremität kann die Therapeutin einen zähen, wächsernen Widerstand spüren, der in alle Richtungen und von Anfang bis Ende der Bewegung gleich stark und geschwindigkeitsunabhängig ist. Manchmal kann dieser Widerstand von dem sog. „**Zahnradphänomen**" begleitet werden. Einem schnellen, ruckartigen Nachlassen, welches durch einen unterliegenden Tremor ausgelöst wird. Von außen erscheinen die Bewegungen mühsam und schleppend, als würden sie sich durch Wasser ziehen.

Der Rigor ist verantwortlich für die parkinsontypische **vornübergebeugte Haltung** und **mangelnde Beweglichkeit im Rumpf**. **Kopf**- und **Rumpfrotation** sind kaum zu beobachten, stattdessen werden **Drehungen en-bloc** durchgeführt. Dies schränkt die Betroffenen bei vielen Betätigungen ein, z. B. Autofahren (Schulterblick), Straße überqueren (rechts-links Blick), soziale Situationen (Ansprache von der Seite), Einkaufen (Einräumen der Ware vom Fließband in Einkaufswagen), **Richtungswechsel beim Laufen**, **Drehen im Bett**. Außerdem sind die Gelenke durch die erhöhte Muskelspannung leicht flektiert, wenn keine aktive Gegenbewegung stattfindet. Dies zeigt sich besonders im Ellenbogen-, Hand-, Finger-, Hüft- und Kniegelenk.Die pathophysiologischen Mechanismen, die zur Entstehung des Rigors beitragen sind komplex und nicht abschließend geklärt.

Komplikationen

Folgen des Rigor sind häufig Schmerzen in den betroffenen Muskelgruppen. Diese können auch schon vor Diagnosebeginn auftreten und missdeutet werden. Im späteren Krankheitsverlauf kann es zu strukturellen Veränderungen kommen, wenn die tendenziell flektierte Haltung nicht regelmäßig aktiv durch Bewegung und Dehnung gelöst wird. So sind Sekundärschäden, wie Muskelverkürzungen bis hin zu Kontrakturen in späteren Krankheitsstadien, nicht selten.

14.2.2 Übungen

Beispiel

Das Ehepaar K. fährt schon seit vielen Jahren jedes Jahr in einem Reisebus nach Kroatien ans Meer. Sie freuen sich schon Monate vorher darauf. Frau K. sagt: „Diese Reise gibt mir wieder für das ganze Jahr die innere Kraft, für meinen Mann zu sorgen." Herr K. benötigt in allen Bereichen Hilfe von seiner Frau, seine Beweglichkeit hat sich seit dem letzten Jahr durch eine Zunahme des Rigors deutlich verschlechtert. Er kann zwar ohne

Unterstützung aus dem Rollstuhl aufstehen, das Ehepaar macht sich jedoch große Sorgen, dass er, auch mithilfe von zwei Personen, die Stufen im Reisebus nicht hinaufkommt. Die Therapeutin erarbeitet ein herausforderndes Übungsprogramm mit Herrn K.: Rotationsübungen, Stehtraining und vor allem tägliches Fahren am Motomed®. Herr K. ist sehr motiviert. ◄

Da der Rigor die Beweglichkeit stark reduziert, ist jede Art der Bewegung förderlich. Klienten äußern sich, sich in ihren Bewegungen danach „freier" zu fühlen. Im Mittelpunkt stehen dabei Rotationsübungen, da der Rigor die Rumpfrotation erheblich einschränkt. Ohne Rotation sind zahlreiche Bewegungen im Alltag nicht mehr, oder nur noch mit großer Anstrengung möglich: Dazu gehören: Drehen im Bett, Transfer aus dem Bett, Kopfdrehung (z. B. im Straßenverkehr), Greifen nach seitlich liegenden Gegenständen … Fahrradfahren und Motomedfahren haben einen positiven Effekt auf den Rigor in den Beinen (s. Abb. 14.18).

► Ein Motomed kann von der Fachfirma vier Wochen kostenlos zur Probe geliehen werden. Anschließend ist eine Verordnung über den Arzt möglich, wenn dieser attestiert, dass es für den Klienten förderlich ist.

Stellt die Therapeutin bei der Betätigungsanalyse fest, dass eine Betätigung aufgrund mangelnder Kopf- oder Rumpfrotation nicht erfolgreich durchgeführt werden kann, können Rotationsübungen als Vorbereitung auf die Betätigung angezeigt sein (s. Abb. 14.19, 14.20, 14.21, 14.22, und 14.23 und Video 14.20, 14.21, und 14.22).

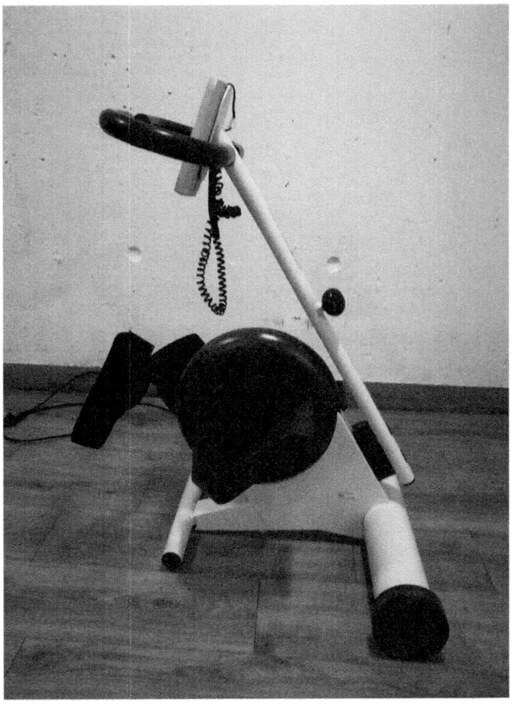

Abb. 14.18 Motomed

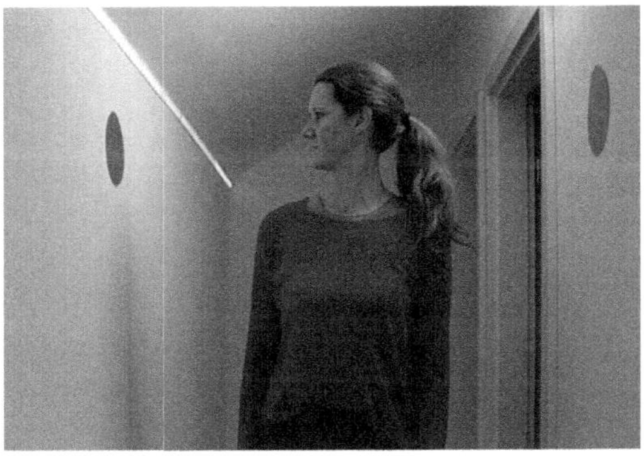

Abb. 14.19 Kopfrotation. Blick abwechselnd auf roten, dann blauen Kreis, damit größtmögliche Rotation erreicht wird

Beispiel

Nach acht Wochen des Trainings in der Ergo- und Physiotherapie, plus dem intensiven Eigenübungsprogramm, geht die Reise los. Herrn K. wird mit viel Hilfe seines Sohnes und seiner Frau Schritt für Schritt, Stufe für Stufe in den Reisebus geholfen. Mit einem Lächeln sinkt er in den Sitz und winkt seinem Sohn aus dem Fenster zu. ◄

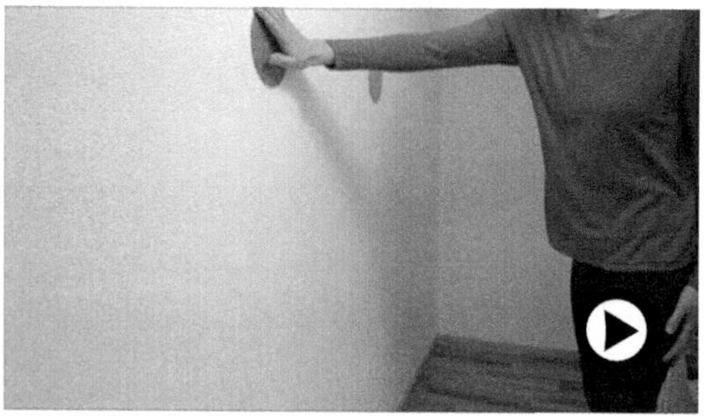

Abb. 14.20 Rumpfrotation mit überkreuzter Armextension (▶ https://doi.org/10.1007/000-2xq)

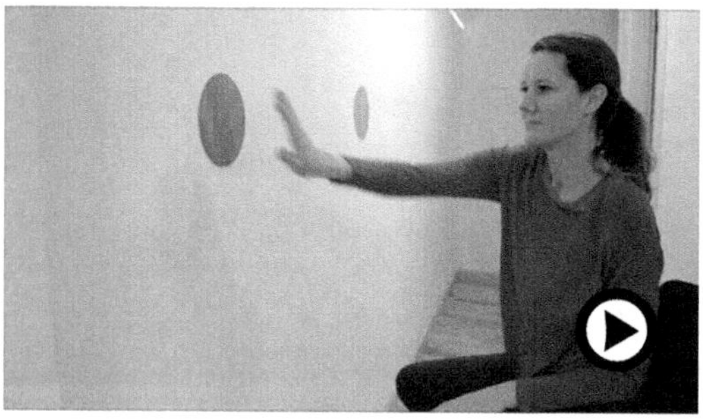

Abb. 14.21 Rumpfrotation mit überkreuzter Armextension im Sitzen (▶ https://doi.org/10.1007/000-2xr)

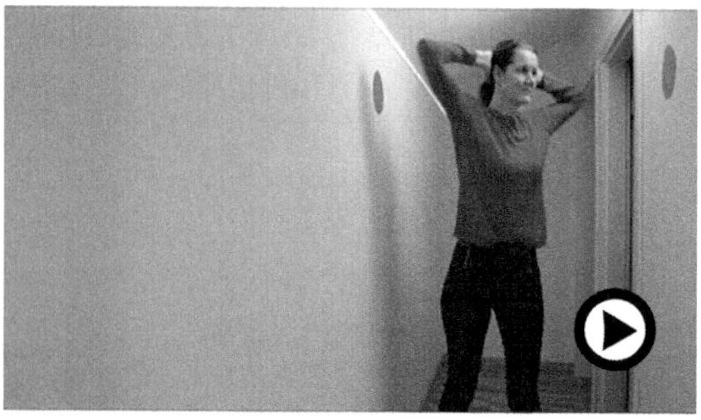

Abb. 14.22 Rumpfrotation mit Dehnung Pektoralis und visueller Nutzung von Referenzkreisen, um möglichst große Rotationsbewegung zu erreichen (▶ https://doi.org/10.1007/000-2xs)

14.3 Tremor

14.3.1 Symptombeschreibung

Der Tremor ist eines der Kardinalsymptome bei M. Parkinson. Der einseitig beginnende, klassische Ruhetremor führt recht zuverlässig zur Diagnose „Morbus Parkinson".

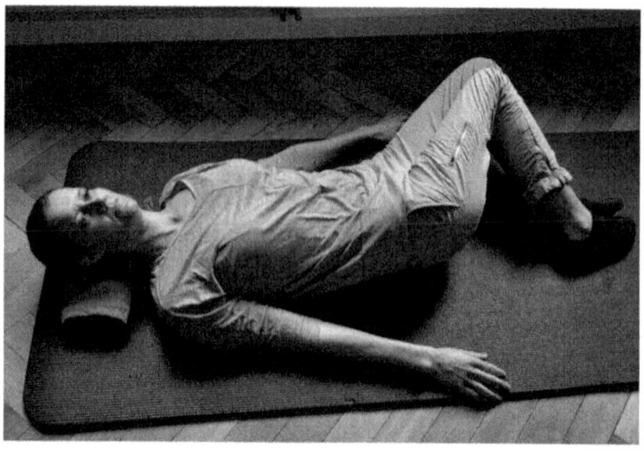

Abb. 14.23 Im Liegen Beine nach rechts und links kippen. Diese Übung ist optimal um die Rumpfrotation isoliert zu üben, wenn der Klient bei der Drehung im Bett die Bewegung en bloc durchführt. Durch die isolierte Übung wird die Körperwahrnehmung auf die, für den Klienten, ungewohnte Bewegung gerichtet, damit er die Bewegung in der Alltagssituation abrufen kann

Definition Man unterscheidet drei Tremorformen bei M. Parkinson:

- Typ I: Isoliert auftretender Ruhetremor oder Ruhetremor wird von Halte-/Bewegungstremor derselben Frequenz begleitet

Ruhetremor ist der typische Parkinson-Tremor. Das rhythmische Zittern tritt bei entspannter Muskulatur meist in den oberen Extremitäten auf, hat eine große Amplitude und eine relativ langsame Frequenz von 4–6 Hz. Meist tritt der Ruhetremor allein auf, es kann jedoch ein Halte-/Bewegungstremor in der gleichen Frequenz auftreten.

- Typ II: Ruhe- und Halte-/Bewegungstremor unterschiedlicher Frequenz

Bei diesem Tremortyp kommt ein Ruhetremor (s. o.) in Kombination mit einem Halte-/Bewegungstremor (s. u.) einer höheren Frequenz vor. Es gibt Vermutungen, dass es sich hierbei um zwei Tremorarten handelt, der Parkinson-Tremor mit dem essenziellen Tremor.

- Typ III: reiner Halte-/Bewegungstremor

Der reine Halte-/Bewegungstremor tritt beim M. Parkinson sehr selten auf. Bei dieser Tremorform wird das rhythmische Zittern bei

Muskelanspannung aktiviert und hat eine höhere Frequenz von >5 Hz. Trotz dieser allgemein anerkannten Unterscheidung der drei Tremorformen sind in der Praxis Mischformen nicht selten und selbst die Abgrenzung zum essentiellen Tremor ist nicht immer eindeutig, zumal es Studien gibt, die auf eine Verknüpfung der beiden Diagnosen hindeuten.

Ätiologie Ursächlich für den Tremor ist eine gestörte Funktion in den komplexen Regelkreisen der Basalganglien. In der Literatur sind unterschiedliche Erklärungsansätze zu finden, wovon jedoch keiner als bestätigt gilt.

Prävalenz Bei um die 70 % der an M. Parkinson Erkrankten tritt im Laufe der Zeit Tremor auf.

Klinik Tremor wird bei ca. 70 % der Menschen im Frühstadium der Erkrankung als erstes Symptom bemerkt. Er beginnt meist unilateral und kann später bilateral auftreten.

Ruhetremor tritt bei komplett entspannter Muskulatur auf, z. B. bei aufgelegten Unterarmen. Er kann durch geistige Beschäftigung (z. B. in Dreierschritten Rückwärts zählen), Stress, Angst und Schlafmangel verstärkt werden. Dabei nimmt die Amplitude zu, nicht die Frequenz. Außerdem ist es Menschen mit M. Parkinson meist möglich, den Tremor kurzzeitig durch Willenskraft zu unterdrücken – abgrenzend zu anderen Tremortypen (z. B. essenzieller Tremor). Sobald die Muskulatur aktiviert wird, hört der Ruhetremor auf. Meist erscheint der Tremor in der oberen Extremität, aber auch der Kopf oder die untere Extremität können betroffen sein. Oftmals tritt er als sog. Pillendreher-Tremor in Erscheinung, bei dem Daumen und Zeigefinger aneinander gerieben werden. Im Gegensatz zum Ruhetremor tritt der **Halte-** und **Bewegungstremor** bei Muskelaktivität auf. Er wird also beim Greifen oder Halten eines Gegenstandes sichtbar und beeinflusst den Alltag und die Selbständigkeit erheblich.

Folgen/Komplikationen Der Tremor wird von Patientinnen als unterschiedlich einschränkend im Alltag empfunden, je nach Ausprägung und begleitenden Symptomen. Viele Klientinnen versuchen den Tremor zu unterdrücken, z. B. durch Festhalten der Hand, oder zu verstecken, z. B. hinter dem Rücken oder in der Tasche, um in der Öffentlichkeit nicht aufzufallen.

Medizinische Möglichkeiten

- Medikamente (L-Dopa beeinflusst Tremor kaum)
- Tiefe Hirnstimulation

Beispiel

Für Herrn P. ist die Familie das Wichtigste – und gutes Essen. Doch seit einiger Zeit zieht er sich lieber von den Familienfeiern zurück. Er schämt sich so. Wegen des Tremors in beiden Händen bleibt nichts auf der Gabel, er verschüttet alles und sein Essensplatz sieht anschließend unansehnlich und fleckig aus. So sollen ihn seine Enkel nicht sehen. ◀

14.3.2 Umgang im Alltag

Eines der Symptome, die Betroffene subjektiv am stärksten einschränkt, ist der Tremor. Er kann sich negativ auf alle Bereiche des täglichen Lebens auswirken und ist kaum kontrollierbar. Außerdem ist er für Außenstehende klar sichtbar, was vielen Betroffenen äußerst unangenehm ist. Tremor ist am effektivsten medikamentös behandelbar. Wenn Medikamente nicht oder nicht mehr anschlagen, gibt es bedauerlicherweise kaum therapeutisch wirksame Methoden. Aus diesem Grund wird der kompensatorische Ansatz am häufigsten verwendet.

Offener Umgang im Alltag
Zunächst ist es wichtig, nicht gegen den Tremor „anzukämpfen". Dies führt zu Anspannung und Stress, was wiederum den Tremor verstärkt. Sich eine gewisse Gelassenheit anzueignen ist für Klientinnen ein lohnendes Ziel beim Umgang mit Tremor in der Öffentlichkeit. Die Umsetzung im Alltag ist allerdings kompliziert, weil Gefühle von Scham oder Wut aufkommen können (s. Abb. 14.24).

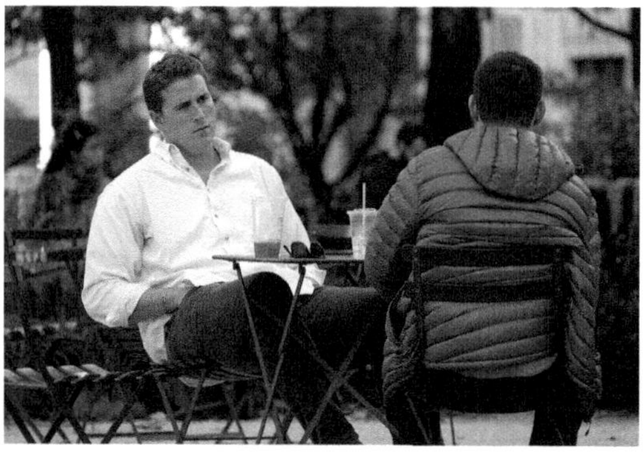

Abb. 14.24 Ein offenes Gespräch über Tremor kann unangenehme Situationen in der Öffentlichkeit entspannen

Einige Betroffene schaffen es, offensiv mit dem Tremor umzugehen, indem sie es zu Beginn der Interaktion kurz ansprechen. Dadurch erlangen sie etwas Kontrolle über die unangenehme Situation.

In Bewegung bleiben
Der parkinsontypische Ruhetremor tritt nur auf, wenn der Körperteil in Ruhe ist, die Muskeln also inaktiv sind. Viele Klientinnen nutzen diese Tatsache aus, und bleiben vor allem in sozialen Situationen, in denen das äußere Erscheinungsbild möglichst normal erscheinen soll, konstant in Bewegung. Bei einem Tremor in der Hand wird beispielsweise viel gestikuliert oder mit einem Stift oder Knetball gespielt.

Entspannung
Bei allen Betroffenen wird der Tremor durch Stress verstärkt, bei manchen Menschen tritt der Tremor nur in Stresssituationen auf. Eine Entspannung kann zu einer Abnahme des Tremors führen. Die effektivste Methode zur Entspannung ist individuell unterschiedlich und sollte mit der Klientin zusammen erarbeitet werden (siehe Abschn. 14.10.4, Entspannung).

Körperhaltung
Die Körperhaltung hat in manchen Fällen einen Einfluss auf die Stärke des Tremors. Folglich kann die Veränderung der Stellung des Körpers bei der Durchführung einer Tätigkeit den Tremor verbessern. Oftmals entdecken die Betroffenen diese Tatsache selbst. Es ist ratsam, in der Therapie verschiedene Stellungen der Körperteile zu probieren, z. B. stärker angewinkelte Beine, festes Aufstellen der Füße auf dem Boden, Nutzen der Rückenlehne, stärkere Beugung des Hüftgelenks, körpernahes oder -fernes Agieren mit Händen.

Ablenkende Faktoren
Bei einigen Klientinnen verstärkt sich der Tremor bei Dual-Tasks oder wenn äußere Faktoren von der durchgeführten Tätigkeit ablenken. Dementsprechend sollte darauf geachtet werden, dass in Situationen, in denen vermehrt Tremor auftritt, die Aufgaben Schritt für Schritt und in einer ruhigen Umgebung durchgeführt werden.

14.3.3 Kompensation

Im Alltag kann ein Tremor äußerst einschränkend sein. Speisen und Getränke werden verschüttet, Stürze provoziert und die soziale Interaktion leidet. Es ist für Ergotherapeuten entscheidend, die genaue Situation zu analysieren, in denen die Klientin sich vom Tremor eingeschränkt fühlt, um geeignete Kompensationsstrategien vorzuschlagen. Dabei sollen die Therapeuten dazu ermutigt werden, ihr ganzes ergotherapeutisches Repertoire zu nutzen, um für die individuelle Betätigung der Klientin eine individuelle Lösung zu finden. Hierbei können folgende Punkte hilfreich sein.

Größe der Auflagefläche
Eine Vergrößerung der Auflagefläche bei einer Tätigkeit kann das Auftreten des Tremors (meist Intensions- oder Haltetremor) unterbinden oder abschwächen. Dazu müssen gewohnte Bewegungsabläufe verändert werden, was vielen Menschen mit M. Parkinson, wegen der reduzierten kognitiven Umstellungsfähigkeit, schwerfällt. Eine ausführliche Erarbeitung mit häufiger Wiederholung der neuen Betätigung ist empfehlenswert. Beispiele Sind in Abb. 14.25, 14.26, 14.27, 14.28, und 14.29, Videos 14.27, Video 14.29) zu finden.

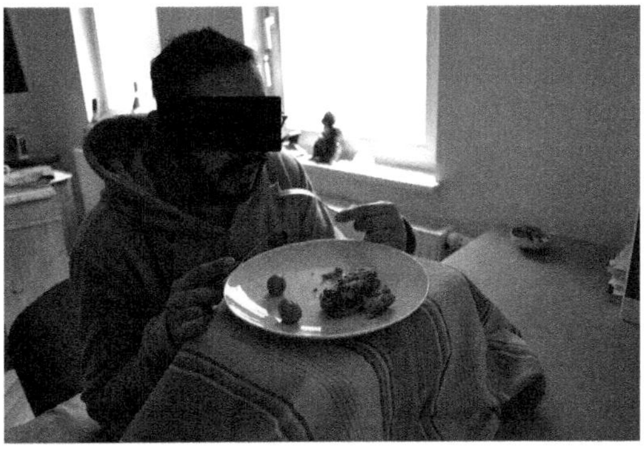

Abb. 14.25 Erhöhung des Tellers, damit der Weg von Teller zu Mund kürzer ist und die Hand konstant aufgelegt bleiben kann

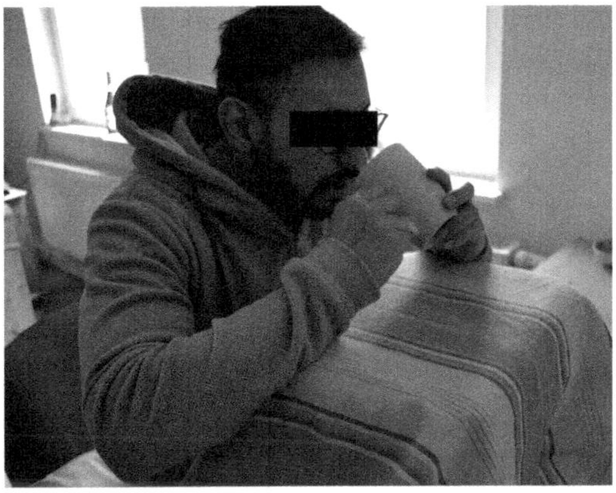

Abb. 14.26 Beim Trinken Hand mit Tasse auf erhobenen Block ablegen und kippen, dabei die Tasse mit beiden Händen umfassen

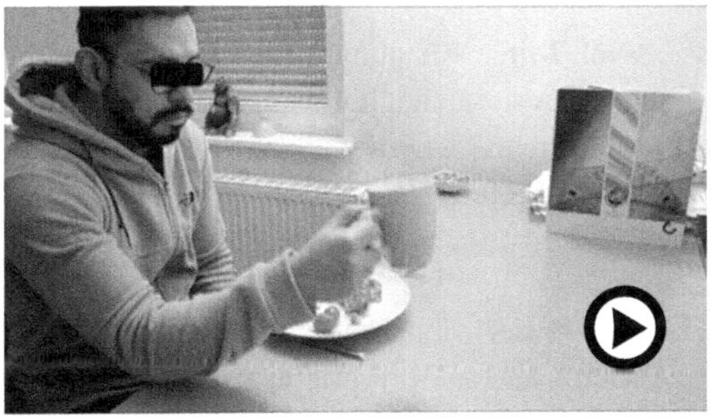

Abb. 14.27 Beim Greifen nach einem Gegenstand mit Arm am Tisch entlangfahren und Ellenbogen aufstützen beim Trinken (▶ https://doi.org/10.1007/000-2xt)

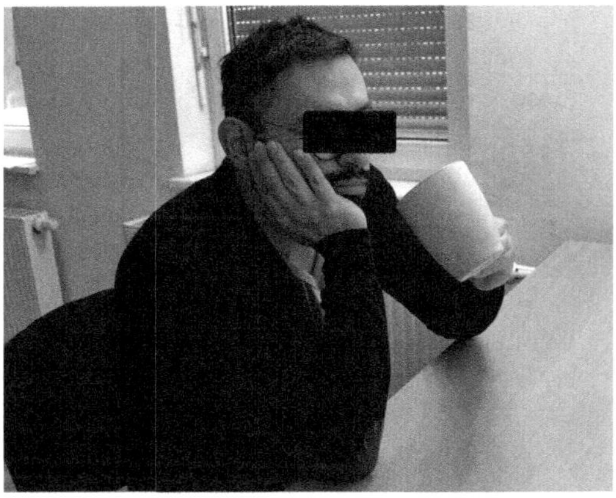

Abb. 14.28 Beim Trinken/Essen mit Kopftremor, Ellenbogen auf Tisch abstützen, Kopf auf Hand ablegen

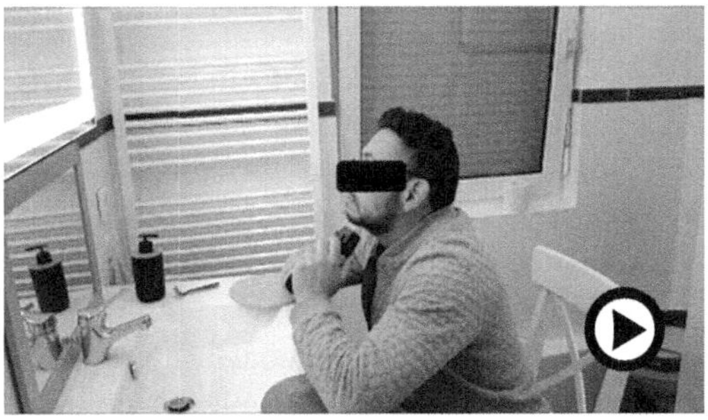

Abb. 14.29 Bei Tremor ist der kompensatorische Therapieansatz meist der effektivste. Nutzung von vergrößerter Unterstützungsfläche bei Betätigungen und Führung des Arms mit eigener Hand, oder Umfassung des Gegenstandes mit beiden Händen (▶ https://doi.org/10.1007/000-2xv)

Hilfsmittel

Vor allem Hilfsmittel können bei Tremor hilfreich sein. In Abschn. 15.3 sind Hilfsmittel aufgeführt, auf die dies zutrifft, z. B. beschwerte Gegenstände, Tremor ausgleichende Utensilien und spezifische Deckel.

Beispiel

An Weihnachten ist Herr P. bestens vorbereitet. Die Partnerin ist darauf eingestellt, ihrem Mann nur eine kleine Portion auf den Teller zu geben. Sein Teller steht auf einer kleinen Kiste, damit der Weg zum Mund nicht so weit ist, und er benutzt eine schwere Gabel, damit sie nicht so durch die Gegend fliegt, und hat einen Strohhalm im Glas. Vor dem Essen spricht er das Thema mit seinem Sohn und seiner Enkelin, die neben ihm sitzen, offen an: „Tut mir leid, wenn gleich etwas danebengeht, der Parkinson und ich geben uns Mühe, euch nicht zu bekleckern. Aber wenn ihr Schutzkleidung braucht, einfach Bescheid sagen …," ergänzt er mit einem Zwinkern. ◀

14.4 Posturale Instabilität und Stürze

14.4.1 Symptombeschreibung

Im späteren Krankheitsverlauf tritt bei den meisten Patienten eine posturale Instabilität auf. Aus dem fehlenden Zusammenspiel von Stellreflexen, Aufrichtung und Kraft in der unteren Extremität resultiert eine erhöhte Stand- und Gangunsicherheit mit akuter Sturzgefahr. Laut der neuesten Definition der MDS (International Parkinson and Movement Disorder Society) gilt die posturale Instabilität nicht mehr als Kardinalsymptom. Die Einschränkung der posturalen Stabilität, ist ein späteres Krankheitszeichen und tritt einige Jahre nach der Diagnosestellung auf. Wenn es schon bei Diagnosestellung auftritt ist es ein „Red Flag" für einen atypischen Parkinson.

Die posturale Stabilität ist die Fähigkeit des Körpers, eine Position nach einem destabilisierenden Reiz wiederzuerlangen. Nicht erkrankte Personen zeigen folgende natürliche Reflexe bei einem destabilisierenden Reiz, z. B. Geschubstwerden:

- Korrektive Strategien, ohne Veränderung der Unterlagefläche
  - Sprunggelenkstrategie (ausgleichende Bewegung in Sprunggelenken)
  - Hüftgelenkstrategie (ausgleichende Bewegung in den Hüftgelenken)
- Protektive Strategien, mit Veränderung der Unterlagefläche
  - Ausfallschritt (vor, zurück oder zur Seite)
  - Greifen oder Abstützen der Arme (Festhalten an festem Gegenstand oder Abstützen am Boden bei Sturz)

Alle o. g. Strategien sind bei Parkinson-Patienten vermindert oder nicht beobachtbar. Als Ursache für die posturale Instabilität bestehen zwei Hauptfaktoren. Zum einen führt die **reduzierte Propriozeption** zu einem **ungenauen Körperschema**, sodass die Notwendigkeit für eine Anpassung der Haltung oder für einen Ausfallschritt nicht registriert wird und auch die Genauigkeit der Ausgleichbewegung oder des Ausgleichschrittes unzureichend ist. Zum anderen führt die **Bradykinese** zu einer **Verzögerung der notwendigen Reaktion**, sodass das Gleichgewicht gegebenenfalls nicht gehalten werden kann.

Die posturale Instabilität kann wechselhaft sein, da sie stark von der Medikamentenwirkung und Aufmerksamkeit abhängig ist. So mag die posturale Stabilität bei der Testung unauffällig sein. Sobald der Klient jedoch nicht seine ganze Aufmerksamkeit auf die korrektiven oder protektiven Strategien fokussiert, treten Stürze auf. Dies sollte bei der therapeutischen Einschätzung einer Sturzgefährdung immer mit bedacht werden.

▶ **Cave!** Mit Abnahme der posturalen Stabilität steigt die Sturzwahrscheinlichkeit rapide an und nach dem ersten Sturz nimmt die Sturzgefahr stetig zu.

Stürze

Etwa 60 % der Menschen mit M. Parkinson haben schon einen Sturz erlebt, ca. 39 % stürzen regelmäßig. Die Ursachen für Stürze bei Parkinson-Betroffenen sind komplex und vielschichtig. Primär sind sie mit folgenden Merkmalen verbunden: Alter, Schwere der Erkrankung, Medikamenteneinnahme, Gang- und Gleichgewichtsdefizite, mangelnde Aktivität und kognitive Einschränkungen (Allen et al. 2013). Sekundär wirken sich Merkmale auf die Sturzwahrscheinlichkeit aus, die als Reaktion nach einem Sturz auftreten: Fallangst, reduziertes Selbstvertrauen, Schwäche und mangelnde Mobilität. Die Folge von Stürzen können Schenkelhalsfraktur, andere Frakturen, Kopftrauma, Prellung und weitere Verletzungen sein. Außerdem ergeben sich in Folge einer häufig auftretenden Fallangst Mobilitätsverlust, Osteoporose, Rückzugstendenzen, soziale Isolation und Depressionen.

Beispiel

Herr Sch. liegt am Boden, der rechte Arm schmerzt. „Verdammt! Schon wieder gefallen." Da kommt auch schon seine Tochter die Treppe herauf gehetzt. „Papa, was ist passiert? Ich habe den Rumms gehört. Lass dir aufhelfen!" Doch Herr Sch. will keine Hilfe. Er schickt die Tochter wieder hinunter, rappelt sich selber auf und sammelt die Socken vom Boden auf, die er sich gerade hatte anziehen wollen. ◀

Vor allem im späteren Verlauf der Erkrankung tritt verstärkt eine posturale Instabilität auf und Stürze nehmen zu. Destabilisierende Reize, wie das Anfahren der Straßenbahn oder angerempelt werden (externer Reiz) sowie plötzliches Freezing (interner Reiz), können nicht ausgeglichen werden. Die Sturzgefahr nimmt stark zu. Eine frühe Intervention, die auf Gang- und Gleichgewichtstraining fokussiert, wird empfohlen und ist auch vorbeugend indiziert. Die Wichtigkeit des frühen Trainings der posturalen Stabilität sollte auch den Klienten und Angehörigen gegenüber hervorgehoben werden, damit das Thema im Eigentraining und Sport angemessen gefördert wird, vor allem auch mit Blick darauf, dass Medikamente wenig Einfluss auf die posturale Stabilität haben.

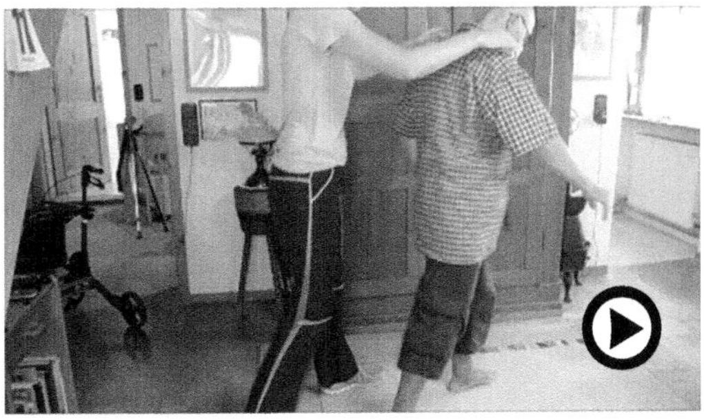

Abb. 14.30 Pulsionstraining zur Sturzprävention (▶ https://doi.org/10.1007/000-2xw)

14.4.2 Übungen zur Sturzprävention

Pulsionstraining

Jöbges et al. beschreibt (2004) folgendes Pulsionstraining: Die Therapeutin zieht wiederholt kurz an den Schultern des Patienten nach hinten oder nach rechts oder links. Wie kräftig gezogen und gestoßen wird, wird dem Grad der posturalen Instabilität des Patienten angepasst und sollte gesteigert oder reduziert werden, je nach Entwicklung der Reaktion des Klienten. Der Patient wird aufgefordert, beim Pulsionstraining einen großen kompensatorischen Schritt zu machen. Das Training wird 20 Minuten lang durchgeführt, es werden etwa 180 bis 230 Schübe und Züge durchgeführt. Die Intensität der Schübe und Züge wird, wenn möglich, im Laufe des Trainings gesteigert (Video 14.30, Abb. 14.30).

Gehen auf unterschiedlichen Untergründen

Im geschützten Rahmen der Therapie kann das Gehen auf unterschiedlichen Untergründen, z. B. Gras, Steine, schräge Ebene, Kissen, weiche Matte zu einer verbesserten Gangsicherheit auf unterschiedlichen Untergründen führen (s. Video 14.31, Abb. 14.31).

14.4.3 Veränderung von gewohnten Betätigungsmustern

Durch die verminderte kognitive Flexibilität fällt es Menschen mit M. Parkinson schwer, ge-

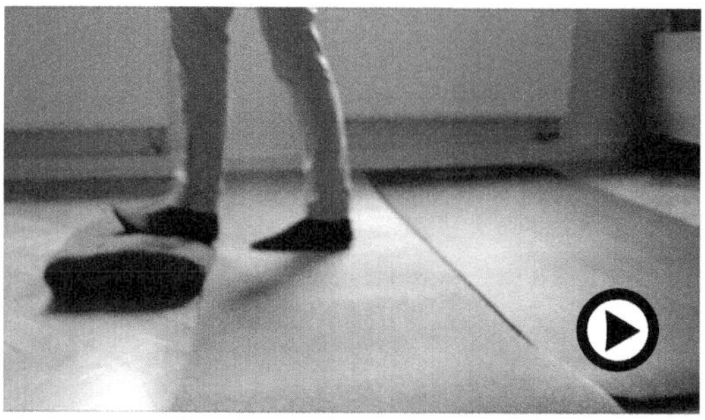

Abb. 14.31 Verbesserung der Gangsicherheit: Gehen auf unterschiedlichen Untergründen (▶ https://doi.org/10.1007/000-2xx)

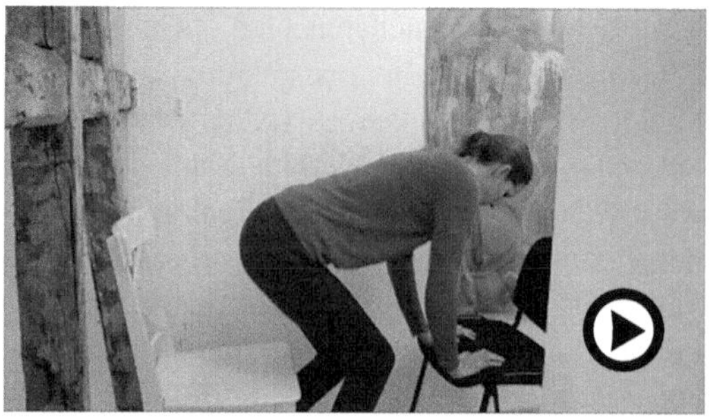

Abb. 14.33 Aufstehen mit notwendiger Oberkörpervorlage, mit Stuhl als Referenzfläche üben (▶ https://doi.org/10.1007/000-2xz)

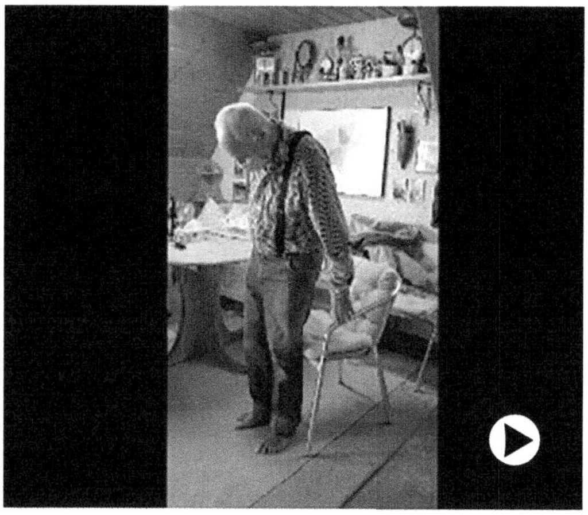

Abb. 14.32 Sturzgefährdung beim Hinsetzen. Veränderung der Betätigung „Hinsetzen": 1. Hand an Armlehne. 2. Visuelle Kontrolle. 3. Sitz an beiden Kniekehlen spüren. 4. Stopp und langsam setzen (▶ https://doi.org/10.1007/000-2xy)

wohnte Betätigungsmuster zu verändern. So kommt es häufig zu Stürzen, weil die ursprüngliche Durchführung der Betätigung nicht mehr sicher ist. Die Therapeutin kann die Umstände des Sturzes durch gezieltes Nachfragen erfahren. Oftmals erkennt sie unmittelbar, was verändert werden muss, um eine sichere Durchführung zu gewährleisten. Daraufhin sollte der Klient die Betätigung wiederholt in der veränderten Form durchführen, damit die Therapeutin Veränderungen ergänzen kann, und damit das neue Betätigungsmuster sich verfestigt. Zwei Beispiele sind in Video 14.32, Abb. 14.32 und Video 14.33 Abb. 14.33 zu sehen. Ein Foto der Betätigung an dem Ort der Durchführung kann als Erinnerungshilfe dienen.

14.4.4 Wieder aufstehen

Regelmäßige Stürze sind der häufigste Auslöser für eine Heimunterbringung bei M. Parkinson. Es ist also äußerst wichtig, zusätzlich zum Training auch die Umwelt des Klienten zu adaptieren und Vorkehrungen zu treffen, um Stürzen vorzubeugen, die Verletzungsgefahr zu minimieren und Notfallabläufe zu besprechen. Bei sturzgefährdeten Klienten ist das Besprechen und Üben des Verhaltens **nach** einem Sturz ein wichtiger Therapieinhalt.

Verhalten nach dem Sturz

- Kurz liegen bleiben, durchatmen
- Abchecken: Ist alles in Ordnung?
- Wenn nein: Notfallknopf drücken/mit Telefon Hilfe anrufen
- Wenn ja: langsam hinsetzen
- Vom Sitz in den Vierfüßlerstand kommen
- Stabile Aufstützmöglichkeit suchen (Stuhl, Kaffeetisch)
- Mit stärkerem Bein einen großen Ausfallschritt machen
- Mit gegenüberliegender Hand oder beiden Händen abstützen
- Gewicht auf aufgestellten Fuß verlagern
- In den Stand kommen

▶ Das Wiederaufstehen sollte in der Ergotherapie mit allen sturzgefährdeten Klienten geübt werden, um ein überlegtes, geplantes Handeln nach einem Sturz zu fördern.

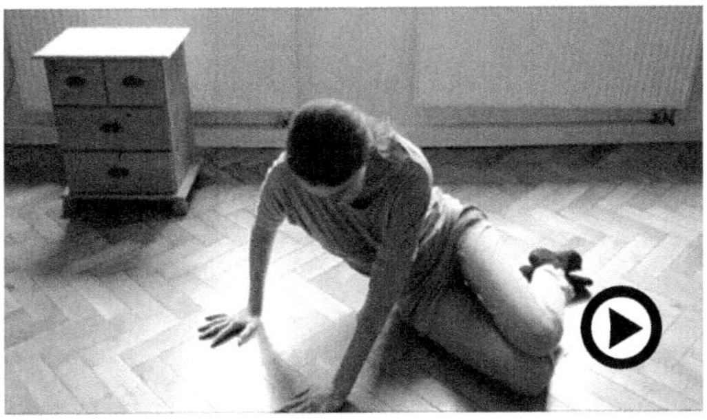

Abb. 14.34 Schritt für Schritt aufstehen nach einem Sturz (▶ https://doi.org/10.1007/000-2y0)

Dieser Ablauf sollte wiederholt geübt werden, damit die Abläufe verinnerlicht werden. Im Ernstfall verfällt der Klient dann nicht in Panik, sondern hat einen eingeübten Handlungsplan. Das Aufstehtraining wird in verschiedenen Räumen durchgeführt, damit der Klient lernt, sich geeignete Festhaltemöglichkeiten zu suchen. Außerdem müssen Angehörige angeleitet werden, dem Betroffenen im Ernstfall aufzuhelfen. Auch hier hilft die Wiederholung dem Helfer, ruhig und besonnen vorzugehen, anstatt hektisch an den Händen des Gestürzten zu ziehen (siehe Video 14.34, Abb. 14.34).

Dabei sollte der Angehörige denselben Ablauf, wie oben beschrieben, anleiten, sodass der Betroffene möglichst viel Gewicht selbst übernehmen kann. Dies entlastet den Angehörigen und stellt die sicherste Möglichkeit dar, den Klienten zu unterstützen. Der Angehörige stellt sich dabei auf die gegenüberliegende Seite des aufgestellten Beins und greift unter dem Arm und seitlich an der Hüfte oder dem Rücken, um den Betroffenen zu stabilisieren.

14.4.5 Kontextfaktoren Verändern

Zur Sturzprävention gehört eine sorgfältige Wohnraumberatung und bei Bedarf eine Hilfsmittelversorgung. Der Wohnraum bietet oftmals eine Vielzahl an Stolperfallen. Das liegt zum einen daran, dass Betroffene eine mangelnde Awareness (Krankheitsbewusstheit) haben und die Stürze nicht mit ihrem Wohnraum in Verbindung bringen, zum anderen haben sie häufig eingeschränkte exekutive Funktionen mit einer reduzierten kognitiven Umstellungsfähigkeit, die sie davon abhalten, Veränderungen in ihrem Heim vorzunehmen. Typisch notwendige Veränderungen sind z. B.:

- Läufer entfernen
- Antirutschstreifen auf Treppen anbringen
- Geländer an Treppen
- Stuhl in jedem Raum, vor allem im Eingangsbereich
- Ausreichende Beleuchtung, vor allem nachts auf dem Weg zur Toilette
- Feste Schuhe in Wohnung tragen
- Haltemöglichkeiten in Bad
- Antirutschbeschichtung in Dusche

Für Hilfsmittel zur Sturzprävention sowie weitere Umweltanpassungen (siehe Abschn. 15.2 und 15.3).

Beispiel

Die Therapeutin hört ihren Anrufbeantworter ab: „Hallo Frau O., hier ist Sch. Ich wollte mich bei Ihnen bedanken. Sie haben gerade einen Sturz verhindert. Ich habe an den großen Schritt gedacht, den wir zusammen geübt haben. Bis nächste Woche!" ◀

14.5 Einschränkung von automatisierten Bewegungen

14.5.1 Symptombeschreibung

Menschen mit der Parkinson-Erkrankung zeigen bei zielgerichteten Bewegungen nur leichte Ungenauigkeiten, wenn sie ein externes Ziel haben. Die Durchführung von automatisierten Bewegungen ist jedoch deutlich eingeschränkt. Die Bewegungen sind ungenau und die Amplitude nimmt mit jeder Wiederholung ab, außerdem kommt es zum Stocken oder Einfrieren der Bewegung, dem sog. Freezing.

Laut Balleine und O'Doherty (2010) ist der **dorso-mediale** Teil des **Striatums** wichtig für die Kontrolle von zielgerichteter Motorik. Für Gewohnheiten und Automatismen sind **laterale** sensomotorische **Bereiche des Striatums** zuständig. Da bei M. Parkinson der caudo-laterale Teil des Striatums durch Dopaminmangel betroffen ist, kann hiermit die deutliche Problematik von automatisierten Bewegungsabläufen erklärt werden.

Im Alltag aller Menschen ist ein großer Teil der Bewegungsabläufe automatisiert. Nur so ist es möglich, mehrere Handlungen gleichzeitig durchzuführen, z. B. Auto fahren, laufen und sprechen, zuhören und schreiben. Bei Parkinson-Betroffenen fallen die Einschränkung der automatisierten Bewegung bei zahlreichen Betätigungen im Alltag auf, z. B. gehen, sprechen, Mimik, Gemüse schälen, schreiben, sprechen, Haare bürsten, Mimik, Armpendeln beim Gehen, Brot schneiden …

Beispiel

Frau Z. setzt zum Sprechen an, ihr Mund geht auf: „Ich finde …" – dann wieder zu. Das Thema hat schon gewechselt. Keiner am Familientisch hat sie gehört oder wahrgenommen, dass sie etwas sagen wollte. Enttäuscht sinkt sie in sich zusammen. Sie nimmt sich vor, beim nächsten Thema laut und betont wie der „Oberlehrer" zu reden, so wie sie es in der Ergotherapie geübt hat. ◀

14.5.2 Nutzung neuer Betätigungsmuster

Die Durchführung von automatisierten Bewegungen wie Gehen oder Schreiben ist bei Menschen mit M. Parkinson eingeschränkt. Bewegungen sind ungenau und mit jeder Wiederholung nimmt die Amplitude ab. Um dem entgegenzuwirken, müssen **Bewegungen „ent-automatisiert"** werden. Bewusste, zielgerichtete Bewegungen sind noch gut möglich. Es müssen neue Betätigungsmuster gesucht werden. Bei einer der Klientin wichtigen Betätigung, die aufgrund des eingeschränkten Automatismus nicht erfolgreich durchgeführt werden kann, sollte der Therapeut versuchen, die Betätigung so abzuändern, dass die Klientin:

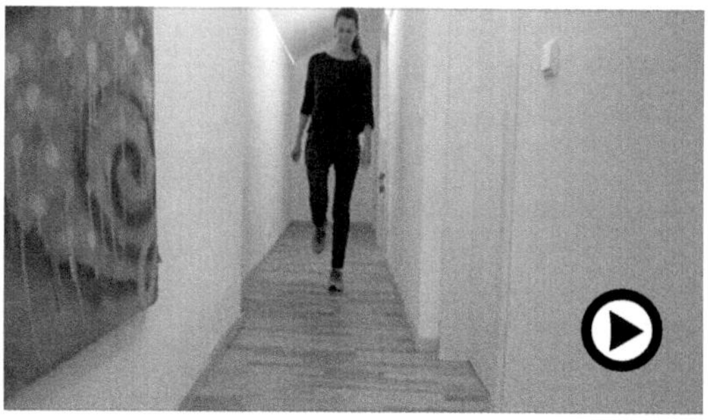

Abb. 14.35 Neue Betätigungsmuster beim Laufen, um Freezing zu vermeiden (▶ https://doi.org/10.1007/000-2y1)

1. ihre volle Aufmerksamkeit auf die Betätigung richtet,
2. Referenzflächen nutzt,
3. neue/nicht automatisierte motorische Abläufe nutzt.

Ein paar Beispiele:

Betätigung Gehen (s. Video 14.35, Abb. 14.35)

- Marschieren
- Knie übertrieben anheben
- Die Abrollbewegung übertreiben
- Auf einer Linie „balancieren"
- Über Kreuz gehen
- Kleine und große Schritte abwechselnd
- Leise Schleichen
- Stampfen
- „Schlittschuhlaufen"

Betätigung Schreiben

- Druckbuchstaben
- Großbuchstaben, siehe Abb. 14.36
- Stift anders halten als gewohnt, z. B. zwischen Zeige und Mittelfinger (Interdigitalgriff) siehe Abb. 14.37.

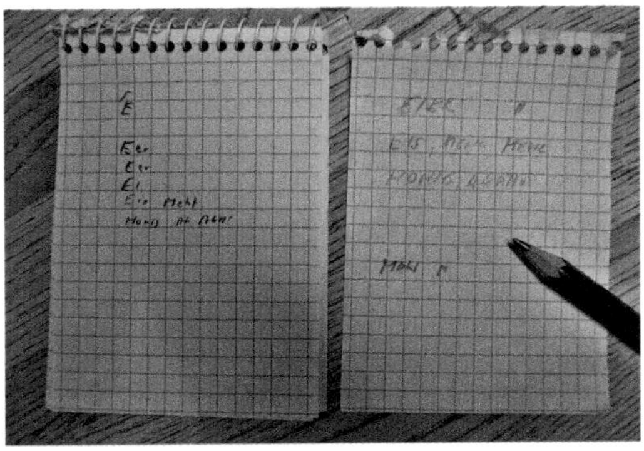

Abb. 14.36 Großbuchstaben, um Mikrografie zu vermeiden

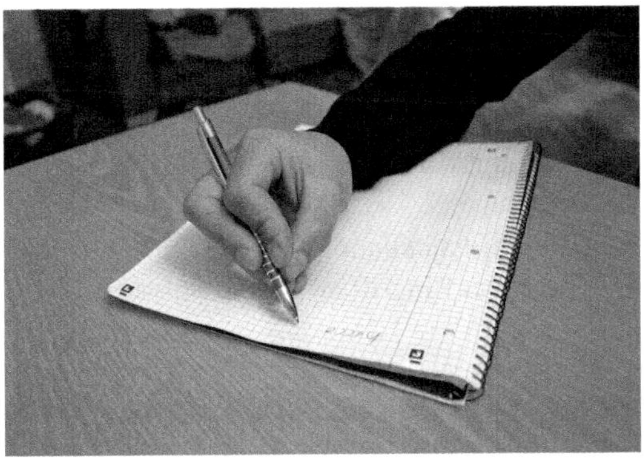

Abb. 14.37 Neues Betätigungsmuster (Interdigitalgriff), um Mikrografie zu vermeiden

Betätigung Tisch abwischen

- Betätigung mit nicht-dominanter Hand durchführen
- Von Kante zu Kante wischen
- Andere Bewegung: statt von rechts nach links – liegende 8

Betätigung Haare bürsten

- Mit nicht dominanter Hand bürsten
- Bürste anders als gewohnt halten
- Sich vorstellen, es wäre eine Pferdemähne o. ä.
- Anderes Kämmutensil verwenden

Betätigung Brot schneiden

- Sich vorstellen, man würde einen Baumstamm sägen
- Brot ungewohnt halten, z. B. auf die Kante stellen
- Haltung ändern z. B. gerade stehen, leichte Schrittstellung

Betätigung Mimik und Sprechen

- Wie ein Clown grimassieren
- Übertriebene Mimik (wirkt nach außen meist nicht übertrieben)
- Übertrieben laut sprechen

Betätigung Körperpflege

- Neue Waschutensilien nutzen, z. B. Schwamm statt Waschlappen
- Bewegungsrichtung ändern, z. B. kreisen statt hoch-runter wischen

Betätigung Autofahren

- Da Autofahren ohne automatisierte Bewegungsabläufe nicht möglich ist, sollten Parkinson-Klientinnen mit Einschränkungen der automatisierten Bewegungen nicht mehr Autofahren. Es besteht die Möglichkeit, bei spezialisierten Fahrschulen die eigene Fahreignung testen zu lassen.

Beispiel

Schon kommt ihr Lieblingsthema zur Sprache: der Garten. Sie hebt den Kopf und gleichzeitig den Zeigefinger (wie der Oberlehrer), nun hat sie die Aufmerksamkeit der Nebensitzer. Mit lauter, „oberlehrerhafter" Stimme verkündet sie: „Meine Kürbisse sind dieses Jahr wunderbar geworden. Die möchte ich euch nachher gerne zeigen." Keiner in der Familie hat bemerkt, dass sie übertrieben gesprochen hat, aber sie war gut hörbar und ist wieder in das Geschehen eingebunden. „Wann gibt's wieder Kürbissuppe, Oma?" fragt die Enkelin. ◄

14.6 Dystonien

14.6.1 Symptombeschreibung

Definition Der Begriff Dystonie bezeichnet eine Bewegungsstörung mit länger anhaltenden, **unwillkürlichen Kontraktionen** der quergestreiften Muskulatur, die häufig zu verzerrenden und repetitiven Bewegungen, abnormen Haltungen oder bizarren Fehlstellungen von Körperteilen führen (Deuschl et al., Leitlinien für Diagnostik und Therapie in der Neurologie 2016).

Ätiologie Dystonien können als primäres Krankheitssymptom des M. Parkinson oder als Folge der Einnahme von L-Dopa auftreten. Die Pathophysiologie im Gehirn ist noch ungeklärt, Untersuchungen kamen sogar zu widersprüchlichen Ergebnissen. Als Primärsymptom tritt die Dystonie früh in der Krankheitsgeschichte, oftmals als erstes wahrgenommenes Symptom auf, z. B. als Fußkrämpfe. Häufiger jedoch tritt die Dystonie mit der Langzeiteinnahme von L-Dopa auf. In diesen Fällen wird die Dystonie meist während Medikamentenwirkungspausen (in der Nacht) oder in der „Wearing-Off-Phase", vor Einnahme der nächsten Medikamentendosis beobachtet. Es ist aber auch eine „Peak-Dose-Symptomatik" möglich, wenn die Medikamentenwirkung am stärksten ist.

Prävalenz Eine Dystonie tritt im Laufe der Parkinson-Erkrankung bei etwa 30 % der Betroffenen auf.

Klinik Bei jedem Betroffenen kann die Dystonie an einer anderen Körperstelle auftreten, bleibt aber nach dem Aufreten an dieser Stelle präsent. Am häufigsten sind ein oder zwei Füße betroffen. Der Fuß wird unwillkürlich flektiert, die Zehen krümmen sich unter den Fuß, manchmal geht der große Zeh in die Extension. Dystonien treten jedoch auch im Nacken (Tortikollis), Kopfbereich (craniale Dystonie), Rumpf (Axiale Dystonie), Augenliedern (Blepharospasmus) und der oberen Extremität auf. Sie halten zwischen wenigen Minuten und zwei Stunden an und sind meist mit Schmerzen verbunden. Typischerweise wird eine Dystonie durch Aktivität herbeigeführt und löst sich bei Ruhe oder im Schlaf wieder.

Folgen/Komplikationen Dystonien führen häufig zu Schmerzen im betroffenen Bereich, beträchtlichen negativen Auswirkungen auf die Ausführung von Alltagsaktivitäten und zur Stigmatisierung durch das Umfeld und folglich einem sozialen Rückzug.

Medizinische Möglichkeiten

- Reduktion der Einnahme von L-Dopa
- Botulinium Toxin Spritze
- Medikamente
- Tiefe Hirnstimulation
- Operativer Eingriff an Muskulatur (früher)

14.6.2 Therapeutische Möglichkeiten

Beispiel

Frau L. legt sich zurück ins Bett – so wird das nichts mit dem Anziehen. Der rechte Fuß ist stark verkrampft und schmerzt, wie jeden Morgen. Frau L. flucht: „Diese ätzende Dystonie!" Verärgert ruft sie ihren Mann, um ihr mit der Hose zu helfen. ◄

Je nach Ausprägung der Dystonie – von einer isolierten Fußdystonie bis hin zu einer Ganzkörperdystonie – kann die Lebensqualität von Klienten erheblich eingeschränkt sein. Sie verlieren einen großen Teil ihrer Selbständigkeit, haben Schmerzen und leiden unter dem Stigma des nicht zu verbergenden, auffälligen Symptoms. Weder die genaue Ursache noch effektive Therapie von Dystonien sind eindeutig nachgewiesen, sodass die Behandlung oftmals von Versuch und Irrtum geprägt und das Ergebnis häufig leider nicht zufriedenstellend ist. Therapeutische Möglichkeiten bei Dystonien sind sehr limitiert.

Physiologische Haltung, Mobilisation und Dehnung

Trotz der starken Muskelkrämpfe können physiologische, endgradige Bewegungen und Haltungen trainiert werden, um die verkürzten Muskelgruppen zu dehnen, die Antagonisten zu kräftigen und die Bewegungskoordination zu fördern. Andernfalls übernehmen die dystonen Muskelgruppen die Kontrolle über die Bewegung, da sie durch die konstante Innervierung extrem kräftig sind.

► Um die allgemeine Beweglichkeit zu erhalten und Kontrakturen vorzubeugen, ist eine regelmäßige Mobilisierung und Dehnung der dystonen Muskeln empfehlenswert.

Um den gewünschten Effekt zu erzielen, muss der Klient ein Eigenübungsprogramm durchführen.

Hilfsmittel

Der Einsatz von Hilfsmitteln kann zur Unterstützung der Durchführung der Betätigung dienen. Beispielhaft sollen hier einige genannt werden, eine ausführliche Auflistung von Hilfsmitteln ist in Abschn. 15.3 zu finden.

- Griffverdickung
- Keilkissen/Lordosekissen
- Armlehnen und hohe Rückenlehne an Stuhl
- Duschstuhl
- …

Stigmatisierung

Die starke Muskelaktivität wirkt befremdlich auf Außenstehende, wodurch es häufig zu einer Stigmatisierung der Betroffenen kommt. Klienten ziehen sich immer mehr zurück und vermeiden Sozialkontakte aus Scham. Die Sekundärkomplikationen durch die vermehrte Immobilität können die Dystonie verstärken. Um aus diesem negativen Zyklus auszubrechen, ist es hilfreich wenn der Klient lernt, entspannt mit der offensichtlichen Einschränkung umzugehen.

In der Therapie dienen Gespräche dazu, Ängste aufzudecken, negative und positive Erfahrungen mit Abstand zu betrachten und neue Verhaltensweisen anzuregen. In Rollenspielen kann der Klient verschiedene Reaktionen und Kommunikationsprozesse ausprobieren, um einen passenden Umgang im Alltag zu finden. Besonders wertvoll ist ein Austausch in der Gruppe. Hier können Betroffene ihre Erfahrungen und erprobten Tipps im Umgang mit Außenstehenden diskutieren.

Entspannung und Erholung

Dystonie wird durch Stress, Fatigue, Angst oder Schlafmangel verstärkt. Es ist zu empfehlen, in der Ergotherapie einen gesunden Schlaf- und Erholungsrhythmus zu besprechen sowie Entspannungstechniken zu trainieren und im Alltag Stresssituationen zu vermeiden. Mehr dazu in Abschn. 14.8 und 14.10.4.

Wahrnehmungsschulung

Durch die dauerhaft veränderte Haltung verschiebt sich die Wahrnehmung der entsprechenden Körperpartie, sodass die physiologische Körperhaltung nicht mehr als solche wahrgenommen wird. Um dem entgegenzuwirken, ist ein Wahrnehmungstraining mit visueller (Spiegel) und sensorischer (Wand, Stuhl) Kontrolle zu empfehlen.

Vermeidung auslösender Reize

Dystonien werden meist durch bestimmte Bewegungen hervorgerufen oder verstärkt. Zur Identifizierung der auslösenden Bewegung oder Haltung analysiert die Therapeutin diese genau. Sobald die auslösende Bewegung oder Haltung eruiert ist, kann diese vom Klienten vermieden und nach Alternativen gesucht werden, um eine kurzfristige Erleichterung zu erfahren, z. B. Ablegen des Kopfes auf Sofarücken statt aufrechtem Sitzen.

Sensorische Trickmanöver (gestes antagonistes)

In einer Studie von Schramm et al. (2003) wurde folgende Einflussweise auf die zervikale Dystonie beschrieben: „In einer ersten Phase bringt leichter manueller Gegendruck bzw. aktive Bewegung den Kopf in eine günstige Ausgangsposition mit bereits leicht reduzierter Muskelaktivität. In einer zweiten Phase kann dann die Kopfposition mithilfe eines vorwiegend sensorische Trickmanövers unter Einwirkung auf zentrale sensomotorische Integrationsprozesse stabilisiert werden.“ Dazu wird z. B. mit dem Finger über die Wange gestrichen oder leicht berührt.

Beispiel

Seit ein paar Wochen macht Frau L. morgens, noch vor dem Aufstehen ihre Entspannungsübungen. Dann setzt sie sich langsam und konzentriert an die Bettkante. Die Kleidung liegt schon bereit, sie muss nicht aufstehen, um sie zu erreichen. Kleidungsstück für Kleidungsstück zieht sie sich langsam über und bleibt dabei in der entspannten Grundstimmung. Geschafft! Stolz setzt sie sich fertig angezogen zu ihrem Mann an den Frühstückstisch. ◀

14.7 Haltungsanomalien

Haltungsanomlien sind beim M. Parkinson häufig feststellbar. Die genauen pathophysiologischen Abläufe sind noch nicht abschließend geklärt, sodass die einzelnen Krankheitsbilder nicht klar definiert werden können. Eine Abgrenzung zu ähnlichen Symptomen erfolgt nicht immer einheitlich, teilweise widersprechen sich die Erklärungsansätze sogar (z. B. Kamptokormie – Rumpf Dystonie, zervikale Dystonie [Tortikollis] – Kortikollis, Pisa-Syndrom – Skoliose).

14.7.1 Symptombeschreibung Kamptokormie

Definition Nach Margraf et al. (2010): „… eine ausgeprägte pathologische Rumpfvorneigung beim Stehen und Gehen, die im Liegen vollständig reversibel ist.“

Ätiologie Studien belegen eine umschriebene Myopathie der paravertebralen Muskulatur als hauptsächlichen pathophysiologischen Mechanismus. Der Ursprung dieser Myopathie ist wahrscheinlich auf eine Dysregulation des propriozeptiven polysynaptischen Reflexbogens im Rückenmark zurückzuführen. Diese wird wiederum vermutlich durch neuronale Veränderungen im Gehirn ausgelöst. Es herrscht also ein Ungleichgewicht zwischen Rückenstreckern und Rückenbeugern, der meist mit einer Schwäche der dorsalen Muskulatur zusammenhängt, in einzelnen Fällen aber auch auf einen erhöhten Tonus der ventralen Muskulatur zurückzuführen ist (Dystonie). Eine knöcherne Veränderung ist nicht der Auslöser.

Prävalenz Die Prävalenz von Kamptokormie bei der an M. Parkinson erkrankten Menschen wurde auf zwischen 6,9 % und 10 % ermittelt. Obwohl die Kamptokormie statistisch gesehen selten auftritt, ist es ein für Therapeuten gegenwärtiges Krankheitsbild, da die Betroffenen in ihrer Lebensqualität stark eingeschränkt sind, soziale Isolierung erleben und häufig starke Schmerzen haben.

Klinik Starke Vorneige des Oberkörpers, mindestens 45°, teilweise kombiniert mit einer Seitneigung. Kamptokormie tritt meist im fortgeschrittenen Stadium der Parkinson-Erkrankung auf, wobei es zu einer langsamen (über mehrere Jahre) oder schnellen (über wenige Wochen) Zunahme der Oberkörpervorneige kommt. Im Durchschnitt wird eine Kamptokormie 7–8 Jahre nach Beginn des M. Parkinson festgestellt. Bei Müdigkeit oder Stress ist eine Verstärkung des Symptoms zu beobachten.

Komplikationen Es kann zu Rückenschmerzen, vermehrten Stürzen, Dyspnoe und Einschränkung der Gehfähigkeit, bis hin zu Rollstuhlnutzung, kommen.

Medizinische Möglichkeiten Die Kamptokormie ist medizinisch nur selten zufriedenstellend behandelbar. Folgende therapeutische Möglichkeiten sind, abhängig von der Ursache, gegeben:

- Orthese
- Hilfsmittel (Rollator, Rollstuhl)
- L-Dopa
- Tiefe Hirnstimulation
- Botuliniumtoxin

14.7.2 Symptombeschreibung Anterocollis

Anterocollis oder Antecollis bei M. Parkinson stellt eine vorwärtsgerichtete Flexion des Nackens dar. Die aktive Aufrichtung des Nackens gegen die Schwerkraft ist eingeschränkt oder nicht möglich, bis hin zu einer Auflage des Kinns auf das Sternum, und erscheint deutlicher ausgeprägt in Relation zur Flexion des Rumpfes.

Prävalenz Ca. 5–8 % der von M. Parkinson betroffenen Patientinnen zeigen eine Anterocollis.

Ätiologie Anterocollis tritt meist einige Jahre nach Diagnosestellung auf. Die Ursache ist nicht abschließend geklärt. Es scheint unterschiedliche Formen zu geben, zudem ist der Zusammenhang von Ursache und Wirkung unklar. Folgende Faktoren wurden im Zusammenhang mit Anterocollis festgestellt: Myopathie, Medikamentenwirkung, Ungleichgewicht von Muskelgruppen. Es kann häufig eine Zunahme des Muskeltonus in den Nackenflexoren ertastet werden. Das Bild unterscheidet sich von einer Dystonie, da keine sensorische Trickmanöver (geste antagoniste) zur kurzzeitigen Verbesserung der Flexion eingesetzt werden können.

Komplikationen Patientinnen berichten von Schmerzen im hinteren Nackenbereich. Außerdem können Schluckstörungen und starker Speichelaustritt sowie Einschränkungen des Visus und eine Kontraktur in der Fehlstellung auftreten.

14.7.3 Symptombeschreibung Pisasyndrom

Das Pisa-Syndrom ist nach dem schiefen Turm von Pisa benannt und stellt eine seitliche Achsenabweichung ab 10° dar. Die Achsenabweichung kann zur mehr oder weniger betroffenen Seite hin auftreten und kann bei passiver Mobilisation oder im Liegen rückgängig gemacht werden. Zur Differenzierung – eine **Skoliose** liegt vor, wenn die Seitneigung durch passive Mobilisation oder im Liegen nicht komplett reversibel ist. Im Klinikalltag werden die Diagnosen „Pisa-Syndrom" und „Skoliose" häufig verwechselt.

Prävalenz Ca. 8,8 % der Menschen mit M. Parkinson sind vom Pisa-Syndrom betroffen.

Ätiologie Das Pisa-Syndrom tritt meist nach mehreren Jahren (durchschnittlich sieben Jahre) der Parkinson-Erkrankung auf. Die genaue Pathophysiologie wird in der Wissenschaft kontrovers diskutiert. Eine einseitige Veränderung im Gehirn scheint in mehreren Untersuchungen darauf hinzuweisen, dass dort die Ursache des einseitig auftretenden Symptoms lokalisiert ist. In ca. 15 % der Fälle tritt das Pisa-Syndrom nach Veränderung der Medikamenteneinnahme auf.

Komplikationen Patientinnen mit dem Pisa-Syndrom geben größere Schmerzen an und haben eine erhöhte Sturzwahrscheinlichkeit. Sowohl Arthrose als auch Osteoporose treten wesentlich häufiger auf.

14.7.4 Diverse Therapieansätze

Beispiel

Frau V. klingelt. Sie setzt sich aufs Bett und wartet. Sie muss sich dringend hinlegen, ihr Rücken tut ihr wahnsinnig weh. Sie weiß, das einzige das hilft, ist sich flach ins Bett legen und eine halbe Stunde ausruhen. Sie klingelt noch mal. Seit sehr vielen Jahren ist Frau V. schief und krumm, und wenn sie steht, hat sie Schmerzen. Sie hat es so akzeptiert und sitzt meistens in ihrem Lieblingssessel. Hier im Heim ist sowieso nicht viel los, das sie interessiert. Nur alleine ins Bett einsteigen, das würde sie gerne wieder können! Sie klingelt noch einmal. Als die Pflege kommt, hat sich Frau V. schon allein ins Bett manövriert. Sie liegt schräg und friert, weil die Bettdecke unter ihr liegt. ◀

Da die Studienlage zur Pathophysiologie der Haltungsanomalien noch nicht abschließend geklärt ist, sind folglich auch die therapeutischen

Ansätze nicht ausgereift, sondern beruhen vielmehr auf Erfahrungswerten und Versuch und Irrtum.

In der Praxis können folgende Ansätze, am besten in Kombination, wirksam sein. Die folgenden therapeutischen Interventionen sind bei allen Haltungsanomalien anwendbar.

Mobilisierung
Sobald sich eine Fehlstellung abzeichnet, sollte direkt und intensiv mit einer aktivierenden Mobilisierung begonnen werden. Sobald eine Chronifizierung mit degenerierter und fettig umgebauter Muskulatur besteht, ist eine therapeutische Intervention kaum noch effektiv. Viele Patienten vermeiden Aktivität, was die Symptomatik verstärkt. Eine Dehnung verkürzter Strukturen, aktive Mobilisierung und Kräftigung des Rumpfes werden empfohlen, um die Aufrichtung zu unterstützen. Beispiele für Übungen zu Mobilisation sind in Abschn. 14.1 und 14.2, zur Dehnung in Abschn. 14.7.6 zu finden.

Wahrnehmungstraining
Die propriozeptive Wahrnehmung der Aufrichtung ist deutlich eingeschränkt. Eine Korrektur der Aufrichtung kann durch eine intensive Wahrnehmungsschulung erreicht werden. Dazu dienen folgende Therapiemittel:

- Wand als Referenzfläche (siehe Abb. 14.38 und 14.39)
- Übergehend zu weniger stabilen Referenzflächen, z. B. Brett, Stock
- Stuhllehne
- Spiegel zur visuellen Kontrolle (Abb. 14.40)
- Videoaufnahmen
- Sitz auf Wackelkissen (Instabilität erhöht Aufmerksamkeit und die tonische Muskulatur wird aktiviert)

Mehr zur Behandlung von Dysfunktion der sensorischen Integration und Propriozeption ist in Abschn. 14.18 zu finden.

Hilfsmittel
Ein hoher **Rollator mit Unterarmschalen** kann im Alltag die Aufrichtung begünstigen, um Mo-

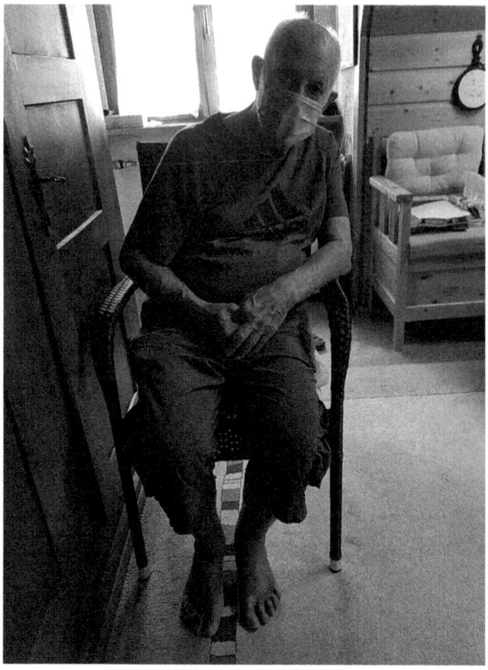

Abb. 14.38 Klient kippt zur linken Seite, was teils große Schmerzen an den Rippen der linken Seite verursacht. Er kann es jedoch nicht selbständig korrigieren

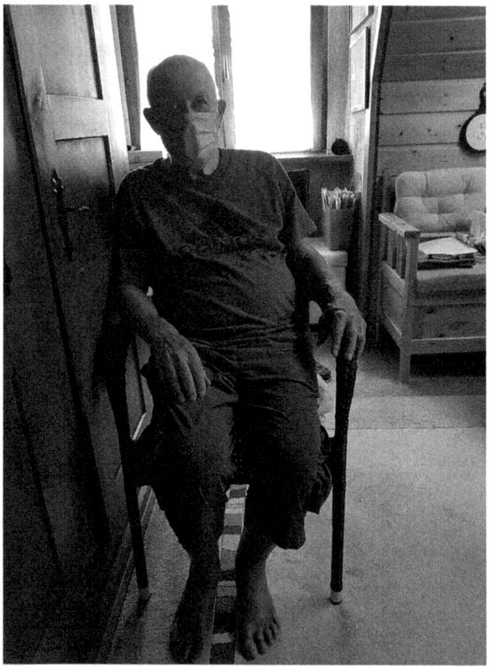

Abb. 14.39 Durch die Nutzung einer stabilen Referenzfläche (Schrank) ist eine selbständige Aufrichtung und Entlastung des Brustkorbs möglich

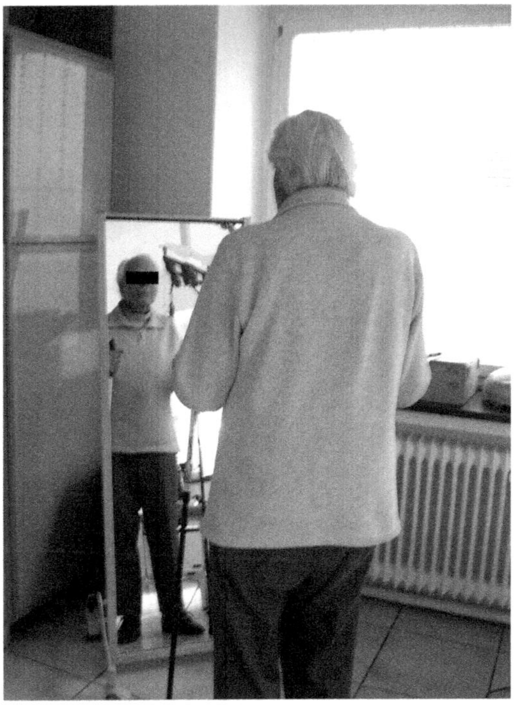

Abb. 14.40 Die visuelle Kontrolle im Spiegel hilft dem Klienten seine Haltung zu kontrollieren

bilität zu ermöglichen und die Sturzgefahr zu verringern. Bei einer chronischen Kamptokormie oder Pisa-Syndrom mit Zunahme der Sturzgefahr ist die Versorgung mit einem **Rollstuhl** meist unumgänglich.

Rucksack oder Tasche tragen
Durch das Tragen einer **Tasche** mit leichtem Gewicht über der Schulter auf Seite der Beugung, kann in einigen Fällen eine reflektorische Gegenbewegung in die Aufrichtung ausgelöst werden. Auch ein **Rucksack** mit leichtem Gewicht auf dem Rücken, kann als eine Art Erinnerungshilfe dienen, um die aktive Aufrichtung zu unterstützen. Sobald Tasche oder Rucksack abgesetzt werden, lässt sich jedoch keine anhaltende Verbesserung feststellen.

Sensorische Trickmanöver (geste antagoniste)
Das Wirken von sensorischen Trickmanövern ist primär für Dystonien charakteristisch (s. o.). Es kann in Einzelfällen jedoch auch bei Kamptokormie, Pisa-Syndrom und Anterocollis-Effekt zeigen.

Studie
Bartolo et al. untersuchten 2010 in einer Studie mit 44 Teilnehmern die rumpfspezifische therapeutische Intervention zur Verbesserung **lateraler** Rumpfflexion bei M. Parkinson. Es wurde eine Verbesserung der Aufrichtung festgestellt, die auch noch sechs Monate nach der Intervention feststellbar war. Folgendes Training wurde durchgeführt:

90-minütiges Training, fünf Mal die Woche, für vier Wochen. Die 90 Minuten bestanden aus kardiovaskulären Aufwärmübungen (10 Minuten), Dehnungsübungen (15 Minuten), Krafttraining (15 Minuten), Gangtraining (20 Minuten), Balancetraining (15 Minuten) und Entspannungsübungen (15 Minuten).

14.7.5 Aufrichtung

Ein typisches „Markenzeichen" der Parkinson-Erkrankung ist die kyphotische, vornübergebeugte Haltung des Oberkörpers. Ab einer Neigung von 45° spricht man von einer Kamptokormie, doch auch bei einer weniger ausgeprägten Vorneigung können Schwierigkeiten bei der Verrichtung von Alltagshandlungen auftreten. Die mangelnde Aufrichtung wirkt sich negativ auf viele Bereiche aus. Häufig berichten Klientinnen von starken Schmerzen im Rücken, die durch die unphysiologische Haltung und Fehlbelastung der Wirbelsäule hervorgerufen werden. Die Schmerzen haben einen großen Einfluss auf die Ausübung von Betätigungen, Sozialkontakte und Selbstwertgefühl.

Auch wenn keine Schmerzen auftreten, kann die mangelnde Aufrichtung von den Klientinnen als starke Beeinträchtigung wahrgenommen werden. Höher gelegene Gegenstände können nicht gut erreicht werden. Die Sturzgefahr nimmt durch den verschobenen Körpermittelpunkt zu. Und auch der ästhetische Aspekt wird von Klientinnen genannt, dessen äußerliches Bild einen hohen Stellenwert hat. Die Aufrichtung nimmt bei den aktivierenden Therapien folglich einen wichtigen Platz ein und findet sich häufig in betätigungsorientierten Zielformulierungen wieder. Ein paar Beispiele sind:

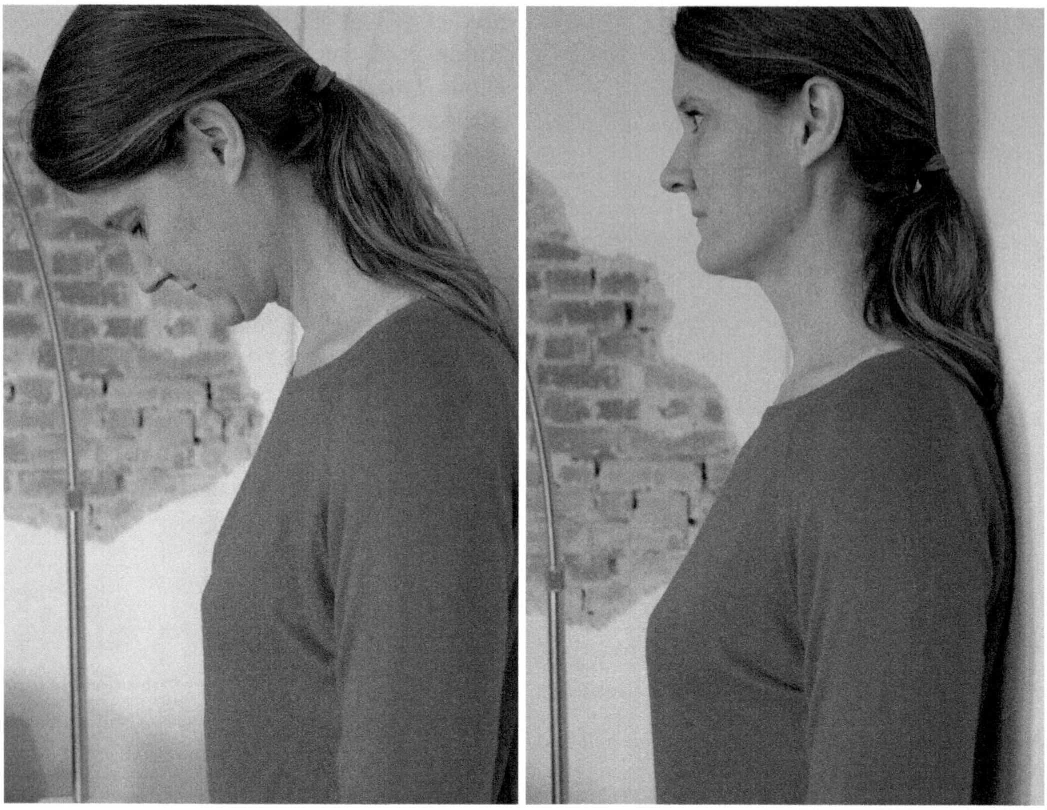

Abb. 14.41 (a, b) Aufrichtung mit der Wand als Referenzfläche. Der Therapeut erarbeitet mit der Klientin, welche Berührungspunkte sie bei der gebeugten Haltung und bei der aufgerichteten Haltung spürt (Wirbelsäule, Gesäß, Schulterblätter)

- „Die Aufrichtung verbessern, um die Jacke vom Haken nehmen zu können."
- „Verbesserung der Aufrichtung, um schmerzfrei am Mittagstisch sitzen zu können."
- „Aufrechtes Laufen zum Briefkasten, um Stürze zu vermeiden."
- „Selbständige Hygiene im Badezimmer."

► Als Hintergrund ist es für Therapeuten hilfreich zu wissen, dass die Ursache für eine mangelnde Aufrichtung bei M. Parkinson eng mit der veränderten Wahrnehmung zusammenhängt. Nur selten liegt eine strukturelle Veränderung vor und wenn eine vorliegt, dann als **Folge** der Kyphose und **nicht** als **Ursache**.

Man geht davon aus, dass die Rückmeldung der Sinneszellen in Gelenken, Knochen, Muskeln und Sehnen sich mit der Zeit an die Fehlhaltung anpassen und ein Gewöhnungseffekt eintritt. Fragt man einen Menschen mit M. Parkinson, ob er aufrecht steht, wird er dies meist bejahen. Stellt man dann einen Spiegel vor ihn, ist er überrascht und kann die Fehlhaltung meist mithilfe der visuellen Kontrolle korrigieren. In Abb. 14.41a, b und 14.42 wird eine hilfreiche Übung zur Verbesserung der Aufrichtung bei M. Parkinson vorgestellt. Hierbei ist zu betonen, dass davon abgeraten wird, solche Übungen als Standard einzusetzen, sondern nur, wenn der Therapeut die mangelnde Aufrichtung als Ursache für das problematische Betätigungsanliegen der Klientin sieht.

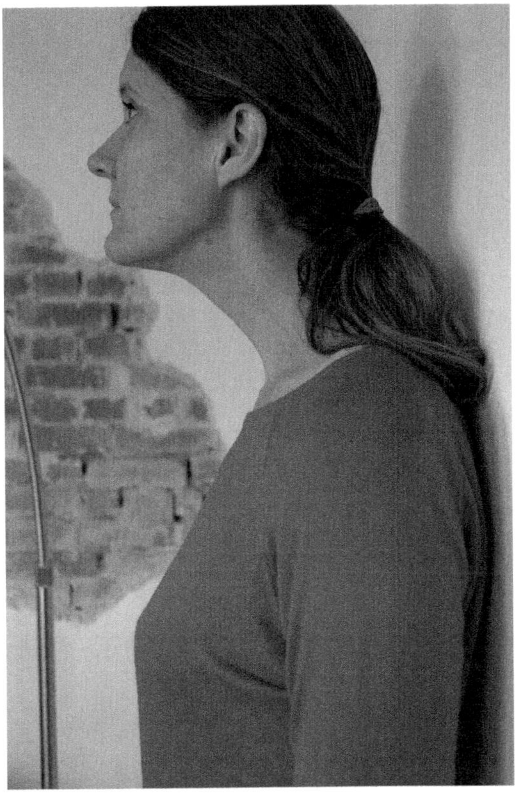

Abb. 14.42 Dabei sollte eine Überstreckung des Nackens vermieden werden. Das Kinn sollte Richtung Brustbein gehen

14.7.6 Dehnung

Eine Dehnung der Muskeln sollte aktiv und passiv geschehen. **Aktives Dehnen** heißt, dass durch aktive Anspannung der Antagonisten die zu verkürzten Muskeln in die Dehnung gezogen werden. Z. B. der Kopf wird gegen einen Widerstand flektiert, damit die Extensoren der Halswirbelsäule gedehnt werden oder aktive Dehnung des Muskulus Pektoralis durch aktive Extension und Retroversion des Arms (siehe auch Abb. 14.47). Dabei ist die Intensität geringer als beim passiven Dehnen und die physiologische Haltung wird durch ein Ausbalancieren von Agonisten und Antagonisten trainiert.

Passives Dehnen geschieht bei entspannter Muskulatur mit Zug gegen einen Widerstand (Wand, Boden, gegenüberliegende Hand). Dabei entsteht ein größerer Zug als bei der aktiven Dehnung. Faszien, Sehnen und Muskeln werden stärker gedehnt, eine Veränderung ist meist sofort spürbar. Es wird dazu geraten, beide Dehnungsformen zu kombinieren, um die Vorteile beider Methoden zu erhalten. Der zusätzliche Einsatz von **Faszienbehandlungen** vorab unterstützen Dehnübungen (verbesserter Stoffwechsel, Schmerzlinderung, erhöhte Propriozeption).

Beispielhaft sind in den Abb. 14.43, 14.44, 14 .45, 14.46, 14.47, 14.48, und 14.49 ein paar Übungen zu finden.

Beispiel

In der Ergotherapie haben Frau V. und ihre Therapeutin mit dem Einsteigen ins Bett begonnen. Doch schnell kamen sie auf das Thema der mangelnden Rumpfaufrichtung und den damit verbundenen Schmerzen zu

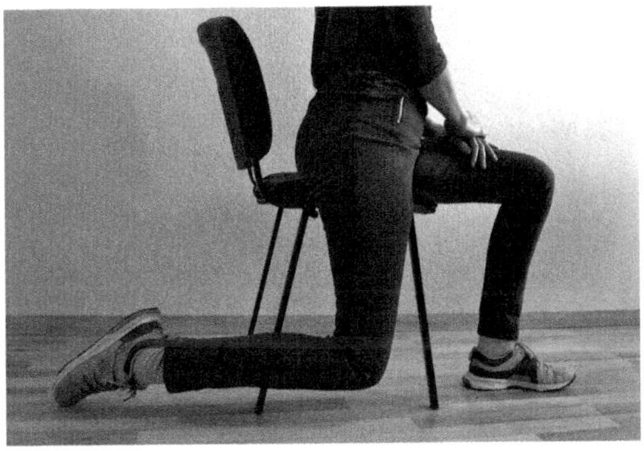

Abb. 14.43 Dehnung der Hüftbeuger (passive Dehnung mit der Schwerkraft). Im Sitzen an Stuhlkante, Bein nach unten und hinten strecken. Variation: Rückenlage, Bein hängt über Seite der Bank

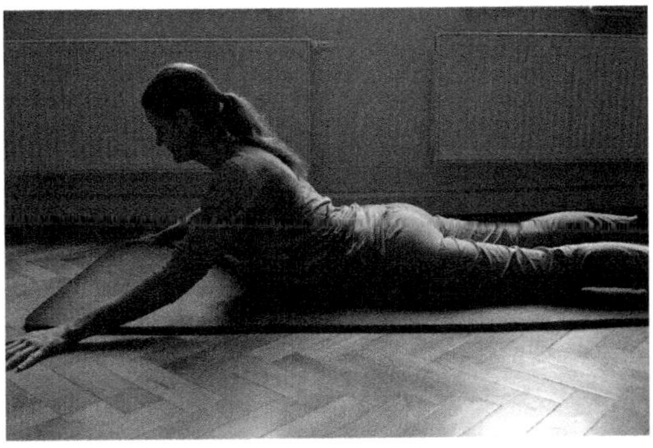

Abb. 14.44 Zur Dehnung der vorderen Muskelkette dient die Yoga-Übung „Kobra“

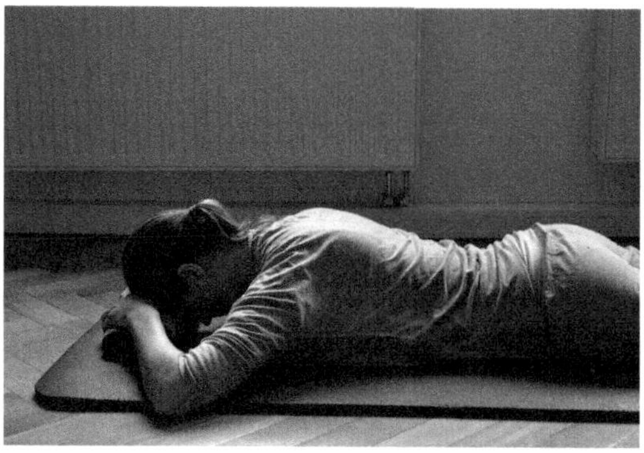

Abb. 14.45 Bei verkürzter ventraler Muskulatur ist das Aufrichten des Oberkörpers in die Extension nicht möglich. Das Liegen auf dem Bauch kann in dem Fall ausreichen, um die ventralen Muskeln zu dehnen

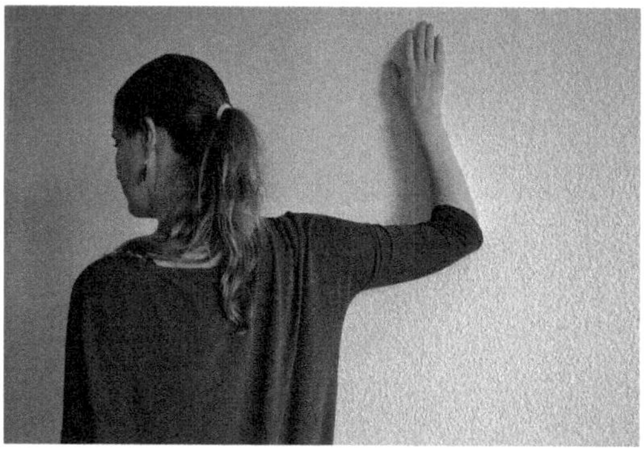

Abb. 14.46 Musculus-Pectoralis-Dehnung, an Wand (passive Dehnung)

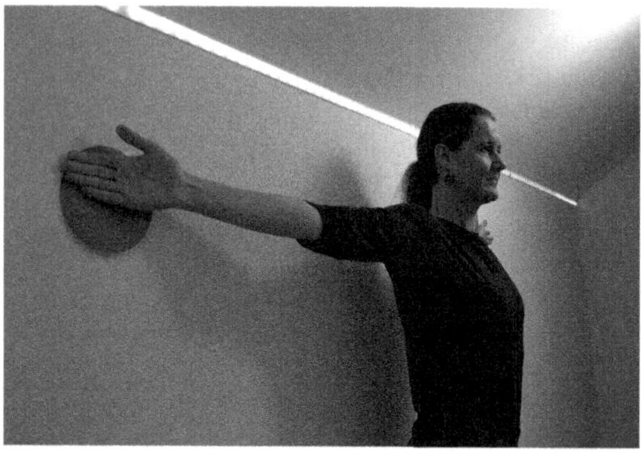

Abb. 14.47 Musculus-Pectoralis-Dehnung mit Referenzfläche (aktive Dehnung). Variation im Sitzen oder Liegen möglich

sprechen. Die Therapeutin erklärte der betagten Dame, dass es nie zu spät ist, um kleine Verbesserungen zu erreichen und eine multi-

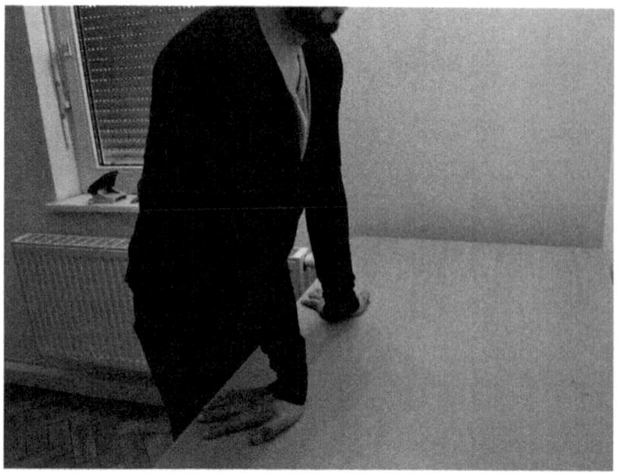

Abb. 14.48 Dehnen der Fingerflexoren im Stehen. Dabei sollte darauf geachtet werden, dass der Klient nicht mit Kraft in die Haltung geht, sondern möglichst eine entspannte Dehnung erreicht. Wenn diese Handhaltung nicht möglich ist, kann auch das Auflegen der Hände auf den Tisch, ohne die Rotation ausreichen

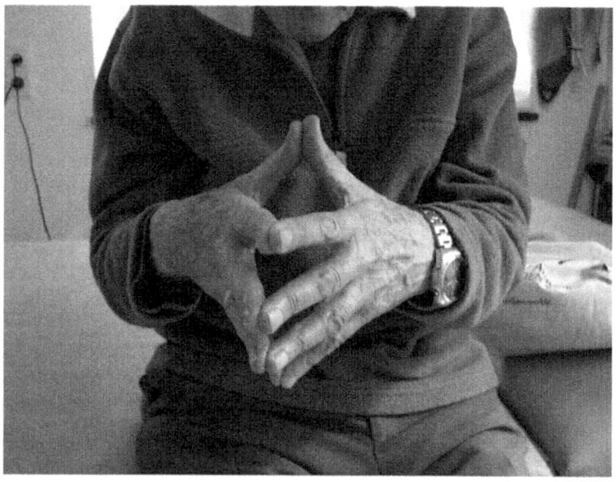

Abb. 14.49 Fingerflexoren Dehnen im Sitzen

modale Therapie mit unterschiedlichen Komponenten zur Mobilisierung, Stärkung, Entspannung und Dehnung, kombiniert mit Gehen und Balancetraining sich laut einer Studie positiv auf die Rumpfausrichtung auswirkt.

Frau V. hat verstanden. Sie achtet nun darauf, regelmäßig an den angebotenen Gruppenübungen des Heims teilzunehmen. Zusätzlich macht sie ihre Morgengymnastik im Bett und dehnt abends Rücken-, Bauch- und Armmuskulatur. Außerdem läuft sie bei jedem Wetter ein, zwei Runden im Garten und setzt Atemübungen ein, wenn sie sich verspannt fühlt

Tab. 14.8 Übersicht der nicht-motorischen Symptome

Kognitiv/psychisch	Vegetativ	Sensorisch/Schmerz
Demenz	Dranginkontinenz	Dysästhesien
Depressionen	Schweißausbrüche	Akathisie
Ängste/Phobien	Dyspnoe	Restless-Legs-Syndrom
Fatigue	Orthostatische Hypotension	Hyposmie
Apathie	Sexuelle Dysfunktion	Schmerzen
Schlafstörungen	Seborrea	
Exzessive Tagesschläfrigkeit	Blasen Dysfunktion	
Psychotische Episoden mit visuellen Halluzinationen	Obstipation	

oder Schmerzen auftreten. Sie fühlt sich agiler und hat wieder ein besseres Körpergefühl. Jetzt denkt sie ohne Erinnerung immer mal wieder daran, sich aufzurichten und es gelingt ihr auch besser. Ins Bett kommt sie noch immer nicht gut ohne Hilfe, aber sie legt sich seltener außerhalb der regelmäßigen Ruhezeiten ins Bett, da sie jetzt aktiver ist. ◀

Übersicht

Neuropsychiatrische Symptome bei M. Parkinson

In der GEPAD-Studie von Reichmann et al. 2010, wurden mit 1449 Menschen mit M. Parkinson in Deutschland klinische Assessments zur Feststellung von Demenz, Depressionen und anderen psychiatrischen Erkrankungen durchgeführt. Dabei wurde festgestellt, dass nur knapp 30 % der Untersuchten **keine** psychiatrischen Symptome zeigten. Bei ca. 29 % konnte eine demenzielle Entwicklung nachgewiesen werden. Ca. 34 % hatten depressive Verstimmungen und 61 % hatten zusätzlich andere neuropsychiatrische Symptome. Die Studienleiter folgerten, dass die neuropsychiatrische Last von Parkinson-Patientinnen im gesamten Krankheitsverlauf, sogar in frühen Stadien, beachtlich ist und eine zentrale Herausforderung für Forschung und klinische Behandlung darstellt. Die Ursachen für die psychischen Symptome sind ein verwobenes Zusammenspiel aus hirnorganischen Veränderungen, sekundär-reaktivem Effekt als Reaktion auf die chronische Erkrankung, Medikamentenwirkungen und -schwankungen (On-Off), Scham über äußeres Erscheinungsbild, Angst (vor Stürzen), sozialem Rückzug und vielem mehr, die faktisch weder auseinanderdividierbar sind, noch genau kategorisiert werden können. Das Wissen über die Vielfalt an Symptomen und komplexen Ursachen hilft Ergotherapeuten, fachlich korrekt zu agieren und gleichzeitig die Klientin als Menschen, gefangen in einer nichtbezwingbaren Krankheit, zu erkennen. Die nicht-motorischen Symptome können in drei Untergruppen eingeteilt werden (siehe Tab. 14.8).

14.8 Umgang mit Stress

Beispiel

„Dieses Jahr gehe ich nicht zur Vereins-Weihnachtsfeier", erzählt Frau T. ihrer Ergotherapeutin. „Ich kann ja nicht mehr Autofahren." Die Therapeutin bietet ihr an, zusammen ein Taxi zu bestellen. „Es ist ja nicht nur das. Ich habe nichts zum Anziehen, meine Frisur ist ausgewachsen und wie soll ich das dann mit meinen Medikamenten machen? Das schaffe ich nie!" Schon beim Gedanken daran gerät Frau T. in Stress. ◀

14.8.1 Auslöser von Stress bei M. Parkinson

Stressauslöser
Viele Menschen mit M. Parkinson sind durch die zunehmende Belastung durch verschiedenste Symptome und die reduzierte kognitive Flexibilität stressanfälliger. Auslöser für Stress können, genau wie bei Nicht-Betroffenen, vielfältig sein. 2016 wurden in einer Studie der Techniker Krankenkasse die häufigsten Stressauslöser in Deutschland erfasst. Die fünf am häufigsten genannten Stressauslöser waren:

1. die Arbeit,
2. hohe Ansprüche an sich selbst,
3. zu viele Termine und Verpflichtungen in der Freizeit,
4. Teilnahme am Straßenverkehr,
5. ständige Erreichbarkeit.

Krankheitsunabhängige Auslösefaktoren werden von an Parkinson-Erkrankten als wesentlich stressreicher empfunden, da Symptome wie Verlangsamung, reduzierte kognitive Flexibilität und Fatigue die Situationen noch verstärken. Hinzu kommen bei Menschen mit M. Parkinson die krankheitsspezifischen Stressauslöser z. B.:

- Angst vor Stürzen,
- Sorge, in der Öffentlichkeit aufzufallen,
- Angst vor Verschlechterung,
- Verlangsamung,
- Belastung der Partnerschaft.

Stressauslöser sind von Person zu Person unterschiedlich und eng an die Persönlichkeit und Ausprägung der Erkrankung geknüpft. Ergotherapeutinnen erleben alle Variationen: von Klienten, die schon vor der Erkrankung gute Stressbewältigungsstrategien aufweisen konnten und eine gewisse Gelassenheit ausstrahlen, bis hin zu Klienten, die vom neuen „Ist-Zustand" völlig überwältigt sind und von einer Stresssituation in die nächste kommen. Es wird als negativer Stresszirkel bezeichnet, wenn Stress zu Anspannung führt, die Anspannung zu verstärkten Parkinson-Symptomen, und diese wiederum negative Gedanken schüren, die den Kreis schließen und den Stress verstärken. Es gilt, in der Therapie oder anhand von gutem Selbstmanagement, diesen Stresszirkel zu unterbrechen.

Auswirkung von Stress
Stress verstärkt die meisten Symptome der Parkinson-Erkrankung. Besonders auffällig ist die negative Auswirkung auf:

- Tremor
- kognitive Funktionen
- Bradykinese
- Freezing
- Rigor
- Depressionen

Zusätzlich deutet die aktuelle Studienlage darauf hin, dass Stress den Krankheitsverlauf negativ beeinflusst (Hemmerle et al. 2012).

14.8.2 Reflexion

Macht und Ellgring (2018) empfehlen, zunächst mit einem Stresstagebuch Stresssituationen zu identifizieren und damit zusammenhängende Gefühle, körperliche Reaktionen, Parkinson-Symptome und negative sowie positive Gedanken schriftlich festzuhalten. Daraufhin können drei konkrete Strategien zur Verbesserung der Stressbewältigung angewandt werden:

- Entspannung (dieses Thema wird ausführlich in Abschn. 14.10.4 behandelt
- Aktivitätsplanung
- gedankliche Veränderung

14.8.3 Umgang mit Zeitdruck

Zeitmanagement
Durch die stetige Zunahme der Verlangsamung nehmen die Klienten häufig nicht wahr, dass sie nun mehr Zeit für eine Tätigkeit benötigen. Sie passen ihre Zeitplanung nicht an und geraten täglich unter Zeitdruck, was wiederum zu Stress führt. Eine einzelne Betätigung muss also kri-

	Montag	Dienstag	Mittwoch	Donnerstag	Freitag	Samstag	Sonntag
06:00							
07:00	Medis Anziehen	Medis Anziehen	Medis Anziehen	Medis Anziehen	Medis Anziehen	Medis Anziehen	Medis Anziehen
08:00	Frahstack	Frahstack	Frahstack	Frahstack	Frahstack	Frahstack	Frahstack
09:00	9:30 Fahrdienst						
10:00	Ergotherapie	Eigenabung	Eigenabung			Eigenabung	Eigenabung
11:00	Fahrdienst			Logopadie			
12:00	Mittagessen	Mittagessen	Mittagessen	Mittagessen	Mittagessen	Mittagessen	Mittagessen
13:00	Pause	Pause	Pause	Pause	Pause	Pause	Pause
14:00	Medis	Medis	Medis	Medis	Medis Fahrdienst	Medis	Medis
15:00				Fahrdienst	Physiotherapie		
16:00				Ergotherapie	Fahrdienst		
17:00	17:30 Mitfahren			Fahrdienst			
18:00	Medis Tai Chi	Medis	Medis	Medis	Medis	Medis	Medis
19:00	Tai Chi	Abendessen	Abendessen	Abendessen	Abendessen	Abendessen	Abendessen
20:00	Mitfahren						
21:00	Abendessen						
22:00							

Abb. 14.50 Bei der stressvermeidenden Tagesstrukturierung sollte im Wochenplan genügend Zeit für An- und Abfahrt, Pausen und auch kleine Betätigungen eingetragen werden

tisch reflektiert und bei Bedarf angepasst werden. Dazu kann das Formular zur Selbstreflexion (siehe Anhang) als Hilfe verwendet werden. Dabei wird häufig festgestellt, dass die Art der Durchführung nicht mehr adäquat ist, oder die Betätigung nicht mehr relevant ist und gestrichen werden kann oder anders in den Tagesablauf integriert werden muss (siehe unten).

Aktivitätsplanung

Das Vorausplanen von Aktivitäten kann den Zeitdruck und den damit verbundenen Stress deutlich reduzieren. Das heißt, anstatt wie vor der Erkrankung ein halbe Stunde vor einem Termin oder einem Treffen benötigte Dinge (Brille, Dokumente, Eintrittskarten, passende Kleidung, Geschenk …) zusammenzusuchen, können strukturierende Maßnahmen helfen, die Aktivität ruhig und bedacht anzugehen. Dafür können folgende Instrumente hilfreich sein:

- Kalender
- To-do Liste
- Erinnerungs-App

Tagesstrukturierung

Im Hinblick auf den Gesamtablauf des Tages und der Woche können Adaptationen sinnvoll sein, wenn zu viele Aktivitäten geplant sind oder sich zu bestimmten Zeiten die Aufgaben häufen und zu Stress führen. Mithilfe des Wochenplans, der im Anhang zu finden ist, erhalten Klient und Therapeutin einen Überblick über alle Aktivitäten in einer Woche. Meist zeigt sich hier schon, wann eine Überlastung auftreten kann (s. Abb. 14.50).

Folgende Punkte sollten Therapeutin und Klient anpassen:

- Aktivitätskluster entzerren
- Anfahrtszeiten fest einplanen
- Erholungszeiten fest einplanen
- Beachtung von On/Off-Phasen
- unnötige oder unbeliebte Aktivitäten streichen oder abgeben
- Zeitpuffer einplanen

Gesundheitsfördernde Aktivitäten planen

Eine pflichtdominierte Wochenstruktur mit Arztterminen, therapeutischen Anwendungen, Haus-

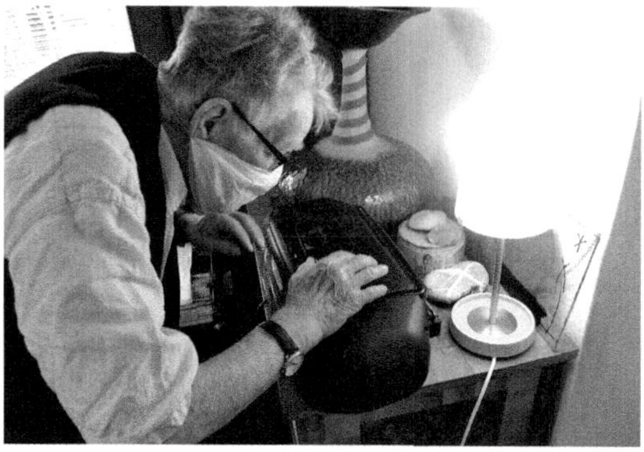

Abb. 14.51 Das Einlegen und Abspielen einer Musik-CD wird geübt, um die wohltuende Betätigung „Musik hören" wieder in den Tagesablauf zu integrieren

halt, Familie und Arbeit kann auf Dauer eine Belastung werden, wenn dadurch die positiven, gesundheitsfördernden Aktivitäten keinen Platz finden.

Das gemeinsame Ausfüllen des Wochenplans kann eine solche Überlastung aufzeigen und die Basis für ein Gespräch über die Wichtigkeit bestimmter Faktoren zur Förderung der Gesundheit bieten. Folgende Aktivitäten sollten im Wochenplan einen festen Platz finden:

- aktive sportliche Betätigung,
- Erholungspausen,
- Schlaf,
- soziale Beziehungen,
- Entspannung (mehr dazu in Abschn. 14.10.4),
- individuelle wohltuende Aktivitäten/Hobbies (z. B. Yoga, Massage, Gartenarbeit, Musik hören (s. Abb. 14.51), Lesen, Dart spielen …).

14.8.4 Gedankliche Veränderung

Negative Gedanken haben einen entscheidenden Einfluss auf das Stressempfinden. Sie laufen meist automatisch ab, ohne bewusst wahrgenommen zu werden, und doch entsteht dadurch häufig eine negative Kettenreaktion aus belastenden Gedanken, Gefühlen, Anspannung, Symptomen und Verhalten. Durch eine bewusste Veränderung der Gedanken verlieren die negativen Gedanken an Kraft, der Klient erlebt sich als selbstwirksam.

Negative Gedanken erkennen

Um sich der Gedanken in Stresssituationen bewusst zu werden, gibt es verschiedene Hilfsmittel:

- **Stresstagebuch**
- **Gedankliche Reflexion**: Nach einer Stresssituation wird, wenn möglich mithilfe der Ergotherapeutin, eine Art „Brainstorming" gemacht, in dem der Klient alle Gedanken und die damit verbundenen Gefühle auflistet.
- **Rollenspiele** können helfen, komplizierte Situationen in einem sicheren Rahmen zu analysieren. Dabei ist der Zugriff auf aufkommende Gedanken evtl. leichter möglich.

Gedanken verändern

Betrachtet der Klient die negativen Gedanken kritisch und prüft sie auf deren objektive Richtigkeit, entdeckt er meist, dass sie so nicht angemessen sind.

Zusammen wird versucht, anstatt der negativen Gedanken andere positive zu formulieren.

Als Beispiel sind ein paar typische negative Gedanken und deren verändertes, positives Gegenüber in Tab. 14.9 zu finden.

Selbstanweisung

Nachdem der Klient die negativen Gedanken in positive umgewandelt hat, kann er sie als sog. Selbstanweisung gedanklich wiederholen. Die Selbstanweisung kann an bestimmte Situationen geknüpft werden, in denen häufig Stress erlebt

Tab. 14.9 Negative Gedanken und Vorschläge für positive Veränderung der Gedanken

„Ich bin zu langsam."	„Ich nehme mir die Zeit, die ich brauche."
„Am Telefon versteht mich keiner."	„Ich gebe mir Mühe, laut und deutlich zu sprechen."
„Es ist peinlich, dass ich beim Essen Hilfe brauche."	„Ich habe eine liebevolle Frau, die mir beim Essen hilft."
„Ich habe tagsüber keine Energie, weil ich nachts so schlecht schlafe."	„Ich lerne meine Energie für das Wichtige zu nutzen und gönne mir mehr Pausen."
„Ich falle meinen Kindern zur Last."	„Ich mache so viel wie möglich selbst und bin meinen Kindern für die Hilfe sehr dankbar."

wird. Dadurch können Situationen entschärft, Stress reduziert und das Selbstvertrauen gestärkt werden.

Einstellung zur Krankheit verändern

- **Positive Glaubenssätze formulieren**: Genau wie Klienten negative Gedanken zu bestimmten Situationen haben, entwickeln sie solche auch zu ihrer Parkinson-Erkrankung. Ein generelles Gefühl von Stress kann sich entfalten. Auch in diesem Fall ist das Erkennen und Aufschreiben der negativen Glaubenssätze ein erster Schritt. Mit dem Wissen, dass die negativen Gedanken einen negativen Stresskreislauf verstärken, sollten positive Glaubenssätze mit dem Klienten erarbeitet werden. Diese sollten nicht willkürlich und ohne Zusammenhang sein, sondern bestenfalls die Ansichten des Klienten repräsentieren und von ihm selbst formuliert werden.

  Dr. med. Schröder (2015), selbst an M. Parkinson erkrankt, beschreibt in seinem Buch „Leben mit Parkinson" seine Beziehung zum M. Parkinson so: „Wir müssen uns aber auf ihn einlassen und man tut gut daran, ihn genauer kennenzulernen … Ein ferner, unbekannter Parkinson-Dämon erscheint uns weitaus gefährlicher als ein gut durchschaubarer und enttarnter Gefährte Parkinson."

  Dagmar: (www.gesundheitsinformation.de) „Ich fand es für mich mit der Zeit wichtig, mich nicht immer zu fragen, ´warum ich?', sondern das Schöne am Leben wieder im Kleinen zu entdecken, mir eine Aufgabe zu suchen und meine Aktivitäten immer wieder an meine Möglichkeiten anzupassen."

  Holger: (www.gesundheitsinformation.de) „Ich finde es wichtig, sich die Freude am Leben und die Neugier zu bewahren. Auch mal etwas Neues zu wagen, etwas zu probieren, was man schon immer mal machen wollte und sich möglichst nicht zu verstecken. Sich für andere, für ein Hobby, für die Arbeit zu engagieren und aktiv zu sein. Das lenkt auch von der Krankheit ab."
- **Positive Seiten der Parkinson-Erkrankung**: Dies mag im ersten Moment sarkastisch klingen. Viele Menschen mit M. Parkinson sind jedoch durchaus fähig, für sich auch positive Seiten des M. Parkinson zu erkennen. Zum Beispiel „endlich mehr Zeit", „verbessertes Einfühlungsvermögen", „neue Hobbies"… Eine solche Liste mit dem Klienten zu erstellen, kann zu einer positiveren Sicht auf die Erkrankung führen.

14.8.5 Angehörigenberatung

Immer wieder kommt es dazu, dass Angehörige den Stresspegel erhöhen, in dem sie sich ungeduldig verhalten. So verständlich das ist, wenn man ständig mit einem verlangsamten Menschen zu tun hat, so kontraproduktiv ist die Ungeduld. Hektik, Ausrufe wie „Beeil dich!", Augen verdrehen und am Arm ziehen, damit der Betroffene schneller aufsteht, bewirken nicht eine schnellere Durchführung, sondern eine Abnahme der Geschwindigkeit oder schlimmstenfalls den Abbruch der Tätigkeit durch ein Auslösen von Freezing durch den erhöhten Stresspegel. Erkennt die Ergotherapeutin diesen Negativkreislauf zwischen Angehörigen und Klienten, sind folgende Therapieansätze möglich:

- **Spiegelung des Verhaltens**: Um eine Verhaltensänderung zu erzielen, reicht oftmals schon das Bewusstmachen des negativen Einflusses, damit der Angehörige weniger Druck ausübt.
- **Gespräche/Rollenspiele**: Zusätzlich können mithilfe von Gesprächen und Rollenspielen unterschiedliche Verhaltensweisen ausprobiert und Änderungen angeregt werden.
- **Räumliche Trennung**: Manchmal ist eine Entspannung der Situation möglich, in dem der Angehörige z. B. in einem anderen Zimmer wartet, während der Betroffene seine Schuhe anzieht.

Beispiel

Frau T. sitzt zwischen all den Menschen, die sie schon jahrelang kennt. Die Weihnachtsfeier ist in vollem Gange. Es wird gelacht, gegessen und auf das Jahr zurückgeblickt. Um teilnehmen zu können, hat Frau T. viel Vorbereitungszeit gebraucht. Die Therapeutin hat es mit ihr zusammen durchstrukturiert, Kleidung ausgesucht und gebügelt, die Handtasche gepackt (eine kleine Medikamentenbox, Inkontinenzeinlage, Telefonnummer des Taxiunternehmens, Geld, Lippenstift) und einen Termin beim Frisör ausgemacht. Aber daran denkt Frau T. jetzt nicht. Sie genießt einfach das Beisammensein und die vorweihnachtliche Stimmung. ◀

14.9 Demenz und kognitive Einschränkungen

Beispiel

Frau K. steht im Flur, irgendetwas wollte sie doch gerade machen. Ist es vielleicht Zeit, die Medikamente einzunehmen? Sie sieht auf dem Zettel nach, der auf ihrem Tisch liegt. 8:00 Uhr, 12:00 Uhr, 16:00 Uhr L-Dopa. Ist es schon 12 Uhr? Hat sie die Medikamente für 8 Uhr schon genommen? Sie ruft ihre Schwägerin an, die ist ungeduldig. Ständig ruft Frau K. an, fragt verwirrende Fragen. Am Telefon kann sie ihr doch auch nicht helfen. Frau K. legt auf und fühlt sich noch nervöser als vorher. Sie läuft hin und her, setzt sich kurz hin und studiert die vielen Zettel auf dem Tisch, auf denen sie sich Erinnerungsstützen notiert hat. Das Zittern in der rechten Hand ist stärker als sonst. Sie läuft wieder hin und her, das hilft gegen das Zittern, aber die innere Unruhe wird noch schlimmer. So oder so ähnlich läuft jeder Morgen bei Frau K. ab, wenn keiner zu Hause ist, um sie zu beruhigen und abzulenken. ◀

14.9.1 Symptombeschreibung

Definition Das idiopathische Parkinson-Syndrom steht häufig mit kognitiven Einschränkungen bis hin zur Demenz in Zusammenhang. Vor allem die Wortflüssigkeit, exekutive Funktionen (z. B. kognitive Flexibilität, Inhibition, Problemlösung) und visuell-räumliche Funktionen (z. B. Längen-, Positions- und Winkeleinschätzung, räumliche Orientierung) sind beeinträchtigt.

Ätiologie Biochemische Veränderungen im Gehirn von an M. Parkinson Erkrankten legen nahe, dass es unterschiedliche Ursachen für eine demenzielle Entwicklung gibt. Das Fronto-Striatal-Syndrom als Folge des Dopaminmangels führt zu Defiziten des Arbeitsgedächtnisses, der Planung, der Inhibition, der Erinnerungsfähigkeit, der Wortflüssigkeit und der psychomotorischen Schnelligkeit. Andererseits treten auch kognitive Einschränkungen auf, die nicht Folge eines Dopaminmangels sind, z. B. Defizite der Aufmerksamkeit (wie etwa Vigilanz und Fluktuation in Wachheit), Sprache, räumlich-visuelle Funktionen und Gedächtnis. In seltenen Fällen wird eine Demenz medikamentös induziert oder durch Depressionen ausgelöst.

Prävalenz Im Verlauf der Erkrankung treten häufig kognitive Einschränkungen auf. Die Prozentangaben zu demenzieller Entwicklung bei M. Parkinson gehen in Studien weit auseinander und werden zwischen 4 % und 93 % angegeben. Das Auftreten einer Demenz wurde in Querschnittsstudien bei 30 % bis 40 % der Parkinson-Erkrankten festgestellt. Es wird davon ausgegangen, dass **alle** Patientinnen im **fortgeschrittenen Stadium** kognitive Einschränkungen oder eine Demenz entwickeln.

Klinik Die Parkinson-Demenz ist klar von der Alzheimer-Demenz zu unterscheiden.

Patientinnen mit IPS haben in der Regel keine oder nur wenig Einschränkung der Sprache, beim Benennen von Gegenständen, dem Gedächtnis und der Praxie, wohingegen Aufmerksamkeit, Exekutivfunktionen und visuell-räumliche Wahrnehmung auffällig sind (siehe Tab. 14.10).

Ob eine Verlangsamung der Informationsverarbeitung, eine sog. **Bradyphrenie**, bei der Parkinson-Erkrankung tatsächlich auftritt, ist nicht abschließend geklärt. Zwar wird ein verlangsamtes Denken offenbar häufig beobachtet, jedoch ist eine klare Abgrenzung zur motorischen Verlangsamung und zu Depressionen kompliziert, da beides auch

Tab. 14.10 In diesen Bereichen entwickeln Parkinson-Betroffene typischerweise kognitive Auffälligkeiten

Häufig Auffälligkeiten	Meist **keine** Auffälligkeiten
• Gedächtnis und lernen - Freies Erinnern **ohne** Abrufhilfe - Neuerlernen von Handlungen	• Gedächtnis und lernen - Erinnern **mit** Abrufhilfe - Orientierung
• Exekutive Funktionen - Intern dirigiertes Verhalten (spontane Initiierung von aufgabenspezifischer Planung) - Geteilte Aufmerksamkeit • Auch „set-shifting" (Anpassung des Verhaltens auf wechselnde Stimuli) - Beibehalten des Aufmerksamkeits-Sets bei gleichbleibendem Stimulus - Verbale Wortflüssigkeit - Tätigkeiten wechseln	• Exekutive Funktionen - Extern dirigiertes Verhalten - Konzeptbildung
• Visuell-räumliche Wahrnehmung	
	• Fähigkeit zum Benennen von Objektdarstellungen
	• Logisches Denken
• Informationsverarbeitung, Denkgeschwindigkeit noch ungeklärt	

zu verzögerter Reaktion und Sprachproduktion führen kann. Deshalb sollte nicht davon ausgegangen werden, dass bei Menschen mit M. Parkinson eine Bradyphrenie vorliegt.

Es kann eine Verlangsamung bei der Bearbeitung von Tests mit hohem kognitiven Anspruch erkannt werden, doch interpretieren die Wissenschaftlerinnen dies nicht definitiv als Verlangsamung des Denkprozesses, sondern geben zu bedenken, dass dies an einer verminderten Fähigkeit zur Findung von Problemlösungsstrategien liegen könnte. Auch eingeschränkte exekutive Funktionen können zu einer kognitiv verzögerten Verarbeitung führen. Im Umgang mit Parkinson-Betroffenen ist dieses Wissen hilfreich. Die Qualität des Denkens kann trotz einer verlangsamten Reaktion sehr hoch sein.

Medizinische Möglichkeiten

- Medikamente
- Absetzen auslösender Medikamente
- Behandlung von Depressionen

14.9.2 Kompensationsstrategien bei Merkschwierigkeiten

Bei Menschen mit der Parkinson-Erkrankung ist die Einschränkung des freien Erinnerns ohne Abrufhilfe charakteristisch. Das bedeutet, dass die Klientinnen ohne externe Hilfe Schwierigkeiten haben, sich an Dinge zu erinnern. Sobald ein Hinweis von außen gegeben wird, ist die Erinnerung wieder präsent. Z. B. auf die Frage „Was haben Sie gestern gemacht?" kann keine Antwort gegeben werden. Auf die Frage „Gestern haben Sie Ihre Enkel ja getroffen, was haben Sie da gemacht?" kommt eine detailreiche Erzählung.

Therapeutischer Ansatz

- **Kalender/Tagebuch**: Zur Unterstützung der Merkfähigkeit werden zu jeder Situation Kurznotizen über Wichtiges und Schönes gemacht, die bei Bedarf nachgeschlagen werden können (Abb. 14.52).
- **Auf Mobiltelefon vom Erlebten Fotos machen**: Um Erinnerungen extern zu triggern, werden Fotos mit dem Mobiltelefon aufgenommen, die später in Gesprächen gezeigt und mit Erzählungen ausgeschmückt werden können (Abb. 14.53).
- **Externe Erinnerungshilfen für Medikamenteneinnahme**: Mithilfe einer Erinnerungsapp, elektrischer Tablettendose, (siehe Abb. 14.54) oder Armbanduhr mit Erinnerungsfunktion können die genauen Einnahmezeiten der Medikamente eingehalten werden.
- **Kalenderführung**: Je nach Fähigkeit wird ein täglicher, wöchentlicher oder monatlicher Kalender genutzt, um Termine im Blick zu behalten.

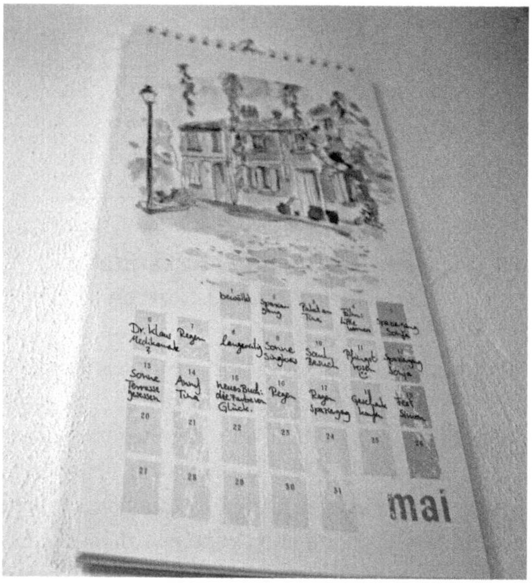

Abb. 14.52 Kalender mit Kurznotizen zu Erlebtem, als Erinnerungshilfe

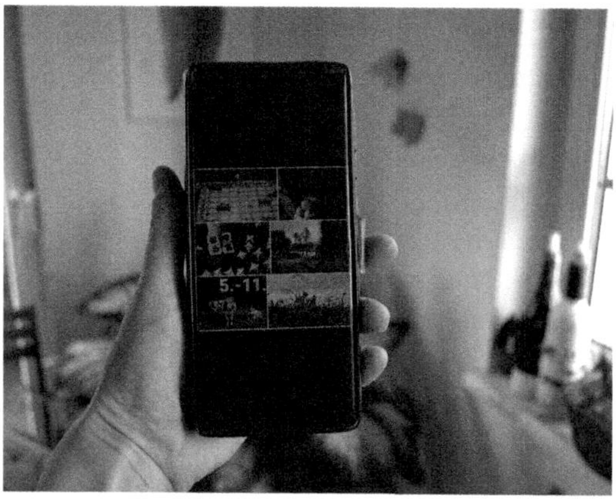

Abb. 14.53 Collage aus Fotos der Woche im Mobiltelefon, als Erinnerungshilfe

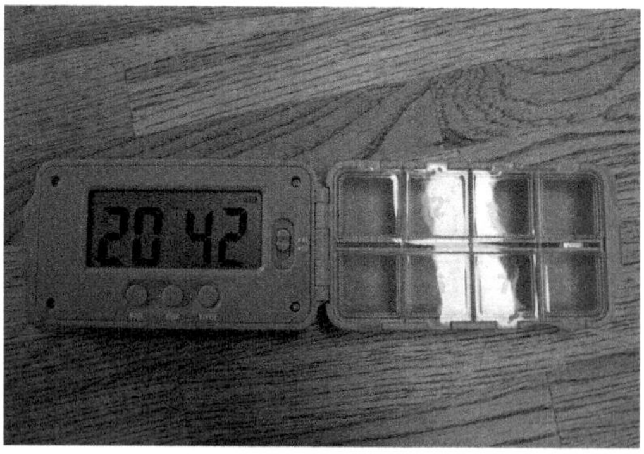

Abb. 14.54 Beispiel einer Tablettendosierhilfe mit Erinnerungsfunktion

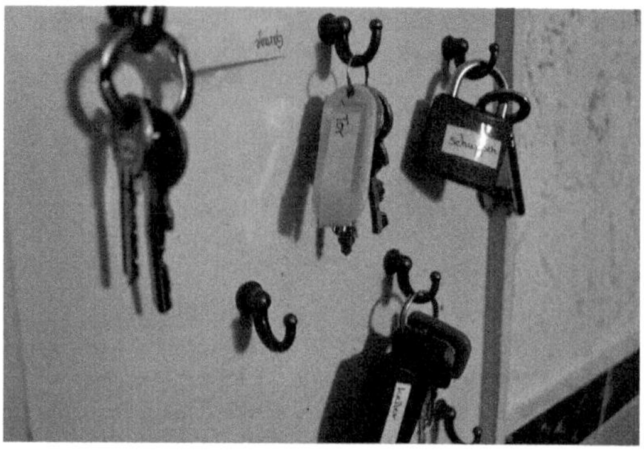

Abb. 14.55 Schlüssel beschriften als Erinnerungshilfe

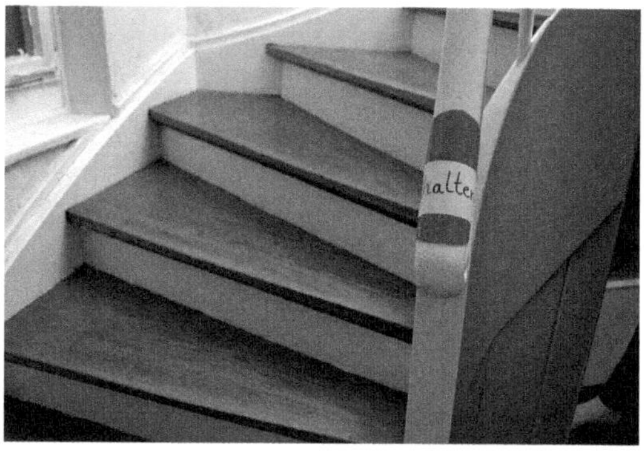

Abb. 14.56 Erinnerung, sich beim Treppensteigen an dem Geländer festzuhalten

- **Beschriftung von Gegenständen**: Schrankinhalte, Schlüssel, Kurzwahltasten auf Telefon bebildern oder beschriften (Abb. 14.55).
- **To-Do-Liste**: Morgens kann als Ritual zusammen mit einem Angehörigen der Tag durchgegangen und eine To-Do-Liste angefertigt werden, die in den Kalender oder an einen anderen gut sichtbaren Ort gehängt wird.
- **Zettel an wichtige Orte**: Zur Erinnerung können an wichtigen Stellen Zettel angebracht werden, z. B. Einstellungen bei Waschmaschine, Herd aus, Schlüssel mitnehmen, Hände waschen, Festhalten am Geländer (siehe Abb. 14.56), Katze füttern …
- **Einkaufsliste** sofort ergänzen, wenn etwas fehlt.
- **Dinge immer am selben Ort platzieren** (Schlüssel, Handy, Geldbörse).
- **Rituale einführen**, z. B. immer beim Fernsehen ein Glas Wasser trinken.

14.9.3 Neuerlernen von Handlungen

Solange alles beim Alten bleibt, sind Menschen mit M. Parkinson kognitiv häufig unauffällig. Sobald sich jedoch etwas verändert (z. B. neues Hilfsmittel, Einführung eines neuen Kalenders …), kann es ihnen schwer fallen, neue Verhaltensweisen und Handlungen zu erlernen.

Therapeutischer Ansatz

Um bei einer Parkinson-Demenz neues Handeln zu lernen, ist eine **Kombination** aus **prozeduralem Lernen** und **deklarativem Lernen** notwendig. Prozedurales Lernen bedeutet, „Lernen durch Tun“ mit häufiger Repetition. Deklaratives Lernen ist die bewusste Aufnahme von Informationen, die dann ebenso bewusst wieder abgerufen werden können.

Menschen mit M. Parkinson können Erklärungen meist gut verstehen, eine Umsetzung in die Praxis ist jedoch meist nur in Kombination mit prozeduralem Lernen möglich.

Zur Einführung der Nutzung eines neuen Hilfsmittels wie eines Rollators macht es Sinn, das Hilfsmittel klar sichtbar in die Nähe des Tätigkeitsbereichs zu platzieren, z. B. im Eingangsbereich des Hauses.

Zusätzlich zur Erklärung der Bedienung sollte der Therapeut es kurz vormachen, um dann sofort in die Aktivität der Klientin zu wechseln. Dabei können knappe Anweisungen vor der Durchführung die Handlungsschritte initiieren.

Eine Videosequenz, in der jemand mit Erklärung des Therapeuten adäquat am Rollator geht, kann einen positiven Einfluss auf die Nutzungsbereitschaft haben.

Das Führen der Hände kann ausprobiert werden. Manche Klientinnen wehren sich gegen das Führen oder die Berührung bringt sie durcheinander.

14.9.4 Exekutive Funktionen

Zu den exekutiven Funktionen gehören fünf kognitive Fähigkeiten:

1. **Intern dirigiertes Verhalten (spontane Initiierung von aufgabenspezifischer Planung):** Menschen mit der Parkinson-Erkrankung zeigen eine zunehmende Passivität mit einer Antriebsstörung. Je nach Ausprägung könnten sie teilweise stundenlang sitzen und nichts tun, wenn von außen kein Impuls kommt (Apathie). Klientinnen vergessen Spaziergänge und nehmen Medikamente und Flüssigkeit nicht mehr ohne Erinnerung ein.
   Therapeutischer Ansatz:
   - Tätigkeiten können an andere, regelmäßig auftretende Tätigkeiten geknüpft werden, z. B.: „Immer, wenn die Uhr zur vollen Stunde schlägt, trinke ich ein halbes Glas Wasser“ oder „Immer nach dem Essen gehe ich eine Runde um den Block“.
   - Es können externe Erinnerungen eingerichtet werden, z. B. Erinnerung über Mobiltelefon, Partner initiiert Handlung
   - Hilfsmittel zur Erinnerung (Medikamentenbox, Übungsapp) (siehe Abschn. 15.3)
   - Aktivitätsgruppen werden gesucht oder gebildet, z. B. Yoga mit Nachbarin, Sportgruppe …
2. **Geteilte Aufmerksamkeit**
   Klientinnen sind in abnehmendem Maße imstande, ein sog. Shifting anzuwenden, also das Verhalten auf wechselnde Stimuli anzupassen. Z. B.: Die Klientin schreibt einen Einkaufzettel, der Ehemann öffnet den Küchenschrank und zählt auf, was fehlt. So muss die Klientin immer wieder zwischen „Schreiben“ und „Zuhören“ wechseln. Diese Interferenz wird vor allem durch drei Faktoren beeinflusst:
   1. dem Schwierigkeitsgrad der Aufgaben,
   2. der Ähnlichkeit der Aufgaben (unter Berücksichtigung der benötigten Sinne) und
   3. der Übung der Durchführung einer Aufgabe.

   Daraus lassen sich die therapeutischen Ansätze ableiten.

Therapeutischer Ansatz:

- Schwierigkeit der Aufgaben reduzieren, z. B. Partner nennt ein fehlendes Lebensmittel, wartet geduldig, bis Klientin es aufgeschrieben hat und geht langsam vor
- Ähnliche Aufgaben vermeiden, z. B. dem Partner zuhören, während das Radio läuft
- Wiederholtes Üben der geteilten Aufmerksamkeit, nicht abstrakt, sondern bezogen auf die spezifische Situation, z. B. Therapeut nennt aufzuschreibende Worte
- Vermeidung der geteilten Aufmerksamkeit

3. **Stark fluktuierende Aufmerksamkeit**
Die Aufmerksamkeit ist häufig im Verlauf der Erkrankung gestört und stark fluktuierend, mit immer wieder luziden (klaren) Momenten. Dies hängt meist mit der wechselnden Medikamentenwirkung zusammen.
Therapeutischer Ansatz:

  - Klientinnen nie unterschätzen
  - Flexibel bleiben bei der Therapie
  - Angehörige aufklären

Therapeuten sollten Klientinnen niemals unterschätzen. Durch die fluktuierende Medikamentenwirkung variieren kognitive Prozesse und die Kommunikationsfähigkeit stark.

4. **Verbale Wortflüssigkeit**
Während des Sprechens kann häufig beobachtet werden, dass Menschen mit M. Parkinson stark verlangsamt und stockend sprechen und teilweise den Faden verlieren. Das Sprechen ist eine kognitive Anforderung durch die Koordination der Mundmotorik mit dem Nachdenken über das, was gesagt werden soll. Durch dieses Dual-Tasking entsteht eine mentale Überforderung, die zum Stocken führen kann.
Therapeutische Möglichkeiten:

  - Ablenkende Faktoren reduzieren
  - Der Betroffenen klar sagen, dass sie sich Zeit lassen darf
  - Trennung von Nachdenken, was gesagt werden soll, und Sprechen
  - Angehörigenschulung (nicht ablenken, Geduld zeigen)
  - Durch Atemübung Entspannung des Kehlkopfes und Reduktion von Stress
  - Pacing: Mithilfe eines Sprechbretts oder Taktgebers Silbe für Silbe sprechen, um schnelles Sprechen zu rhythmisieren (z. B. zwei aufgemalte Punkte: Mit dem Finger wird abwechselnd ein Punkt berührt und jeweils eine Silbe gesprochen)
  - Reduktion von Stress durch Aufklärung der Kommunikationspartner, dass die Sprache verlangsamt ist
  - Am Anfang des Satzes bewusst laut und deutlich ansetzen
  - Mimik bewusst einsetzen, um Kommunikation zu unterstützen
  - Zeichen vereinbaren, wenn Klientin Unterstützung benötigt (Wortfindung)

5. **Tätigkeiten wechseln**
Das Wechseln von einer Tätigkeit zur anderen fällt den betroffenen Menschen zunehmend schwer, z. B. einen Anruf während des Kochens entgegenzunehmen. Es kann zu einer Unterbrechung des Bewegungsflusses, Akinese, Unsicherheit bei der Handlungsplanung oder -durchführung und kurzzeitiger kognitiver Desorientierung kommen.
Therapeutische Möglichkeiten:

  - Wenn möglich, sollte die Klientin dazu angehalten werden, einen Wechsel von Tätigkeiten erst vorzunehmen, wenn die vorherige Tätigkeit beendet ist, z. B. das Telefon nicht abzuheben, sondern zurückzurufen, sobald die Tätigkeit beendet ist.
  - Wenn ein Wechsel der Tätigkeiten unumgänglich ist, ist eine Einübung des Tätigkeitswechsels möglich. Dabei muss betätigungsspezifisch trainiert werden, da ein Übertrag von abstrakter Situation auf eine spezifische Situation nicht gelingt, z. B. wenn das sofortige Beantworten des Telefons ein notwendiger Teil des Jobs ist (Sekretärin).

14.9.5 Visuelle-Räumliche Wahrnehmung

Bei Menschen mit M. Parkinson kann die visuell-räumliche Wahrnehmung eingeschränkt sein. Da eine Reihe von visuellen und okulomotorischen Einschränkungen (z. B. Blickparese, Doppelbilder) sowie visuelle Verarbeitungsstörungen mit M. Parkinson einhergehen können, ist nicht immer klar erkennbar, welche Ursache bei visuellen Auffälligkeiten der Auslöser ist. Klientinnen berichten häufig von Doppelbildern, Schwierigkeiten zu fokussieren und Abstände einzuschätzen. Es kann teilweise beobachtet werden, dass Patientinnen danebengreifen, Möbel anrempeln oder beim Lesen Probleme haben.

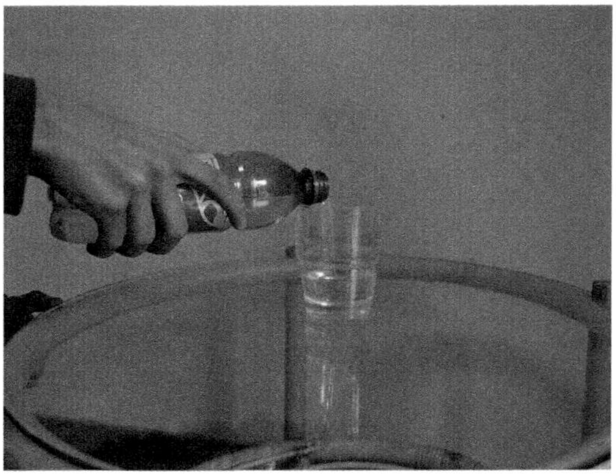

Abb. 14.57 Um visuell-räumliche Wahrnehmungsstörung zu kompensieren, die sensorischen Referenzflächen nutzen und beim Einschenken Flasche auf den Glasrand auflegen

Therapeutische Möglichkeiten

- Übung
  - Wichtige Betätigungen, bei denen räumlich-visuelle Wahrnehmung unabdingbar ist, trainieren, z. B. Schreiben, Besteck einräumen, Laufen in der Wohnung, Kalendernutzung, Schachspielen
- Kompensationsstrategien
  - Betätigungen langsamer durchführen, um Fehlwahrnehmung auszugleichen
  - Gegenstände (z. B. Stühle, Küchenutensilien, Geschirr beim Essen) immer gleich positionieren, damit keine visuelle Kontrolle notwendig
  - Klare sensorische Zielpunkte und Referenzflächen nutzen, z. B. Kaffeepulver erst in den Filter füllen, wenn Filter innen mit dem Löffel berührt wird, beim Wassereinschenken Flasche auf Glas auflegen (siehe Abb. 14.57)
- Vermeidung
  - Autofahren einstellen
  - Fahrradfahren einstellen
  - Angehörige Überweisungen durchführen lassen

Kognitives Training

In einer Studie von Reuter et al. (2012) war eine multimodale Therapie zur Verbesserung der Kognition am effektivsten. Dabei erhielten die Klientinnen eine **kognitive Therapie** und zusätzliche **Lehreinheiten zur Übertragung in das Alltagsleben** sowie ein zusätzliches **Bewegungstraining**.

Cruise et al. (2011) konnten eine Verbesserung der Kognition nach einem zwölfwöchigen Fitness- und Krafttraining feststellen. Weitere Informationen zu Kraft- und Ausdauertraining für Menschen mit M. Parkinson sind in Abschn. 10.3 zu finden.

Beispiel

Frau K. freut sich jetzt auf die Ergotherapie. Sie weiß, dass die Therapeutin Struktur in ihren Tagesablauf bringt. Jede Woche gehen sie die gesammelten Zettelchen durch, tragen wichtige Termine zusammen in den Kalender ein und werfen unnötige Notizen in den Müll. Sie haben gemeinsam den veralteten Geburtstagskalender aktualisiert und nun mit einer Überarbeitung des Adressbuchs begonnen, damit beides übersichtlich ist. Außerdem nutzt sie jetzt eine Medikamentenbox mit Erinnerungsfunktion. Sie ruft nicht mehr so häufig ihre Schwägerin an, wodurch auch diese weniger gestresst ist. Dadurch ist die Beziehung entspannter, was sich wiederum positiv auf die Ausgeglichenheit von Frau K. auswirkt. ◀

14.10 Depressionen und Ängste

Beispiel

Irgendwo muss doch diese blöde Spritze sein. Gerade noch hatte Herr B. sie in der Hand. Hektisch dreht er sich, sucht auf dem Tisch, im Regal und auf dem Boden – nichts. Wenn er sie nicht gleich findet, kommt er vielleicht in eine Unterzuckerung, das darf nicht passieren, außerdem kommt der ganze Tagesablauf durcheinander. Herr B. beschimpft sich selbst, er beschimpft die Spritze, er beschimpft den Diabetes und den Parkinson. ◀

14.10.1 Symptombeschreibung

Bei einer depressiven Episode zeigt der Patient einen reduzierten Antrieb, Aktivität und Konzentrationsfähigkeit. Seine Stimmung ist niedergeschlagen und die Fähigkeit Freude zu empfinden ist vermindert. Außerdem können Müdigkeit, Schlafstörungen, Appetitverlust, Schuldgefühle, Gefühle der Wertlosigkeit und Libidoverlust hinzukommen.

Ätiologie Die Unfähigkeit, Freude und Lust zu empfinden (**Anhedonie**) ist auf zwei Ursachen zurückzuführen. Zum einen ist Dopamin im Gehirn u. a. für die Motivation und den Antrieb zuständig und hat in Verbindung mit Noradrenalin einen wesentlichen Einfluss auf unser Glücksempfinden. Deswegen wird es als Belohnungshormon bezeichnet. Ist die Dopaminausschüttung reduziert, nimmt das Glücksempfinden folglich auch ab.

Die zweite Ursache für Depressionen bei M. Parkinson ist die mangelnde Krankheitsverarbeitung.

Prävalenz Etwa 33,6 % der Menschen (Riedel et al. 2010), die die Diagnose M. Parkinson bekommen, erleben im Laufe der Erkrankung eine Depression. Die Diagnostik von Depressionen ist durch die Überschneidung von Symptomen mit kognitiven und motorischen Einschränkungen (Antriebsarmut, reduzierte Mimik, leise Stimme, Konzentrationsschwierigkeiten ...) nicht immer eindeutig. Aus diesem Grund schwanken die angegebenen Prävalenzzahlen teilweise erheblich und in der Praxis werden etwa die Hälfte der Betroffenen nicht erkannt.

Klinik Folgende Beschwerden können bei Depressionen auftreten:

- Innere Leere
- Hoffnungslosigkeit
- Anhedonie (Unfähigkeit, Freude zu empfinden, s. o.)
- Müdigkeit
- Bedrückte Grundstimmung
- Gereiztheit
- Pessimismus
- Traurigkeit
- Reizbarkeit
- Suizidgedanken

Es gibt Untersuchungen, die nahelegen, dass Depressionen bei der Parkinson-Erkrankung von einer primären Depression abgegrenzt werden können. Diese Studien kommen jedoch zu teils widersprüchlichen Ergebnissen und haben keine Auswirkung auf die ergotherapeutische Arbeit. Eine wichtige Abgrenzung gibt es bei reaktiven Depressionen oder depressiven Symptomen, die aufgrund der eingeschränkten Krankheitsbewältigung auftreten. Außerdem muss von affektiven Schwankungen im Zusammenhang mit Wirkungsfluktuationen der Medikamente unterschieden werden. Diese treten (teils sehr stark) in den Off-Phasen auf, verschwinden jedoch, sobald die nächste Medikamentendosis eingenommen wird.

Folgen/Komplikationen Depressionen wirken sich erheblich auf die Lebensqualität aus. Außerdem verschlechtert sich häufig der Allgemeinzustand der Patienten und soziale Kontakte nehmen durch die Antriebslosigkeit stark ab.

Therapeutische Möglichkeiten:

- Optimierung der dopaminergen Therapie
- Antidepressive Medikamente
- Medikamentenpumpe
- Tiefe Hirnstimulation
- Psychotherapie
- Verhaltenstherapie
- Psychoedukation
- Schlafentzug

Ängste/Phobien

Definition Ängste und Phobien treten im Zusammenhang mit dem idiopathischen Parkinson-Syndrom gehäuft auf. Dabei scheint die soziale Phobie, mit oder ohne **Agoraphobie**, im Vordergrund zu stehen. Agoraphobie ist die Angst vor sozialen Situationen, besonders wenn der Betroffene im Fokus der Aufmerksamkeit ist, wie beim Bezahlen an der Kasse oder Essen im Restaurant.

Ätiologie Gegenwärtig ist der genaue Mechanismus der angstauslösenden Abläufe im Gehirn noch unklar. Man geht von einem defizitären Zusammenspiel zwischen komplexen dopaminergen, noradrenergen und serotonergen Systemen aus.

Prävalenz Die Häufigkeit von Angststörungen bei M. Parkinson wird auf 30–40 % beziffert. Wobei von einer Unterdiagnostizierung ausgegangen wird.

Klinik Ängste sind vielen Menschen mit M. Parkinson bekannt. Nicht immer werden sie als Angststörung diagnostiziert, denn der Übergang von normaler Sorge zu einer einschränkenden Angsterkrankung ist fließend, vor allem bei einer degenerativen Erkrankung mit ausgeprägten Symptomen. Das Auftreten von Angst- und Panikattacken ist in den Off-Phasen deutlich erhöht und wird von Betroffenen als erhebliche Einschränkung erlebt, oftmals mehr als die physischen Symptome des Offs. Es wird von Gefühlen elementarer Angst und stark behindernder Panik berichtet. Auch ein Zusammenhang von demenzieller Entwicklung und Angst konnte nachgewiesen werden, die oftmals von allgemeiner Ängstlichkeit und innerer Unruhe geprägt ist.

Folgende Symptome können auftreten:

- Erröten
- Händezittern
- Übelkeit
- Herzklopfen
- Brustschmerz
- Erstickungsgefühle
- Schwindel
- Entfremdungsgefühle
- Nervosität
- Zittern
- Muskelspannung
- Schwitzen

Folgen/Komplikationen
Menschen mit Angststörungen vermeiden meist die auslösenden Situationen (z. B. soziale Kontakte, Präsenz in der Öffentlichkeit), wodurch es zu einer zunehmenden Isolation kommen kann. Leider wird dies von Angehörigen und Ärzten oftmals verkannt und nicht entsprechend behandelt.

Medizinische Möglichkeiten

- Anpassung der Medikamenteneinnahmezeiten, um Wirkungsfluktuationen zu reduzieren
- Medikation
- Medikamentenpumpe
- Tiefe Hirnstimulation
- Psychotherapie
- Verhaltenstherapie
- Psychoedukation

14.10.2 Erkennen von depressiven Verstimmungen und Ängsten

Zunächst ist es wichtig, als Therapeutin die Eventualität einer Depression oder Phobie zu kennen, um Anzeichen erkennen zu können. Da sich die Symptome von M. Parkinson und Depressionen oder Ängsten teilweise überschneiden, ist eine Abgrenzung auch für Ärzte häufig schwierig. Nur weil der Klient leise spricht, antriebsarm ist, wenig Mimik und Gestik zeigt und Schlafstörungen hat, lässt sich nicht auf eine Depression schließen. Mit wachsendem Vertrauen sind es jedoch oftmals die Therapeutinnen, die zuerst den Verdacht auf eine Depression oder Angstsymptomatik aussprechen, da die Klienten sich zunehmend öffnen und ihre Gefühle kommunizieren.

Äußert der Klient negatives Gedankenkreisen, bedrückte oder niedergeschlagene Stimmung, Ängste und sogar Suizidgedanken, sind dies klare Hinweise für eine depressive Verstimmung. Ängste zeigen sich oftmals in Vermeidung der angstauslösenden Situationen. Eine Sturzangst führt zur Reduktion der Mobilität, eine soziale Phobie verhindert die Teilnahme an sozialen Situationen oder das Bewegen in der Öffentlichkeit.

Rücksprache mit Arzt

Erkennt die Therapeutin o. g. Symptome, die auf Depressionen oder Ängste hinweisen, empfiehlt es sich, die Ärztin darüber zu informieren, damit diese weitere Therapiemöglichkeiten (Medikamente und/oder psychologische Behandlung) verordnen kann. Bei Suizidgedanken oder -absichten besteht eine akute Dringlichkeit. In diesem Fall ist eine telefonische Informierung des Arztes ratsam. Unter diesen Umständen ist die Therapeutin zum Selbstschutz des Klienten von der Schweigepflicht entbunden.

14.10.3 Umgang mit Gedankenkreisen/negativen Gedanken

Gespräche

Es kann für den Klienten eine Entlastung sein, mit der Therapeutin über seine depressiven Gedanken zu sprechen. Dabei müssen Ergotherapeutinnen mit Vorsicht vorgehen, da sie nicht die notwendige Ausbildung haben, um eine Gesprächstherapie professionell führen zu können. Empathisches Zuhören kann für den Klienten schon eine große Erleichterung bringen. Dabei sollte das Gedankenkreisen des Klienten nicht verstärkt werden.

Aktiv werden

Erkennt die Therapeutin die negative Gedankenspirale, kann sie das Gespräch in eine andere Richtung lenken und durch Aktivität und die Arbeit an den Klientenzielen das Gedankenkreisen unterbrechen. Dieselbe Umgangsweise kann mit dem Klienten geübt werden, damit er eine Handhabe für Zeiten hat, in denen er allein ist.

Negative Gedanken bewusst machen → Gedanken stoppen → aktiv werden

Selbstreflexion

Mit der Ergotherapeutin kann der Klient kritische Situationen besprechen und seine Gefühle, Gedanken und Reaktionen reflektieren. Daraufhin sollten alternative Reaktionsmöglichkeiten besprochen werden, die der Klient bei Wiederauftreten der Situation ausprobieren kann. Dazu sind in Abschn. 10.1 (Selbstmanagement) viele weitere Ideen zu finden, wie der Klient erlernen kann, mit seiner Erkrankung und den damit einhergehenden Schwierigkeiten selbstbestimmt umzugehen (Abb. 14.58, 14.59, und 14.60).

In Abschn. 14.10.3, Umgang mit Stress, Gedankliche Veränderung, sind hierzu weitere hilfreiche Therapieansätze zu finden.

14.10.4 Entspannung

Es gibt zahlreiche Techniken und Methoden, um Entspannung zu erreichen. Der positive Effekt auf motorische und nicht-motorische Symptome

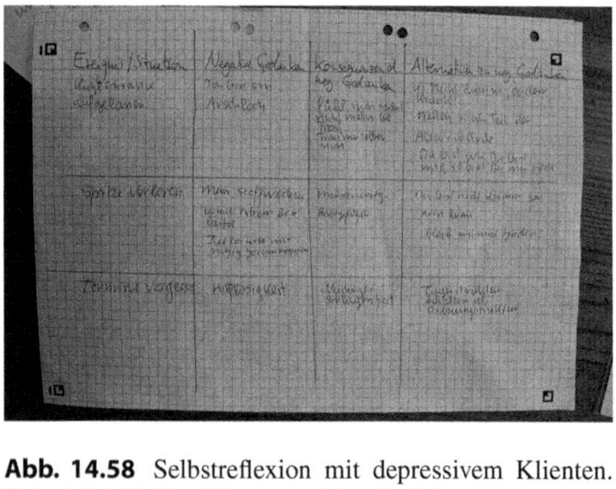

Abb. 14.58 Selbstreflexion mit depressivem Klienten. Beispiel 1. Zeile: Klient beschimpft sich selbst, wenn er den Kühlschrank aus Versehen offenstehen lässt

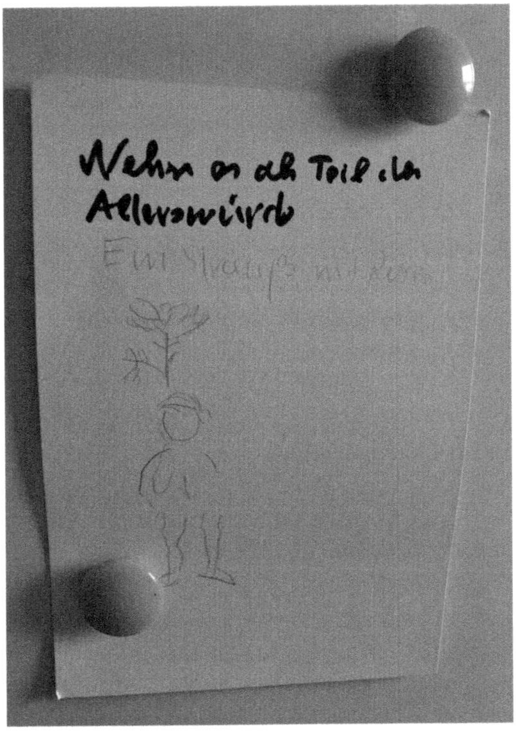

Abb. 14.59 Eine Alternative zu negativen Gedanken wird erarbeitet. Der Klient schreibt in eigenen Worten auf eine Karte: „Nimm es als Teil der Alterswürde. Ein Strauß mit Rosen"

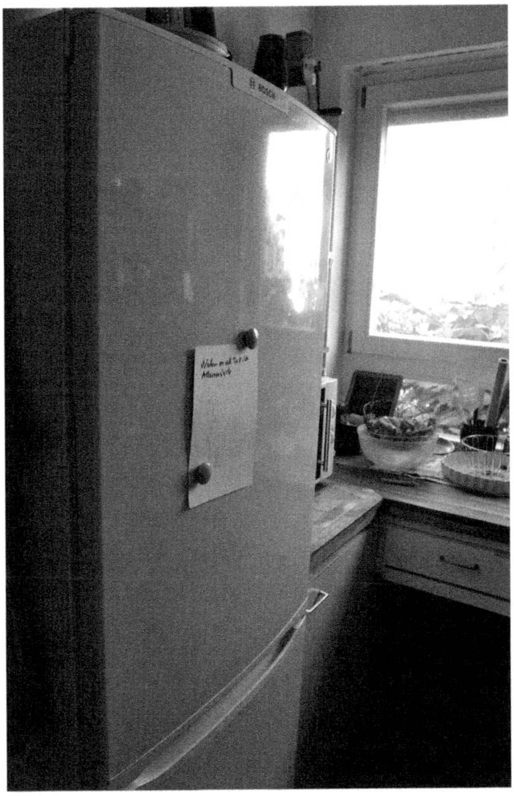

Abb. 14.60 Ein veränderter Gedanke wird an Kühlschrank geheftet, als Erinnerung an einen positiven Umgang mit sich selbst

sowie auf die Lebensqualität wird zunehmend durch Studien bestätigt (van der Heide et al. 2021 [Achtsamkeit]; McLean et al. 2017 [Mindfullness-based Stress Reduction]; Schlesinger et al. 2009 [geführte Entspannungsübungen]; Son und Choi 2018 [Meditationsgestützte komplexe Bewegungsübungen]; Arzu et al. 2012 [tiefe Atmung]).

Hier kann die Ergotherapeutin, basierend auf eigenen Fortbildungen und Erfahrungen, nach eigener Einschätzung auswählen, welche Entspannungsmethode angewandt werden kann. Das können z. B. sein:

- Feldenkrais,
- Progressive Muskelentspannung nach Jakobsen,
- Autogenes Training,
- Erholungspausen (Schlafen, Hinsetzen),
- Atemübungen,
- Achtsamkeitstraining.

Beispielhaft werden hier die letzten beiden Techniken vorgestellt.

▶ Atemübungen

Atemübungen bestechen durch ihre Einfachheit. Durch die tiefe Atmung wird der Parasympathikus stimuliert, der eine beruhigende Wirkung auf die Organe und das Stressempfinden hat.

Atemübung
Zeit: ca. 5 Minuten

Ort: ruhiger Ort, an dem keine Unterbrechung zu erwarten ist

Ausgangsposition: liegend oder aufrecht sitzend (wenn möglich ohne Anlehnen)

Augen: geschlossen oder auf den Boden blickend

Anleitung: Atmen Sie ein und aus, in Ihrem eigenen Rhythmus.

Die Luft fließt durch die Nase ein und durch den Mund wieder aus.

Beim Ausatmen achten Sie auf das Ende des Ausatmens. Drücken Sie den letzten Rest der Luft stetig hinaus, bis wirklich nichts mehr in den Lungen ist.

Dann fließt der Atem automatisch wieder über die Nase ein

und lange und stetig aus

und durch die Nase wieder ein.

Diesen Rhythmus führen Sie fort, in Ihrem eigenen Tempo.

(Die Übung kann kurz oder lang dauern. Die Therapeutin kann die Anleitung zwischendurch aussetzen oder weiterführen, wenn der Klient eine Erinnerung benötigt.)

Atemübung mit Visualisierung
Zeit: ca. 30 Sekunden

Ort: immer und überall einsetzbar (gerade in unruhigen, stressauslösenden Situationen unauffällig und schnell)

Ausgangsposition: alle möglich

Augen: geschlossen, oder auf den Boden blickend

Anleitung (in Therapie) oder Visualisierung (in Alltagssituation):

Beim Einatmen stellen Sie sich vor, Sie würden an einer Blume riechen.

Beim Ausatmen stellen Sie sich vor, Sie hätten eine Kerze vor sich und wollten die Flamme stetig zum Flackern bringen (nicht auspusten), (3–5 x wiederholen).

- Die Therapeutin kann Entspannungsübungen als Audiodatei auf das Smartphone des Klienten aufsprechen und abspeichern.

Achtsamkeitsübungen
Kabat Zinn entwickelte schon 1979 eine Methode, um Stress abzubauen. Die Methode heißt MBSR (mindfulness-based stress reduction). Hierzu werden Kurse angeboten, um die Umsetzung zu erlernen und zu üben. Es wird zwischen formellen Übungen (verschiedenen Meditationen) und Achtsamkeitsübungen im Alltag unterschieden. Regelmäßiges Meditieren senkt den Stresspegel und hat nachgewiesenermaßen positive Auswirkungen auf die Gesundheit (Schmerzen, Konzentration, Ängste …). Diese kurze Meditation kann zur Anregung dienen. Den Wortlaut kann die Therapeutin nach Bedarf verändern.

Achtsamkeitsübung für Parkinson-Betroffene
Setzen Sie sich bequem und entspannt hin. Lehnen Sie sich am besten nicht an, sondern sitzen Sie aufrecht. Die Füße stehen fest nebeneinander auf dem Boden. Legen Sie die Hände auf die Oberschenkel oder in den Schoß.

Nun schließen Sie die Augen oder suchen Sie einen Punkt auf dem Boden, an dem der Blick entspannt ruhen kann. Nehmen Sie sich einen Moment, um an diesem

Ort anzukommen. Wir machen jetzt zusammen eine Achtsamkeitsübung. Sie müssen dafür nichts tun, versuchen Sie einfach, im Moment zu sein und meinen Worten zu folgen.

Richten Sie Ihre Aufmerksamkeit auf Ihren Atem. Spüren Sie, wie er ein und wieder ausfließt. Nehmen Sie den ganzen Weg des Einatmens wahr. Wie die Luft die Nasenflügel streift, den Rachen hinunterfließt, die Lunge füllt und dann wieder den Weg nach draußen findet. Der Atem gleitet von selbst. Sie müssen nichts tun, einfach nur spüren.

An welchem Punkt im Körper spüren Sie den Atem am klarsten? An den Nasenflügeln? Im Brustkorb? Im Bauch oder Rücken? Verbinden Sie sich mit diesem Punkt einige Atemzüge lang. (*Pause*) Spüren Sie nun in Ihren Körper hinein! Welche Empfindungen nehmen Sie in den Muskeln, Knochen und Gelenken wahr? Nehmen Sie jeden Bereich des Körpers nach und nach wahr. Wo spüren Sie Entspannung? Wo spüren Sie Kraft und Stärke? Wo Ruhe oder Unruhe? Wo spüren Sie vielleicht nichts? Spüren Sie irgendwo etwas Unangenehmes? Schmerzen? Anspannung? Tremor? Wenn Sie einen solchen Punkt finden, nehmen Sie ihn ganz bewusst wahr. Und bewerten Sie nicht! Wie fühlt es sich an? Sehen Sie sich den Punkt mit dem inneren Auge von allen Seiten in Ruhe an. Und dann gehen Sie weiter im Körper. Gibt es noch weitere Punkte, die Probleme machen? Sehen Sie sie wieder von allen Seiten an, ohne zu bewerten. Einfach wahrnehmen. Und dann drehen Sie Ihre Aufmerksamkeit wieder weg.

Nun nehmen Sie den Körper als Ganzes wahr. Betrachten Sie ihn mit Neugierde und Bewunderung. Dieser Körper, der Ihnen manchmal Probleme und Sorgen bereitet – er leistet auch sehr viel. Das Zusammenspiel von Muskeln, Knochen, Gefühlen, Organen, Augen und vielem mehr. Ihr Körper verdient Wertschätzung und Achtung. Betrachten Sie Ihren Körper mit Wertschätzung! Vielleicht möchten Sie sich auch bei ihm bedanken. Lassen Sie die Augen geschlossen. Und nehmen nun Ihre Umgebung wahr. Welche Geräusche hören Sie? Spüren Sie die Luft an Ihrer Haut? Und die Kleidung? Nehmen Sie den Boden unter den Füßen wahr. Wie er Ihnen festen Untergrund bietet.

Nehmen Sie nun auch die anderen Personen im Raum wahr. Und langsam kommen Sie wieder ins Hier und Jetzt. Wenn Sie bereit sind, öffnen Sie langsam die Augen und strecken sich, so wie es sich gerade gut anfühlt.

Achtsamkeit im Alltag

Im Alltag kann Achtsamkeit dazu dienen, den Moment zu erleben und Dinge mit mehr Gelassenheit zu akzeptieren. Diese Fähigkeit ist für Menschen mit neurodegenerativen Erkrankungen sehr wertvoll. Durch die zunehmende Verschlechterung neigen Klienten häufig dazu, mit ihren Gedanken in der Vergangenheit („Vor einem Jahr konnte ich das noch.") oder der Zukunft („Hoffentlich muss ich nicht ins Heim.") zu verweilen. Den Moment bewusst wahrzunehmen – den winzigen Augenblick in seiner Fülle zu erleben –, ist eine Bereicherung für jeden Menschen, für einen Parkinson-Erkrankten kann es jedoch wie eine Befreiung sein. Achtsamkeitsübungen im Alltag können in der Ergotherapie in vielen Settings eingesetzt werden, z. B.:

- **Trainingspausen**: Während der therapeutischen Intervention kann eine Achtsamkeitsübung den Fokus wiederherstellen oder in angespannten Momenten die Situationen entschärfen.
- **Eigenübung**: Die kleinen Übungen eignen sich optimal als Eigenübungen für zu Hause.
- **Körperwahrnehmung**: Durch die Zentrierung wird auch der Körper bewusst wahrgenommen.

- **Selbstmanagement**: Zur Unterstützung des Selbstmanagements ist die Achtsamkeit eine hilfreiche Unterstützung. Durch die Wahrnehmung der eigenen Bedürfnisse, Gefühle und Gedanken können Ziele treffender formuliert und Problemlösungsstrategien entwickelt werden.
- **Angehörige**: Durch die hohe Belastung, der Angehörige meist ausgesetzt sind, erleben sie häufig einen ständigen Stresszustand. Betrachtet die Therapeutin die Angehörigen als erweiterten Klienten, kann eine Anleitung von Achtsamkeitsübungen mit dem Ziel der Gesundheitserhaltung ein wichtiger Teil der Intervention sein.

Achtsamkeitsübung Körperwahrnehmung

Anleitung: Besprechen Sie mit Ihrer Therapeutin, in welchen Situationen es wichtig ist, gut auf Ihren Körper zu hören. Das können z. B. Momente sein, in denen Ihre Symptome, wie Tremor oder Unbeweglichkeit, verstärkt auftreten. Wann immer Sie eine solche Situation erleben, wenden Sie folgende Achtsamkeitsübung an: Halten Sie kurz inne. Spüren Sie genau nach, was in Ihrem Körper passiert. Gehen Sie gedanklich ihren Körper durch. Fangen Sie bei Ihren Füßen an und wandern langsam nach oben. Wenn Sie etwas spüren, nehmen Sie es wahr, aber bewerten Sie es nicht. Einfach mit dem inneren Auge ansehen, dann gedanklich weiter im Körper nach oben wandern. Wenn Sie am Scheitel angekommen sind, lenken Sie die Aufmerksamkeit auf Ihre Atmung. Ein paar Atemzüge lang.

Achtsamkeitsübung im Moment

Anleitung: Manchmal kann es passieren, dass sich im Alltag mit Terminen, Einschränkungen und Sorgen die Gedanken vor allem um Ereignisse in der Vergangenheit und der Zukunft drehen. Das löst ein Gefühl von Stress und innerer Unruhe aus. Nehmen Sie sich vor, im täglichen Leben häufiger im Moment zu leben. Kehren Sie Ihre Aufmerksamkeit zunächst nach innen. Spüren Sie den Atem ein- und ausströmen, nehmen Sie ihren Körper, so wie er gerade ist, wahr. Dann richten Sie alle Sinne nach außen. Was können Sie hören? Was spüren Sie? Gibt es Gerüche? Und was sehen Sie? Reagieren Sie nicht. Kommen Sie von einem Zustand des „Tuns“ in einen Zustand des „Seins“.

Achtsamkeitsübung in Stressmomenten

Anleitung: In Momenten, in denen Ihnen alles zu viel wird und Sie spüren, wie der Stress aufsteigt, nehmen Sie sich ein paar Augenblicke Zeit. Atmen Sie ruhig ein und aus und spüren Sie Ihren Atem. Dann richten Sie Ihre Aufmerksamkeit auf Ihren Körper. Wo spüren Sie den Stress? Im Kopf, im Nacken, im Gesicht oder ziehen Sie die Schultern vielleicht hoch? Spüren Sie genau nach, wie es sich anfühlt. Dann atmen Sie nochmals drei Mal bewusst ein und aus.

14.10.5 Krankheitsverarbeitung

Menschen, die an M. Parkinson erkranken, erfahren eine mehr oder weniger starke Belastung. Wie stark diese erlebt wird, hängt wesentlich mit der Krankheitsverarbeitung (**Coping**) zusammen. Diese Fähigkeit, die Krankheit nicht als dominierend wahrzunehmen, sondern selbstwirksam agieren und entscheiden zu können, ist bei jedem Klienten unterschiedlich ausgeprägt. Auch durchläuft jeder Klient im Laufe der Jahre selbstverständlich unterschiedliche Phasen des Copings, weshalb eine Auseinandersetzung damit immer wieder indiziert sein kann. Für eine gelingende Krankheitsverarbeitung können bestimmte Faktoren förderlich sein, jedoch gibt es nicht den einen Weg, sondern es muss ein individuell passender Umgang gefunden werden.

Analyse

Zunächst sollte zusammen mit dem Klienten herausgefunden werden, in welchen Situationen er sich als selbstwirksam, und wann er sich als machtlos erlebt. Die Krankheitsverarbeitung wird von drei Ebenen beeinflusst: den Einstellungen, Gefühlen und dem Verhalten. Diese drei Bereiche beeinflussen sich wiederrum gegenseitig (siehe Abb. 14.61).

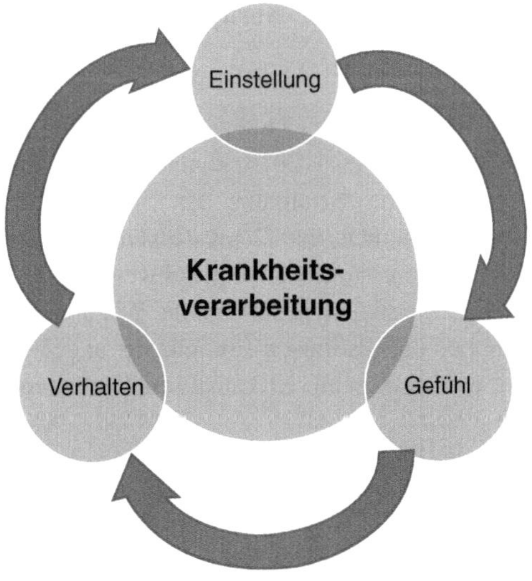

Abb. 14.61 Coping oder Krankheitsverarbeitung werden von drei Ebenen beeinflusst

Mithilfe der Abbildung kann der Klient seine Krankheitsverarbeitung reflektieren. Der Klient macht sich Gedanken darüber, wie er sich in bestimmten Situationen verhält, welche grundsätzliche Einstellung dahintersteckt und wie das subjektive Gefühl dabei ist. Z. B. in der Situation: „Einladung zum Ausflug des Turnvereins."

- **Einstellung**: „Da kann ich sowieso nicht mithalten."
- **Gefühl**: „Scham vor alten Sportfreunden."
- **Verhalten**: Absage.

Veränderung

Sobald der Zusammenhang von Einstellung zur Krankheit, Gefühl und Verhalten analysiert wurde, kann eine Veränderung begonnen werden. Dazu setzt der Klient an einem der drei Ebenen an und verändert diese bewusst.

Beispiel:

- **Ansatz an Einstellung**: „Ich mache mit, so gut es geht."
- **Ansatz an Gefühl**: „Ich freue mich, meine alten Sportfreunde nach langer Zeit wieder zu treffen."
- **Ansatz an Verhalten**: Klient kommuniziert vorher mit dem Organisator, dass eine Teilnahme erfolgt und fragt an, wie weit die Laufstrecke sein wird. Dann entscheidet er, ob er nur am Kaffeetrinken oder auch an der Wanderung teilnehmen wird. Dadurch entsteht eine positive Dynamik.

Ansprüche senken

Ein wiederkehrendes Thema in der Ergotherapie ist der Umgang der Klienten mit den Ansprüchen an sich selbst. Obwohl den Klienten bewusst ist, dass sie eine schwere und progrediente Krankheit haben, gelingt es ihnen oftmals nicht, sich zuzugestehen, Pausen zu machen, schwere Arbeiten zu delegieren und generell ihren Perfektionismus abzulegen. Dadurch entstehen jedoch ein konstanter Stress und das Gefühl, „nicht gut genug" zu sein. In dem Prozess des Akzeptierens der Parkinson-Erkrankung und der abnehmenden Leistungsfähigkeit sind Ergotherapeutinnen wertvolle Begleiterinnen. Mit empathischer Unterstützung sollte die Therapeutin den Klienten dazu anregen, wohlwollend seine Betätigungen zu reflektieren und in Anbetracht der aktuellen Möglichkeiten mit zustimmendem Blick das Ergebnis zu betrachten. Durch die reduzierte Eigenwahrnehmung der Menschen mit M. Parkinson kann das für sie ein wahres „Aha"-Erlebnis sein und mit großer Dankbarkeit angenommen werden.

14.10.6 Soziale Interaktion

Menschen, die sozial gut eingebunden sind, erleben wesentlich seltener depressive Verstimmungen und Ängste und können sich schneller daraus befreien, wenn sie niedergeschlagen sind. Ein stabiles soziales Netzwerk ist also eine ideale Unterstützung für Menschen mit progredienten Krankheiten wie dem M. Parkinson. Je nach Situation des Klienten ist es sinnvoll, die sozialen Kontakte zu erhalten, wiederzubeleben oder neue zu suchen.

Ist der Klient sozial eingebunden, gilt es im Rahmen der Therapie die Bedeutung von sozialen Interaktionen hervorzuheben und zu erhalten. Außerdem sind familiäre Kontakte äußerst wertvoll und sollten gefördert werden. Folgende Maßnahmen zur Förderung der sozialen Kontakte können in der Ergotherapie Anwendung finden:

- Briefe, E-Mails, Grußkarten etc. an Bekannte, Freunde und Familie schreiben
- Über moderne Medien Videotelefonie nutzen (siehe Abb. 14.62
- Geburtstage und andere Festtage zur Kontaktaufnahme nutzen (Geburtstagskalender anlegen, Karten gestalten …)
- Konkrete Planung der Teilnahme an Feiern und Ausflügen (Kleidung, Geschenk, Transport, Rückzugsmöglichkeit, Berücksichtigung spezieller Bedürfnisse wie ruhiger Raum oder Medikamenteneinnahme)
- Feste Einplanung in Wochenplanung, z. B. Gymnastikgruppe oder Frauenkreis in Kalender eintragen
- Planung von Einladung der Freunde, Enkel, Nachbarn …

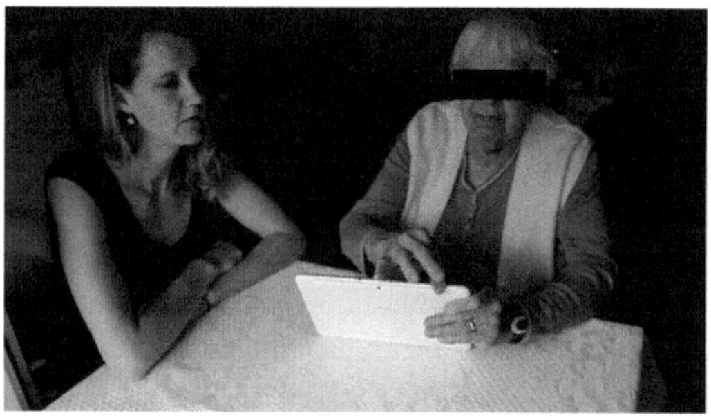

Abb. 14.62 Anbahnung oder Wiederaufnahme von sozialer Interaktion ist bei Menschen mit depressiver Symptomatik eine wertvolle ergotherapeutische Tätigkeit, z. B. über Videotelefon

- Anregung und Initiierung von neuen Kontakten über Selbsthilfegruppen, Seniorengruppen, Sitzgymnastik, Singkreis, Gehirnjogging, Frühstückstreff, kirchliche oder andere Gruppenangebote.

Bei der Planung von sozialen Interaktionen sollte die Therapeutin sich auf die individuellen Wünsche des Klienten einstellen. Wann, wie oft, wie und mit wem sich Klienten in soziale Situationen begeben, ist eine sehr persönliche Entscheidung und kann von außen nicht bestimmt werden.

14.10.7 Weitere Therapieansätze

Sport

In mehreren Studien (Kwok et al. 2019; Wu et al. 2017; Reynolds et al. 2016) konnte belegt werden, dass sportliche Betätigung ein Schlüsselfaktor beim Management von Depressionen ist, und bei leichten Depressionen sogar gleichwertig wirksam wie eine Medikamenteneinnahme. Welche Sportarten bei der Parkinson-Erkrankung angebracht sind, wird in Abschn. 10.3 ausführlich erläutert.

Tagesstrukturierung

Mit der Depression gehen oftmals Antriebsstörungen einher. Die Klienten stehen morgens spät auf, übernehmen wenig Eigeninitiative bei der Tagesgestaltung und die Hürde, aktiv zu werden, ist sehr hoch. Dagegen hilft häufig eine klare Tagesstruktur.

Dazu setzt man sich mit dem Klienten und, wenn vorhanden, zusammenlebenden Angehörigen zusammen und füllt den Wochenplan gemeinsam aus, der im Anhang zu finden ist. Dabei wird die für den Klienten ideale Balance zwischen Aktivität und Entspannung, Pflichten und Erholung gesucht. Einen ausgeglichenen Wochenplan zu erstellen bedarf mehrerer Versuche über ein paar Wochen hinweg, in denen immer wieder etwas angepasst wird. Die Therapeutin kann von Beginn an mehrere Kopien des leeren Wochenplans machen, um diesem Umstand gerecht zu werden.

Eine andere Einsatzweise ist, dass Klient und Angehörige wöchentlich ihre Woche gemeinsam planen. Dies kann ein stabilisierendes Ritual sein, bei dem Stress und Überlastung vorgebeugt und in einem klaren Rahmen dafür gesorgt wird, dass z. B. Sport und soziale Interaktionen eingeplant werden.

Beispiel

Mitten in der innerlichen Schimpftirade fällt ihm sein Positivspruch ein: „Du bist, wie du bist. Und so bist du gut!" Es erinnert ihn an seine guten Freunde, die ihn akzeptieren, auch mit seinen Macken. Er setzt sich hin und atmet durch. Dieses Vorgehen hat er nun verinnerlicht. Atmen und auf den Atem achten. Langsam entspannt er sich. „Die Spritze ist weg," denkt er. „Sie wird schon wieder auftauchen. Und ich habe ja noch Ersatzspritzen." ◀

14.11 Fatigue

Beispiel

Schon morgens beim Aufstehen fühlt sich Herr G. unglaublich ausgelaugt. Es kostet ihn Überwindung aufzustehen: Am liebsten würde er einfach im Bett bleiben. Aber heute hat er so viel zu tun. Die Kinder kommen zu Besuch. Er will aufräumen, einkaufen, kochen und der Hund muss vorher natürlich noch raus. Doch nach dem Frühstück merkt er – es geht wirklich nicht. Sein Körper ist schwer, der Kopf fühlt sich an wie leergefegt und die Augen wollen sich schließen. So kann er seine Kinder nicht empfangen. ◀

14.11.1 Symptombeschreibung

Definition Fatigue, oder auch **Erschöpfungssyndrom**, ist eine überwältigende körperliche, geistige oder psychische Erschöpfung, die sich negativ auf die Alltagsfähigkeit und Lebensqualität auswirkt und sich durch Schlaf oder Erholung nicht wesentlich bessert.

Ätiologie Die Ursache für Fatigue bei M. Parkinson ist ungeklärt. Man geht von einer Kombination von diversen pathophysiologischen Einflussfaktoren aus.

Prävalenz Ca. 50 % der Menschen mit M. Parkinson haben Fatigue, wobei die Angaben in verschiedenen Studien stark divergieren, da es an einer einheitlichen Untersuchungsmethode mangelt und teilweise Überschneidungen mit anderen Krankheitszeichen (Apathie, Depression, Tagesschläfrigkeit) bestehen.

Klinik Patientinnen mit Fatigue-Syndrom erleben eine erdrückende Erschöpfung und haben keine Energie, um aktiv zu werden. Die Erschöpfung kann körperlicher, psychischer oder kognitiver Natur sein oder eine Kombination der drei. Dabei tritt die Fatigue, abgrenzend von der exzessiven Tagesschläfrigkeit, nicht zu einer bestimmten Tageszeit auf und ist auch nicht mit vorangegangener körperlicher oder geistiger Verausgabung verbunden. Vielmehr kann die Fatigue immer auftreten, auch schon morgens nach dem Aufstehen. In manchen Fällen kann eine Verbindung zu einer depressiven Verstimmung bestehen.

Folgen/Komplikationen Fatigue beeinflusst die Lebensqualität negativ und die Selbständigkeit bei Alltagsbetätigungen ist herabgesetzt. Auch für die Beziehung mit Angehörigen ist die Fatigue eine Belastung, da wesentlich mehr von diesen übernommen werden muss, obwohl die körperliche Einschränkung evtl. nicht allzu ausgeprägt ist. Durch Unkenntnis über das Krankheitsbild der Fatigue entstehen so Missverständnisse und das Gefühl, ausgenutzt zu werden.

Medizinische Möglichkeiten:

- Medikamente
- Sportliche Aktivität
- Energiemanagement

Da die Fatigue von betroffenen Klientinnen als stark einschränkend wahrgenommen wird und gleichzeitig Medikamente selten zufriedenstellende Wirkung zeigen, ist ein gezieltes Energiemanagement, in Kombination mit aktiver Bewegung, eine interessante therapeutische Intervention.

14.11.2 Körperliche Aktivität

Der natürliche Impuls bei Fatigue ist oftmals, sich zu schonen, um die Energiereserven nicht aufzubrauchen. Die Effektivität von Bewegungstherapie zur Verbesserung von Fatigue bei Multipler Sklerose ist eindeutig nachgewiesen. Die Studienlage bei M. Parkinson ist noch uneindeutig, zeigt jedoch auch Daten, die zu einer Empfehlung von Bewegungstherapie zur Verbesserung von Fatigue führen (Henning et al. 2017). Mit dem Wissen, dass sich physische Aktivität förderlich auf die gesamte Gehirngesundheit auswirkt, scheint eine Empfehlung zur körperlichen Aktivität bei Fatigue alternativlos, da der Auslöser des Fatigue-Syndroms auf eine Dysbalance im Gehirn zurückzuführen ist.

Intensität und Länge des Trainings sollte individuell angepasst werden. Die Klientin sollte durch Selbstbeobachtung und Reflexion ihr Körpergefühl verbessern, sodass sie selbst erkennt, welche Art des Trainings förderlich ist, und sowohl Intensität als auch Häufigkeit des Trainings auf ihre Bedürfnisse adaptieren kann. Im Allgemeinen sind kurze intensive Trainingsintervalle besser als ein langes Training. Mehr dazu in Abschn. 10.3 allgemeines Kraft- und Ausdauertraining.

14.11.3 Energiemanagement

Der zweite wichtige Aspekt bei der Behandlung von Fatigue ist das Energiemanagement. Dabei lernen Betroffene mit den reduzierten Energiereserven umzugehen und zu haushalten. Packer et al. (1995) und Signer und Weise (2020) entwickelten und untersuchten Gruppenprogramme für Menschen mit Fatigue und Multipler Sklerose. Es ist gut belegt, dass sich Gruppenkonzepte förderlich auf Lebensqualität und Wohlbefinden auswirken sowie die negativen Auswirkungen von Fatigue auf den Alltag der Teilnehmerinnen reduzieren. In der Gruppe entsteht eine unterstützende Dynamik, durch die sich die Teilnehmerinnen verstanden und gestärkt fühlen. Für deren Implementierung wird zu einer entsprechenden Fortbildung geraten. Es wird zurzeit eine erkrankungsunabhängige Version der Energiemanagementmethode entwickelt.

Energieprofil
Um einen Perspektivwechsel anzuregen und den Blick auf Handlungsmöglichkeiten zu richten, wird der Fokus nicht mehr auf die Fatigue (Defizit), sondern auf die zur Verfügung stehende Energie (Ressource) gerichtet. Dafür wird das Bild eines „Energiekontos" verwendet (siehe Abb. 14.63).

Jeder Mensch hat morgens ein gewisses Level an Energie auf seinem Konto. Durch bestimmte Betätigungen nimmt die Energie ab, durch andere kann das Konto wieder aufgefüllt werden. Die bewusste Wahrnehmung des Energielevels und absichtsvolle Entscheidung dafür oder dagegen, die Energie auszugeben oder zu sparen, kann einen ausgeglichenen und erfüllten Alltag ermöglichen.

Achtsamkeit
Den meisten Menschen ist nicht bewusst, welche Betätigungen wie viel Energie kosten oder wieder aufladen. Diese Wahrnehmung ist die Voraus-

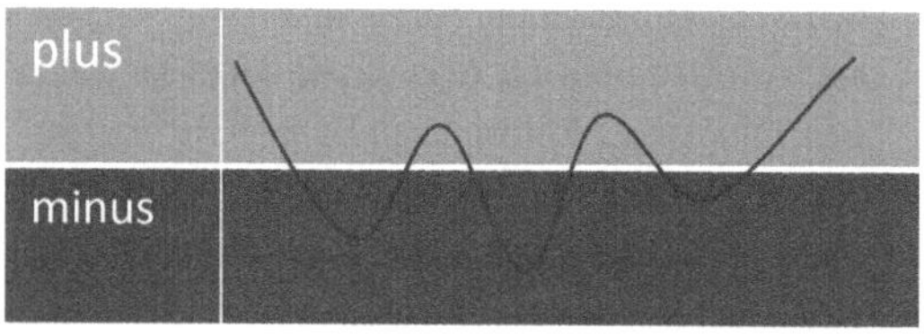

Abb. 14.63 Energiekonto. Visualisierung der vorhandenen Energiereserven über den Tag verteilt. (In Anlehnung an Hersche et al. 2017)

setzung für ein gutes Energiemanagement. Dafür sollte zunächst ein Achtsamkeitstraining (siehe Abschn. 14.10.4) durchgeführt werden, um zu erspüren, in welcher Körperregion die Energie und der Mangel an Energie wahrgenommen werden und wie genau es sich anfühlt. Durch die feinere Wahrnehmung kann die Klientin auch im Alltag besser spüren, ob eine Betätigung ihre Energiereserven aufstockt oder abträgt.

Tagebuch
Außerdem kann Tagebuch geführt werden. Mithilfe eines Tagesprotokolls wird in Bezug auf die Uhrzeit und durchgeführten Betätigungen das Energielevel eingetragen. So kann z. B. über eine Woche hinweg beobachtet werden, wie sich die zur Verfügung stehende Energie verändert. Dazu kann das Parkinson-Tagebuch (siehe Anhang) verwendet werden. So können Energiegeber und Energiefresser identifiziert und bei Bedarf auch eine Veränderung über die Therapiedauer hinweg erfasst werden.

Prioritäten
Anschließend erstellt die Klientin ihre individuelle Prioritätenliste. Dort werden alle Betätigungen aufgelistet, die im Alltag durchgeführt werden und nach persönlicher Wichtigkeit geordnet. Menschen mit Fatigue erledigen unbewusst erst alles, was getan werden „muss“, z. B. Haushalt, Arbeit und Kinderversorgung. Angenehme Betätigungen, soziale Kontakte und Hobbies werden häufig vernachlässigt, da dafür keine Energie mehr übrig ist. Durch die Priorisierung kann diese Tatsache reflektiert werden.

Pausenmanagement
Häufig nutzen Menschen mit Fatigue die energievollen Zeiten, um größere Projekte umzusetzen oder schwere körperliche Aktivitäten zu verrichten. Dabei kann es dazu kommen, dass die Energiereserven komplett aufgebraucht werden und die Klientin einen Zusammenbruch erlebt. Deswegen ist vorausschauendes Einplanen von Pausen und Ruhephasen unabdingbar. Die Klientin soll lernen einzuschätzen, wann welche Art von Pause (Schlaf, hinsetzen, hinlegen) angebracht ist und große Projekte in kleine Schritte aufzuteilen.

Betätigungsplan
Mit einer vorsichtigen Planung des Tages und der Woche, unter Berücksichtigung der o. g. Faktoren, erreicht die Klientin ein ausgewogenes Energiemanagement. Dies mag der Betroffenen zunächst ungewohnt oder unnötig erscheinen, bei einer konsequenten Umsetzung lernt sie jedoch eine Menge über sich selbst und es wird einer Überlastung vorgebeugt. Dazu kann der Wochenplan (siehe Anhang) hilfreich sein. Schon beim Ausfüllen erkennt man, an welchen Tagen eine Überlastung droht oder wo keine ausreichende Ruhezeit eingeplant ist, und kann dies anpassen. Mit der Zeit lernt die Klientin durch das Vorausplanen, eigenverantwortlich mit ihrer Energie zu haushalten und für ihre Bedürfnisse einzustehen.

14.11.4 Strategien und Hilfsmittel

Durch Veränderung von Arbeitsabläufen und Einsatz von Hilfsmitteln oder Technologien kann die körperliche Belastung im Alltag deutlich reduziert werden, sodass mehr Energie für andere Tätigkeiten zur Verfügung steht. Es ist hilfreich, die täglichen Arbeitsabläufe im Haushalt oder bei der Arbeit bewusst zu überdenken. Der Ergotherapeut erfasst anhand einer Betätigungsanalyse, von Fotos der Arbeitsumgebung und Berichten der Klientin den Ist-Zustand. In Zusammenarbeit mit der Klientin werden anschließend mögliche Vereinfachung der Arbeitsabläufe, Entlastungen durch Strategien und einsetzbare Hilfsmittel besprochen.

Der Ergotherapeut H. Lorenzen empfiehlt (2010) dafür „Aktivitätsinseln“ einzurichten. Dabei wird ein umgrenzter Arbeitsplatz (wie Werkstatt, Waschküche) identifiziert und in a) festgelegte Strukturen (z. B. bauliche Strukturen, große Möbel) und b) flexible Strukturen (z. B. Anordnung von Gegenständen auf der Arbeitsfläche, Beleuchtung) unterteilt. Anschließend werden die festgelegten und flexiblen Strukturen analysiert, um festzustellen, welche sich ungünstig auf das Fatigue-Management auswirken und ob und wie Anpassungen möglich sind. Durch Experimentieren mit verschiedenen Möglichkeiten entsteht die ideale Arbeitsumgebung – die Aktivitätsinsel.

Jede Arbeitssituation ist individuell zu beurteilen und entsprechend anzupassen, hier einige Vorschläge für **Arbeitserleichterungen**:

- Sitzgelegenheiten schaffen
- Wege verkürzen oder effizienter organisieren (z. B. Geschirr, Besteck und Co. in Nähe des Esstisches)
- Häufig benötigte Gegenstände in Reichweite
- Übersichtliche Organisation
- Aufgaben an Familienmitglieder delegieren
- Haushaltshilfe

Hilfsmittel

- Stehhilfe
- Saug-/Mähroboter (s. Abb. 14.64)
- Servierwagen
- Hilfsmittel zur Erleichterung des Öffnens von Deckeln
- Digitale Steuerung (z. B. über Smartphone) von Licht, Radio, Heizung, Rollläden, ...
- Einkaufstrolley
- Elektromobil
- E-Fahrrad
- Spracherkennung statt Tippen

Weitere Hilfsmittel werden in Abschn. 15.3 vorgestellt.

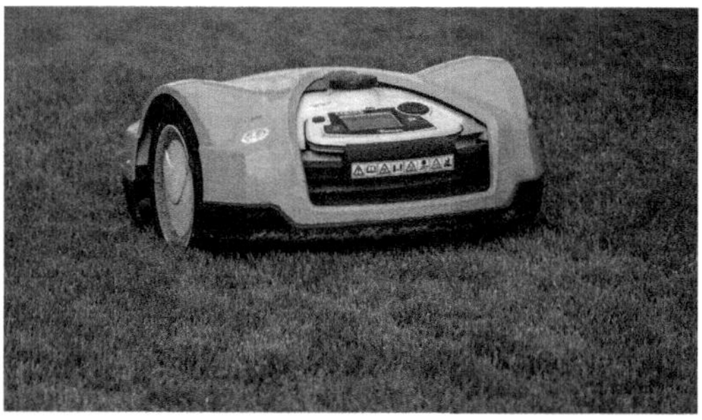

Abb. 14.64 Ein Mähroboter und andere technische Hilfsmittel können Menschen mit Fatigue entlasten und die Energiereserven auffüllen

14.11.5 Kommunikation

Da Fatigue von außen nicht sichtbar ist, erkennen Außenstehende oftmals nicht, dass die Betroffene darunter leidet. Dazu ist das Krankheitsbild recht unbekannt, was dazu führen kann, dass die Energielosigkeit als Faulheit oder Unlust interpretiert wird. Aus diesem Grund ist eine offene Kommunikation über das bei M. Parkinson häufig auftretende Symptom wichtig. Je nach Beziehung zum Gegenüber können folgende Punkte hilfreich sein:

- Fatigue – ein häufig auftretendes Symptom bei M. Parkinson
- Beschreibung – wie fühlt sich Fatigue an?
- Auswirkungen auf den Alltag
- Hilfreiche Unterstützung, Entlastungsmöglichkeiten

Mit nahen Angehörigen und Lebenspartner sollten konkrete Absprachen getroffen werden.

- Aufgabenverteilung, z. B. Wäsche waschen, aufhängen und abnehmen sowie falten übernimmt Klientin, vollen Wäschekorb die Treppe hoch tragen übernimmt Partner.
- Klare Kommunikation bei unerwartet auftretender Fatigue, z. B. „Es würde über mein Limit gehen, jetzt Autozufahren. Lass uns lieber eine Pause machen."
- Feste Ruhezeiten einhalten.
- Klare Grenzen besprechen, z. B. nur eine Aktivität am Tag.

14.11.6 Innere Einstellung (Ansprüche senken)

Schafft die Klientin es, obige Punkte umzusetzen, wird sie feststellen, dass sich die Fatigue positiv beeinflussen lässt. Diese Erfahrung führt dazu, dass sich die innere Haltung ändert. Die in westlichen Kulturen typische Einstellung, dass maximaler Aufwand zu maximalen Ergebnissen führt, kann kritisch hinterfragt werden. Durch vorsichtiges Abwägen, Priorisierung und Senkung der Ansprüche an sich selbst kann auch mit Fatigue eine hohe Lebensqualität erreicht werden. Die eigene Akzeptanz der Umstände, wie sie sind, führt zu Entspannung und innerer Zufriedenheit. Dies ist ein Prozess, der in der Ergotherapie angestoßen und begleitet werden kann, wenn die Klientin dafür offen ist. Sicherlich ist es in der komplexen Situation der Klientin jedoch auch verständlich, wenn sie mit ihrem Zustand hadert und ihn nicht ohne weiteres annimmt. Auch dies sollte vom Therapeuten empathisch begleitet werden.

Beispiel

Zuerst geht er mit dem Hund eine kleine Runde spazieren. Durch reflektiertes Energiemanagement weiß er, dass ihm dies wieder neue Energie gibt. Bewegung an der frischen Luft mit seinem lebhaften Hund tut ihm immer gut. Dann ruft er seinen Sohn an und erklärt ihm: „Ich habe in der Ergotherapie über meine Dauermüdigkeit gesprochen und gelernt, meine Ansprüche herunterzuschrauben, Hilfe einzufordern und eine Prioritätenliste zu machen. Meine Prioritätenliste für heute sieht so aus:

- Kinder sehen,
- mit Hund raus,
- ordentliche Wohnung,
- selber kochen.

Die Fatigue hat mich leider heute wieder überkommen, aber ich möchte unbedingt euch Kinder sehen." Der Sohn schlägt vor, beim thailändischen Restaurant Essen zu bestellen. Damit fallen das Einkaufen und Kochen weg. Nun macht sich Herr G. ans Aufräumen. Er konzentriert sich auf das Wohnzimmer und die Gästetoilette und macht alle zehn Minuten eine kurze Verschnaufpause. Eine halbe Stunde bevor die Gäste kommen, legt er sich zu einem Nickerchen hin. Jetzt ist er bereit. ◀

14.12 Apathie

Beispiel

Frau F. erkennt ihren Mann kaum wieder. Er sitzt schon seit zwei Stunden im selben Sessel. Er tut nichts, einfach nur sitzen. Sein Mobiltelefon liegt ungenutzt neben der ungelesenen Tageszeitung, daneben ein unberührtes Glas Wasser. „Wollen wir heute etwas zusammen unternehmen?" fragt sie ihn. „Ja," antwortet er. „Worauf hast du Lust?" möchte Frau F. wissen. „Eis essen? Oder wir gehen zum See, Enten füttern? Oder wir fragen Gabi und Klaus, ob sie sich im Café Villa mit uns treffen!" Herr F. hebt die Schultern: „Was du möchtest." Frau F. wird ungeduldig: „Was ist nur mir dir los? Früher warst du doch an allem interessiert. Die Politik war dir wichtig und der Umweltschutz. Du hast immer deine Freunde angerufen und Nachrichten geschrieben. Und du saßt nie länger als 15 Minuten, dann warst du schon wieder aktiv. Und jetzt? Dir ist alles egal. Ich vermisse deine Lebenslust." Ihr Mann sieht sie nachdenklich an: „Ja, ich weiß auch nicht warum." ◀

14.12.1 Symptombeschreibung

Definition Apathie ist die Abnahme der Initiierung von zielgerichtetem Verhalten aufgrund von abgeflachten Gefühlen, reduziertem Interesse und herabgesetzter emotionaler Reaktivität und Motivation (s. Abb. 14.65).

Ätiologie Das Zusammenwirken unterschiedlicher, hoch komplexer pathophysiologischer Prozesse im Gehirn führt zur Apathie. Dabei scheint überwiegend der Dopaminmangel im dopaminergen mesocorticolimbischen System auslösend zu sein. Das mesolimbische System wird auch als positives Belohnungszentrum bezeichnet, da bestimmtes Verhalten Glücksgefühle auslöst und so auch das Lernen positiv verstärkt. Im Rückschluss ist klar: Entfällt dieser positive Kreislauf,

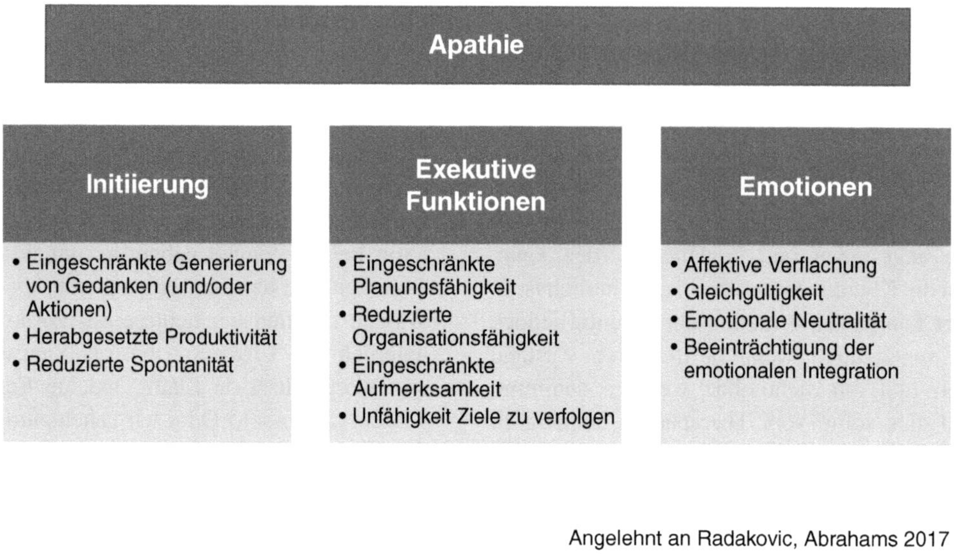

Abb. 14.65 Apathie wirkt sich auf drei Bereiche aus. (Angelehnt an Radakovic und Abrahams 2018)

nimmt die Motivation ab, aktiv zu werden – der Mensch bleibt passiv, apathisch.

Prävalenz Apathie tritt bei etwa 40 % der Menschen mit M. Parkinson auf. Apathie korreliert nicht mit der Erkrankungsschwere. Es gibt häufig einen Zusammenhang mit depressiven und demenziellen Symptomen.

Klinik Das Symptom der Apathie ist häufig bei Menschen mit der Parkinson-Erkrankung zu beobachten und nicht immer von anderen Symptomen klar abgrenzbar, vor allem, weil es oft in Kombination mit weiteren nicht-motorischen Symptomen, wie Depressionen und Demenz, auftritt. Apathie wirkt sich auf drei Bereiche aus: **Initiierung, exekutive Funktionen, Emotionen**. Klienten mit Apathie können teilweise über Stunden ohne Beschäftigung oder Aktivität sitzen, sie zeigen kein Interesse an der Umgebung oder daran, aus **Eigeninitiative** etwas zu beginnen. Die Fähigkeit Ziele zu fassen oder etwas zu planen ist eingeschränkt (**exekutive Funktionen**). Dabei wirken sie nicht niedergeschlagen oder unzufrieden, und auch auf Nachfrage äußern sie kein Bedauern über die Inaktivität, sondern zeigen sich oft gefühlsarm oder neutral (**emotionale Abflachung**). Bei der Nachfrage nach Befinden, Wünschen oder Zielen fällt es Menschen mit Apathie oft schwer, Gedanken zu formulieren, was im therapeutischen Zielfindungsprozess eine große Hürde sein kann. Typische Sätze sind: „Ich bin zufrieden.", „Soll mir recht sein." und „Es ist mir gleich, was wir heute machen.".

Folgen/Komplikationen Die Betroffenen selbst leiden unter dem Symptom der Apathie kaum, den Angehörigen jedoch fällt der Umgang mit der Passivität meist sehr schwer. Es kommt zu Konflikten und Unverständnis („Du könntest doch, wenn du wolltest."). Klienten mit Apathie bewegen sich wesentlich seltener und kürzer als andere Menschen mit M. Parkinson. Dadurch verschlechtert sich der Allgemeinzustand häufig und es können Sekundärschäden wie verkürzte Strukturen, Verschlechterung der posturalen Stabilität und damit eine erhöhte Sturzgefahr, Verschlimmerung der Verdauungsprobleme, Abnahme von sozialen Kontakten und Abbau der kognitiven Fähigkeiten entstehen.

Medizinische Möglichkeiten

- Medikamente

14.12.2 Angehörigenarbeit

In vielen Fällen kann es schwer sein, bei einer festgestellten Apathie einen therapeutischen Ansatz zu finden, da die Mehrzahl der Klienten nur einen geringen Leidensdruck hat und selten als eigenes Ziel „wieder aktiv sein“ oder die Aufnahme eines Hobbies nennt. Teil der Apathie ist eine gewisse Akzeptanz oder Gleichgültigkeit in der Situation, sodass für eine Therapeutin, die klientenzentriert arbeitet, kein Handlungsbedarf besteht. Expandiert man jedoch den Blick und betrachtet die Angehörigen als erweiterte Klienten, kann meist ein Konfliktfeld erkannt werden, aus dem eine klare Zielformulierung entstehen kann, z. B. „vermehrte Mithilfe beim Anziehen“, „Wahrnehmen von gemeinsamen Interessen“ oder „Verbesserung der Kommunikation in der Beziehung“.

Aufklärung von Angehörigen
Bei Konfliktsituationen mit Angehörigen kann die Aufklärung über den Zusammenhang der Apathie mit dem Krankheitsbild des M. Parkinson förderlich sein. Mit dem Wissen, dass Apathie häufig Teil des Symptomkomplexes ist, und der Betroffene sich nicht absichtlich „stur stellt“ oder lustlos ist, kann bei den Angehörigen ein Verständnis für das Verhalten und damit eine wohlwollende Akzeptanz eintreten. Dazu können Artikel über das Thema, Erfahrungen anderer Betroffener oder Angehörige in Selbsthilfegruppen oder Onlineforen und die persönliche Darstellung der Therapeutin dienen.

14.12.3 Aktivierung

Der Begriff „Aktivierung“ ist kritisch zu betrachten, da die Klienten meist nicht „aktiviert“ werden möchten, sondern mit der Passivität zufrieden sind. Das Interessante ist, dass die Klienten oftmals genauso zufrieden sind, wenn sie zu Aktivitäten mitgenommen werden, obwohl die Initiative nicht von ihnen ausgegangen ist. Mit dem Wissen, dass sich „aktiv sein“ positiv auf das Allgemeinbefinden und zahlreiche Symptome auswirkt, kann eine Aufforderung zur Teilnahme an Unternehmungen ohne die ausdrückliche Zustimmung des Klienten gerechtfertigt sein. Sperrt sich der Klient während der Aktivität oder äußert sich danach negativ, sollte im Gespräch eine Alternative gesucht werden. Beispiele können sein:

- Ehefrau nimmt ihren Mann mit zum Gottesdienst/Selbsthilfegruppe/Theater.
- Klient wird zur Gymnastikgruppe gebracht.
- Gäste werden zum Essen eingeladen.
- Der Bruder nimmt den Betroffenen mittwochs zu einem Einkaufsbummel mit.

So können die Bedürfnisse von Angehörigen oder Freundinnen, mit dem Klienten gemeinsame Erlebnisse zu haben, ernst genommen werden und der Klient hält seine sozialen Kontakte aufrecht.

Aktivitätsplan
Mit dem Wissen, dass körperliche und geistige Betätigung sich auf die motorischen und nicht-motorischen Symptome M. Parkinsons positiv auswirkt, ist eine regelmäßige Betätigung wichtig, um einem schnellen Abbau vorzubeugen. Zur Strukturierung der Tätigkeiten ist ein Wochenplan hilfreich. Hier kann zum Beispiel besprochen werden, dass täglich eine Betätigung im Haushalt vom Klienten übernommen wird (kochen, Betten machen, Tisch decken) und drei Mal die Woche außerhäusliche Betätigungen rhythmisiert sind (Spaziergang zum Friedhof, Literaturkreis, Chor). Auch soziale Kontakte können hier fest eingeplant werden (Anruf bei Mutter, Mittagessen bei Freunden). Durch das Führen eines Kalenders entsteht eine Verbindlichkeit, die von den meisten Klienten eingehalten wird.

In einer Studie entwickelte und untersuchten Butterfield et al. (2017) ein Programm zur Unterstützung von Menschen mit Apathie und M. Parkinson. Dabei wurde ein **Aktivitätsplan** in Zusammenarbeit mit dem Klienten festgelegt und wöchentlich (per Telefon) besprochen. Dabei wurde die Wichtigkeit der konkreten Zielsetzung (fünf Aktivitätsziele), des externen Cueings (Erinnerung durch Plan) und der Verbindlichkeit/Kontrolle (Anruf der Therapeutin) beachtet.

Ablauf des Programms:

1. Einmaliges persönliches Treffen zur Vorstellung des Programms
2. Brainstorming zur Formulierung von fünf Aktivitätszielen für die Dauer des Programms
3. Jede Aktivität konkret mit Tag und Uhrzeit planen
4. Ende jeder Woche ein Telefonanruf des Coachs, bei dem die Anzahl der erreichten Aktivitätsziele in der Woche berichtet wird. Außerdem werden Probleme bei der Einhaltung der Ziele besprochen und bei Bedarf Anpassungen vorgenommen.

Die Ergebnisse zeigten eine signifikante Verbesserung der Apathie. Sekundär wurde auch die Wirkung auf weitere Faktoren untersucht:

- Depressivität – signifikant verbessert
- Lebensqualität – kurzfristig verbessert
- Alltagsfähigkeit – keine Verbesserung
- Belastung der Pflegeperson – keine Verbesserung

14.12.4 Sportliche Aktivität und Ausdauertraining

Ob sportliche Aktivität und Ausdauertraining einen positiven oder sogar negativen Effekt auf Apathie bei der Parkinson-Erkrankung hat, wird kontrovers diskutiert, und es gibt keine eindeutigen Studien dazu. Das liegt zum einen daran, dass in Untersuchungen nicht immer der kausale Zusammenhang zwischen Apathie und Übungshäufigkeit feststellbar ist. Trainiert der Klient mehr, weil die Apathie weniger ausgeprägt ist, oder ist die Apathie weniger ausgeprägt, weil der Betroffene mehr trainiert? Zum anderen gibt es Überschneidungen mit anderen Symptomen (Demenz, Depression), die bei der Diagnostik nicht immer klar getrennt werden. Es wird empfohlen, mit den Klienten, bei denen die Apathie im Vordergrund steht, wie oben beschrieben, einen wöchentlichen Aktivitätsplan auszuarbeiten. Dabei sollte vor allem auf regelmäßige und angenehme Aktivitäten Wert gelegt werden, die die körperliche Betätigung, kognitive Anregung und soziale Interaktion begünstigen, ohne ambitionierte sportliche Ziele zu verfolgen. In Absprache mit dem Klienten können Intensität und Häufigkeit der Aktivitäten individuell angepasst werden.

Beispiel

„Gleich kommen Gabi und Klaus. Gabi und ich trinken zusammen einen Kaffee, und Klaus nimmt dich eine Runde mit in den Park und danach will er mit dir das Fußballspiel gucken. Gehst du dich bitte fertig machen.“ Frau F. zeigt in Richtung Garderobe. Der Ergotherapeut hat ihr erklärt, dass die Trägheit Teil der Parkinson-Erkrankung ist, und ihr Tipps für einen Umgang damit gegeben. Gabi und Klaus kommen jetzt jeden Mittwoch. Sie haben sich gefreut, als ihre Freundin auf sie zukam und um Unterstützung gebeten hat. Bisher fühlten sie sich etwas hilflos, doch jetzt ist der Kontakt mit ihren Freunden wieder so eng wie früher. ◀

14.13 Schlafstörungen und exzessive Tagesschläfrigkeit

Beispiel

Mitten im Gespräch mit dem Sohn nickt Herr W. ein und fängt an, nach vorne aus dem Stuhl zu kippen. In letzter Sekunde fängt ihn sein Sohn auf. „So kann das nicht weitergehen!“ stellt der Sohn fest. Jede Nacht passiert das Gleiche. Herr W. wacht um Mitternacht auf, die Blase drückt, er schlurft zur Toilette und wieder zurück. Dann liegt er eine Weile wach, findet keine bequeme Schlafposition. Das Gleiche wiederholt sich um drei Uhr morgens und dann gegen fünf. Tagsüber fühlt er sich dann unausgeschlafen und unkonzentriert. ◀

14.13.1 Symptombeschreibung verschiedener Schlafstörungen

Symptombeschreibung Insomnie

Definition Eine Schlafstörung (Insomnie) wird als nächtliche Beschwerde definiert, die eine ungenügende Menge an Schlaf oder das Gefühl nach dem Schlaf, nicht genug ausgeruht zu sein, bezeichnet.

Ätiologie Die Ursachen für Schlafstörungen bei M. Parkinson sind vielfältig und komplex. Neben einer primären Schlafstörung können sich auch folgende Faktoren negativ auf den Schlaf auswirken:

- REM-Schlaf-Verhaltensstörung
- Restless-Legs-Syndrom
- Depression
- Schlechte Schlafhygiene
- Nykturie (nächtliches Wasserlassen)
- Schmerzen
- Dystonien
- Akinese
- Schwierigkeiten, sich im Bett zu drehen
- Medikamentennebenwirkungen
- Lebhafte Träume

Prävalenz Etwa 80 % der Menschen mit IPS sind von Schlafstörungen betroffen.

Klinik Schlafstörungen werden unterteilt in Probleme einzuschlafen (Schlafinitiierung), Probleme durchzuschlafen (Durchschlafstörung) und zu frühes Aufwachen am Morgen. Alle drei Probleme können bei Menschen mit M. Parkinson auftreten, am häufigsten wird jedoch von Durchschlafstörungen berichtet (74–88 %). Das Symptom der Schlafstörungen lässt sich häufig schon lange vor Diagnosestellung beobachten (s. u., RBD).

Außerdem wird das (auch bei gesunden Menschen auftretende) nächtliche Aufwachen als wesentliche Einschränkung erlebt, da die Hypokinese ein Wenden im Bett einschränkt. Hinzu kommt ein häufiges nächtliches Wasserlassen, was die nächtliche Ruhe zusätzlich unterbricht.

Folgen/Komplikationen Schlafstörungen wirken sich gravierend auf die Tagesmüdigkeit, Konzentrationsfähigkeit und Stimmung aus. Oftmals kommt der Tag-Nacht-Rhythmus aus dem Gleichgewicht, sodass Klientinnen sich tagsüber entweder bewusst ins Bett legen oder z. B. im Sessel plötzlich einschlafen. Sogar ad hoc auftretende „Schlafattacken" können auftreten.

- Schlafstörungen führen in der Regel zu exzessiver Tagesschläfrigkeit, was von der Fatigue abzugrenzen ist (siehe Tab. 1.2 in Abschn. 1.5)
- Verminderte Konzentrationsfähigkeit
- Schlechte Allgemeinbefindlichkeit

Medizinische Möglichkeiten:

- Medikamente
- Anpassung der Medikamentendosis
- Psychotherapie

Symptombeschreibung RBD (REM-Schlaf-Verhaltensstörung)

Definition Bei RBD (**R**apid Eye Movement-sleep-**b**ehaviour-**d**isorder) erschlaffen die Muskeln im Schlaf nicht wie bei Gesunden, sondern die Träume werden ausgelebt.

Ätiologie RBD ist ein weit verbreitetes Frühzeichen für M. Parkinson und tritt durch die Neurodegeneration im Gehirn auf. 60–70 % der Menschen, die darunter leiden, entwickeln nach 10–30 Jahren IPS oder Multisystematrophie (MSA), eine seltene neurodegenerative Erkrankung.

Prävalenz Etwa 40 % der Parkinson-Patientinnen haben ein RBD.

Klinik Träume werden vor allem in der zweiten Nachthälfte, der sog. REM-Phase, aktiv ausgelebt. Die Betroffenen bewegen sich, treten und schlagen um sich. Dabei sind die Träume lebhafter und aggressiver als bei Gesunden.

Folgen/Komplikationen Es besteht die Gefahr der Eigen- oder Fremdverletzung durch Angreifen des Bettpartners oder Stürze aus dem Bett.

Medizinische Möglichkeiten:

- Stark limitierte Möglichkeiten
- Evtl. Anpassung der Medikamente
- Sicherung des Bettes zur Verletzungs- und Sturzvermeidung

Symptombeschreibung exzessive Tagesschläfrigkeit
Etwa ein Drittel der Menschen mit M. Parkinson leidet unter exzessiver Tagesschläfrigkeit. Die Ursache kann eine Schlafstörung oder eine ungünstige Medikamenteneinstellung sein. Die Patientinnen fühlen eine vermehrte Müdigkeit, bis hin zu plötzlich auftretenden Schlafattacken. Dies kann negative Auswirkungen auf die Alltagsfähigkeit haben und besonders gefährlich für das Führen eines Fahrzeugs sein.

Symptombeschreibung Restless-Legs-Syndrom
Siehe Abschn. 14.16

14.13.2 Ergotherapeutische Intervention bei Schlafstörungen

Schlafstörungen sind kein primärer Tätigkeitsbereich der Ergotherapie. Da sie bei Klientinnen mit IPS jedoch häufig auftreten und als stark belastend empfunden werden, ist die Auseinandersetzung damit empfehlenswert.

Anpassung des therapeutischen Anspruchs
Mit dem Wissen, dass die Klientin unter Schlafstörungen leidet, entsteht beim Therapeuten ein verbessertes Verständnis für das Befinden der Betroffenen. So ist die Klientin nach einer besonders unruhigen Nacht meist physisch und kognitiv weniger leistungsfähig, was sowohl beim Assessment als auch bei der therapeutischen Intervention berücksichtigt werden sollte.

Therapeutische Möglichkeiten (Tab. 14.11)

Tab. 14.11 Je nach Ursache der Schlafstörung können verschiedene therapeutische Ansätze geeignet sein

Mögliche Ursachen für Schlafstörungen	Mögliche therapeutische Ansätze
RBD (REM-Schlaf-Verhaltensstörung)	Bei Verletzungsgefahr: Bett abpolstern, Matte auf Boden
Restless-Legs-Syndrom	Kalte oder warme Wickel, warme Fußbäder, Massieren, Bürsten der Beine oder Bewegungsübungen, Dehnen
Depression (siehe Abschn. 14.10) Schlechte Schlafhygiene	Gesunden Schlafrhythmus etablieren, feste Schlafenszeiten einhalten, tagsüber ausreichend körperliche Bewegung, ruhiges Abendritual (z. B. Buch lesen, Katze streicheln, Entspannungsübungen …), abends keine Bildschirmnutzung
Nykturie (nächtliches Wasserlassen)	Abendliche Trinkmenge reduzieren, Toilettenstuhl oder Urinflasche, um nächtliche Aktivität zu reduzieren und Stürze zu vermeiden, indem Weg zu Toilette erspart wird
Schmerzen	Schlafstellung besprechen, evtl. Lagerung
Dystonien (vor allem im Fuß)	Siehe Abschn. 14.6.2, nächtliches einnehmen von Medikamenten
Schwierigkeiten, sich im Bett zu drehen (Akinese)	Üben der physiologischen Drehung im Bett Beine anstellen, Beine zur Seite kippen, mit Arm über Körper greifen, Kopf in Richtung der Drehung rotieren evtl. Hilfsmittel zur Unterstützung: Bettgitter, Haltegurt an Seite befestigt Glatte Bettwäsche (z. B. Seide)
Medikamentennebenwirkungen	Kommunikation mit Ärztin

Beispiel

Herr W. atmet ein und aus. Er liegt flach auf dem Rücken und tut nichts anderes, nur atmen. Dann lässt er den Tag gedanklich Revue passieren. Er hat seine Abende mit seinem Ergotherapeuten umgestellt. Der Fernseher wird ab 21 Uhr ausgeschaltet. Stattdessen macht er eine letzte Runde Dehnungsübungen, liest ein Buch und vermeidet die Tasse Tee am Abend, die er früher so gerne trank. Jetzt schläft er bis etwa zwei Uhr durch. Den Weg zur Toilette hat er nun nicht mehr, da er eine Urinflasche am Bett hat. So schläft er schneller wieder ein. ◀

14.14 Psychotische Episoden mit visuellen Halluzinationen

Beispiel

Frau R. sieht besorgt aus, als die Therapeutin in das Patientenzimmer kommt. „Ich habe wieder etwas gesehen," erzählt sie. „Mein Bruder war hier. Ich konnte ihn wirklich sehen und ich habe auch nicht geschlafen. Ich saß da am Tisch und er kam zur Tür herein, genau wie Sie gerade. Aber ich wusste, dass es nicht wahr ist, obwohl es so schien. Das macht mir Angst." ◀

14.14.1 Symptombeschreibung

Definition Die Psychose bei IPS ist ein Oberbegriff für ein klinisches Spektrum von verschiedenen kognitiven und Wahrnehmungsstörungen, insbesondere illusionäre Verkennungen, Halluzinationen meist visueller Natur, Wahnvorstellungen, Verwirrtheit und paranoide Wahrnehmungsverarbeitung.

Ätiologie Es gibt einen klaren Zusammenhang zwischen psychotischen Syndromen und Demenz, Dauer der Erkrankung, Depression und Schlafstörungen. Im Vordergrund stehen jedoch die Nebenwirkungen der Parkinson-Medikamente. Dopaminagonisten können, laut Studienergebnissen auslösend wirken, selten auch L-Dopa.

Prävalenz Psychotische Symptome treten bei weniger als 10 % der unbehandelten Parkinson-Patienten auf, aber bei bis zu 40 % der mit Parkinson-Medikamenten behandelten Patienten mit IPS.

Klinik Psychotische Symptome bei IPS haben unterschiedliche Erscheinungsbilder. Bei einer illusionären Verkennung handelt es sich um eine Sinnestäuschung. So wird zum Beispiel in einem Baum das Gesicht eines Angehörigen gesehen. Halluzinationen sind meist visueller, seltener akustischer oder sensibler Art. Es werden z. B. Menschen oder Tiere gesehen, die auf den Patienten selten bedrohlich wirken, eine Einsicht ist oft vorhanden. Bei einer paranoiden Psychose, oft mit Verfolgungswahn, fürchtet der Patient z. B. um sein Leben oder meint, bestohlen zu werden.

Folgen/Komplikationen

- Nach Demenzen sind psychotische Symptome bei Parkinson-Patienten der häufigste Grund für eine stationäre Behandlung in einer psychiatrischen Klinik.
- Starke Belastung der Angehörigen.
- Psychotische Episoden gelten als Meilenstein – einhergehend mit schlechter Prognose.

Medizinische Möglichkeiten

- Anpassung der Medikamentenzusammensetzung.
- Absetzen potenziell auslösender Medikamente.
- Medikamentengabe.

14.14.2 Ergotherapeutische Intervention

Wahnvorstellungen und Halluzinationen können den Klienten tief verunsichern. Auch wenn die Einsicht, dass das Wahrgenommene nicht real ist, vorhanden ist, reagieren die Betroffenen meist irritiert und verängstigt.

Um die Psychose nicht zu verstärken, sollte die Therapeutin nicht direkt nach Halluzinationen fragen. Berichtet der Klient spontan davon, ist eine genaue Dokumentation des Zeitpunktes und der Art wichtig. Anschließend kann die Therapeutin in Absprache mit dem Klienten, dem behandelnden Arzt das Symptom kommunizieren, da Betroffene sich im Allgemeinen schämen, Wahnvorstellungen zu erleben, und ihrem Arzt nicht sofort davon berichten. Da Menschen mit psychotischen Episoden meist tief verunsichert sind, ist eine gutes Vertrauensverhältnis essenziell. Spürt der Klient die Offenheit und Empathie der Therapeutin, wird es ihm leichter fallen, z. B. über Halluzinationen zu sprechen.

Des Weiteren sind Maßnahmen zur Unterstützung der Selbständigkeit, Förderung des Selbstwertgefühls und Verbesserung der sozioemotionalen Kompetenz und Kommunikationsfähigkeit Teil der ergotherapeutischen Behandlung. Inhalte können sein:

- Rollenspiele (zum Umgang mit Halluzinationen)
- Tagesstrukturierung
- Gespräche mit Angehörigen
- Anleitung zur Vereinfachung des Alltags (um Überforderung zu vermeiden)
- Tagebuch führen, zum verbesserten Verständnis der Erkrankung
- Kognitive Verhaltenstherapie (nach entsprechender Fortbildung)
- Psychoedukation (nach entsprechender Fortbildung)

▶ **Cave!** Bei psychotischen Episoden oder Halluzinationen, keine Gedankenreise oder Fantasiereise durchführen, da sie auslösend wirken kann.

Beispiel

„Das kann von den Medikamenten kommen, Frau R.", die Therapeutin lässt die verunsicherte Dame sich bei ihr einhaken und begleitet sie wieder an den Sitzplatz. Sie bringt ihr ein Glas Wasser und notiert sich, dass sie die Halluzinationen in der Teambesprechung nochmal erwähnt. Dann geht sie zur Therapie über. „Heute wollten wir doch zusammen eine große Runde mit den Walkingstöcken laufen, Frau R. Sind Sie bereit?" ◀

14.15 Vegetative Symptome

Beispiel

Nach ein paar Übungen in der Therapie ist Herr J. nassgeschwitzt. Er wischt sein Gesicht mehrfach mit einem Taschentuch trocken. Am Ende der Therapie hat er große Schweißflecken unter den Achseln und am Rücken. Es ist ihm sehr unangenehm. Schnell zieht er seine Jacke über und verabschiedet sich. ◀

Das vegetative Nervensystem reguliert die Funktion der inneren Organe und Gefäße. Es wird nicht bewusst gesteuert, sondern autonom reguliert, weshalb es auch „autonomes Nervensystem" heißt. Das vegetative Nervensystem unterteilt sich in zwei Anteile, den Sympathikus und den Parasympathikus, die eine gegensätzliche Wirkung auf die Organe haben. Der Sympathikus wirkt energiemobilisierend und aktivitätssteigernd, der Parasympathikus dagegen konserviert und baut Körperenergien wieder auf. Bei M. Parkinson kann es auch zu einer Störung des vegetativen Nervensystems kommen. Dies führt zu einer Vielzahl an Symptomen der inneren Organe und des Blutkreislaufs.

14.15.1 Verschiedene Symptome

Dranginkontinenz
Störungen des Harntrakts sind ein vielfach festgestelltes Symptom bei Menschen mit M. Parkinson und schränken die Lebensqualität erheblich ein. Ca. 70 % der Patientinnen berichten von Blasenfüllsymptomen mit häufigem Wasserlassen, Nykturie (vermehrtes nächtliches Wasserlassen) und Dranginkontinenz.

Hautveränderungen
Vermehrtes Schwitzen
Ein häufig frühes Symptom ist das vermehrte Schwitzen. Es kann in abgegrenzten Körperbereichen, einseitig oder am gesamten Körper auftreten. Oft tritt das Schwitzen nachts auf, sodass das Schlafbekleidung und Bettwäsche durchnässt ist.

Seborrhoische Dermatitis
Dies ist ein scharf markiertes, rot gefärbtes, juckendes Ekzem mit fettigen Schuppen. Meist im Gesicht oder auf der Kopfhaut aber auch auf Brust oder Extremitäten zu finden.

Fettige Haut
Die Talgproduktion der Haut verändert sich bei einigen Menschen mit M. Parkinson. Die Haut wird zu trocken oder (häufiger) fettig. Tritt dies im Gesicht auf, wird von einem „Salbengesicht" gesprochen.

Dyspnoe
Etwa 40 % der Parkinson-Erkrankten leiden unter Dyspnoe mit vermehrter Atemarbeit, Kurzatmigkeit und Atemnot. Die Ursache kann Parkinson-unabhängig sein (z. B. Herzinsuffizienz) oder mit der Parkinson-Erkrankung zusammenhängen, z. B. kyphotische Haltung, Rigor, Angst-/Panikattacken oder Dystonie.

Orthostatische Hypotension
Setzt sich oder steht die Patientin plötzlich aus dem Liegen auf, fällt aufgrund einer fehlerhaften Blutdruckregulation der Blutdruck ab. Es kann zu Schwindel, Synkopen mit plötzlichem „Schwarzwerden vor Augen", Schwäche und/oder Abgeschlagenheit kommen. Orthostatische Hypotension tritt bei jeder zweiten Parkinson-Betroffenen auf.

Sexuelle Dysfunktion
Rund 60 % der Männer und 40 % der Frauen mit M. Parkinson sind mit ihrem Sexualleben unzufrieden. Dazu können beim Mann erektile Dysfunktion und vorzeitiger Samenerguss gehören, bei der Frau vaginale Trockenheit. Bei Mann und Frau können reduzierte Erregung, Schwierigkeiten, einen Orgasmus zu erreichen und herabgesetztes sexuelles Verlangen, entstehen.

Parkinson-Medikamente können eine Hypersexualität bewirken. Zusätzlich können andere Symptome die Sexualität negativ beeinflussen, z. B. Depressionen, eingeschränkte Fingerfeinmotorik, Dystonien, Apathie.

Verstopfung
Etwa zwei Drittel der Menschen mit M. Parkinson sind von Verstopfung (Obstipation) betroffen. Dazu gehört langsame Stuhlweiterleitung im Darm, harter Stuhl, unregelmäßiger Stuhlgang und Stuhlentleerung nur durch starkes Pressen.

14.15.2 Ergotherapeutische Intervention (Tab. 14.12)

Beispiel

In der nächsten Ergotherapiestunde spricht der Therapeut gleich zu Beginn das Thema des Schwitzens an: „Ich habe letzte Woche gesehen, dass Sie schnell anfangen zu schwitzen." Herr J. ist es peinlich: „Ja, das tut mir leid. Ich kann nichts dagegen tun." Der Therapeut erwidert: „Sie brauchen sich nicht zu entschul-

Tab. 14.12 Ergotherapeutische Interventionsmöglichkeiten bei vegetativen Symptomen

Vegetatives Symptom		Ergotherapeutische Möglichkeiten
Dranginkontinenz		• Einplanung von regelmäßigen Toilettenpausen in Therapie und im Alltag • Hilfsmittel (Toilettenstuhl/Bettflasche) direkt am Bett, um nächtlichen Weg zur Toilette zu vermeiden • Nachts leichte Hochlagerung des Oberkörpers vermindert Harndrang • Hoseneinlagen/Windel zur eigenen Entspannung z. B. in Öffentlichkeit • Beckenbodentraining (z. B. Tanzberger-Konzept)
Hautveränderungen	Vermehrtes Schwitzen	• Wechselkleidung bei Ausflügen • Kühlende Kleidungsmaterialien aus Naturfasern • Mehrere Lagen anziehen, wie Jacke/Weste, die Hals und Unterarme schnell offen legen können (wirkt abkühlend) • Vermehrte Flüssigkeitszufuhr • Stofftaschentuch, um Gesicht zu trocknen • Lüften des Therapieraums
	Seborrhoische Dermatitis	• Vermittlung zu Hautarzt • Spezifische Hautpflegegrundsätze recherchieren und im Alltag umsetzen
	Fettige Haut	• Spezifische Hautpflegegrundsätze recherchieren und im Alltag umsetzen
Dyspnoe/Atemnot (evtl. in Verbindung mit Dyskinensien/Dystonie)		• Atemtherapie • Haltungstraining (wenn ursächlich) • Lagerung • Für Frischluft sorgen • Atemstimulierende Einreibung (ASE)
Orthostatische Hypotension		• Vermehrte Flüssigkeitsaufnahme • Edukation (Aufklärung über Symptom) • Schrittweises Aufsetzen
Sexuelle Dysfunktion		• Offenheit und Gesprächsbereitschaft seitens des Therapeuten • Kommunikation mit Partner • Sexualhilfsmittel, z. B. Vibrator, Gleitmittel • Anpassung der Zeit der Medikamenteneinnahme
Obstipation (Verstopfung)		• Ausreichende Flüssigkeitszufuhr • Körperliche Bewegung • Ballaststoffreiche Ernährung

digen. Sie können nichts dafür, das ist ja leider eins der Parkinson-Symptome."

„Ach, das wusste ich gar nicht."

„Deswegen wollte ich es heute mit Ihnen besprechen. Sehen Sie, heute habe ich das Fenster aufgemacht, damit die Luft frischer ist, und Sie nicht so schnell schwitzen. Außerdem wollte ich Ihnen anbieten, sich für die Therapie umzuziehen, wie für den Sport. Bringen Sie einfach extra Trainingskleidung mit und ziehen sich 10 Minuten vor der Therapie in der Toilette um. Würde Ihnen das helfen?"

„Ja," lächelt Herr. J., „das ist eine sehr gute Idee, danke." ◀

14.16 Dysästhesien/Restless-Legs-Syndrom und Akathisie

14.16.1 Symptombeschreibung

Beispiel

Herrn P. fallen im Gespräch mit der Ergotherapeutin immer wieder die Augen zu. „Es tut mir wirklich leid. Ich war in der Nacht wieder zwei Stunden wach. Meine Restless Legs gehen nur weg, wenn ich um den Tisch laufe." ◀

Dysästhesien
Viele Patientinnen berichten von Hypästhesie oder Parästhesie in den Extremitäten. Dieses Symptom steht bei M. Parkinson selten im Vordergrund, kann jedoch, vor allem in Kombination mit dem Restless-Legs-Syndrom, als störend empfunden werden. Bei Überprüfung der Oberflächensensibilität kann bei den meisten Menschen mit der Parkinson-Erkrankung eine leichte bis mittlere Einschränkung festgestellt werden, die nicht immer im Alltag auffällt.

Restless-Legs-Syndrom
Das Restless-Legs-Syndrom tritt meist nachts oder bei Entspannung auf. Es manifestiert sich mit Bewegungsdrang und großer Unruhe in den Beinen und starken Parästhesien, wie Kribbeln, Ziehen, Stechen oder Schmerzen. Durch Bewegen der Beine oder Umherlaufen werden die Missempfindungen etwas reduziert. Aus diesem Grund treten sekundär Schlafstörungen und folglich exzessive Tagesschläfrigkeit auf.

Akathisie
In seltenen Fällen kann aufgrund des fehlenden Dopamins eine Akathisie ausgelöst werden. Es äußert sich als eine starke Unruhe, die die Betroffenen ständig in Bewegung hält. Stillsitzen ist nicht mehr möglich, Beine und Arme werden überkreuzt, wieder auseinandergenommen und bewegt. Im Stehen verlagern Betroffene konstant das Gewicht von einem Bein auf das andere. Dazu kommen innere Unruhe und ein starkes Gefühl der Anspannung. Das äußere Erscheinungsbild ist kaum vom Restless-Legs-Syndrom zu unterscheiden, es fehlen jedoch die Missempfindungen.

14.16.2 Ergotherapeutische Intervention

Gewichtsdecken können tagsüber und nachts eine Erleichterung der Dysästhesien bewirken und einen ruhigeren Schlaf ermöglichen (Achtung: verstärkt eingeschränktes Drehen im Bett). Auch andere klare sensorische Reize können angewandt werden. Dazu zählen: fester Druck mit den Händen auf die betroffene Körperstelle geben, festes Abreiben mit einem Handtuch, Zucker-Öl-Einreibungen und die Anwendung von Kälte oder Wärme.

Kalte oder warme Wadenwickel können Restless Legs beruhigen. Außerdem können Entspannungsübungen helfen, die Fokussierung von den Missempfindungen weg zu verlagern. Auch wenn bei Akathisie keine Missempfindungen auftreten, können klare Reizsetzungen in Einzelfällen eine Linderung bewirken.

Beispiel

Nun hat Herr P. neben dem Bett einen nassen Waschlappen liegen. Statt aufzustehen, macht er damit eine Beinmassage, anschließend eine Meditation. „Es hilft nicht immer, aber immer wieder," erklärt er der Therapeutin. ◀

14.17 Schmerzsyndrome

Beispiel

Frau F. kommt jede Woche in die Ergotherapie. Bei der Begrüßung berichtet die Klientin regelmäßig von belastenden Rückenschmerzen. Die Therapeutin erkennt die Schmerzen der Klientin an, geht dann jedoch zur geplanten Intervention zur Verfolgung der Betätigungsziele über. ◀

14.17.1 Symptombeschreibung

Schmerzen
Zwischen 40–85 % der Menschen mit M. Parkinson erleben Schmerzen. Die Ursachen hierfür sind vielfältig und können nicht immer abschließend geklärt werden. In den Phasen, in denen die Medikamente nicht wirken (Off-Phase), ist die Schmerzempfindlichkeit oftmals deutlich erhöht, sodass schon normale Berührungen als Schmerz wahrgenommen werden. Die Ursache hierfür wird in einer Störung der Schmerzverarbeitung in den Basalganglien gesehen. Zusätzlich zu dieser „zentralen" Schmerzursache gibt es beim Parkinson-Syndrom zahlreiche Symptome, die

Schmerzen verursachen können. Dazu zählen: Rigor, Dystonie, Haltungsanomalien (Pisa-Syndrom, Kamptokormie, Anterocollis), Restless-Legs-Syndrom, myofasziale Verkürzungen, Neuropathien, Bewegungsmangel.

Schmerzen werden meist im Schulter- oder unteren Rückenbereich angegeben, sie können jedoch überall im Körper auftreten. Teilweise, aber nicht immer, ist eine Korrelation mit der Wirkungsfluktuation der Medikamente nachzuweisen, z. B. bei der morgendlichen Dystonie oder „peak-dose"-Dyskinesien. Ein bekanntes Problem ist, dass Parkinson-Klienten die Schmerzsymptomatik nicht mit der Erkrankung in Zusammenhang bringen und folglich ihrer Neurologin nicht davon berichten. Da Schmerzen sich erheblich auf die Lebensqualität auswirken, ist dies extrem ungünstig.

Die Schmerzen können so dominant sein, dass sie alle Betätigungen beeinträchtigen und die Teilhabe deutlich einschränken, sodass die Lebensqualität vom Klienten als sehr gering eingestuft wird. Aus diesen Gründen kann das primäre Ziel der ergotherapeutischen Behandlung die Schmerzreduktion sein. Beispiele für ergotherapeutische Ziele sind:

- „Reduktion der Schmerzen im Rücken, um wieder Freude am Tanzen zu haben."
- „Schmerzmanagement, um eine konzentrierte Kommunikation mit Enkelkindern zu ermöglichen."

Das Thema Schmerzmanagement ist sehr komplex, da die subjektive Schmerzwahrnehmung einige sehr unterschiedliche Einflussfaktoren hat. Dazu gehören:

- strukturelle Probleme (z. B. Muskelverkürzungen, Faszien Verklebungen),
- individuelle Schmerzempfindlichkeit,
- Bewertung des Schmerzes.

Die Schmerzbehandlung kann in dieser Publikation nicht umfassend vermittelt werden. Aus diesem Grund werden die unterschiedlichen Therapiemethoden nur genannt und kurz beschrieben, sodass der Therapeut sich bei Bedarf weiteres Wissen aneignen kann.

14.17.2 Bewegungsanalyse und -veränderung

Der primäre Ansatz der Schmerzbehandlung in der Ergotherapie ist die Ergründung der Schmerzursache. Bei M. Parkinson liegt die Ursache oftmals in der Fehlhaltung, die wiederum zur einseitigen Überlastung bestimmter Muskelgruppen führt. Zunächst erfragt der Ergotherapeut, bei welcher Tätigkeit oder nach welcher Tätigkeit die Schmerzen typischerweise auftreten, z. B. Schlafen, Laufen, Spülmaschine ausräumen … und bei welchen Tätigkeiten sie verbessert sind. Dabei müssen vor allem die Schlafgegebenheiten betrachtet werden. Die Schlafposition und die Unfähigkeit, sich im Bett zu wenden, führen häufig zu schmerzhaften Verspannungen. Beim sog. Kopfkissenphänomen ist es den Klienten durch den starken Rigor in der Halsmuskulatur nicht möglich, den Kopf abzulegen; er wird in der Luft gehalten, was zu starken Schmerzen in Nacken und Rücken führen kann.

Anschließend führt der Therapeut eine Bewegungsanalyse durch, um zu erkennen, ob Fehl- oder Schonhaltungen oder unphysiologische Bewegungen sichtbar sind. Er analysiert den Bewegungsablauf, bei dem die Schmerzen auftreten oder verstärkt werden. In Zusammenarbeit mit dem Klienten wird experimentiert, wie die Betätigung verändert werden kann, um eine Fehlbelastung zu verhindern. Dabei sollten folgende Faktoren beachtet werden:

- effizienter Einsatz von Energie,
- Hilfsmittel,
- Pausen,
- physiologische Bewegung,
- Kräftigung notwendiger Muskelgruppen,
- störende Faktoren (Tremor, Dystonien, Dyskinesien).

14.17.3 Passive Schmerzbehandlung

Besitzt der Therapeut Kenntnisse zu passiven Behandlungen wie Triggerpunkt-Therapie, Gua Sha und Dehnungsübungen (siehe Abschn. 14.7.6), können diese zur zeitweisen Schmerzlinderung eingesetzt werden. Für eine langfristige Verbesserung des Schmerzes ist eine oben beschriebene Bewegungsveränderung notwendig. Ein typischer Schmerzbereich bei Menschen mit M. Parkinson ist die Rückenmuskulatur. Beispielhaft wird hier ein mögliches therapeutisches Vorgehen für diese Problematik beschrieben.

Beispiel

Nachdem Frau F. das Thema Schmerzen immer wieder erwähnt, verändert die Therapeutin in Absprache mit der Klientin das therapeutische Vorgehen. Zu Beginn jeder Behandlung steht nun der Schmerz im Rücken im Vordergrund. In einem kurzen Interview stellt die Therapeutin fest, dass die Klientin zwei Mal wöchentlich mehrere Schubkarren mit gehacktem Holz füllt, diese ins Haus karrt und dort neben dem Holzofen aufstapelt. Danach sei sie „erledigt" und müsse sich erst mal ausruhen. Diese Tätigkeit wird von der Klientin klar mit den Rückenschmerzen in Verbindung gebracht. Außerdem vermutet die Therapeutin, dass die kyphotische Oberkörperhaltung der Klientin zu den Schmerzen beiträgt.

Die Therapeutin fordert Frau F. auf, die Bewegungsabläufe zu erklären. Es wird schnell klar, dass eine wesentliche Vereinfachung der Betätigung nicht möglich ist und auch eine Aufteilung in Teilschritte mit Pausen nicht die gewünschte Entlastung bringen würde. Die Therapeutin schlägt vor, sich Hilfe dafür zu holen, und dabei größere Mengen an Holz zu transportieren, damit es nur zweiwöchentlich durchgeführt werden muss. Der Klientin fällt sofort ein junger Nachbar ein, den sie für ein Trinkgeld darum bitten könnte.

Außerdem macht die Therapeutin die Klientin auf ihre gebeugte Körperhaltung aufmerksam. Frau F. ist sichtlich überrascht, dass es der Therapeutin auffällt und möchte sich selbst im Spiegel überprüfen. Sie korrigiert die Aufrichtung mit visueller Kontrolle selbst. Sobald der Spiegel entfernt wird, geht Frau F. unbewusst wieder zu ihrer gewohnt gebeugten Haltung über. Die Körperwahrnehmung stimmt nicht mehr mit der wirklichen Körperphysiologie überein. Mit einer Aufrichtungsübung, mit der Wand als Referenzfläche, wird die Wahrnehmung mit und ohne visuelle Kontrolle erarbeitet. Sobald Frau F. die Aufrichtung in der Therapiesituation ohne visuelle Kontrolle umsetzen kann, wird der Übertrag in den Alltag geübt. Zunächst macht die Klientin verschiedene Bewegungsübergänge mit dem Fokus auf der Aufrichtung (Liegen zum Sitzen, Sitzen zum Stehen, Gehen, Gehen mit Richtungswechsel). Später werden Betätigungen aus dem Alltag simuliert (Einkäufe in den Schrank einräumen, Gartenarbeit ...). Durch die für die Parkinson-Erkrankung charakteristischen Schwierigkeiten mit Dual-Tasks verfällt die Klientin regelmäßig in eine kyphotische Haltung. Deshalb erarbeitet die Therapeutin ein neues Bewusstsein für den Zusammenhang der Haltung mit den Schmerzen im Rücken. Sie leitet die Klientin an, in jeder Betätigung kurze Pausen einzuschieben, in denen sie ihre Aufmerksamkeit auf die Aufrichtung lenkt, sodass zwar keine konstante Aufrichtung stattfindet, jedoch regelmäßig die Rückenmuskulatur aktiviert wird. Erinnerungszettel in der Wohnung machen Frau F. im Alltag darauf aufmerksam auf die Aufrichtung zu achten.

Parallel dazu zeigt die Therapeutin der Klientin Kräftigungsübungen für den Rücken und Dehnungsübungen mit Referenzflächen für die ventrale Muskelkette, die Frau F. als Eigenübungen zu Hause durchführen kann (siehe Abschn. 14.7.5 und 14.7.6). Zur Schmerzlinderung führt die Therapeutin am Rücken der Klientin eine Triggerpunkt-Behandlung durch. ◄

14.18 Dysfunktion der sensomotorischen Integration und Propriozeption

Beispiel

Am Esstisch kippt Herr W. Stück für Stück nach rechts, bis er regelrecht über der Armlehne hängt. Seine Frau erinnert ihn immer wieder: „Schatz, du fällst nach rechts. Setz dich wieder aufrecht." Daraufhin kommt er ein paar Zentimeter in die Aufrichtung. Die Tochter drückt ihren Vater nach links und stopft ein Sofakissen in die rechte Seite. „So Papa, jetzt bleib doch mal so sitzen. Du kannst doch aufrecht sitzen." Zwei Minuten später hängt Herr W. über dem Kissen. ◀

14.18.1 Symptombeschreibung

Aufgrund der eingeschränkten Funktion der Basalganglien werden sensorische Reize inkorrekt organisiert und die Bewegungsführung beeinträchtigt. In mehreren Studien konnte festgestellt werden, dass die Propriozeption deutlich eingeschränkt war.

So zeigten Adamovich et al. (2001) in einer Studie, dass Menschen mit M. Parkinson im zielgenauen Erreichen eines Punktes mit dem Finger, **ohne** visuelle Kontrolle des Fingers, wesentlich eingeschränkter waren. **Mit** visueller Kontrolle wich ihre Zielgenauigkeit jedoch kaum von den gesunden Kontrollpersonen ab.

So empfinden Klientinnen selbst ihre Haltung als aufrecht und ihre Bewegungsamplitude als weit ausladend. Von außen betrachtet kann jedoch eine kyphotische Haltung und minimierte Bewegungsamplitude festgestellt werden. Es wird davon ausgegangen, dass dies einen wesentlichen Faktor bei der eingeschränkten motorischen Bewegungsfähigkeit darstellt, da die sensorische Kontrolle der Bewegungsamplitude defizitär ist.

Bei nicht betroffenen Menschen wird die Motorik konstant mithilfe der Propriozeption abgeglichen. Tiefensensorische Reize werden von Rezeptoren in den Muskelspindeln, Sehnen und Gelenkkapseln wahrgenommen. Durch Druck und Zug werden Informationen über Muskellänge, Geschwindigkeit der Muskelkontraktion, Muskelzug und Gelenkposition aufgenommen. Im Gehirn wird die Bewegung dementsprechend angepasst und ausgerichtet. Diese konstante Kalibrierung geschieht zeitgleich und meist unbewusst. Die innere Kalibrierung ist durch das dysfunktionale Limbische System bei M. Parkinson fehlerhaft. Auf neuronaler Ebene konnten Forschende in Untersuchungen zeigen, dass im Limbischen System eines gesunden Gehirns die Neuronen bei passiver Mobilisierung eines Gelenks **spezifisch** erregt werden. In dem von M. Parkinson veränderten Gehirn werden die Neuronen **unspezifisch** erregt und geben somit weniger differenzierte propriozeptive Informationen an die kortikalen Motoneuronen weiter. In mehreren Studien konnte nachgewiesen werden, dass Menschen mit der Parkinson-Erkrankung ihre Bewegungen weniger genau wahrnehmen als eine Kontrollgruppe von nicht betroffenen Menschen. Dadurch ist die Amplitude der Bewegungen deutlich reduziert, zielgerichtete Bewegungen sind ungenau und posturale Stellreflexe sind verändert, was zu Gleichgewichtsstörungen und Gangunsicherheit führt.

14.18.2 Ergotherapeutische Intervention

Um die mangelnde Verarbeitung von propriozeptiven Reizen auszugleichen, sind äußere Referenzflächen notwendig. Der Therapeut gibt der Klientin also nicht die Anweisung „große Bewegungen", sondern konkrete Zielvorgaben, z. B. „bis zur Wand", „Berühren Sie mit der Hand die Tischkante", „Kommen Sie mit dem Kopf bis zu meiner Hand". Dadurch gelingen der Klientin weitaus größere Amplituden und diese können auch mehrfach ohne Amplitudenreduktion wiederholt werden.

Referenzflächen sollten vom Therapeuten klar beschrieben werden. Sie müssen visuell und sensorisch gut wahrnehmbar sein, z. B. feste Flächen, klare Kanten und Ecken, oder ersatzweise laminierte, farbige Punkte, um der Klientin die klare Rückmeldung zu geben: „Die Bewegung wurde korrekt durchgeführt“, die bei Gesunden durch die funktionierende Propriozeption geschieht. Das wichtige Instrument der Referenzflächen bei M. Parkinson wird in einigen Kapiteln mit weiteren Therapieideen und Beispielen für den Einsatz in der ergotherapeutischen Praxis dargelegt. (siehe Abschn. 13.4, 14.1.6, 14.7.4, und 14.7.5)

Beispiel

Seit neuestem sitzt Herr W. auf der anderen Seite des Tisches. Dort ist die Wand auf seiner linken Seite. Die Tochter zweifelt: „Aber Mama, er fällt doch nach rechts, da müsste die Wand besser sein.“ „Nein,“ erklärt die Mutter. „Die Ergotherapeutin hat uns erklärt, dass die Tiefensensibilität nicht mehr gut funktioniert. Er spürt also nicht gut, wenn er kippt. Und wenn du ihm sagst, er solle sich aufrichten, dann weiß er nicht genau, wann er aufgerichtet ist. Dabei hilft die Wand. Sie ist eine klare feste Fläche, das kann der Papa gut spüren.“ Die Tochter ist nicht überzeugt: „Papa, war das nicht besser mit dem Kissen?“ „Nein, meine Rippen haben immer wehgetan.“ Und tatsächlich, während des Essens lehnt sich Herr W. entspannt an die Wand. Zwei Mal passiert es, dass er zu kippen beginnt. Dann genügt eine kurze Aufforderung der Frau: „Denk an die Wand!“ Schon richtet er sich wieder auf. ◀

14.19 Off-Phasen

Beispiel

Frau P. räumt die Spülmaschine aus. Sie beeilt sich, sie hat nur noch 20 Minuten, bis sie in die Off-Phase kommt. Das kennt sie schon. Doch schon bei den ersten Gläsern merkt sie – irgendetwas stimmt nicht. Die Bewegungen sind nicht flüssig, beim Loslassen der Gläser stockt die Hand. Und schon fällt ihr eins aus der Hand und zerbricht. Sie will die Scherben schnell aufkehren, doch auch hier fühlt sie sich steif und unbeweglich. Das Off ist schon früher da! ◀

14.19.1 Auslöser und Erscheinungsbild

Im Verlauf der Parkinson-Erkrankung treten bei vielen Klienten regelmäßige Off-Phasen auf. Die Off-Phase ist gekennzeichnet durch starke Akinese und Rigor. Je nach Ausprägung der Erkrankung können sich auch weitere Symptome verstärken, z. B. kognitive Einschränkung, Speichelaustritt, Tremor, … Sie dauern von wenigen Sekunden bis zu einer Stunde an und sind meist zur gleichen Uhrzeit zu beobachten. Die Ärztin wird versuchen, die Off-Phasen durch Erhöhung der Einnahmefrequenz oder Veränderung der Medikamentenart oder -dosis zu beseitigen. Ab einer gewissen Erkrankungsdauer ist dies oftmals nicht mehr möglich oder die Medikamente verursachen starke Nebenwirkungen, die zu große Belastungen mit sich bringen. Für weitere Informationen zu Medikamentenfluktuationen und der Entstehung von Off-Phasen (siehe Abschn. 3.1).

14.19.2 Umgang mit Off-Phasen im Tagesablauf

Ist eine medikamentöse Veränderung nicht hilfreich, muss der Klient lernen, damit umzugehen und die Off-Phase in seinen Tagesablauf zu integrieren.

► Off-Phasen sind die Realität bei den meisten Menschen mit IPS im fortgeschrittenen Stadium. Es gilt, einen akzeptierenden Umgang damit zu finden.

Anstatt sich darüber zu ärgern und zu versuchen, den Alltag normal weiterlaufen zu lassen, ist es sinnvoll, die benötigte Zeit einzuplanen und so angenehm wie möglich zu gestalten. Einige Ideen zur Gestaltung der Off-Phase zu Hause:

- **Gemütliche Ecke einrichten**: Es kann ein bequemer Sessel an einen schönen Ort gestellt werden, zum Beispiel mit Blick ins Grüne oder zum Fernseher gerichtet. Der Sessel sollte hoch sein, um das Aufstehen zu erleichtern. Es können Dinge bereitgelegt werden, die in der Off-Phase griffbereit sein sollen, wie die Fernbedienung, ein Getränk, Essen, Buch, Lesebrille, Notizblock mit Stift, Radio, Notknopf, Telefon, Medikamente, Decke, … (s. Abb. 14.66)

- **Schlafen**: Da die Nächte meist unruhig sind, sind Schlafpausen am Tag oft notwendig. Eine solche kann absichtlich in die Off-Phase gelegt werden, in der Aktivsein ohnehin schwerfällt.
- **Entspannung**: Diese ruhige Phase kann ideal dazu genutzt werden, gelernte Entspannungstechniken anzuwenden oder zu meditieren. Dazu ist ein ruhiger Raum mit gedimmtem Licht und einer CD oder App zur Führung ideal.

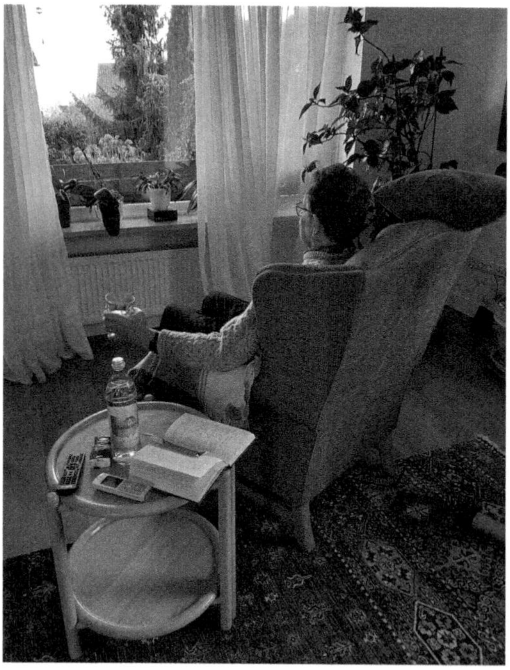

Abb. 14.66 Für die Off-Phasen kann ein gemütlicher Sitzplatz mit nützlichen und angenehmen Gegenständen bereitstehen

- **Gedankliche Einstellung**: Gelingt es dem Klienten, die Off-Phase positiv zu betrachten, ist die Gefahr geringer, ein psychisches Tief zu erleben. Betrachtet man die Off-Phase als einen Teil der Krankheit, die einem die Chance bietet, neue Erlebnisse zu erfahren, können die kleinen Dinge bewusst wahrgenommen werden. Ein Vogel auf dem Balkon, die Spur der Regentropfen auf dem Fenster oder der Text eines Liedes – plötzlich ist Zeit und Ruhe, um diese Dinge intensiv zu erleben.
- **Aktivitätsabbruch**: Bei überraschendem Eintreten in einen Off-Zustand ist ein Abbruch der aktuellen Tätigkeit meist sinnvoll. Auch wenn dies im ersten Moment eine Enttäuschung ist, gelingt eine erfolgreiche Durchführung von aktiven Betätigungen durch die Unbeweglichkeit schließlich selten und ist häufig mit Sturzgefahr verbunden. In sozialen Situationen kann es vorher angesprochen werden, dass ein plötzlicher Rückzug nötig sein könnte, um Missverständnisse zu vermeiden.

14.19.3 Off-Phase in Therapie

Wie in Abschn. 10.4 besprochen, ist die therapeutische Intervention in der On-Phase wesentlich effektiver und sollte, wenn möglich, immer in dieser Zeit geplant werden. Trotzdem kann es vorkommen, dass der Klient durch veränderte Medikamenteneinnahme oder Umstellung der Therapiezeit im Off zur Behandlung erscheint.

- **Betätigungsanalyse**: Nicht immer hat die Therapeutin die Chance, die Betätigung auch in der Off-Phase zu analysieren und muss sich mit Erzählungen und Beschreibung der Situation begnügen, z. B. wenn das morgendliche Aufstehen aus dem Bett eingeschränkt ist, die Therapie jedoch am Nachmittag durchgeführt wird. In dem Fall, dass der Klient in einer Off-Phase zur Therapie erscheint, kann die Betätigungsanalyse nachgeholt werden. Auch eine Intervention zum Thema „Welche Betätigungen fallen allgemein häufig in die Off-Phase und wie wird damit umgegangen?“ ist denkbar (für eine genaue Beschreibung der Durchführung der Betätigungsanalyse siehe Kap. 6).

- **Off-Management**: Dies bietet eine ideale Gelegenheit, über das Off-Management zu Hause zu sprechen. Eine Liste mit wichtigen Veränderungen für zu Hause kann erstellt werden, um ein angenehmeres Erlebnis im Off zu haben.
- **Entspannung**: Eine Entspannungs- oder Achtsamkeitsübung ist eine schöne Möglichkeit, die Off-Phase in der Therapie positiv zu nutzen.
- **Handmassage**: Eine Handmassage dient der Entspannung und stellt einen Kontakt zwischen Therapeutin und Patient her. Sensible und propriozeptive Reize wirken meist detonisierend (entspannend), dies hat überwiegend auch eine positive Wirkung auf die Stimmungslage.
  Anleitung: Zunächst sollte nachgefragt werden, ob beim Patienten Komorbiditäten in den Händen, wie Arthritis, Carpaltunnelsyndrom oder Nervenläsionen, bestehen, um die Massage adäquat anpassen zu können. Die Massage kann mit einem Aromaöl, einer festen Creme oder ohne durchgeführt werden. Der Patient sitzt in einer ihm angenehmen Haltung, der Arm wird locker auf einen Tisch, eine Armlehne oder das Bein der Therapeutin abgelegt. Es sollte darauf geachtet werden, dass die Schulter des Klienten entspannt ist.

  - Die Handfläche wird mit moderat festem Druck spiralförmig von der Mitte nach außen massiert, anschließend von außen nach innen. Die Bewegung sollte langsam erfolgen.
  - Dann streicht man, am Daumenballen beginnend, die Handfläche von innen zu den Fingern hin aus. Dabei sollte mit stetigem Druck gearbeitet werden.
  - Anschließend werden die Finger umfasst und vorsichtig einzeln nach distal ausgestrichen. Dabei kann etwas Zug ausgeübt werden, wenn es dem Klienten angenehm ist. Dies kann drei Mal wiederholt werden.
  - Danach werden mit mäßigem Druck die Endglieder der Finger und die Fingerkuppen kreisend massiert.
  - Zum Abschluss wird die Hand gedreht, sodass der Handrücken nach oben zeigt, und die Fingerzwischenräume werden mit dem Pinzettengriff ausgestrichen (siehe Video 14.67, Abb. 14.67).

- **Lagerung**: Eine angenehme Lagerung während des Offs kann zusammen mit den Angehörigen erarbeitet, besprochen und ausprobiert werden, um Schmerzen vorzubeugen und eine wohltuende Körperausrichtung zur Entspannung zu finden.
- **Angehörigenberatung**: Scheint der Klient sich in der Off-Phase nicht auf die Therapie einlassen zu können, bietet dies eine günstige Gelegenheit, mit den Angehörigen ins Gespräch zu kommen und sich gezielt Zeit für ihre Wünsche und Bedürfnisse zu nehmen.
  Nichtstun: Therapeutinnen sind liebend gerne im „Tun". Aktivität, Betätigung und Förderung – sind alles Begriffe, die in der Ergotherapie gelebt werden. So kann es große Überwindung kosten, „Nichtstun" als ergotherapeutisches Vorgehen umzusetzen (s. Abb. 14.68). In der Parkinson-Therapie ist dies ein wichtiges therapeutisches Werkzeug, das gut dosiert eingesetzt werden sollte, und umso wertvoller ist, je überzeugter es angewandt wird.
- Dazu gehört:
  – Gemeinsamkeit erleben
  – Die Natur genießen
  – Kaffee/Tee trinken

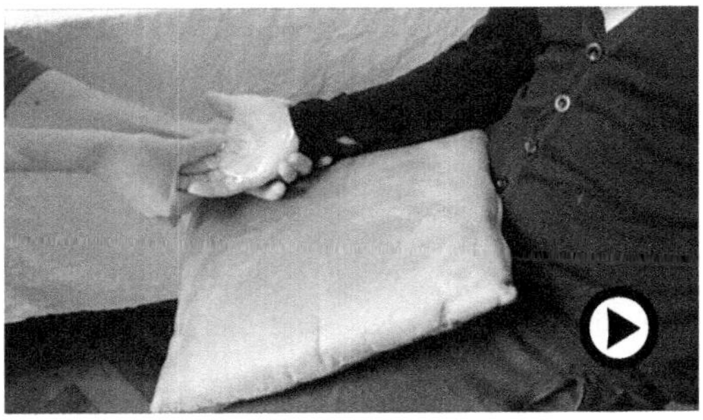

Abb. 14.67 Eine Handmassage kann eine gute Möglichkeit sein, dem Klienten etwas Angenehmes zu bieten, wenn dieser in der Off-Phase zur Therapie erscheint (▶ https://doi.org/10.1007/000-2y2)

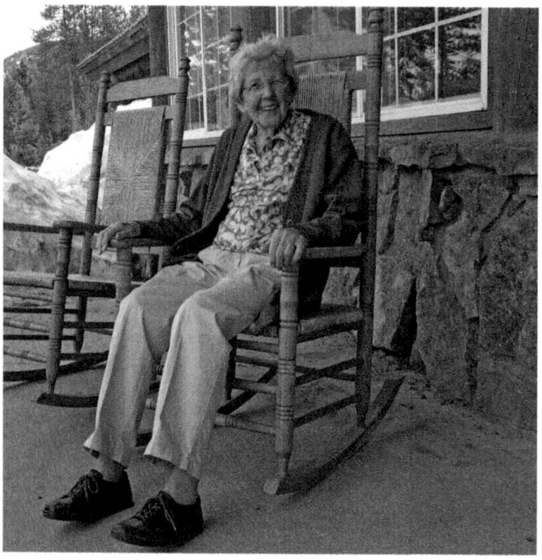

Abb. 14.68 In der Off-Phase können ruhige Momente des „Nichtstun" die optimale Therapie sein

- Fotos von lieben Menschen oder schönen Orten ansehen
- Lieblingsmusik hören
- Menschen beobachten
- …

Off-Phasen kommen nie gelegen. Sie unterbrechen den Fluss der Therapie, bremsen den Fortschritt und sind allgemein unerwünscht. Und doch sind sie eine Realität der Parkinson-Erkrankung, vor allem im fortgeschrittenen Stadium. Genauso wie es wichtig ist, dass der Patient diese Phasen akzeptiert, ist es auch für die Therapeutin vorteilhaft, entspannt damit umzugehen. Gelingt es der Therapeutin, einen Schritt zurück zu machen und die Off-Phase als Perspektivwechsel und Chance zu sehen, entlastet das Klient und Therapeutin gleichermaßen und neue Wege können entdeckt werden.

Beispiel

Jetzt bringt's nichts mehr aufzuräumen. Frau P. lässt das Kehrblech und die Scherben auf dem Boden liegen. Langsam hangelt sie sich an der Küchenzeile entlang zur Wand, von dort in Zeitlupe zu ihrem Off-Sessel. Endlich! Angekommen! Normalerweise versucht sie noch in der On-Phase den Sessel zu erreichen. Zu oft ist sie auf dem Weg gestürzt. Sie entspannt sich – macht den CD-Player an und lässt Tschaikowskis „Süßer Traum" über sich hinweg plätschern. Ein Saft und ein Schälchen mit Nüssen stehen schon bereit und auch das Telefon steht in greifbarer Nähe. ◀

14.20 Schreiben

Beispiel

Frau S. war immer stolz auf ihre gleichmäßige schöne Schrift und bekam häufig Komplimente. Das Schreiben fand sich in allen Bereichen ihres Alltags wieder – in ihrem Beruf als Sekretärin, in den langen Briefen, die sie leidenschaftlich gern an Familie und Freundinnen verfasste, und fast jeden Tag ihres Lebens in ihrem persönlichen Tagebuch, wo sie Erlebtes festhielt und Gedanken ordnete. Seit der Parkinson in ihr Leben trat, nahm nicht nur die Lust am Schreiben ab, sondern vor allem die Enttäuschung am Resultat zu. Diese ungelenke Mini-Schrift sollte ihre sein? Also ließ sie es einfach sein. ◀

14.20.1 Schreiben mit M. Parkinson

Die Betätigung „Schreiben" wird im COPM sehr häufig von Klientinnen als Ziel gewählt. Das Schreiben mit Stift und Papier ist vielen Menschen ein persönliches Anliegen. Darin sind Erinnerungen ans Briefe schreiben an Freunde und Familie geknüpft sowie die Notwendigkeit, Formulare auszufüllen, Einkaufszettel oder andere Notizen zu schreiben und Verträge u. Ä. zu unterschreiben. Nicht selten erschrecken Klientinnen mit M. Parkinson, wenn sie etwas soeben Geschriebenes ansehen. „Früher hatte ich eine schöne Schrift." oder „Das kann man ja kaum noch lesen." sind häufige Aussprüche.

▶ Obwohl sie im Nachhinein erkennen, dass ihre Schrift unleserlich ist, ist es für die meisten Betroffenen während des Schreibprozesses nicht möglich, ihre Schrift zu verändern.

Bestenfalls gelingt das „Großschreiben" beim ersten Wort noch, danach, wenn der Automatismus des Schreibens im gesunden Gehirn einsetzt, ist das Parkinson-Gehirn überfordert. Dies wirkt sich negativ auf das Schriftbild aus. Es kommt zu drei Parkinson-typischen Merkmalen:

1. Im Anfangsstadium ist die reduzierte Flüssigkeit des Schreibens beobachtbar. Der **Schreibfluss** wird unterbrochen, die Schrift wirkt ungleichmäßig.
2. Außerdem nimmt die **Schreibgeschwindigkeit** ab.
3. Die **Mikrografie** ist am bekanntesten und tritt meist in späteren Stadien des M. Parkinsons auf. Sie besteht aus immer kleiner werdenden Buchstaben, bis hin zur Unleserlichkeit, und endet manchmal in einem Strich, ohne jegliche Schwünge.

In einer Studie von Nackaerts (2016) konnte gezeigt werden, dass ein **Amplitudentraining** sich positiv auf die Schriftgröße, jedoch negativ auf Schnelligkeit und Schreibfluss auswirkt. Es kommt zu einem sog. Trade-off. Anders als bei gesunden Versuchspersonen verbessert sich nur einer der drei Faktoren (Schnelligkeit, Schreibfluss oder Schriftgröße). Je nachdem, auf welchen Faktor der Fokus während des Trainings und des Schreibens gelegt wird, verbessert sich dieser Faktor, die anderen beiden bleiben gleich oder verschlechtern sich etwas. Die Schriftgröße wurde als der Faktor identifiziert, der sich am meisten auf die Leserlichkeit des Geschriebenen auswirkt. Aus diesem Grund setzt das Schreibtraining an diesem Punkt an. Die Flüssigkeit und Schnelligkeit sollten bewusst **nicht** trainiert werden, weil es sich sonst negativ auf die Leserlichkeit auswirkt.

14.20.2 Vorbereitung des Kontexts

Um das bestmögliche Resultat beim Schreiben zu erhalten, ist es vorteilhaft, den Kontext vorzubereiten.

- **Realer Kontext**: Das Schreibtraining sollte möglichst im Kontext (Büro, Küchentisch …) der Klientin durchgeführt werden, um die realen Kontextfaktoren sofort mit einbeziehen zu können (Höhe des Stuhls, Ordnung auf Schreibfläche, Lichteinfall …) (siehe Abb. 14.69).

- **Sitzposition**: Der Stuhl sollte fest und so nah am Tisch stehen, dass die Klientin die Unterarme entspannt auf dem Tisch ablegen kann. Die Sitzhöhe sollte mindestens einen 90° Winkel in Knie- und Hüftgelenk gewährleisten. Die Füße stehen fest auf dem Boden. Der Oberkörper ist aufgerichtet,

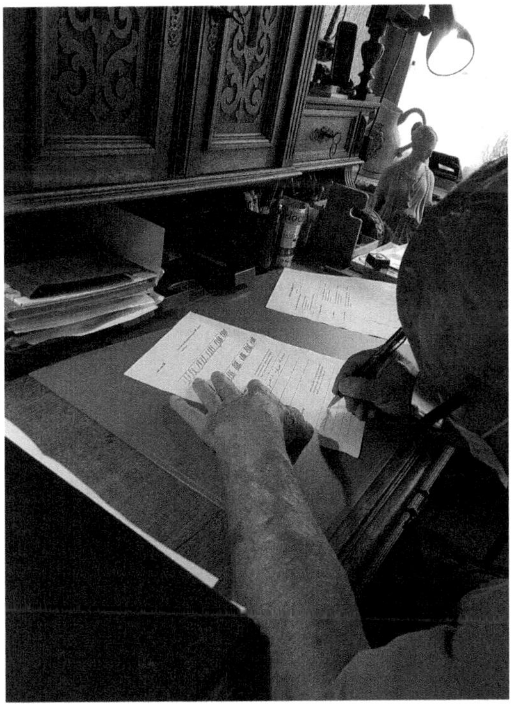

Abb. 14.69 Schreibtraining wird im realen Kontext des Klienten, seinem Büro, durchgeführt

wenn möglich, sollte die Rückenlehne nicht genutzt werden.

- **Tischhöhe**: Die Höhe des Tisches sollte sicherstellen, dass sich die Unterarme locker auf den Tisch ablegen lassen.
- **Beleuchtung**: Eine ausreichende Beleuchtung sollte gewährleistet sein, da viele Parkinson-Klientinnen verschiedenartige Einschränkungen des Visus zeigen, welche durch mangelnde Beleuchtung noch verstärkt werden.
- **Keine Ablenkung**: Der Schreibprozess stellt für viele Menschen mit der Parkinson-Erkrankung eine große Herausforderung dar. Wenn noch ablenkende Faktoren dazukommen, scheitert die Betätigung häufig daran. Folgende potenzielle Ablenkungen sollten vermieden und mit Angehörigen besprochen werden:
  - Radio/Musik
  - Laufender Fernseher
  - (Mobil-) Telefon
  - Gespräche
  - Andere Personen im Raum
  - Zeitdruck durch Termin

14.20.3 Schreibtraining

Im Allgemeinen führen intensive Übungen mit einer großen Amplitude zu einer Verbesserung der Bradykinese und auch im Alltag zu einer Vergrößerung der Amplitude beim Schreiben. Deswegen sind Schwungübungen mit Referenzflächen eine sinnvolle Vorbereitung für das Schreibtraining (s. Tab. 14.13).

Prinzipien des Schreibtrainings bei M. Parkinson

1. Größe trainieren, nicht Schnelligkeit
2. Nach jeder Übung – Pause
3. Keine Ablenkung
4. Täglich drei Mal wiederholen (hohe Repetition)
5. Möglichst in realem Kontext (Büro, Küchentisch …)

14.20.4 Schreiben im Alltag

Prinzipien für das Schreiben bei M. Parkinson

1. Auf Größe der Schrift konzentrieren, nicht auf Schnelligkeit
2. Kurze Schreibblöcke – Pause (Chunking)
3. Liniertes Papier (nicht kleiner als 1 cm Abstand)
4. Evtl. Druckschrift besser lesbar
5. Keine Ablenkung

Linien als visuelle Cues
Jedes Papier, auf dem die Klientin schreibt (Einkaufszettel, Tagebuch, Brief), sollte liniert sein. Der Linienabstand muss 1 cm oder mehr betragen.

Tab. 14.13 Schreibtraining

Schreibtraining			
Vorbereitung	Durchführung	Wiederholungen	
1. **Hand-Arm Transport** Referenzflächen mit Tape auf Tisch markieren, links und rechts 50 cm von Körpermitte.	Mit Schreibhand von links nach rechts über Tisch fahren bis zu den Referenzflächen. Therapeut zählt laut mit	20 Mal	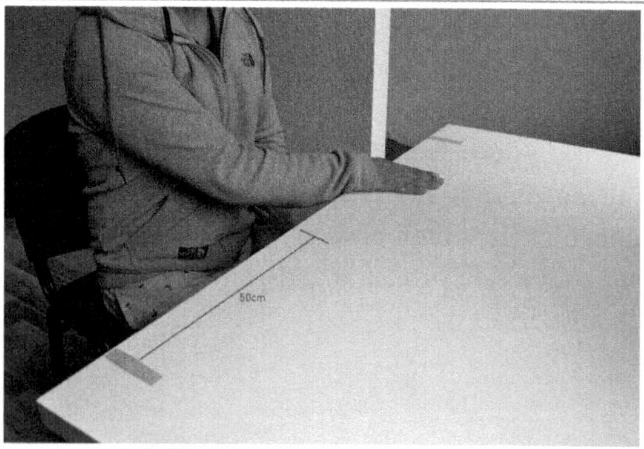

Tab. 14.13 (Fortsetzung)

Schreibtraining			
2. **Handgelenk Flex.-Ext.** Unterarm auf Tisch ablegen, Schreibhand auf äußere Handkante stellen. Zwei Referenzflächen (z. B. Bücher) neben Hand aufstellen, sodass sie bei Palmarflexion (ca. 90°) bzw. Dorsalextension (ca. 45°) berührt werden.	Mit Schreibhand die Referenzflächen abwechselnd berühren. Therapeut zählt laut mit	20 Mal	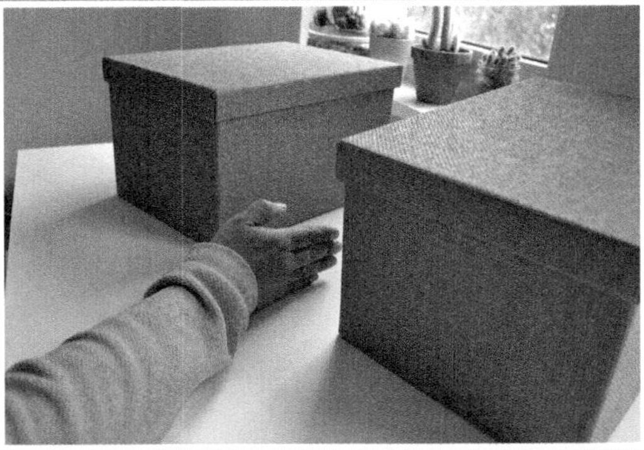
3. **Finger vor – zurück** Bleistift, Blatt mit zwei Punkten (2 cm Durchmesser) senkrecht übereinander (4 cm voneinander entfernt)	Stift zwischen Punkten hin- und herführen. Bewegung kommt aus den Fingern	20 Mal	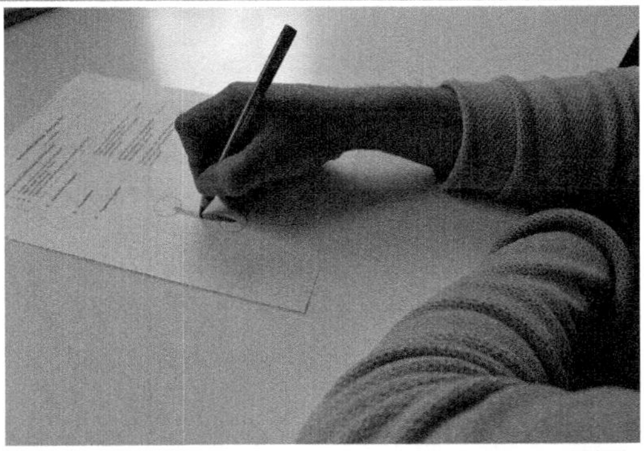
4. **Zwei Zeilen** llll Bleistift, Blatt mit Linien (3 cm Abstand)	Vier zusammen-hängende l schreiben, absetzen, wiederholen	2 Zeilen	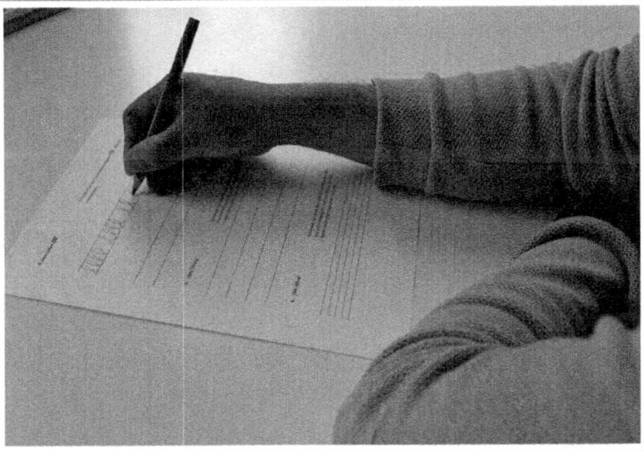
5. **Satz-Übung** Bleistift, Blatt mit Linien (3 cm Abstand)	Beliebiger Satz aus Alltag der Klientin (mit 4–8 Wörtern) schreiben, dabei strikt auf Linienberührung achten. z. B. „mit freundlichen Grüßen *Name*“	Je nach Länge des Satzes	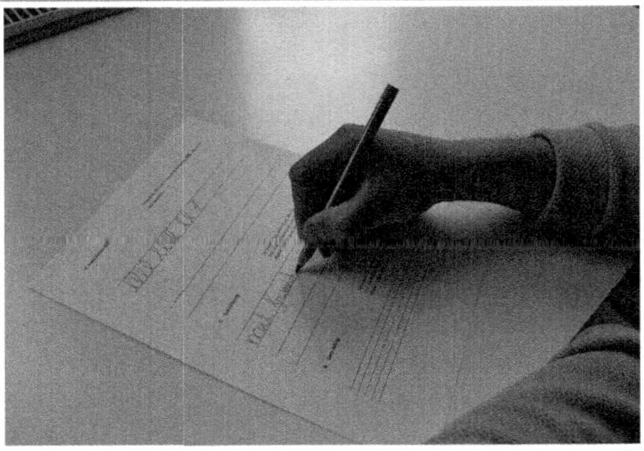

Tab. 14.13 (Fortsetzung)

Schreibtraining			
6. **Satz Alltag** Stift der Klientin (Kugelschreiber, Tintenroller …), Blatt mit Linien (1 cm Abstand)	Beliebiger Satz aus Alltag der Klientin (mit 4–8 Wörtern) schreiben, dabei strikt auf Linienberührung achten	Je nach Länge des Satzes	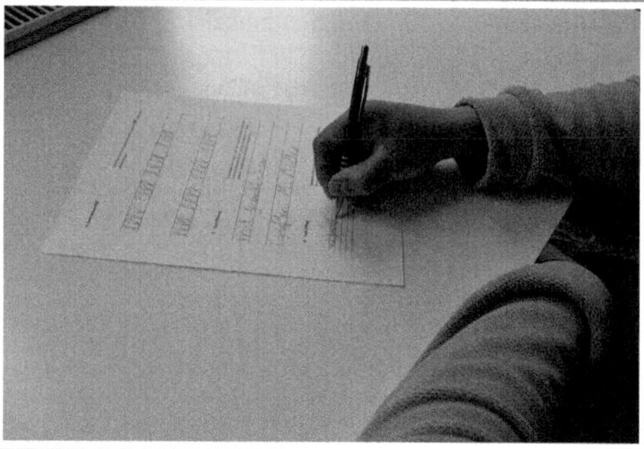

Beim Schreiben wird die Klientin dazu aufgefordert, die Buchstaben immer oben und unten an die Linien „stoßen" zu lassen (siehe Abb. 14.70).

Nackaerts et al. stellten in einer Studie (2015) fest, dass sich beim Schreiben mit Linien mit einem kleinerem Abstand als 1 cm die Schrift sogar verschlechterte. In diesem Fall wirkt sich das Cueing also negativ aus.

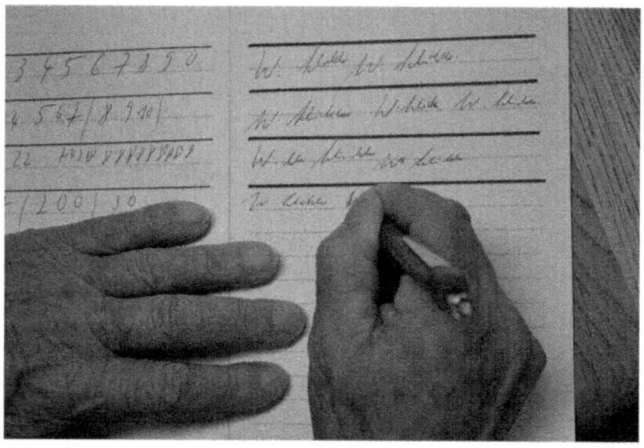

Abb. 14.70 Liniertes Papier oder sogar verstärkte Linien dienen dem Klienten als Cueing oder Referenzfläche, um größer und dadurch leserlicher zu schreiben

Druckschrift

Da die Betätigung „Schreiben" automatisiert ist, was bei Parkinson-Betroffenen zu Problemen führt, kann ein neues Betätigungsmuster genutzt werden. Auf diese Weise wird die Bewegungsdurchführung etwas anders initiiert und es kommt nicht zur Mikrografie. Zwei mögliche Arten eines neuen Betätigungsmusters beim Schreiben sind Großbuchstaben und das Halten des Stiftes in einer ungewohnten Haltung (z. B. zwischen 3. Und 4. Finger) (siehe Video 14.71, Abb. 14.71 und 14.72).

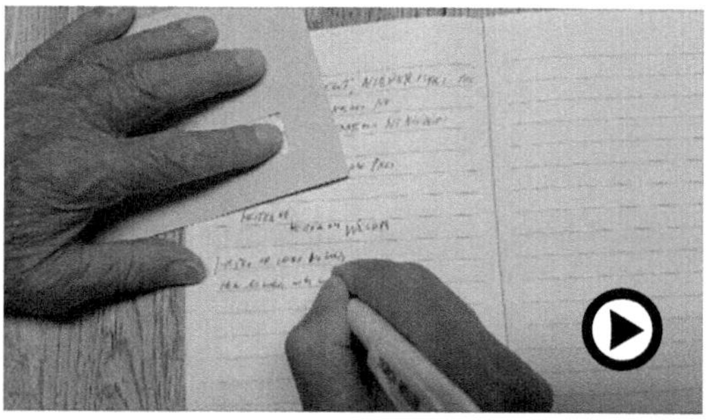

Abb. 14.71 Die Schrift des Klienten ist unleserlich, wenn weder die Linien, noch Druckschrift genutzt werden (▶ https://doi.org/10.1007/000-2y3)

Chunking/Entkoppelung, um Dual-Tasking zu vermeiden

Beobachtet der Therapeut, dass die Klientin beim Schreiben vermehrt ins Stocken gerät, zur Mikrografie neigt oder viele Schreibfehler macht, kann dies mit einer Überlastung durch Dual-Tasking zusammenhängen. Das Schreiben ist nicht nur eine motorisch sehr anspruchsvolle Tätigkeit, sondern verlangt auch, gleichzeitig ein Wort korrekt niederzuschreiben und das nächste zu planen. Dieses Multitasking verlässt sich in hohem Maße auf die Automatisierung der Schreibbewegung. Um dieses Problem zu beheben, kann durch Chunking das Dual-Tasking vermieden werden. Zunächst werden wenige Wörter oder

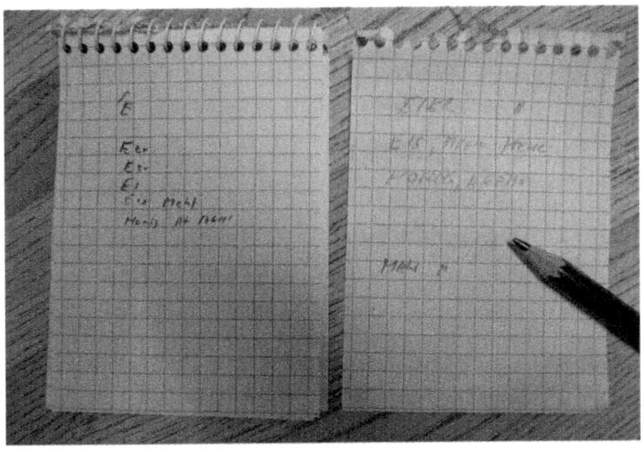

Abb. 14.72 Einkaufszettel ohne und mit Großbuchstaben

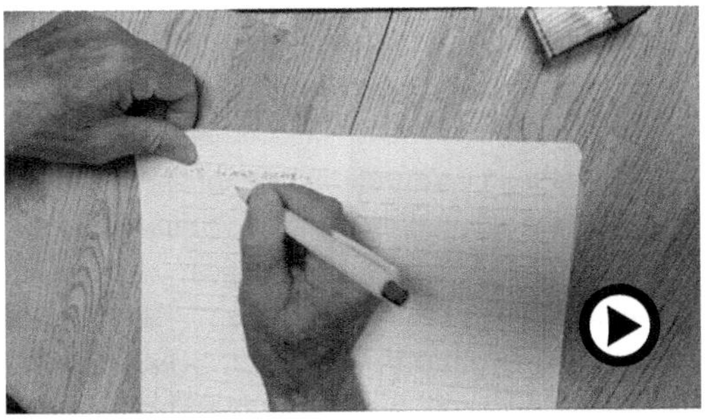

Abb. 14.73 Chunking: Nach wenigen Buchstaben setzt der Klient den Stift ab, pausiert kurz, schreibt dann weiter (▶ https://doi.org/10.1007/000-2xb)

Buchstaben geplant, dann erst wird der Stift aufgenommen, die Wörter werden geschrieben, anschließend werden die nächsten Wörter oder Buchstaben geplant (siehe Abb. 14.73). Auf diese Weise wird der kognitive Prozess teilweise von der motorischen Umsetzung entkoppelt. Zur Vereinfachung der Unterbrechung kann die **Fenstermethode** genutzt werden. Es wird ein Fenster in ein Stück Tonpapier geschnitten, in das die entsprechende Anzahl von Buchstaben oder Wörtern passen. Die Klientin muss zum Weiterschreiben kurz pausieren, um das Fenster weiterzurücken. Der Automatismus wird unterbrochen (s. Video 14.73/Abb. 14.73, Video 14.74/Abb. 14.74).

LSVT BIG als Vorbereitung

Laut einer Untersuchung ist ein intensives Amplitudentraining nach LSVT BIG als Vorbereitung zum Schreiben sinnvoll, da die Schrift auch sechs Wochen später größer ist als ohne das Training.

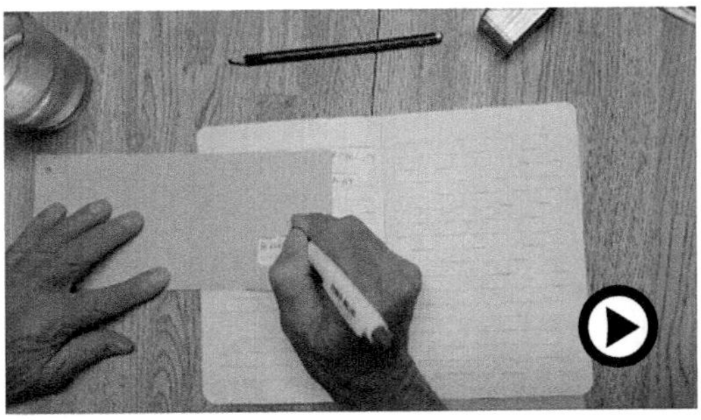

Abb. 14.74 Mit der Fenstermethode kann das Chunking unterstützt werden (▶ https://doi.org/10.1007/000-2y5)

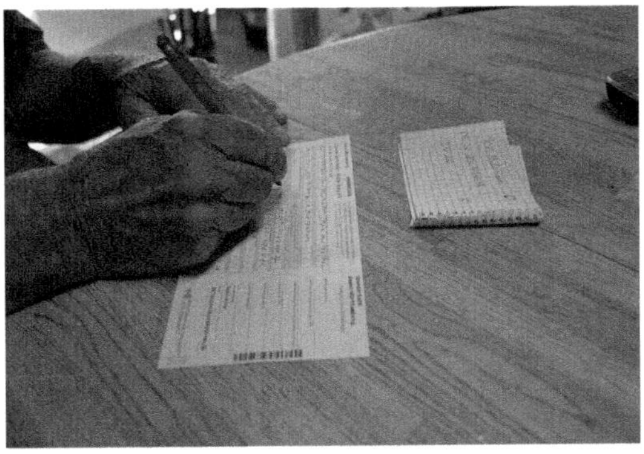

Abb. 14.75 Überweisungen ausfüllen, als Teil des Schreibtrainings

Das LSVT BIG darf nur von Therapeuten durchgeführt werden, die an der Fortbildung dazu teilgenommen haben (für weitere Informationen siehe Abschn. 14.1.6).

Übertrag in Alltag

Nach dem Schreibtraining muss das Schreiben grundsätzlich in die wichtige Betätigung der Klientin übertragen werden. War das Ziel der Klientin, wieder selbständig Überweisungen ausfüllen zu können, muss dies umgesetzt werden. Dabei fallen oftmals neue Schwierigkeiten auf, zum Beispiel die sehr kleinen Kästchen einer Überweisung (siehe Abb. 14.75).

Unterschrift

Viele Klientinnen mit M. Parkinson zeigen eine stark verkleinerte Unterschrift. Da die Unterschrift wohl die wichtigste Betätigung beim Schreiben darstellt, ist es sinnvoll, diese bei Schreibproblemen immer gezielt zu üben. Dazu

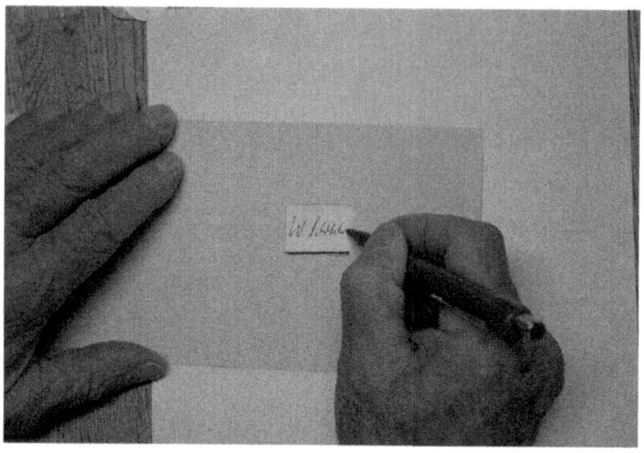

Abb. 14.76 Fenstermethode um Unterschrift größer zu schreiben

können verstärkt nachgezogene Linien hilfreich sein. In der Situation, in der die Unterschrift ohne Hilfslinien geleistet werden muss, kann die Fenstermethode helfen (siehe Abb. 14.76). Es wird ein Fenster in ein Stück Tonpapier geschnitten. Die Klientin nutzt die Ränder als Referenzlinien, um die Unterschrift größer durchführen zu können.

Schreiben mit Tremor

Mit einem Tremor zu schreiben ist in vielen Fällen nicht möglich. Je nach Ausprägung des Tremors können folgende Tipps ausprobiert werden.

- **Vergrößerung der Auflagefläche**: Durch Abstützen des gesamten Unterarms kann der Tremor evtl. abgeschwächt werden.
- **Entspannung**: Da Stress und Anspannung den Tremor verstärken, kann eine Entspannungsübung vor dem Schreiben und eine allgemein entspannte Atmosphäre die Leserlichkeit verbessern.
- **Gewichtsmanschetten/beschwerter Stift**: Das Tragen von Gewichtsmanschetten oder die Nutzung eines beschwerten Stifts, kann die Schrift leserlicher machen.
- **Festhalten mit anderer Hand**: Auch eine Stabilisierung, durch Festhalten des Unterarms der Schreibhand, kann unterstützend sein.

Hilfsmittel

Dickere und **schwerere Stifte**, die besser in der Hand liegen, können für Menschen mit M. Parkinson eine große Hilfe sein. Adaptationen (siehe Abschn. 15.3) erleichtern das Halten des Stifts und der Tonus lässt nach, wodurch häufig flüssigeres Schreiben ermöglicht wird. **Tintenroller** wirken sich meist positiv auf den Schreibfluss aus, da auch bei leichtem Druck ein klarer Strich gezogen wird. Durch die Nutzung einer **Griffverdickung** wird eine Erhöhung des Tonus vermieden.

Beispiel

Jetzt schreibt Frau S. wieder täglich. Natürlich nicht so viel wie früher, aber sie hat mithilfe der Ergotherapeutin herausgefunden, was ihr am wichtigsten ist – das Tagebuchschreiben. Um sich nicht zu überfordern, beginnt sie damit, zunächst täglich nur ein bis zwei „Stimmungswörter" in das Tagebuch einzutragen, z. B. „alles blüht", „langweilig", „Kreislauf", „hoffnungsvoll". Täglich macht sie jetzt ihr Schreibtraining und achtet darauf, generell aktiv zu bleiben, weil sie jetzt weiß, dass ihre allgemeine Beweglichkeit sich positiv aufs Schriftbild auswirkt. Und tatsächlich – ihr Mann kann die Einkaufszettel wieder gut lesen, die sie ihm schreibt. ◄

Literatur und weiterführende Literatur

Aarsland D, Creese B, Politis M, Chaudhuri KR, Ffytche DH, Weintraub D, Ballard C (2017) Cognitive decline in Parkinson disease. Nat Rev Neurol 13(4):217–231. https://doi.org/10.1038/nrneurol. Epub 3. PMID: 28257128; PMCID: PMC5643027

Adamovich SV, Berkinblit MB, Hening W, Sage J, Poizner H (2001) The interaction of visual and proprioceptive inputs in pointing to actual and remembered targets in Parkinson's disease. Neuroscience 104(4):1027–1041. https://doi.org/10.1016/s0306-4522(01)00099-9. PMID: 11457588

Allen NE, Schwarzel AK, Canning CG (2013) Recurrent falls in Parkinson's disease: a systematic review. Parkinsons Dis 2013:906274, 16 pages. https://doi.org/10.1155/2013/906274j

Aman JE, Elangovan N, Yeh IL, Konczak J (2015) The effectiveness of proprioceptive training for improving motor function: a systematic review. Front Hum Neurosci 28(8):1075. https://doi.org/10.3389/fnhum.2014.01075. PMID: 25674059; PMCID: PMC4309156

Angelopoulou E, Anagnostouli M, Chrousos GP, Bougea A (2020) Massage therapy as a complementary treatment for Parkinson's disease: a systematic literature review. Complement Ther Med 49:102340. https://doi.org/10.1016/j.ctim.2020.102340. Epub 2020 Feb 6. PMID: 32147033

Arzu G, Colakoglu B, Bilge K, Cakmur R (2012) Evaluation of the effects of home-based deep breathing exercises in Parkinson's disease patients. Arch Neuropsychiatry 49:59–62. https://doi.org/10.4274/npa.y6209

Asano M, Finlayson ML (2014) Meta-analysis of three different types of fatigue management interventions for people with multiple sclerosis: exercise, education, and medication. Mult Scler Int 2014:798285. https://doi.org/10.1155/2014/798285. Epub 14. PMID: 24963407; PMCID: PMC4052049

Baille G, Chenivesse C, Perez T, Machuron F, Dujardin K, Devos D, Defebvre L, Moreau C (2018) Dyspnea: an underestimated symptom in Parkinson's disease. Parkinsonism Relat Disord 60. https://doi.org/10.1016/j.parkreldis.2018.09.001

Balleine B, O'Doherty J (2010) Human and rodent homologies in action control: corticostriatal determinants of goal-directed and habitual action. Neuropsychopharmacology 35:48–69. https://doi.org/10.1038/npp.2009.131

Bartolo M, Serrao M, Tassorelli C, Don R, Ranavolo A, Draicchio F, Pacchetti C, Buscone S, Perrotta A, Furnari A, Bramanti P, Padua L, Pierelli F, Sandrini G (2010) Four-week trunk-specific rehabilitation treatment improves lateral trunk flexion in Parkinson's disease. Mov Disord 25(3):325–331. https://doi.org/10.1002/mds.23007. PMID: 20131386

Benatru I, Vaugoyeau M, Azulay JP (2008) Postural disorders in Parkinson's disease. Neurophysiol Clin 38(6):459–465. https://doi.org/10.1016/j.neucli.07.006. Epub 2008 Aug 21. PMID: 19026965

Blakemore R, MacAskill M, Myall D, Anderson T (2019) Volitional suppression of Parkinsonian resting tremor. Mov Disord Clin Pract 6:470–478. https://doi.org/10.1002/mdc3.12801

Braak H, Del Tredici K, Rüb U, de Vos R, Jansen Steur E, Braak E (2003) Staging of brain pathology related to sporadic Parkinson's disease. Neurobiol Aging 24(2):197–211. https://doi.org/10.1016/s0197-4580(02)00065-9. PMID: 12498954

Bronner G, Royter V, Korczyn A, Giladi N (2004) Sexual dysfunction in Parkinson's disease. J Sex Marital Ther 30(2):95–105. https://doi.org/10.1080/00926230490258893

Brown R, Jahanshahi M (1995) Depression in Parkinson's disease: a psychosocial viewpoint. Adv Neurol 65:61–84. PMID: 7872153

Butterfield L (2013) Apathy in Parkinson's disease: a behavioral intervention study. Graduate theses and dissertations. https://scholarcommons.usf.edu/etd/4873

Butterfield LC, Cimino CR, Salazar R, Sanchez-Ramos J, Bowers D, Okun MS (2017) The Parkinson's Active Living (PAL) program: a behavioral intervention targeting apathy in Parkinson's disease. J Geriatr Psychiatry Neurol 30(1):11–25. https://doi.org/10.1177/0891988716673467

Caballos-Baumann AO, Ebersbach G, George S, Mainka S, Mallien G, Pichler K, Schroeteler F, Tuschkan S, Wagner-Sonntag E, Ziegler K (2018) Aktivierende Therapien bei Parkinson-Syndromen. Thieme, Stuttgart/New York

Calne D, Stoessl A (1986) Early parkinsonism. Clin Neuropharmacol Suppl 2:S3–S8. PMID: 3297316

Canning CG (2005) The effect of directing attention during walking under dual-task conditions in Parkinson's disease. Parkinsonism Relat Disord 11(2):95–99. https://doi.org/10.1016/j.parkreldis.2004.09.006. ISSN 1353-8020

Cochen De Cock V, Bayard S, Jaussent I, Charif M, Grini M, Langenier M, Yu H, Lopez R, Geny C, Carlander B, Dauvilliers Y (2014) Daytime sleepiness in Parkinson's disease: a reappraisal. PLoS One 9(9):e107278. https://doi.org/10.1371/journal.pone.0107278

Contreras A, Grandas F (2012) Risk of falls in Parkinson's disease: a cross-sectional study of 160 patients. Parkinsons Dis 2012:362572. https://doi.org/10.1155/2012/362572. Epub 15. PMID: 22292126; PMCID: PMC3265111

Cruise KE, Bucks RS, Loftus AM, Newton RU, Pegoraro R, Thomas MG (2011) Exercise and Parkinson's: benefits for cognition and quality of life. Acta Neurol Scand 123(1):13–19. https://doi.org/10.1111/j.1600-0404.2010.01338.x. PMID: 20199518

Csoti I (2002) Restless Legs und Morbus Parkinson. Der Multimorbide Parkinsonpatient:17–27. https://doi.org/10.1007/978-3-642-57512-9_2

Cummings JL (1988) Intellectual impairment in Parkinson's disease: clinical, pathologic, and biochemical correlates. J Geriatr Psychiatry Neurol 1(1):24–36. https://doi.org/10.1177/089198878800100106. PMID: 2908099

Cury R, Galhardoni R, Fonoff E, Perez Lloret S, Dos Santos Ghilardi M, Barbosa E, Teixeira M, Ciampi de Andrade D (2016) Sensory abnormalities and pain in Parkinson disease and its modulation by treatment of motor symptoms. Eur J Pain 20(2):151–165. https://doi.org/10.1002/ejp.745. Epub 2015 Jul 6. PMID: 26147660

Cusso ME, Donald KJ, Khoo TK (2016) The impact of physical activity on non-motor symptoms in Parkinson's disease: a systematic review. Front Med (Lausanne) 3:35

Deuschl G, Bain P, Brin M (1998) Consensus statement of the movement disorder society on tremor. Ad hoc scientific committee. Mov Disord 13(Suppl 3):2–23. https://doi.org/10.1002/mds.870131303. PMID: 9827589

Deuschl G, Oertel W, Reichmann H (2016) Leitlinien für Diagnostik und Therapie in der Neurologie Idiopathisches Parkinson-Syndrom Entwicklungsstufe: S3 Kurzversion, DGN

Dixon L, Duncan D, Johnson P, Kirkby L, O'Connell H, Taylor H, Deane KH (2007) Occupational therapy for patients with Parkinson's disease. Cochrane Database Syst Rev 2007(3):CD002813. https://doi.org/10.1002/14651858.CD002813.pub2. PMID: 17636709; PMCID: PMC6991932

Doherty KM, van de Warrenburg BP, Peralta MC, Silveira-Moriyama L, Azulay JP, Gershanik OS, Bloem BR (2011) Postural deformities in Parkinson's disease. Lancet Neurol 10(6):538–549. https://doi.org/10.1016/S1474-4422(11)70067-9. Epub 2011 Apr 22. PMID: 21514890

Ebersbach G (2008) Depressive Störungen bei der Parkinson Erkrankung, Definition – Diagnose – Behandlung NeuroGeriatrie 5(4):146–153. Hippocampus, Bad Honnef

Ebersbach G, Ebersbach A, Edler D, Kaufhold O, Kusch M, Kupsch A, Wissel J (2010) Comparing exercise in Parkinson's disease – the Berlin LSVT®BIG study. Mov Disord 25(12):1902–1908. https://doi.org/10.1002/mds.23212. Erratum in: Mov Disord.;25(14):2478. PMID: 20669294

Ehgoetz Martens KA, Ellard CG, Almeida QJ (2014) Does anxiety cause freezing of gait in Parkinson's disease? PLoS One 9(9):e106561. https://doi.org/10.1371/journal.pone.0106561. PMID: 25250691; PMCID: PMC4175083

Fernandez L, Huys R, Issartel J, Azulay JP, Eusebio A (2018) Movement speed-accuracy trade-off in Parkinson's disease. Front Neurol 9:897. https://doi.org/10.3389/fneur.2018.00897. PMID: 30405521; PMCID: PMC6208126

Foster ER, Bedekar M, Tickle-Degnen L (2014) Systematic review of the effectiveness of occupational therapy-related interventions for people with Parkinson's disease. Am J Occup Ther 68(1):39–49. https://doi.org/10.5014/ajot.2014.008706. PMID: 24367954; PMCID: PMC4413458

Frenkel-Toledo S, Giladi N, Peretz C, Herman T, Gruendlinger L, Hausdorff JM (2005) Effect of gait speed on gait rhythmicity in Parkinson's disease: variability of stride time and swing time respond differently. J Neuroeng Rehabil 2:23. Published 2005 Jul 31. https://doi.org/10.1186/1743-0003-2-23

GBD (2016) Parkinson's Disease Collaborators. Global, regional, and national burden of Parkinson's disease, 1990–2016: a systematic analysis for the Global Burden of Disease Study 2016. Lancet Neurol 17(11):939–953. https://doi.org/10.1016/S1474-4422(18)30295-3. Epub 2018 Oct 1. PMID: 30287051; PMCID: PMC6191528

Giuffrida R, Vingerhoets FJ, Bogousslavsky J, Ghika J (2005) Syndromes douloureux de la maladie de Parkinson [Pain in Parkinson's disease]. Rev Neurol (Paris) 161(4):407–418. https://doi.org/10.1016/s0035--3787(05)85070-2. PMID: 15924076

Glosser G, Wolfe N, Kliner-Krenzel L, Albert ML (1994) Cross-cultural cognitive examination performance in patients with Parkinson's disease and Alzheimer's disease. J Nerv Ment Dis 182(8):432–436. https://doi.org/10.1097/00005053-199408000-00002. PMID: 8040652

Goldman JG, Postuma R (2014) Premotor and nonmotor features of Parkinson's disease. Curr Opin Neurol 27(4):434–441. https://doi.org/10.1097/WCO.0000000000000112. PMID: 24978368; PMCID: PMC4181670

Grossmann J, Pirker W (2004) Klinik und Therapie der Parkinson-Psychose. J Neurol Neurochir Psychiatr 5:42–49

Hacke W, Mair J, Berg D (2019) Neurologie. Springer, Berlin, S 47–51, 96, 589–604

Harrison EC, Horin AP, Earhart GM (2018) Internal cueing improves gait more than external cueing in healthy adults and people with Parkinson disease. Sci Rep 8:15525. https://doi.org/10.1038/s41598-018-33942-6

van der Heide A, Speckens A, Meinders M, Rosenthal L, Bloem B, Helmich R (2021) Stress and mindfulness in Parkinson's disease – a survey in 5000 patients. npj Parkinsons Dis 7:1–10. https://doi.org/10.1038/s41531-020-00152-9

Hemmerle AM, Herman JP, Seroogy KB (2012) Stress, depression and Parkinson's disease. Exp Neurol 233(1):79–86. https://doi.org/10.1016/j.expneurol.2011.09.035. Epub 2011 Oct 6. PMID: 22001159; PMCID: PMC3268878

Henning M, Myers S, Ooton C, Semaan J, Xia R (2017) EC NEUROLOGY review article effectiveness of exercise on reducing fatigue in Parkinson's disease: a systematic review. EC Neurol 9:12–19

Hersche R, Weise A, Barbero M, Kool J (2017) Menschen mit MS-bedingter Fatigue: Entwicklung und Evaluation einer Energiemanagement-Schulung (EMS) bei Menschen mit MS-bedingter Fatigue. Ein Forschungsprojekt. Ergotherapie (10):S.20–22

van Hilten J, Weggeman M, van der Velde E, Kerkhof G, van Dijk J, Roos R (1993) Sleep, excessive daytime sleepiness and fatigue in Parkinson's disease. J Neural Transm Park Dis Dement Sect 5(3):235–244. https://doi.org/10.1007/BF02257678. PMID: 8369103

Hubbard IJ, Parsons MW, Neilson C, Carey LM (2009) Task-specific training: evidence for and translation to clinical practice. Occup Ther Int 16(3–4):175–189. https://doi.org/10.1002/oti.275. PMID: 19504501

ICD-10-GM Version (2018) Kapitel V, Psychische und Verhaltensstörungen (F00-F99) Affektive Störungen (F30-F39)

Isaacson S, Skettini J (2014) Neurogenic orthostatic hypotension in Parkinson's disease: evaluation, management, and emerging role of droxidopa. Vasc Health Risk Manag 10:169–176. https://doi.org/10.2147/VHRM.S53983. Published 2014 Apr 3

Jacobs JV, Nutt JG, Carlson-Kuhta P, Stephens M, Horak FB (2009) Knee trembling during freezing of gait represents multiple anticipatory postural adjustments.

Exp Neurol 215(2):334–341. https://doi.org/10.1016/j.expneurol.2008.10.019

Jankovic J (2005) Motor fluctuations and dyskinesias in Parkinson's disease: clinical manifestations. Mov Disord 20(Suppl 11):11–16. https://doi.org/10.1002/mds.20458. PMID: 15822109

Jöbges M (2008) Physiotherapie bei Patienten mit idiopathischem Parkinson-Syndrom. NeuroGeriatrie 5(4):169–173

Jöbges M, Heuschkel G, Pretzel C, Illhardt C, Renner C, Hummelsheim H (2004) Repetitive training of compensatory steps: a therapeutic approach for postural instability in Parkinson's disease. J Neurol Neurosurg Psychiatry 75(12):1682–1687. https://doi.org/10.1136/jnnp.2003.016550. PMID: 15548482; PMCID: PMC1738854

Jobst E, Melnick M, Byl N, Dowling G, Aminoff M (1997) Sensory perception in Parkinson disease. Arch Neurol 54(4):450–454. https://doi.org/10.1001/archneur.1997.00550160080020. PMID: 9109747

Joshi N, Singh S (2018) Updates on immunity and inflammation in Parkinson disease pathology. J Neurosci Res 96(3):379–390. https://doi.org/10.1002/jnr.24185

Jost W, Koschel J (2015) Die Parkinsonpsychose. Der Neurologe Psychiater, Ausgabe 3, S. 48/49

Kamsma YPT, Brouwer WH, Lakke JPWF (1995) Training of compensational strategies for impaired gross motor skills in Parkinson' disease. Physiother Theory Pract 11(4):209–229. https://doi.org/10.3109/09593989509036407

Karlsen K, Larsen J, Tandberg E, Jørgensen K (2001) Fatigue in patients with Parkinson's disease. Mov Disord. https://doi.org/10.1002/1531-8257(199903)14:2<237::AID-MDS1006>3.0.CO;2-X

Kehagia AA, Barker RA, Robbins TW (2013) Cognitive impairment in Parkinson's disease: the dual syndrome hypothesis. Neurodegener Dis 11(2):79–92. https://doi.org/10.1159/000341998. Epub 2012 Oct 3. PMID: 23038420; PMCID: PMC5079071.Keus SHJ

Kidron D, Melamed E (1987) Forms of dystonia in patients with Parkinson's disease. Neurology 37(6):1009–1011. https://doi.org/10.1212/wnl.37.6.1009. PMID: 3587617

Klamroth S, Steib S, Devan S, Pfeifer K (2016) Effects of exercise therapy on postural instability in Parkinson disease: a meta-analysis. J Neurol Phys Ther 40(1):3–14. https://doi.org/10.1097/NPT.0000000000000117. PMID: 26655098

Klockgether T, Dichgans J (1994) Visual control of arm movement in Parkinson's disease. Mov Disord 9:48–56. https://doi.org/10.1002/mds.870090108

Konczak J, Corcos D, Horak F, Poizner H, Shapiro M, Tuite P, Volkmann J, Maschke M (2009) Proprioception and motor control in Parkinson's disease. J Mot Behav 41(6):543–552. https://doi.org/10.3200/35-09-002. PMID: 19592360

Kwok JYY, Kwan JCY, Auyeung M, Mok VCT, Lau CKY, Choi KC, Chan HYL (2019) Effects of mindfulness yoga vs stretching and resistance training exercises on anxiety and depression for people with Parkinson disease: a randomized clinical trial. JAMA Neurol 76(7):755–763. https://doi.org/10.1001/jamaneurol.2019.0534. PMID: 30958514; PMCID: PMC6583059

de Lau L, Giesbergen P, de Rijk M, Hofman A, Koudstaal P, Breteler M (2004) Incidence of parkinsonism and Parkinson disease in a general population: the Rotterdam Study. Neurol Okt. https://doi.org/10.1212/01.WNL.0000140706.52798.BE

Law M (2002) Participation in the occupations of everyday life. Am J Occup Ther 56(6):640–649. https://doi.org/10.5014/ajot.56.6.640

Law M, Baptiste S, Mills J (1995) Client-centred practice: what does it mean and does it make a difference? Can J Occup Ther 62(5):250–257. https://doi.org/10.1177/000841749506200504. PMID: 10152881

Law M, Steinwender S, Leclair L (1998) Occupation, health and well-being. Can J Occup Therapy 65(2):81–91. https://doi.org/10.1177/000841749806500204

Lemke M (2002) Depression und Morbus Parkinson – Klinik, Diagnose, Therapie. UNI-MED AG, Bremen/London/Boston

Lemke M, Ceballos-Baumann A (2002) Depression bei Parkinson-Patienten: Diagnostische, pharmakologische und psychotherapeutische Aspekte. Dtsch Arztebl 99(40):A-2625/B-2237/C-2100

Leung IH, Walton CC, Hallock H, Lewis SJ, Valenzuela M, Lampit A (2015) Cognitive training in Parkinson disease: a systematic review and meta-analysis. Neurology 85(21):1843–1851. https://doi.org/10.1212/WNL.0000000000002145. Epub PMID: 26519540; PMCID: PMC4662707

Lord S, Galna B, Yarnall AJ, Morris R, Coleman S, Burn D, Rochester L (2017) Natural history of falls in an incident cohort of Parkinson's disease: early evolution, risk and protective features. J Neurol 264(11):2268–2276. https://doi.org/10.1007/s00415-017-8620-y. Epub 2017 Sep 25. PMID: 28948348; PMCID: PMC5656700

Lorenzen H (2010) Fatigue Management, Umgang mit chronischer Müdigkeit und Erschöpfung. Schulz-Kirchner GmbH, Idstein

Ma HI, Hwang WJ, Fang JJ, Kuo JK, Wang CY, Leong IF, Wang TY (2011) Effects of virtual reality training on functional reaching movements in people with Parkinson's disease: a randomized controlled pilot trial. Clin Rehabil 25(10):892–902. https://doi.org/10.1177/0269215511406757. Epub 2011 Jun 1. PMID: 21632652

Macht M, Ellgring H (2018) Verhaltenstherapie bei der Parkinson-Erkrankung, Elsevier GmbH, München

Majsak MJ, Kaminski T, Gentile AM, Flanagan JR (1998) The reaching movements of patients with Parkinson's disease under self-determined maximal speed and visually cued conditions. Brain 121(Pt 4):755–766. https://doi.org/10.1093/brain/121.4.755. PMID: 9577399

Mañanas M, García-Sanchez C, Kulisevsky J (2014) Apathy in Parkinson's disease: neurophysiological evidence of impaired incentive processing. J Neurosci

Off J Soc Neurosci 34(17):5918–5926. https://doi.org/10.1523/JNEUROSCI.0251-14.2014

van der Marck MA, Klok MP, Okun MS, Giladi N, Munneke M, Bloem BR (2014) NPF Falls Task Force. Consensus-based clinical practice recommendations for the examination and management of falls in patients with Parkinson's disease. Parkinsonism Relat Disord 20(4):360–369. https://doi.org/10.1016/j.parkreldis.2013.10.030. Epub 2013 Dec 30. PMID: 24484618

Margraf NG, Wrede A, Rohr A, Schulz-Schaeffer WJ, Raethjen J, Eymess A, Volkmann J, Mehdorn MH, Jansen O, Deuschl G (2010) Camptocormia in idiopathic Parkinson's disease: a focal myopathy of the paravertebral muscles. Mov Disord 25:542–551. https://doi.org/10.1002/mds.22780

Maricle R, Valentine R, Carter J, Nutt J (1998) Mood response to levodopa infusion in early Parkinson's disease. Neurology 50:1890–1892

Martínez-Horta S, Riba J, de Bobadilla RF, Pagonabarraga J, Pascual-Sedano B, Antonijoan RM, Romero S, Mañanas MÀ, García-Sanchez C, Kulisevsky J (2014) Apathy in Parkinson's disease: neurophysiological evidence of impaired incentive processing. The Journal of neuroscience : the official journal of the Society for Neuroscience, 34(17), 5918–5926. https://doi.org/10.1523/JNEUROSCI.0251-14.2014

Martinez-Martin P, Rojo-Abuin J, Rizos A, Rodriguez-Blazquez C, Trenkwalder C, Perkins L, Sauerbier A, Odin P, Antonini A, Ray Chaudhuri K (2017) Distribution and impact on quality of life of the pain modalities assessed by the King's Parkinson's disease pain scale. npj Parkinsons Dis 3. https://doi.org/10.1038/s41531-017-0009-1

Mazzoni P, Hristova A, Krakauer J (2007) Why don't we move faster? Parkinson's disease, movement vigor, and implicit motivation. J Neurosci 27(27):7105–7116. https://doi.org/10.1523/JNEUROSCI.0264-07.2007. PMID: 17611263; PMCID: PMC6794577

McLean G, Lawrence M, Simpson R, Mercer S (2017) Mindfulness-based stress reduction in Parkinson's disease: a systematic review. BMC Neurol 17. https://doi.org/10.1186/s12883-017-0876-4

Menza M, Dobkin R, Marin H, Bienfait K (2010) Sleep disturbances in Parkinson's disease. Mov Disord 25(Suppl 1):S117–S122. https://doi.org/10.1002/mds.22788

Munneke M, Graziano M et al (2014) Europäische Physiotherapie Leitlinie beim idiopathischen Parkinson-Syndrom. KNGF/ParkinsonNet, die Niederlande. https://www.parkinsonnet.info/euguideline

Muratori LM, McIsaac TL, Gordon AM, Santello M (2008) Impaired anticipatory control of force sharing patterns during whole-hand grasping in Parkinson's disease. Exp Brain Res 185(1):41–52. https://doi.org/10.1007/s00221-007-1129-3. Epub 2007 Oct 2. PMID: 17909770

Murphy S, Tickle-Degnen L (2001) The effectiveness of occupational therapy – related treatments for persons with Parkinson's disease: a meta-analytic review. Am J Occup Ther 55(4):385–392. https://doi.org/10.5014/ajot.55.4.385

Nackaerts E, Vervoort G, Heremans E, Smits-Engelsman B, Swinnen S, Nieuwboer A (2013) Relearning of writing skills in Parkinson's disease: a literature review on influential factors and optimal strategies. Neurosci Biobehav Rev 37(3):349–357. https://doi.org/10.1016/j.neubiorev.2013.01.015. ISSN 0149-7634

Nackaerts E, Nieuwboer A, Broeder S, Smits-Engelsman B, Swinnen S, Vandenberghe W, Heremans E (2015) Opposite effects of visual cueing during writing-like movements of different amplitudes in Parkinson's disease. Neurorehabil Neural Repair 30. https://doi.org/10.1177/1545968315601361

Nackaerts E, Heremans E, Vervoort G, Smits-Engelsman BC, Swinnen SP, Vandenberghe W, Bergmans B, Nieuwboer A (2016) Relearning of writing skills in Parkinson's disease after intensive amplitude training. Mov Disord 31(8):1209–1216. https://doi.org/10.1002/mds.26565. Epub 2016 Mar 17. PMID: 26990651

Nieuwboer A, Weerdt W, Dom R, Truyen M, Janssens L, Kamsma Y (2001) The effect of a home physiotherapy program for persons with Parkinson's disease. J Rehabil Med 33:266–272

Nieuwboer A, Vercruysse S, Feys P, Levin O, Spildooren J, Swinnen S (2009) Upper limb movement interruptions are correlated to freezing of gait in Parkinson's disease. Eur J Neurosci 29(7):1422–1430. https://doi.org/10.1111/j.1460-9568.2009.06681.x. Epub 2009 Mar 20. PMID: 19309319

Nieuwboer A, Kwakkel G, Rochester L, et al (2007) Cueing training in the home improves gait-related mobility in Parkinson's disease: the RESCUE trial Journal of Neurology, Neurosurgery & Psychiatry 78:134–140

Nonnekes J, Snijders AH, Nutt JG, Deuschl G, Giladi N, Bloem BR (2015) Freezing of gait: a practical approach to management. Lancet Neurol 14(7):768–778. https://doi.org/10.1016/S1474-4422(15)00041-1. Epub 24. PMID: 26018593

Nonnekes J, Ružicka E, Nieuwboer A, Hallett M, Fasano A, Bloem BR (2019) Compensation strategies for gait impairments in Parkinson disease: a review. JAMA Neurol 76(6):718–725. https://doi.org/10.1001/jamaneurol.2019.0033. PMID: 30907948

Ocampo C, Wan Y, van Wamelen D, Batzu L, Boura I, Titova N, Leta V, Qamar M, Martinez-Martin P, Ray Chaudhuri K (2020) Identifying and responding to fatigue and apathy in Parkinson's disease: a review of current practice. Expert Rev Neurother 20. https://doi.org/10.1080/14737175.2020.1752669

Oertel WH, Deuschl, G, Poewe, W (2012) Parkinson-Syndrome und andere Bewegungsstörungen. https://doi.org/10.1055/b-002-41833

Packer TL, Brink N, Sauriol A (1995) Managing fatigue: a six-week course for energy conservation. Therapy Skill Builders, Tucson

Pagonabarraga J, Kulisevsky J, Strafella AP, Krack P (2015) Apathy in Parkinson's disease: clinical features, neural substrates, diagnosis, and treatment. Lancet

Neurol 14(5):518–531. https://doi.org/10.1016/S1474-4422(15)00019-8. Epub 2015 Apr 12. PMID: 25895932

Pana A, Saggu BM (2020) Dystonia. [Updated 2020 Sep 10]. In: StatPearls [Internet]. StatPearls Publishing, Treasure Island. Available from: https://www.ncbi.nlm.nih.gov/books/NBK448144/

Peterson DS, King LA, Cohen RG, Horak FB (2015) Cognitive contributions to freezing of gait in Parkinson disease: implications for physical rehabilitation. Phys Ther 96(5):659–670. https://doi.org/10.2522/ptj.20140603. PMID: 26381808; PMCID: PMC 4858659

Pfeiffer R (2016) Non-motor symptoms in Parkinson's disease. Parkinsonism Relat Disord 22(Suppl 1):S119–S122. https://doi.org/10.1016/j.parkreldis.2015.09.004. ISSN 1353-8020

Phillips JG, Schiffter T, Nicholls ME, Bradshaw JL, Iansek R, Saling LL (1999) Does old age or Parkinson's disease cause bradyphrenia? J Gerontol A Biol Sci Med Sci 54(8):M404–M409. https://doi.org/10.1093/gerona/54.8.m404. PMID: 10496546

Postuma R, Gagnon J, Bertrand J, Génier Marchand D, Montplaisir J (2015) Parkinson risk in idiopathic REM sleep behavior disorder: preparing for neuroprotective trials. Neurology 84(11):1104–1113. https://doi.org/10.1212/WNL.0000000000001364

Radakovic R, Abrahams S (2018) Multidimensional apathy: evidence from neurodegenerative disease. Curr Opin Behav Sci 22:42–49. https://doi.org/10.1016/j.cobeha.2017.12.022

Radder DLM, Sturkenboom IH, van Nimwegen M, Keus SH, Bloem BR, de Vries NM (2017) Physical therapy and occupational therapy in Parkinson's disease. Int J Neurosci 127(10):930–943. https://doi.org/10.1080/00207454.2016.1275617

Redgrave P, Rodriguez M, Smith Y, Rodriguez-Oroz MC, Lehericy S, Bergman H, Agid Y, DeLong M, Obeso JA (2010) Goal-directed and habitual control in the basal ganglia: implications for Parkinson's disease. Nature reviews. Neuroscience 11(11):760–772. https://doi.org/10.1038/nrn2915

Von Reichmann H, Deuschl G, Riedel O, Spottke A, Förstl H, Henn F, Heuser I, Oertel W, Riederer P, Trenkwalder C, Dodel R, Wittchen HU (2010) Die „German study on the epidemiology of Parkinson's disease with dementia" (GEPAD): mehr als nur Parkinson [The German Study on the Epidemiology of Parkinson's Disease with Dementia (GEPAD): more than Parkinson]. MMW Fortschr Med 8;152 Suppl 1:1–6. German. PMID: 20942300

Reuter I, Mehnert S, Sammer G, Oechsner M, Engelhardt M (2012) Efficacy of a multimodal cognitive rehabilitation including psychomotor and endurance training in Parkinson's disease. J Aging Res 2012:235765. https://doi.org/10.1155/2012/235765. Epub 2012 Sep 12. PMID: 23008772; PMCID: PMC3447352

Reynolds GO, Otto MW, Ellis TD, Cronin-Golomb A (2016) The therapeutic potential of exercise to improve mood, cognition, and sleep in Parkinson's disease. Mov Disord (1):23–38. https://doi.org/10.1002/mds.26484. Epub 2015 Dec 30. PMID: 26715466; PMCID: PMC4724300

Richard I, Justus A, Kurlan R (2001) Relationship between mood and motor fluctuations in Parkinson's disease. J Neuropsychiatr Clin Neurosci 13: 35–41

Riedel O, Heuser I, Klotsche J, Dodel R, Wittchen HU (2010) GEPAD Study Group. Occurrence risk and structure of depression in Parkinson disease with and without dementia: results from the GEPAD Study. J Geriatr Psychiatry Neurol 23(1):27–34. https://doi.org/10.1177/0891988709351833. Epub 2009 Dec 30. PMID: 20042544

Sacheli MA, Murray DK, Vafai N, Cherkasova MV, Dinelle K, Shahinfard E, Neilson N, McKenzie J, Schulzer M, Appel-Cresswell S, McKeown MJ, Sossi V, Jon Stoessl A (2018) Habitual exercisers versus sedentary subjects with Parkinson's disease: multimodal PET and fMRI study. Mov Disord 33(12):1945–1950. https://doi.org/10.1002/mds.27498. PMID: 30376184

Sacheli MA, Neva JL, Lakhani B, Murray DK, Vafai N, Shahinfard E, English C, McCormick S, Dinelle K, Neilson N, McKenzie J, Schulzer M, McKenzie DC, Appel-Cresswell S, McKeown MJ, Boyd LA, Sossi V, Stoessl AJ (2019) Exercise increases caudate dopamine release and ventral striatal activation in Parkinson's disease. Mov Disord 34(12):1891–1900. https://doi.org/10.1002/mds.27865. Epub PMID: 31584222

Schlesinger I, Benyakov O, Erikh I, Suraiya S, Schiller Y (2009) Parkinson's disease tremor is diminished with relaxation guided imagery. Mov Disord 24:2059–2062. https://doi.org/10.1002/mds.22671

Schneider J, Diamond S, Markham C (1987) Parkinson's disease, sensory and motor problems in arms and hands. Neurology 37(6):951. https://doi.org/10.1212/WNL.37.6.951

Schrag A, Jahanshahi M, Quinn N (2000) What contributes to quality of life in patients with Parkinson's disease? J Neurol Neurosurg Psychiatry 69:308–312

Schramm A, Reiners K, Naumann M (2003) Die Wirksamkeit sensibler Trickmanöver bei zervikalen Dystonien ist winkelabhängig. Klin Neurophysiol 34:133. https://doi.org/10.1055/s-2003-816536

Schröder H (2015) Leben mit Parkinson, Achterbahn für Fortgeschrittene. Trias, Stuttgart, S 26

Schulz-Schaeffer W (2016) Camptocormia in Parkinson's disease: a muscle disease due to dysregulated proprioceptive polysynaptic reflex arch. Front Aging Neurosci 8:128. https://doi.org/10.3389/fnagi.2016.00128. PMID: 27445789; PMCID: PMC4914504

Shetty A, Bhatia K, Lang A (2019) Dystonia and Parkinson's disease: what is the relationship? Neurobiol Dis 132. https://doi.org/10.1016/j.nbd.2019.05.001

Signer T, Weise A (2020) Betätigungsorientierte Patientenedukation und Kompensation im stationären Rehabilitations-Alltag: die „Energiemanagement-Schulung" – ein Fallbeispiel. Schulz-Kirchner Verlag GmbH, Rheinsbreitbach, S 135–152

Skorvanek M, Bhatia K (2016) The skin and Parkinson's disease: review of clinical, diagnostic, and therapeutic issues. Mov Disord Clin Pract 4(1):21–31. https://doi.org/10.1002/mdc3.12425. Published 2016 Sep 8

Son HG, Choi E (2018) The effects of mindfulness meditation-based complex exercise program on motor and nonmotor symptoms and quality of life in patients with Parkinson's disease. Asian Nurs Res 12(2):145–153. https://doi.org/10.1016/j.anr.2018.06.001. ISSN 1976-1317

Spillantini M, Schmidt M, Lee VY, Trojanowski J, Jakes R, Goedert M (1997) α-Synuclein in Lewy bodies. Nature 388:839–840. https://doi.org/10.1038/42166

Sporrer W (2016) Ergotherapeutisches Schreibtraining bei Morbus Parkinson – Groß und lesbar schreiben. ergopraxis 9:34–37. https://doi.org/10.1055/s-0042-116770

Strouwen C, Molenaar EALM, Münks L, Keus SHJ, Zijlmans JCM, Vandenberghe W, Bloem BR, Nieuwboer A (2017) Training dual tasks together or apart in Parkinson's disease: results from the DUALITY trial. Mov Disord 32(8):1201–1210. https://doi.org/10.1002/mds.27014. Epub 2017 Apr 25. PMID: 28440888

Sturkenboom I, Thijssen M, Gons-van Elsacker J, Jansen I, Maasdam A, Schulten M, Vijver-Visser D, Steultjens E, Bloem B, Munneke M (2008) Guidelines for occupational therapy in Parkinson's disease rehabilitation. ParkinsonNet/NPF, Nijmegen/Miami

Tarakad A, Jankovic J (2019) Essential tremor and Parkinson's disease: exploring the relationship. Tremor Other Hyperkinet Mov (N Y). https://doi.org/10.7916/D8MD0GVR. PMID: 30643667; PMCID: PMC6329774

Temlett JA, Thompson PD (2006) Reasons for admission to hospital for Parkinson's disease. Intern Med J 36(8):524–526. https://doi.org/10.1111/j.1445-5994.2006.01123.x. PMID: 16866658

Tenison E, Smink A, Redwood S, Darweesh S, Cottle H, van Halteren A, Haak P, Hamlin R, Ypinga J, Bloem B, Ben-Shlomo Y, Munneke M, Henderson E (2020) Proactive and integrated management and empowerment in Parkinson's disease: designing a new model of care. Parkinson's Disease 2020:1–11. https://doi.org/10.1155/2020/8673087

Thompson T, Gallop K, Correll CU, Carvalho AF, Veronese N, Wright E, Stubbs B (2017) Pain perception in Parkinson's disease: a systematic review and meta-analysis of experimental studies. Ageing Res Rev 35:74–86. https://doi.org/10.1016/j.arr.2017.01.005. Epub 2017 Feb 4. PMID: 28179128

Thümler R (2002) Akathisie. In: Morbus Parkinson. Springer, Berlin/Heidelberg. https://doi.org/10.1007/978-3-642-56392-8_12

Tiple D, Fabbrini G, Colosimo C, Ottaviani D, Camerota F, Defazio G, Berardelli A (2009) Camptocormia in Parkinson disease: an epidemiological and clinical study. J Neurol Neurosurg Psychiatry 80(2):145–148. https://doi.org/10.1136/jnnp.2008.150011. Epub 2008 Oct 17. PMID: 18931011

Trepel M (2008) Neuroanatomie, Struktur und Funktion. Urban und Fischer, München

Voermans S (2016) Entspann dich, Deutschland – TK-Stressstudie, herausgegeben von der Techniker Krankenkasse, Hamburg

Winter Y, von Campenhausen S, Gasser J, Seppi K, Reese JP, Pfeiffer KP, Bötzel K, Oertel WH, Dodel R, Poewe W (2010) Social and clinical determinants of quality of life in Parkinson's disease in Austria: a cohort study. J Neurol 257(4):638–645. https://doi.org/10.1007/s00415-009-5389-7. Epub 2009 Nov 28. PMID: 19946784

Wu PL, Lee M, Huang TT (2017) Effectiveness of physical activity on patients with depression and Parkinson's disease: a systematic review. PLoS One 12(7):e0181515. https://doi.org/10.1371/journal.pone.0181515. Published 2017 Jul 27

www.gesundheitsinformation.de. Zugegriffen am am 05.02.2021. Erfahrungsberichte von Patienten, Institut für Qualität und Wirtschaftlichkeit im Gesundheitswesen (IQWiG).

Yeo L, Singh R, Gundeti M, Barua J, Masood J (2012) Urinary tract dysfunction in Parkinson's disease: a review. Int Urol Nephrol 44(2):415–424. https://doi.org/10.1007/s11255-011-9969-y. Epub 2011 May 7. PMID: 21553114

Yoritaka A, Shimo Y, Takanashi M, Fukae J, Hatano T, Nakahara T, Miyamato N, Urabe T, Mori H, Hattori N (2013) Motor and non-motor symptoms of 1453 patients with Parkinson's disease: prevalence and risks. Parkinsonism Relat Disord 19(8):725–731. https://doi.org/10.1016/j.parkreldis.2013.04.001. ISSN 1353-8020

15 Kontextfaktoren verändern – Adaptation

(siehe Abb. 4.4 Spalte 4)

So sehr in den vorgehenden Kapiteln Wert auf intensives Training, Wiederholungszahl und fokussierte Aufmerksamkeit im Alltag gelegt wurde, so wichtig ist es bei der ergotherapeutischen Intervention mit Parkinson-Klienten, die Grenzen des realistisch Erreichbaren zu erkennen. Das idiopathische Parkinson-Syndrom ist eine progrediente Krankheit, die unaufhaltsam voranschreitet. Medikamente und aktive Therapie können den Verlauf positiv beeinflussen, die Lebensqualität steigern und für eine Weile auch die Symptome verbessern. Auf längere Sicht wird es jedoch immer eine Verschlechterung geben. Das auszuhalten und damit umgehen zu lernen ist Aufgabe des Klienten (Krankheitsverarbeitung Abschn. 14.10.5) und der Therapeutin (Entscheidung für Intervention Kap. 12). Im Idealfall geschieht dies in enger Zusammenarbeit zwischen Therapeutin und Klient.

▶ Je nach Krankheitsphase, prognostischer Einschätzung der Therapeutin, kognitiven Kompetenzen und Grad der Motivation des Klienten und je nach Wünschen des Klienten und seiner Angehörigen sowie zeitlichem Rahmen wird die Entscheidung für Kompensation und Adaptation – statt aktivem Training – im Krankheitsverlauf zunehmen.

Aus diesem Grund stellt die Anpassung des Kontexts/Adaptation eine bedeutende Säule in der effektiven Behandlung von Menschen mit M. Parkinson dar.

15.1 Angehörigenberatung

Beispiel

„Lass dir doch helfen!" Genervt schneidet er das Fleisch auf dem Teller seiner Frau klein. Was für eine Sauerei, auf dem ganzen Tisch sind Erbsen und Soße verteilt. Er muss kurz raus auf die Terrasse, frische Luft holen. Er weiß ja, dass sie es nicht mit Absicht macht. Er kann einfach nicht mehr. Seit Jahren stemmt er alles allein. Er macht es ja auch gern, aber es ist einfach viel. Und seine Frau ist nicht mehr dieselbe. Früher waren sie zusammen aktiv, sind gereist und haben viel gelacht. Heute kann er froh sein, wenn sie seine Hand tätschelt. Seine Kinder haben ihm ein Wellnesswochenende geschenkt. Sie wollten in der Zeit alles zu Hause schmeißen. Sie wissen aber gar nicht, wie das geht. Deshalb hängt der Gutschein schon seit einem Jahr an der Pinwand. ◀

Ergänzende Information Die elektronische Version dieses Kapitels enthält Zusatzmaterial, auf das über folgenden Link zugegriffen werden kann https://doi.org/10.1007/978-3-662-62583-5_15. Die Videos lassen sich durch Anklicken des DOI Links in der Legende einer entsprechenden Abbildung abspielen, oder indem Sie diesen Link mit der SN More Media App scannen.

A. Orellana, *Betätigungsorientierte Ergotherapie bei Morbus Parkinson*,
https://doi.org/10.1007/978-3-662-62583-5_15

Mit dem Fortschreiten der Krankheit und zunehmender Schwere der Symptome nimmt die Bedeutsamkeit der Einbindung der Angehörigen in die Therapie zu. Durch ihren ganzheitlichen Ansatz haben Ergotherapeutinnen die Lebenswelt der Klienten konstant im Blick und wissen um die Vorteile, die positive soziale Interaktionen, eine stabile Partnerschaft und liebevolle Fürsorge auf die Lebensqualität von allen Menschen und insbesondere chronisch erkrankter Menschen haben. Leider fühlen sich viele Angehörige im Umgang mit dem Betroffenen überfordert. Gleichzeitig fällt es ihnen oftmals außerordentlich schwer, Aufgaben zu delegieren und sich um sich selbst zu kümmern.

Belastung der Angehörigen

Carter et al. untersuchten (1998) in einer groß angelegten Studie mit 380 Ehepartnern von betroffenen Parkinson-Patienten die Belastung der Angehörigen (speziell der Partner) im Verlauf der Krankheit.

Sie stellten fest, dass die Belastung der Ehepartnerinnen in Korrelation mit dem Krankheitsstadium (von 1 bis 5) nach Hoehn und Yahr stetig zunahm. In Stadium 1 und 2 gaben Angehörige im Durchschnitt in allen Bereichen „keine" oder „nur geringe" Belastung an. Mit jedem Stadium nahm die angegebene Belastung zu. In Stadium 4 und 5 wurden in acht Bereichen der abgefragten zehn, signifikant höhere Belastung angegeben: Sorge, Anspannung, Frustration durch Kommunikationsprobleme, Anstrengung durch Pflege, allgemeine Belastung, finanzielle Belastung, Ressourcenmangel und das Gefühl, manipuliert zu werden. Im Anfangsstadium der Erkrankung veränderte sich der Lebensstil nicht wesentlich, erst ab Stadium 2,5 zeigte sich ein negativer Effekt auf den Lebensstil. Hilfe von anderen wurde in den Stadien 1-2,5 nicht in Anspruch genommen. Bis zum Stadium 4/5 hatten die Angehörigen etwas mehr Hilfe von anderen. Es wurde erstaunlicherweise auch im Endstadium im Schnitt „ein wenig" Hilfe von anderen angegeben.

Interessanterweise gaben die Partnerinnen, auch bei steigender Belastung durch vermehrte Pflege, kaum körperliche Gesundheitsfolgen an. Für die Ehepartner lag das Risiko, an Depressionen zu erkranken, in Stadien 4/5 der Erkrankung bei 27 %. Die Qualität der Beziehung zwischen dem Pflegenden und dem Betroffenen nahm ab Stadium zwei stetig ab. Der Grad, zu dem sich die Pflegenden auf ihre Rolle vorbereitet fühlten, veränderte sich nicht im Verlauf der Krankheit. Sie fühlten sich meist „einigermaßen vorbereitet" bis „recht gut vorbereitet". Die Forschungsgruppe gibt zu bedenken, dass die wahrgenommene Belastung der Betreuer stark variiert. So ist es möglich, dass die Angehörige eines Betroffenen in Stadium 1 schon eine starke Belastung erlebt, eine andere, trotz Stadium 4/5 des Betroffenen, wenig Belastung spürt.

Kommunikation Therapeutin – Angehörige

Bei Aufnahme des Klienten ist es sinnvoll, von Beginn an die Zuständigkeiten und Aufgaben der Ergotherapie zu kommunizieren.

▶ Die Bedeutsamkeit der Zusammenarbeit von Betroffenen, Angehörigen und Therapeutin sollte hervorgehoben werden, damit auch die Angehörigen wissen, dass eine Zusammenarbeit gewünscht und für alle Seiten vorteilhaft ist.

Vielfach kann beobachtet werden, dass der Partner sich vor Therapiebeginn schnell zurückzieht und die Therapeutin „machen lässt". Dies kann in bestimmten Situationen zwar indiziert sein (s. u.), meist ist jedoch zumindest eine kurze Interaktion am Anfang oder Ende der Therapieeinheit – oder sogar durchgehend – förderlich für den therapeutischen Fortschritt. Abhängig vom therapeutischen Setting sind die Angehörigen bei der Therapie nicht präsent (z. B. Klinik, Pflegeheim). Auch hier ist eine Kontaktaufnahme meist angezeigt. Dazu hat sich eine kurze persönliche Notiz am Nachtkästchen bewährt, z. B.:

Liebe Frau Z.,
ich bin die Ergotherapeutin Ihres Mannes. Unsere Therapie findet täglich um 10 Uhr auf dem Zimmer statt. Ich lade Sie ein, einmal dazuzukommen, damit Sie sehen, an welchen Zielen wir arbeiten, und um den Hilfsmittelbedarf/die Handhabe beim Transfer… zu besprechen.
Mit freundlichen Grüßen,
Amy Orellana (Ergotherapeutin)

Für wichtige, persönliche oder komplizierte Absprachen ist natürlich eine Kontaktaufnahme per Telefon oder E-Mail möglich.

Assessment

Ein Fragebogen zur Erfassung der Belastung der Angehörigen von Parkinson-Betroffenen wurde von Ellgring et al. (1990) entwickelt und später weiterentwickelt und mehrfach validiert. Der **BELA-A-k** ist ein einfach durchführbarer Kurzfragebogen mit Fragen zu körperlicher und psychischer Belastung und Auswirkungen auf Alltag, Finanzen, Gesundheit und Zeit für sich. Das **COPM** (siehe Abschn. 5.4) kann auch bei Angehörigen eingesetzt werden, um deren Einschränkungen in ihrem Leben und daraus resultierende Wünsche und Ziele zu erfassen.

Fokusveränderung

Mit Verschlechterung der Symptome und zunehmender Abhängigkeit des Klienten von der Pflegenden tritt die Angehörige in der Ergotherapie zunehmend in den Fokus. Einerseits, wenn die Angehörige verstärkt vulnerabel und hilfsbedürftig erscheint, andererseits, wenn die Klient-Angehörige-Konstellation als eine Einheit wahrgenommen wird und jedes Thema, welches den Klienten betrifft, gleichzeitig immer die Angehörige betrifft. In diesem Fall ist das Miteinbeziehen der Angehörigen in den therapeutischen Prozess unumgänglich und für eine erfolgreiche Intervention ausschlaggebend. In welchem Maße die Angehörige während der Therapie anwesend ist und aktiv teilnimmt, liegt im Ermessen der Therapeutin und hängt sowohl von der Zielsetzung als auch vom Bedarf und der Bereitschaft zur Mitarbeit der Angehörigen ab.

Krankheitsinformationen vermitteln

Erfahrungsgemäß ist der Informationsstand der Angehörigen über die Parkinson-Erkrankung sehr unterschiedlich. Viele Angehörigen sind über fachlich korrekte Informationen zu Symptomen und Prognose sehr dankbar. Fällt der Therapeutin im Laufe der Therapie eine Fehl- oder Unterinformation auf, ist es sinnvoll, das entsprechende Wissen in die Therapie einfließen zu lassen. Ist die Therapeutin unsicher, können Fachbücher oder -artikel Abschnitt für Abschnitt zusammen durchgenommen und besprochen werden. Auch das Hinweisen auf Informationsquellen reicht vielfach aus, wenn der Angehörige sich lieber allein damit beschäftigen möchte.

Handhabe bei pflegerischen Tätigkeiten und Transfer

Die Handhabe des Betroffenen durch den Pflegenden ist im Anfangsstadium meist noch unsicher. Im Laufe der Erkrankung spielt sich das Paar ein. Manche Tipps können dennoch hilfreich sein, wenn die Angehörigen dafür offen sind. Folgende Punkte können mit dem Angehörigen gelesen und bei Bedarf direkt ausprobiert werden.

Tipps für Angehörige

Diese Grundsätze sind beim Umgang mit Menschen mit M. Parkinson immer wichtig:

- **Nicht hetzen!** Stress verstärkt alle Parkinson-Symptome. Deswegen sollte darauf geachtet werden, dass in Pflegesituationen und bei der Unterstützung des Betroffenen genügend Zeit eingeplant wird und eine ruhige, geduldige Atmosphäre herrscht.
- **Cueing**: Unterschiedliche Cueing-Methoden (auditiv, visuell, sensorisch und kognitiv) sollten Betreuern bekannt sein. Cueing kann in vielen schwierigen Situationen eine einfache Lösung sein. Dazu gehören: Freezing, Startschwierigkeiten, Drehen im Bett, Aufstehen, Transfer.
- **Kinästhetik**: Pflegende Angehörige erleben häufig eine körperliche Überlastung mit Verspannung und Schmerzen. Die Anwendung von Kinästhetik bei Transfers aller Art entlastet den Helfenden. Dabei werden Pflegebedürftige zur aktiven Mithilfe angeregt und die Bewegung mit minimalem Kraftaufwand des Pflegenden unterstützt. Bitten Sie die

Therapeutinnen um Tipps zur praktischen Handhabe oder besuchen Sie einen Kinästhetik-Kurs für Angehörige.

- **Hilfsmittel**: Hilfsmittel können nicht nur für den Betroffenen notwendig sein, sondern auch zur Entlastung der Pflegenden. Ihre Ergotherapeutin kann Sie hierzu fachkundig beraten.
- **Weniger ist mehr**: Dual-Tasking, also das Durchführen von zwei Tätigkeiten zur selben Zeit, überlastet das Parkinson-Gehirn. Trotzdem versuchen es die Betroffenen oftmals, weil sie es so gewöhnt sind. Betreuer können darauf achten, dass immer eine Tätigkeit nach der anderen durchgeführt wird. Außerdem sollte während Aktivitäten (z. B. Essen) nicht gesprochen werden, da auch dies zu Problemen (z. B. Verschlucken) führen kann. Anweisungen müssen am Anfang einer Bewegung gegeben werden und sehr kurz sein, z. B. „hoch" statt „Jetzt stehen wir auf, ich helfe dir dabei."
- **Aktivität/Ruhe**: Sowohl regelmäßige körperliche Aktivität und Sport als auch fest eingeplante Ruhezeiten sind für das Wohlbefinden und den körperlichen Gesundheitszustand von Menschen mit M. Parkinson entscheidend.

Stressbewältigung

Selbstbeobachtung

Angehörige betreuen ihren Partner, ihr Elternteil oder ein anderes Familienmitglied oftmals über viele Jahre. Dabei steigt der Anspruch langsam an. Die Anzahl der durchgeführten Pflegetätigkeiten verdreifacht sich nahezu von Stadium 1 (11 Tätigkeiten) bis Stadium 4/5 (fast 30 Tätigkeiten) (Carter et al. 1998). Weil dies jedoch allmählich geschieht, wird es von den Angehörigen selbst häufig nicht wahrgenommen. In der Ergotherapie kann der Angehörige sich die Zeit nehmen, in Ruhe über seine momentane Situation zu reflektieren. Hilfreiche Fragen an sich selbst können sein:

- Welche Rolle habe ich in der Beziehung (mit dem Betroffenen)?
- Wenn ich etwas verändern könnte, was wäre es?
- Genieße ich das Leben – trotz allem – oder „arbeite" ich nur noch?
- Was gibt mir Energie zurück und mache ich das genug?
- Welche Menschen könnten mich in der Betreuung unterstützen?

Die Fähigkeit, im gegenwärtigen Augenblick präsent zu sein und Achtsamkeit zu praktizieren, kann für Angehörige ein hilfreiches Werkzeug sein, um sich nicht überwältigt zu fühlen. Dazu können die Atem- und Achtsamkeitsübungen von Abschn. 14.10.4 verwendet werden. Weitere Strategien zum Umgang mit Stress sind in Abschn. 14.8 nachzulesen.

Entlastung der Angehörigen – Zeit für sich

Die Erfahrung zeigt, dass (Ehe-)Partner oft völlig in der Betreuerrolle aufgehen. Sie entwickeln sich zu Spezialisten für die Besonderheiten des Betroffenen, kennen sowohl die Symptome als auch seine Persönlichkeit und Vorlieben, sodass ein Abgeben an andere Familienmitglieder oder Pflegepersonen unmöglich scheint. Obwohl äußere Anzeichen auf eine Überforderung des Angehörigen deuten (körperliche Einschränkungen, Abnahme der eigenen sozialen Beziehungen, kaum Zeit für eigene Interessen), fällt es ihnen häufig sehr schwer, die Zügel aus der Hand zu geben und Hilfe anzunehmen. Für eine gute psychische und körperliche Gesundheit kann eine **frühzeitige** Einbindung von weiteren Angehörigen oder Freundinnen essenziell sein. Je besser auch entferntere Verwandte und Freundinnen den Klienten mit seinen Symptomen kennenlernen, desto eher sind sie in der Lage, damit umzugehen. Dies ist im weiteren Verlauf der Krankheit eine gute Basis für eine hilfreiche Unterstützung des nächsten Angehörigen.

▶ Besonders positiv wird von allen Seiten eine Aufteilung verschiedener Aufgaben auf unterschiedliche Personen bewertet. So wird keiner überlastet und jeder einzelne kennt sich auf seinem „Spezialgebiet" aus (z. B. Einkaufen, Behördengänge, Haushalt)

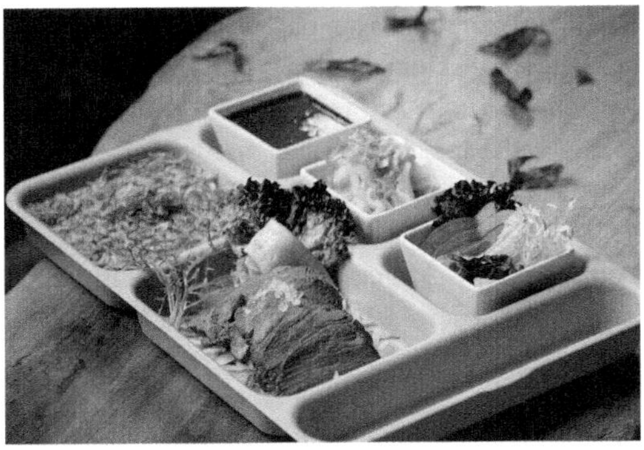

Abb. 15.1 Eine Essenslieferung kann eine große Entlastung von Angehörigen bedeuten. Die Hilfe beim Recherchieren oder der Organisation fällt in den Tätigkeitsbereich der Ergotherapeutin

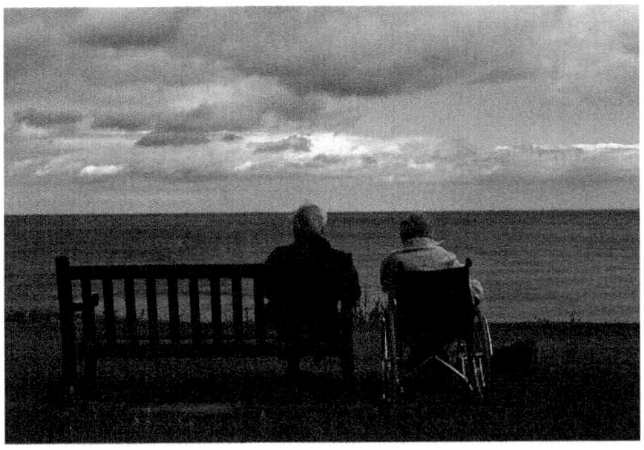

Abb. 15.2 Reisen können für die Angehörigen wieder mit mehr Leichtigkeit gemacht werden, wenn die Reisen zum Beispiel speziell für Menschen mit Behinderung und ihren Angehörigen organisiert werden

Auch die Nutzung von externen Angeboten ist sinnvoll. Einige Beispiele sind:

- Essenslieferung von Essen auf Rädern oder privaten Anbietern (s. Abb. 15.1)
- Pflegedienst für Bereiche, in denen der Klient Unterstützung benötigt (z. B. Medikamentengabe, Duschen, Morgenhygiene, Anziehen, ins Bett gehen)
- 24-Std.-Betreuung im eigenen Heim
- Pflegeheim
- Wöchentliche Angebote, z. B. Singkreis, Bibelkreis, Seniorengymnastik, Sonntagsfrühstück, Walken für Senioren, Selbsthilfegruppe (z. B. bei AWO, Rotes Kreuz, Sportverein, Kirchen, Arbeiter Samariter Bund …)
- Tageweise oder wochenweise Betreuung in der Kurzzeitpflege
- Reisen für Menschen mit Behinderung und ihre Angehörigen (s. Abb. 15.2)
- Tagesbetreuung in Tagespflege
- Nachbarschaftshilfe oder kirchliche Einrichtungen (Hilfe bei Einkaufen, kleine Erledigungen und Gespräche)

Beziehung

Durch den Rollenwechsel von Partner/Kind/Schwester … zu Betreuer und Pfleger verändert sich unweigerlich auch die Beziehung zu demjenigen mit der Parkinson-Erkrankung. Dieser Prozess kann schmerzlich sein, da es einen Abschied von dem Menschen, wie man ihn kannte, beinhaltet. Die Ergotherapeutin kann diesen Schmerz des Angehörigen validieren. Den Verlust zu benennen und den Betreuenden oder Pflegenden wissen zu lassen, dass es normal ist, über diesen Verlust zu trauern, kann für den Betroffenen und seinen Angehörigen befreiend sein. Gelingt es dem Betroffenen und dem Angehörigen, die veränderte Beziehung aktiv zu gestalten, damit beide Seiten wertvolle Aspekte erleben, kann die Beziehung auf eine neue Art und Weise gelebt werden, die für beide Partner positiv ist. Dazu können gemeinsame Erlebnisse beitragen (s. Abb. 15.3). Sie sollten gut vorbereitet sein, damit beide Freude daran haben, ohne überfordernd oder langweilig zu sein. In der Ergotherapie kann diese Vorbereitung schrittweise begleitet werden:

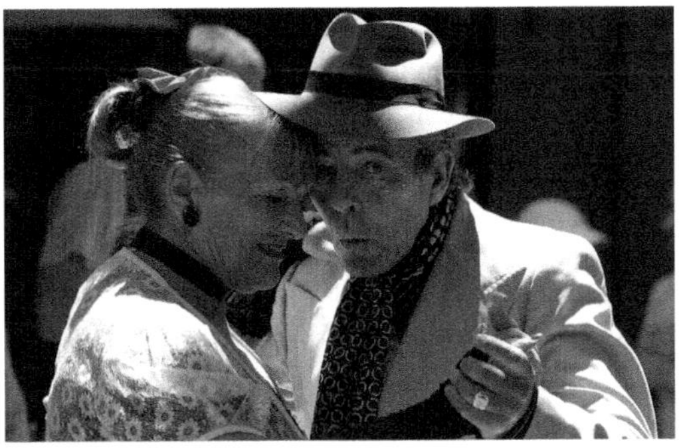

Abb. 15.3 Gemeinsame Erlebnisse sind bei einer veränderten Rollenverteilung im Verhältnis zwischen Betroffenem und Angehörigen wichtig, um die Beziehung aktiv zu gestalten

- **Sammlung**: Klient und Angehöriger sammeln jeder für sich Aktivitäten, die sie früher und heute gern gemacht haben, ohne auf die Möglichkeit der Umsetzung zu achten. „Wenn Sie einen Zauberstab hätten, was würden Sie gerne machen?"
- **Besprechung**: Im zweiten Schritt wird abgeglichen, wo Überschneidungen sind. Oftmals fokussieren sich Klient und Angehörige auf die Unvereinbarkeit der Wünsche. Die Therapeutin kann zur Verständigung beitragen und Gemeinsamkeiten aufzeigen. Dabei ist es wichtig ins Gespräch zu kommen. Möchte der Angehörige z. B. eine Bergwanderung machen, geht es ihm eher um die körperliche Betätigung, um die Aussicht oder um das Naturerlebnis?
- **Lösungen finden**: Nun sollten praktische Lösungswege gesucht werden. Die Therapeutin kann mit ihrem fachlichen Wissen über Hilfsmittel (z. B. unauffälliger Trinkbecher), Angebote (z. B. Reisebusse für Rollstuhlfahrer) und Tipps und Tricks (z. B. Notfalleinlage in Unterwäsche, falls keine Toilette in der Nähe) helfen, praktische Möglichkeiten der Ausführung finden.
- **Umsetzen**: Auch bei der praktischen Umsetzung kann die Ergotherapeutin unterstützen (z. B. Telefonnummern herausfinden, Rollenspiele, üben der Handhabe von neuen Situationen, wie Einsteigen in Reisebus).

Ein weiterer wichtiger Faktor, um eine wertschätzende Beziehung zu gewährleisten, ist die Kommunikation zwischen dem Parkinson-Erkrankten und der Angehörigen.

Umgang mit hadernden Angehörigen

Außenstehende erkennen oft ein Muster der negativen Entwicklung: Der Partner wird zum Betreuer – und schließlich selbst zum Patienten. Der Angehörige erkennt die Situation selbst nicht, gerade weil er mittendrin steckt. Er ist so sehr eingebunden, dass sein eigenes Leben immer an zweiter Stelle steht. Dies führt zu innerer Unzufriedenheit und auf Dauer zu Überforderung. Am Beispiel von typisch geäußerten Sätzen von Angehörigen werden unten Fragen und Gedankenanstöße für ein ergotherapeutisches Beratungsgespräch vorgeschlagen. Um eine Eigenreflexion darüber in Gang zu bringen und dem Angehörigen zu helfen, Lösungswege zu entwickeln, können folgende Gedanken und Fragen hilfreich sein:

Aussage des Angehörigen: „Ich fühle mich nicht überfordert, sondern gut vorbereitet auf die Zukunft."

Gedanken und Fragen der Therapeutin:

1. Therapeutin beschreibt den typischen Veränderungsprozess von Partnerinnen Betroffener mit neurodegenerativen Erkrankungen: von der **Partnerin** zur **Betreuerin** schließlich selbst zur **Patientin.**
2. „Welche Anzeichen würden bei Ihnen eine beginnende Überforderung anzeigen?"
3. „Sehen Sie Aspekte in Ihrer Beziehung, die darauf hinweisen, dass dieser Prozess bei Ihnen begonnen haben könnte?"
4. „In Ihrer Persönlichkeit/Beziehung, welche Punkte sehen Sie, die dafürsprechen, dass es dazu kommen könnte?"
5. „Welche Wünsche haben Sie für sich selbst? (nicht für Ihren Partner)"

Aussage des Angehörigen: „Nur ich kann meinem Mann/Vater/Bruder … helfen."

Fragen der Therapeutin zur Reflexion:

- „Wie hilft Ihnen dieser Gedanke? Inwiefern könnte Ihnen dieser Gedanke vielleicht Probleme bereiten?"
- „Was sind die Vor- und Nachteile dieser Art des Denkens?"
- „Ich verstehe/höre Sie sagen, dass nur Sie ihrem Partner helfen können. Aber Sie sagen auch, dass Sie sich manchmal mehr Zeit für sich wünschen/Rückenschmerzen haben/viel Streit mit Ihrem Partner haben. Stimmt das?" Dann: „Was würden Sie einem Freund sagen, der Ihnen das sagt?" (Widersprüche aufzeigen, neue Sichtweise ermöglichen).

Aussage der Angehörigen: „Hilfe ins Haus holen möchte ich nicht."

Zunächst ist es wichtig, dass die Therapeutin möglichst neutral bleibt, denn wenn der Angehörige das Gefühl hat, in eine Richtung geschoben zu werden, kann er mehr Widerstand geben.

Fragen der Therapeutin zur Reflexion:

- „Was wären Anzeichen, dass es Zeit ist, sich Hilfe zu holen?"
- „Wie wäre es, wenn jemand ins Haus käme? Lassen Sie uns gemeinsam die Nachteile und dann die Vorteile aufschreiben." (Nachteile und Vorteile validieren (z. B. „Ja, verstehe."). Nachteile können weniger schwerwiegend sein, wenn sie gedanklich vorweggenommen werden, oder Lösungen können schon vorher angedacht werden.
- „Lassen Sie uns zusammen ein Brainstorming machen: Welche Art der Hilfe könnten Sie holen?" (z. B. Haushaltshilfe, sporadische Putzhilfe im Frühling/vor Feiern …, Pflege, Unterstützung für einen Abend, um eigenem Interesse nachzugehen …).

Frageserie:

1. „Auf einer Skala von 0–10, wie bereit fühlen Sie sich, Hilfe ins Haus zu holen?" „Wenn 0 = überhaupt nicht bereit, Hilfe zu bekommen ist und 10 = bereit, sofort Hilfe kommen zu lassen ist, wie würden Sie Ihr Bereitschaftsniveau einschätzen?" „Was müsste sich ändern, damit Sie eine Zahl näher an 10 herankommen?" (Zum Beispiel von 2 auf 3)
2. „Was spricht dagegen, Hilfe ins Haus zu holen?" (validieren: „Ja, verstehe.") „Was spricht dafür, Hilfe ins Haus zu holen?"
3. „Wann würden Sie jemanden ins Haus holen? Was müsste sich verändern?"

► Da Ergotherapeutinnen keine psychotherapeutische Ausbildung haben, wird es in manchen Fällen sinnvoll sein, eine Empfehlung für einen Termin bei einer Psychotherapeutin zu geben.

Obige Beispiele zeigen, wie Ergotherapeutinnen Angehörigen helfen können, ihre Gedanken und Gefühle zu der Situation zu verarbeiten. Zusätzlich wird so ein Bewusstsein geschaffen, sodass die Wahrscheinlichkeit steigt, dass die Pflegende oder Betreuende Hilfe sucht.

Beispiel

Nun hat er es doch gewagt. Gemeinsam mit der Ergotherapeutin hat er einen Plan geschrieben, was alles getan werden müsste, wenn er ein Wochenende weg wäre. Von „Medikamente geben", über „beim Aufstehen helfen" bis „Toilettengang". Die Kinder haben in der Ergotherapie fleißig Transfers und Umgang mit Freezing geübt. Und jetzt geht es los. Herr G. küsst seine Frau und nimmt die Koffer. Sein Kumpel steht am Auto und winkt. „Das wird schön," denkt er und tritt durch die Tür. ◄

15.2 Wohnraumberatung

Beispiel

Alles tut weh. „Jetzt muss ich bestimmt doch ins Heim," denkt Frau K., als sie auf den Notknopf an ihrem Handgelenk drückt. Frau K. lebt alleine. Sie möchte hier noch lange bleiben, da sie schon 35 Jahre in ihrer stilvollen Wohnung lebt und ihr Bruder mit Partnerin nebenan wohnt. Ein wenig unsicher läuft sie zwar immer, normalerweise bewegt sie sich deswegen vorsichtig in der Wohnung umher und hält sich, wenn nötig, fest. Doch immer, wenn die Medikamentenwirkung nachlässt, kommt die Angst und sie ist ganz durcheinander. Dann denkt sie nicht daran, vorsichtig zu sein, ist fahrig und bleibt an der Ecke des Teppichs mit dem Fuß hängen. Sie stolpert und landet mit der Seite auf dem Boden. ◄

Die Wohnraumberatung, obgleich eine zentrale Aufgabe der Ergotherapie, ist doch ein sensibles Thema, da in die Privatsphäre der Bewohner eingegriffen wird. Aus diesem Grund ist ein einfühlsames Gespräch mit dem Klienten und Angehörigen notwendig. Änderungen sollten als Ideen vorgeschlagen werden, zwar mit Klarheit und Begründung, aber nie mit Druck. Für viele Klienten ist die

Wohnung ein Stück Kontinuität in ihrem Leben mit einer, sich fortwährend verändernden, Krankheit. Eine Veränderung der Wohnung bedeutet eine Verunsicherung, da es eine Manifestation der konstanten Verschlechterung des Zustandes darstellt. Außerdem fällt es Menschen mit M. Parkinson durch die abnehmende kognitive Flexibilität schwer, Veränderungen vorzunehmen

Bei Sturzgefahr

- Sturzprävention
  - Gute Ausleuchtung
    - Helle Lampen
    - Mehr Lampen
    - Nachtleuchten mit Sensoren, z. B. LED-Leiste
  - Entfernung von Läufern und Teppichen (s. Abb. 15.4)
  - Entfernung von losen Kabeln
  - Stabile Möbel
  - Antirutschbeläge (Bad, Treppe) (s. Abb. 15.5)
  - Sitzgelegenheit in jedem Zimmer, inkl. Eingangsbereich und Bad (s. Abb. 15.6)
  - Anbringen von Haltegriffen
  - Stabile Geländer an Treppen
  - Stufen visuell hervorheben
  - Häufig genutzte Schrankinhalte gut erreichbar organisieren

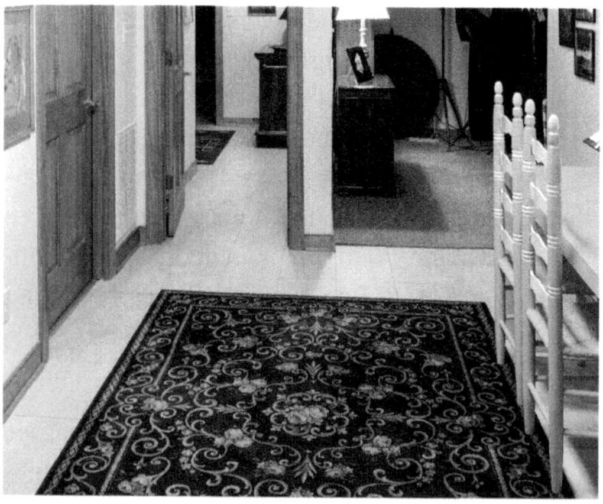

Abb. 15.4 Die Entfernung von Läufern trägt erheblich zur Sturzprophylaxe bei. Jede Veränderung des Wohnraums muss von der Therapeutin behutsam angegangen werden, da es der persönliche Bereich des Klienten ist

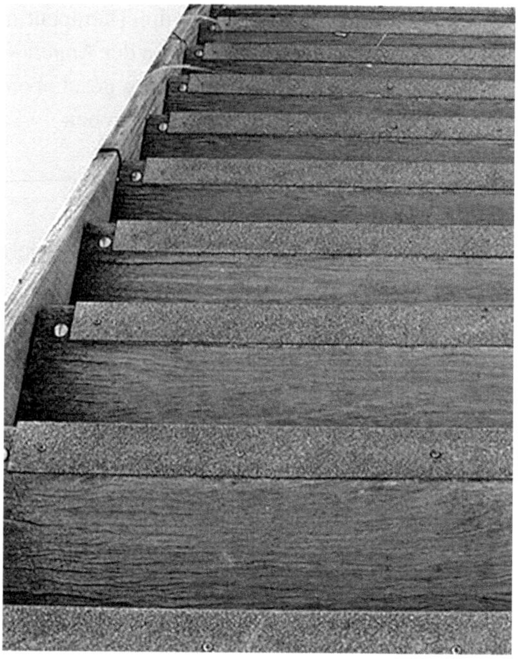

Abb. 15.5 Antirutschstreifen auf den Treppenstufen geben Trittsicherheit beim Treppe Laufen

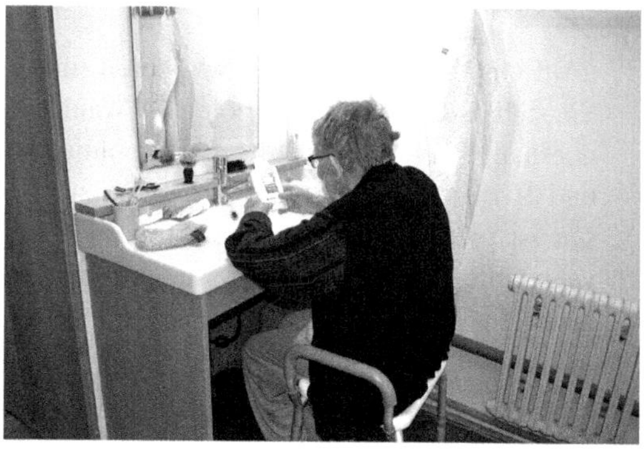

Abb. 15.6 Eine Sitzmöglichkeit im Bad erscheint vielen Klienten zunächst abwegig, wird jedoch meist akzeptiert, wenn der Sicherheitsaspekt von der Therapeutin gut erklärt wird

- Reduzierung des Verletzungsrisikos bei Stürzen
  - Abgerundete Ecken
  - Vitrinen entfernen
  - Tragen von Hüftprotektoren
  - Tragen von Kopfschutz (Helm)

Ermöglichung der größtmöglichen Selbständigkeit

- Gewährleistung der Zugänglichkeit zu notwendigen Räumen
  - Türrahmenverbreiterung (Rollstuhl/Rollatorbreite)
  - Treppenlift
  - Schwellen abflachen
  - Platzierung von Hilfsmitteln (z. B. ein Rollator pro Ebene)
- Erreichbar machen von Haushaltsgeräten
  - Waschmaschine in Bad, statt Keller
  - Staubsauger griffbereit

Vorbeugung von Fatigue

- Reduzierung der Wege im Wohnbereich
  - Nutzung nur einer Wohnebene
  - Umräumen von Möbeln und Geräten (s. Abb. 15.7)

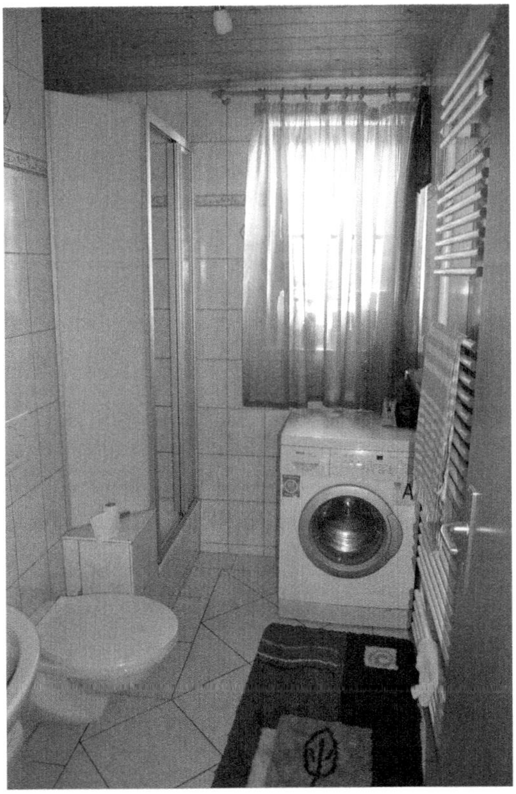

Abb. 15.7 Das Umstellen von Haushaltsgeräten (hier Waschmaschine im Bad, statt im Keller) erleichtert die Haushaltsführung und der Klient spart Energie

- Ausruhmöglichkeiten schaffen
  - Stühle in jedem Raum
  - Stehhilfe in Küche

Reduzierung von Freezing

- Anbringung von visuellen Cues in notwendigen Bereichen
  - Kreuz vor Toilette
  - Striche im Flur
- Freimachen von Wegen
  - Entfernung von herumstehenden Gegenständen, z. B. Dekoration und Unordnung
  - Auseinanderrücken von Möbeln, um Durchgänge zu vergrößern

Kognitive Defizite kompensieren

- Vereinfachung von Abläufen
  - Reduzierung von Schrankinhalten
  - Reorganisation von Schrankinhalten (z. B. Kaffeeutensilien in Schrank bei Kaffeemaschine)
- Beschriftung
  - Schränke
  - Gerätebedienung (s. Abb. 15.8)
  - Schlüssel (s. Abb. 15.9)

Bei Umkippen zur Seite im Sitzen

- Brett an Gegenseite anbringen
- Stuhl seitlich an Wand stellen

Transfer und Aufstehen erleichtern

- Erhöhung von Toilette
- Erhöhung von Stühlen und Sesseln

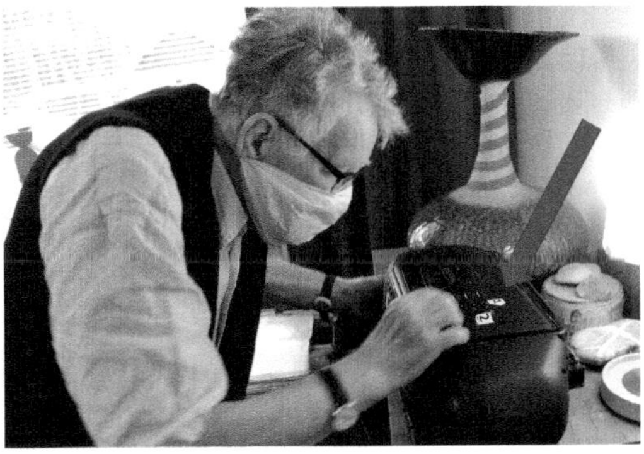

Abb. 15.8 Beschrifteter CD-Player

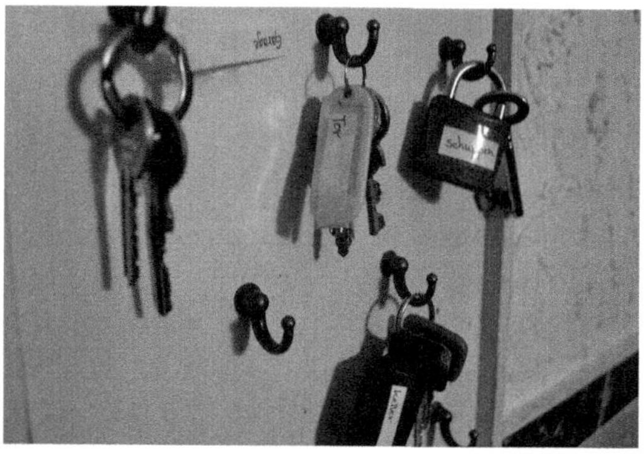

Abb. 15.9 Beschriftete Schlüssel

  - Sitzkissen, Keilkissen
  - Blöcke unter Sesselfüße
- Haltegriffe an Bett und in Bad
- Satinbettlaken, um Drehen im Bett zu erleichtern
- höhenverstellbares Bett
- höheres Auto

Beispiel

Tatsächlich beginnt Frau K., sich verschiedene Heime anzusehen. Die Verletzungen durch die Stürze sind dauerpräsent und die zuständige Schwägerin überlastet. Bis ein Heim ausgesucht und ein Platz gefunden ist, bleibt Frau K. in ihrer Wohnung und es wird eine Ergotherapie verschrieben. Sobald die Therapeutin eintritt, sieht sie einige Stolperfallen – mehrere Teppichläufer, Schlappen an den Füßen sowie eine erhebliche Verletzungsgefahr durch eine Vitrine neben dem Weg zur Küche. Zusätzlich diese Fahrigkeit. Es fällt schwer, Frau K. beim Laufen in der Wohnung zuzusehen, ohne einzugreifen.

Trotzdem geht die Therapeutin die ersten beiden Male wieder, ohne einen einzigen Gegenstand verändert zu haben – zuerst muss die therapeutische Beziehung stimmen.

Frau K. erzählt die Geschichte, wie sie die wunderschönen handgeknüpften Perserteppiche gekauft hat – nach einem Syrienurlaub von einem Tür-zu-Tür-Händler, der zufällig auch aus Syrien kam. Danach rollt sie den Teppich, der die größte Sturzgefahr darstellt und direkt vor der Vitrine liegt, schweren Herzens auf. Die Schwägerin schlägt vor, den schönen Teppich im Flur an die Wand zu hängen, wo er Frau K. seitdem an ihren schönen Urlaub erinnert. ◀

15.3 Hilfsmittel

Beispiel

Schon wieder hat Frau H. eine Wunde am Kopf. „Ich hab mich schon daran gewöhnt." Sie zuckt mit den Schultern. Der Ergotherapeut schüttelt den Kopf. „Das sollten Sie aber nicht, Frau H. Das kann auch mal richtig schiefgehen. Da mache ich mir Sorgen." Er lässt sich den Ort des Sturzes zeigen: das Bad. ◀

Hilfsmittel sind im Verlauf der Erkrankung zunehmend nötig, um die Selbständigkeit weiterhin zu erhalten und Teilhabe zu ermöglich. Zum Aufgabenbereich der Ergotherapie gehört die Recherche, Beratung und das Training der Anwendung der Hilfsmittel. Im folgenden (Tab. 15.1, 15 .2, 15.3, 15.4, 15.5, 15.6 und 15.7, Video 15.10/ Abb. 15.10) sind einige mögliche Hilfsmittel aufgeführt, die für Parkinson-Klienten hilfreich sein können. Eine individuelle Anpassung an die Bedürfnisse und Situation des Klienten ist immer notwendig.

Tab. 15.1 Hilfsmittel zur Erleichterung des Essens

Essen		
Hilfsmittel	Mögliche Anwendungen	
• Adaptiertes Besteck (Griffverdickung)	• Herabgesetzte Feinmotorik • Tremor	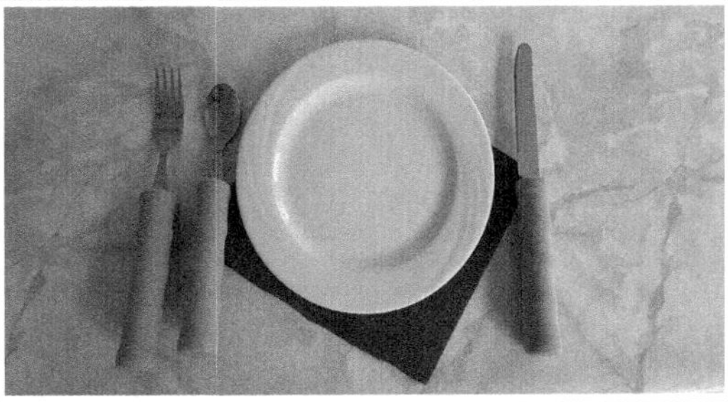
• Schweres Besteck	• Tremor	
• Gewicht für Hand, oder Unterarm-manschette	• Tremor (Achtung, kein Übungsgerät, nur zur Anwendung bei Betätigung)	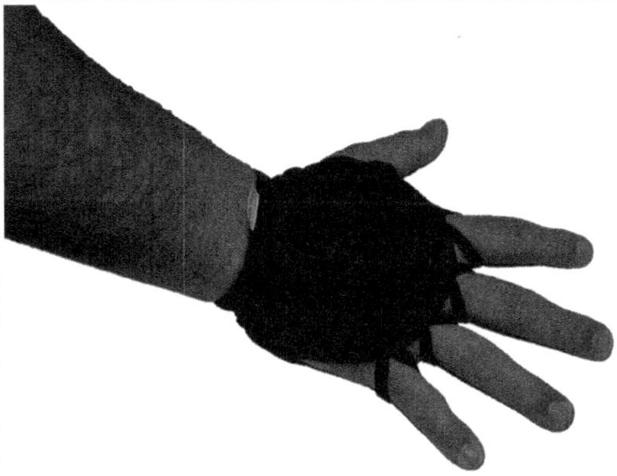 z. B. Handgewicht von Fa. Handithings.
• Anti-Tremor-Löffel	• Tremor, durch entgegengesetztes Schwingen des Löffels wird die Tremorbewegung aufgehoben.	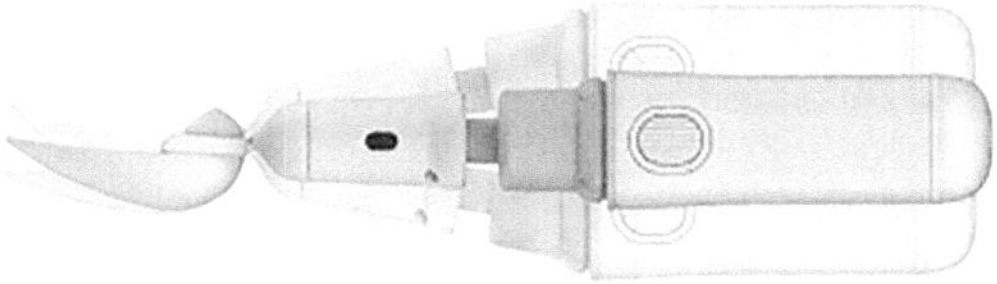 z. B. Bravo Twist ® von Fa. Pro Walk
• Tremor-Löffelaufsatz	• Tremor	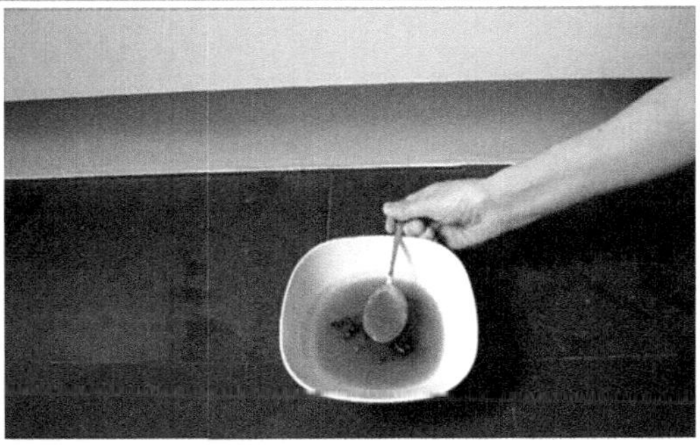 S. auch Video 15.10/Abb. 15.10

(Fortsetzung)

Tab. 15.1 (Fortsetzung)

Essen		
• Antirutschfolie/-unterlage	• Tremor • Herabgesetzte Koordination	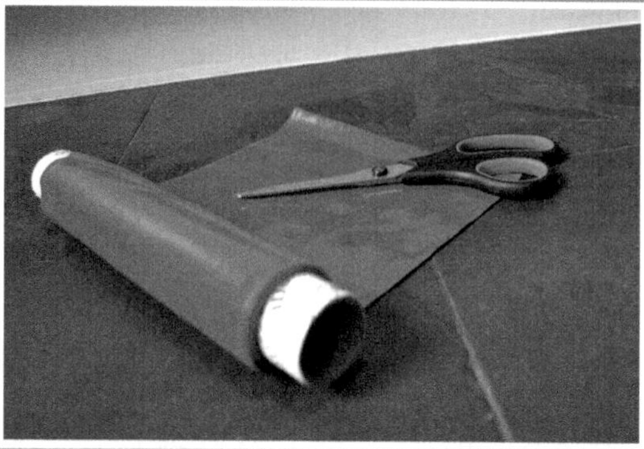
• Trinkbecher mit Deckel, hier spezieller „Trinklernbecher“ mit 360°-Trinkrand, Silikon-dichtscheibe, auslaufsicher	• Tremor • Schluckstörung (zum Trinken muss leicht gesaugt werden, dadurch erhöhte Mundspannung)	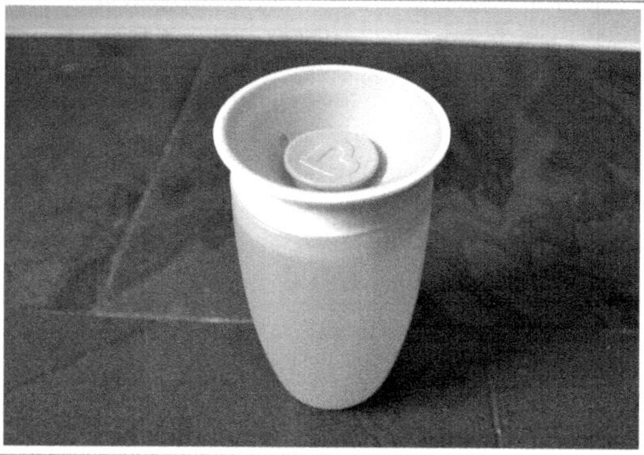
• Trinkbecher mit speziellen Henkeln und beschwert	• Herabgesetzte Koordination	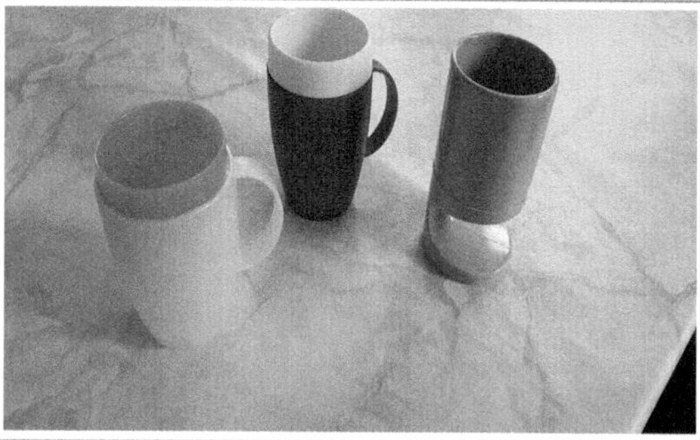
• Thermobecher (unauffällig)	• Tremor • Herabgesetzte Koordination	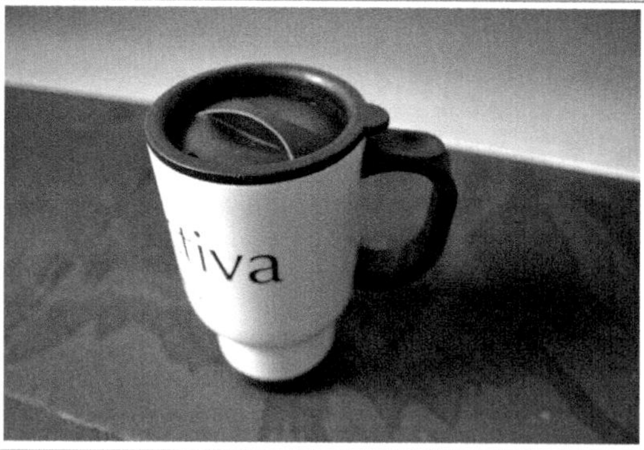

Tab. 15.1 (Fortsetzung)

Essen		
• Tellerranderhöhung (integriert oder aufsteckbar)	• Herabgesetzte Koordination • Tremor	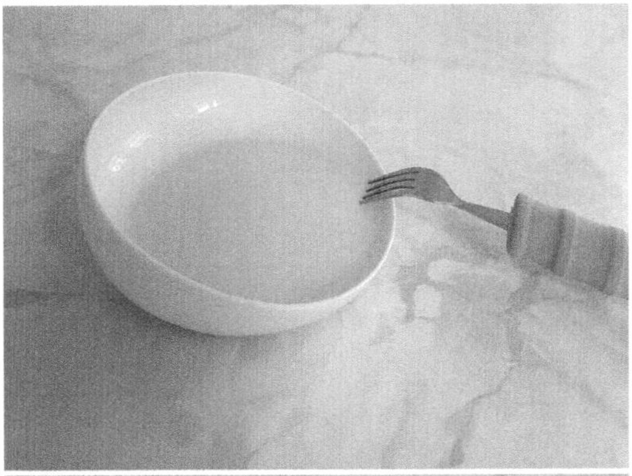 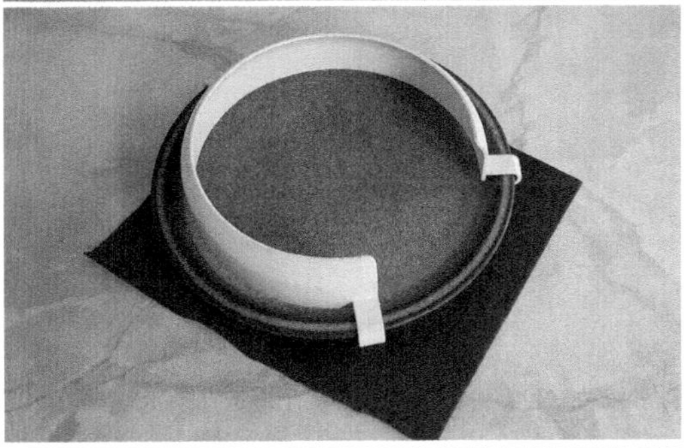

Tab. 15.2 Badhilfsmittel

Bad		
• Badewannenbrett	• Sturzgefahr • Verminderte Kraft	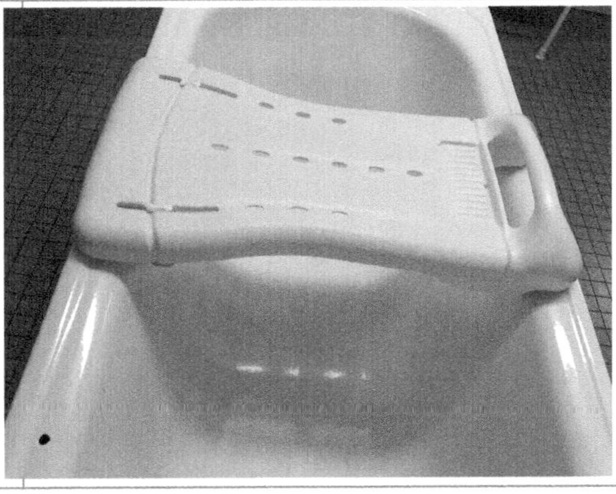

(Fortsetzung)

Tab. 15.2 (Fortsetzung)

Bad		
• Badewannenlifter	• Sturzgefahr • Verminderte Kraft	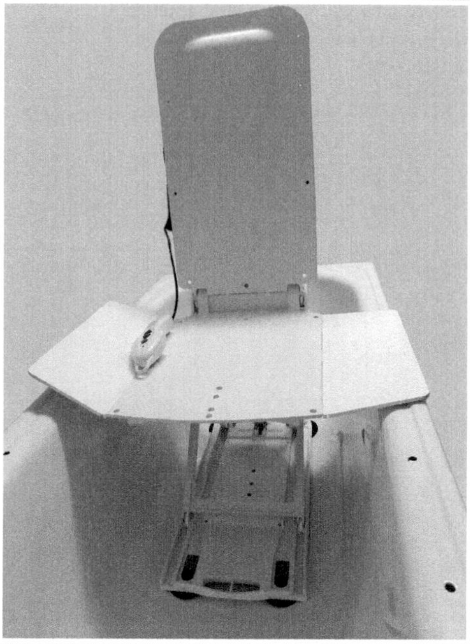
• Duschhocker/ Duschstuhl	• Sturzgefahr • Verminderte Kraft	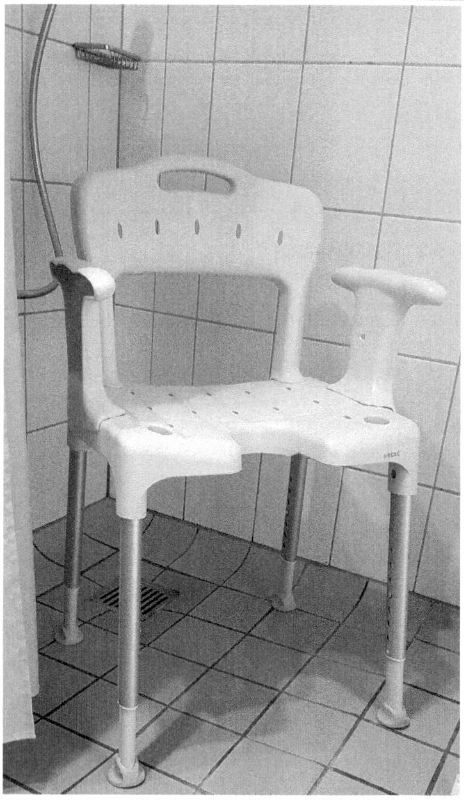

Tab. 15.2 (Fortsetzung)

Bad		
• Toilettenstuhl	• Nächtliche Dranginkontinenz • Nächtliche Sturzgefahr	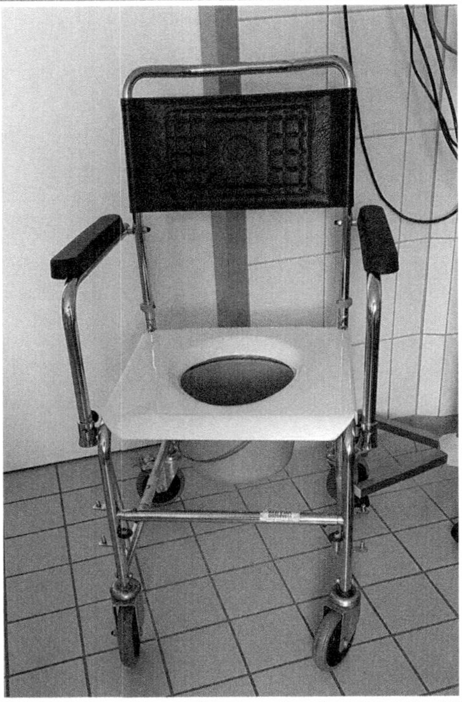
• Urinflasche	• Nächtliche Dranginkontinenz • Nächtliche Sturzgefahr	
• Toilettensitzerhöhung	• Verminderte Beinkraft • Sturzgefahr • Haltungsanomalien	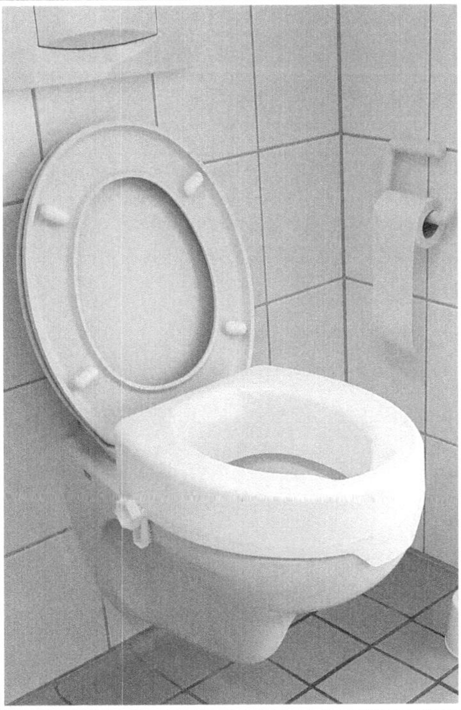
• Haltegriffe	• Sturzgefahr	

Tab. 15.3 Bürohilfsmittel

Büro		
• Adaptierte Stifte, dicke Stifte, Schreibkugel, schwere Stifte	• Eingeschränkte Feinmotorik • Eingeschränkte Handkraft	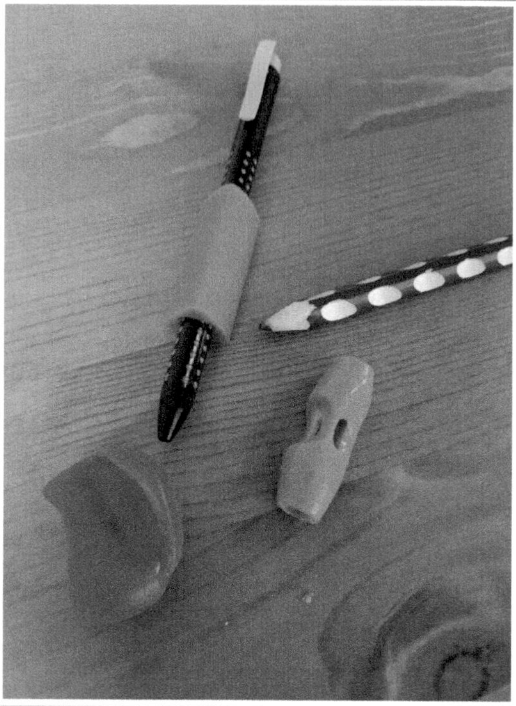
• Antitremor-Maus	• Tremor	
• Computermaus mit Kopfsteuerung	• Tremor	

Tab. 15.4 Küchenhilfsmittel

Küche		
• Öffnungshilfen für Gläser, Flaschen und Dosen	• Verminderte Handkraft • Herabgesetzte Koordination	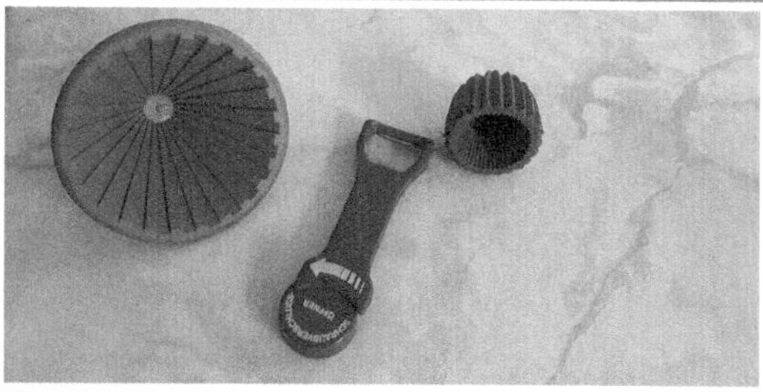

Tab. 15.5 Anziehhilfsmittel

Anziehen		
• Elastische Schnürsenkel	• Feinmotorische Einschränkungen	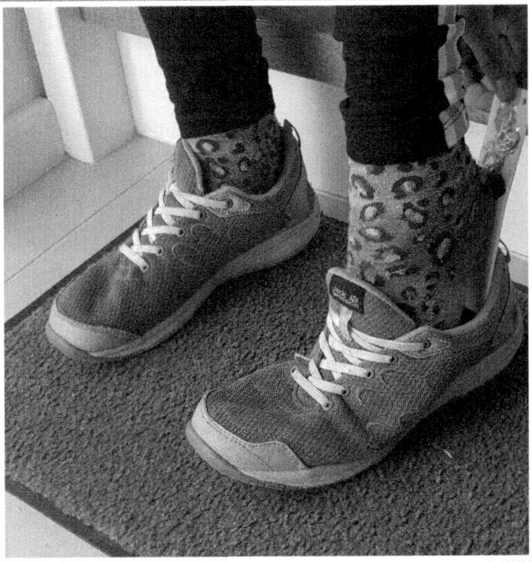
• Schuhlöffel	• Eingeschränkte Vorneigung • Reduzierte Kraft • Eingeschränkte Feinmotorik	
• Knöpf- und Reißverschlusshilfe	• Feinmotorische Einschränkungen	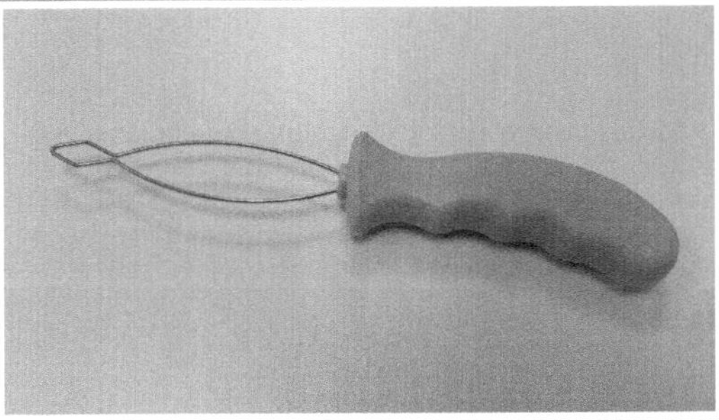

Tab. 15.6 Hilfsmittel zur Erleichterung des Alltags

Alltag		
• Telefon mit großen Tasten und Kurzwahltasten mit Fotos von Familie.	• Kognitive Einschränkungen • Feinmotorische Einschränkungen	
• Türcode statt Schlüssel, elektronische Türschlösser (per App bedienbar)	• Kognitive Einschränkung • Feinmotorische Einschränkung	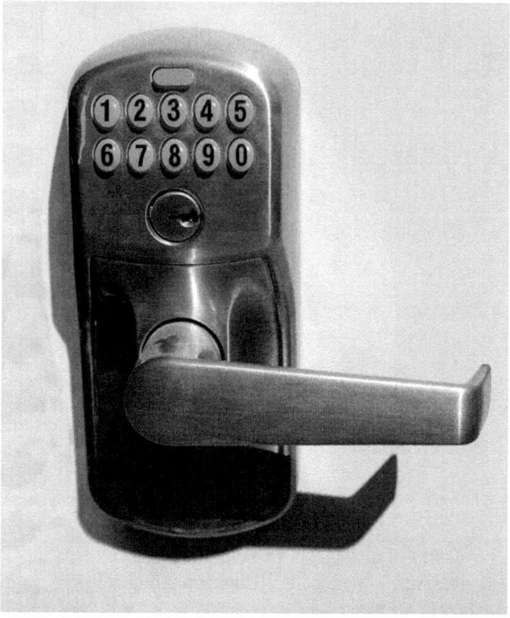
• Medikamentenbox mit Erinnerungsfunktion	• Kognitive Einschränkungen	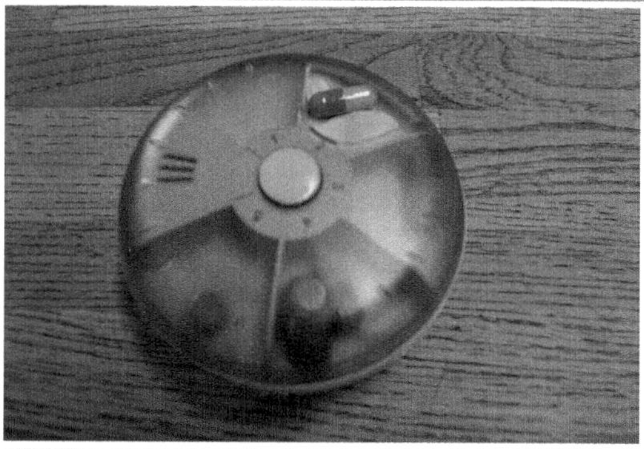
• Schlüsseldrehhilfe	• Feinmotorische Einschränkungen • Verminderte Handkraft	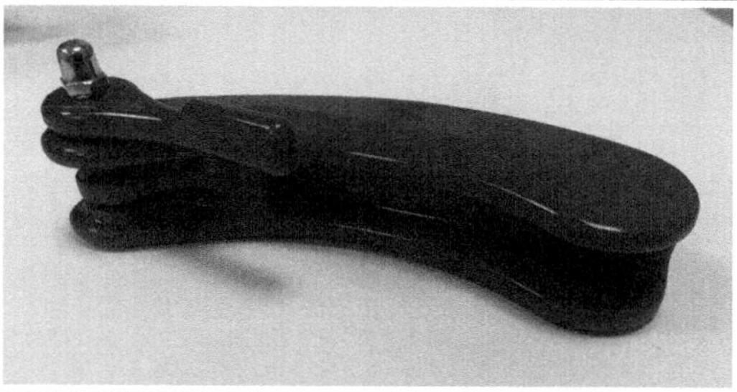
• Buchhalterung	• Tremor • Verminderte Handkraft	

Tab. 15.7 Mobilitätshilfsmittel

Mobilität		
• Rollator	• Sturzgefahr • Freezing	
• Rollator mit reversiblen Bremsen (zum Fortbewegen – Ziehen, zum Stehen – Loslassen)	• Freezing	
• Rollator mit einstellbarer Schleppbremse um schnelles „davonfahren" zu vermeiden	• Festination	
• Rollator mit Laser	• Freezing • Startschwierigkeiten	
• Walkingstöcke	• Aufrichtung • Sturzprävention durch Rhythmus	
• Laserstock (Laserstrahl wird auf Boden projiziert, als Cue)	• Freezing	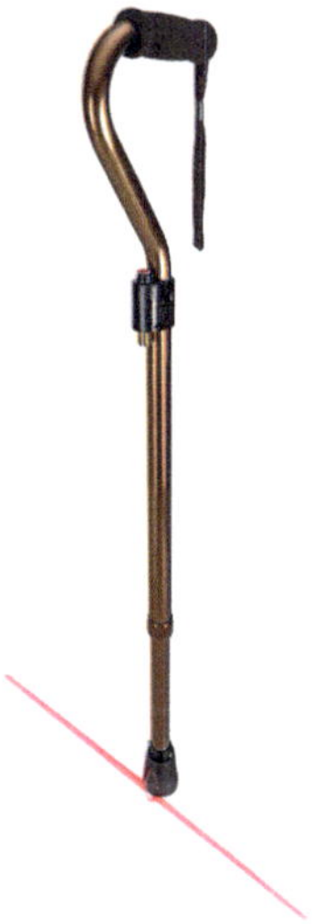 Z. B. Parkinsonstock mit ergonomischer Schaumstoffgriff und Laser Licht von Fa. Ossenberg
• Laserschuhe (Laserstrahl wird abwechselnd auf Boden projiziert, als Cue)	• Freezing	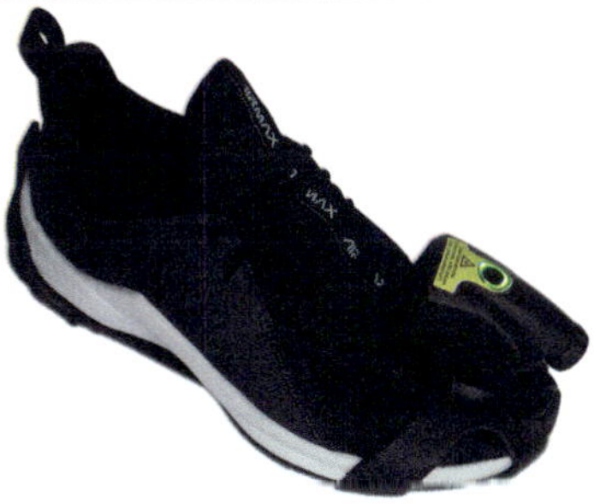 Path finder ® von der Fa. Walk With Path
• Rollstuhl	• Eingeschränkte Gehfähigkeit • Sturzgefahr • Längere Ausflüge	

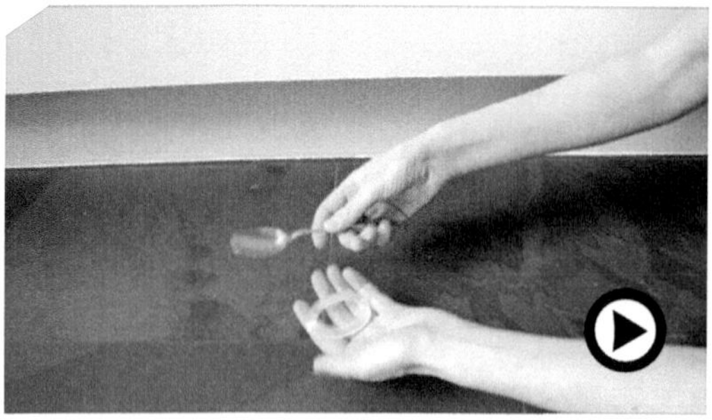

Abb. 15.10 Antitremoraufsatz für Löffel (▶ https://doi.org/10.1007/000-2y6)

Beispiel

Mittlerweile hat sich Frau P. daran gewöhnt, einen Duschhocker im Bad zu haben. Anfangs wollte Sie es aus ästhetischen Gründen nicht, doch der Ergotherapeut hat ein schlichtes Modell für sie gefunden. Und endlich: Sie fühlt sich sicher beim Duschen und Abtrocknen. ◀

Literatur und weiterführende Literatur

Carter JH, Stewart BJ, Archbold PG, Inoue I, Jaglin J, Lannon M, Rost-Ruffner E, Tennis M, McDermott MP, Amyot D, Barter R, Cornelius L, Demong C, Dobson J, Duff J, Erickson J, Gardiner N, Gauger L, Gray P, Kanigan B, Kiryluk B, Lewis P, Mistura K, Malapira T, Zoog K (1998) Living with a person who has Parkinson's disease: the spouse's perspective by stage of disease. Parkinson's Study Group. Mov Disord 13(1):20–28. https://doi.org/10.1002/mds.870130108. PMID: 9452321

Ellgring H, Seiler S, Nagel U, Perleth B, Gasser T, Oertel WH (1990) Psychosocial problems of Parkinson patients: approaches to assessment and treatment. Adv Neurol 53:349–53. PMID: 2239476

Foster ER, Bedekar M, Tickle-Degnen L (2014) Systematic review of the effectiveness of occupational therapy-related interventions for people with Parkinson's disease. Am J Occup Ther 68(1):39–49. https://doi.org/10.5014/ajot.2014.008706. PMID: 24367954; PMCID: PMC4413458

Law M (2002) Participation in the occupations of everyday life. Am J Occup Ther 56(6):640–649. https://doi.org/10.5014/ajot.56.6.640

Law M, Baptiste S, Mills J (1995) Client-centred practice: what does it mean and does it make a difference? Can J Occup Ther 62(5):250–257. https://doi.org/10.1177/000841749506200504. PMID: 10152881

Law M, Steinwender S, Leclair L (1998) Occupation, health and well-being. Can J Occu Ther 65(2):81–91. https://doi.org/10.1177/000841749806500204

Radder DLM, Sturkenboom IH, van Nimwegen M, Keus SH, Bloem BR, de Vries NM (2017) Physical therapy and occupational therapy in Parkinson's disease. Int J Neurosci 127(10):930–943. https://doi.org/10.1080/00207454.2016.1275617

Signer T, Weise A (2020) Betätigungsorientierte Patientenedukation und Kompensation im stationären Rehabilitations-Alltag: die „Energiemanagement-Schulung" – ein Fallbeispiel. Schulz-Kirchner GmbH, Rheinsbreitbach, S 135–152

Sturkenboom I, Thijssen M, Gons-van Elsacker J, Jansen I, Maasdam A, Schulten M, Vijver-Visser D, Steultjens E, Bloem B, Munneke M (2008) Guidelines for occupational therapy in Parkinson's disease rehabilitation. ParkinsonNet/NPF, Nijmegen/Miami

Komplette Betätigung trainieren 16

Beispiel

Herr K. klammert sich mit beiden Händen an die Armlehnen seines Stuhls: „Ich falle!"

„Keine Angst, ich bin hier, Herr K." Die Therapeutin hockt vor seinem Stuhl und gibt ihm über die Knie Input nach unten in die Füße, die fest am Boden stehen. „Jetzt nehmen Sie eine Hand von der Lehne und legen Sie sie mir auf die Schulter." Herr K. hält die Schulter der Therapeutin fest. „Nun die zweite Hand!", fordert die Therapeutin ihn auf. Stück für Stück arbeiten sie sich voran. Herr K. will seine Hose wieder ohne Hilfe anziehen können. Motorisch ist es möglich. Nach einem Sturz aus dem Stuhl beim Hose Anziehen hat er jedoch große Angst. ◀

16.1 Entscheidung für komplette Betätigung trainieren

Die Betätigung kann entweder in Teilen trainiert werden, am problematischen Performance-Skill (siehe Kap. 13) oder es wird die komplette Betätigung trainiert. Die Entscheidung, ob die ganze Betätigung oder nur der „Break-Down-Point" als therapeutische Intervention gewählt wird, hängt mit folgenden Faktoren zusammen:

- **Komplexität der Betätigung**: Bei einer komplexen Betätigung wie „Frühstück zubereiten" wird es meist nicht notwendig sein, die gesamte Betätigung als Training durchzuführen. Sinnvoller ist es, ein Performance-Skill, z. B. Kaffeepulver einfüllen, welches vom Therapeuten als „Break-Down-Point" erkannt wurde, zu beüben. Eine kurze und simple Betätigung, z. B. „Aufstehen aus einem tiefen Sessel", kann als komplette Betätigung trainiert werden, da alle Performance-Skills direkt miteinander zusammenhängen und eine isolierte Beübung meist zielführend ist.
- **Kognition**: Bei Klientinnen mit demenzieller Entwicklung kann es hilfreich sein, die gesamte Betätigung zu trainieren. Die Isolierung eines Performance-Skill, um intensiv daran zu arbeiten, ist für die Klientin evtl. nicht nachvollziehbar, da sie den Zusammenhang mit der Betätigung nicht erkennt.
- **Geschwindigkeit**: Eine hohe Geschwindigkeit ist beim repetitiven Training einer Betätigung von Vorteil (s. u.). Um dies zu ermöglichen, muss häufig ein Teil der Betätigung zunächst ausgeklammert werden. Er soll z. B. soll beim Schließen des Reißverschlusses das Hochziehen geübt werden. Dazu wird das Einfädeln nicht wiederholt geübt, da es die Schnelligkeit der Übung erheblich reduzieren würde und nicht das primäre Problem darstellt.
- **Vorbereitung der Betätigung durch Veränderung der Betätigung, Training einer Körperfunktion oder Adaptation**: War der Inhalt der Therapie auf ein Training oder die Veränderung eines Aspektes der Betätigung konzen-

A. Orellana, *Betätigungsorientierte Ergotherapie bei Morbus Parkinson*,
https://doi.org/10.1007/978-3-662-62583-5_16

triert, ist es wichtig, im Anschluss ein Carry-Over (Übertrag) in den Alltag der Klientin zu schaffen, indem die komplette Betätigung durchgeführt wird.

Es gibt zwei denkbare Fälle:
Entweder, die Klientin übt die Betätigung sofort nach der Assessment-Phase, mit Beginn der therapeutischen Interventionsphase, als Ganzes. Oder (und dieser Fall tritt wohl häufiger auf) es erfolgt zuerst eine andere Art der Intervention, um konkret am festgestellten Problem zu arbeiten, und im Anschluss wird dazu übergegangen, die komplette Betätigung zu üben.

Sofort komplette Betätigung trainieren
Wie oben beschrieben gibt es verschiedene Gründe, die komplette Betätigung zu üben. In diesem Fall kann der Ergotherapeut sofort mit der Vorbereitung des Trainings beginnen (s. u.).

Zunächst andere Intervention, dann komplette Betätigung
In vielen Fällen ist eine sofortige Beübung der ganzen Betätigung nicht zielführend. In einer punktuellen Intervention kann fokussiert am identifizierten Ursprung des Problems gearbeitet werden, um diesen dann später in die Gesamtbetätigung zu integrieren. Im „Perfect fit" (siehe Abb. 4.4) ist dieser Ablauf übersichtlich dargestellt. Hier einige Beispiele:

- Nach dem **repetitiven und intensiven Training eines Performance-Skill** muss immer noch einmal die gesamte Betätigung einige Male durchgeführt werden.
- Wurden **Kompensationsstrategien** mit der Klientin geübt (z. B. Cueing, Aufmerksamkeit fokussieren, Umgang mit Stress, Merkstrategien), sollte nach dem isolierten Einüben zunehmend das selbständige Einsetzen der Strategie im Alltag anhand der Übung der Betätigung als Ganzes trainiert werden.
- Beim Training einer **Körperfunktion** (z. B. Körperausrichtung, Dehnung, Schmerzreduzierung, große Amplitude) ist es meist sinnvoll, noch in derselben Therapieeinheit die Verknüpfung zur Betätigung herzustellen, um die Übertragung in den Alltag sicherzustellen.
- Wurden **Kontextfaktoren** verändert (z. B. Hilfsmittel, Tagesstrukturierung, externe Gedächtnishilfen, Wohnraumanpassung), ist ein Training des Umgangs im Alltag der Klientin notwendig, um eine Verinnerlichung zu gewährleisten. Durch das Üben der kompletten Betätigung wird die Adaptation ganz natürlich in den Handlungsablauf integriert.

Alle o. g. therapeutischen Interventionen werden in Kap. 11 zusammenfassend und den Kap. 13, 14 und 15 ausführlich erläutert.

▶ Eine isolierte Interventionsart ist selten sinnvoll. Erst durch die Kombination der verschiedenen Interventionsmöglichkeiten wird der Therapeut der Komplexität der Betätigung im individuellen Kontext der Klientin gerecht.

16.2 Durchführung

Wurde die Entscheidung getroffen, die komplette Betätigung zu trainieren, wird folgendermaßen vorgegangen:

1. Vorbereitung des Kontexts: Je näher am wirklichen Kontext trainiert wird, desto höher ist die Wahrscheinlichkeit, dass die Klientin das Trainierte später umsetzt. Oder andersherum formuliert – je abstrakter und weiter weg vom Kontext, desto unwahrscheinlicher wird es sein, dass ein Übertrag in den Alltag stattfindet. Um über eine möglichst reale Situation für die Betätigung zu verfügen, kann der Kontext, in dem die Betätigung normalerweise stattfindet, simuliert werden oder es wird bestenfalls direkt im Umfeld der Klientin trainiert. Dabei sind alle Elemente des Kontexts zu beachten:
   - zeitlich – gewohnte Tageszeit und Länge der Durchführung,
   - materiell – gewohnte Umgebung (Raum, Möbel, Hilfsmittel),
   - sozial – normalerweise anwesende Personen (welche Rolle? Helfend, sichernd, beobachtend),
   - soziokulturelle Elemente (Rituale, Glaube, Einstellungen, politische Einflüsse).

Bei körpernahen Betätigungen (z. B. Anziehen, Zähneputzen) hat der Kontext weniger Einfluss auf die Umsetzung. Bei komplexeren, körperfernen Betätigungen (z. B. Tagesplanung, Kochen) ist eine Simulation, besonders in Institutionen, meist unumgänglich. Hier ist die möglichst genaue Kenntnis der gewohnten Umgebung der Klientin eine hilfreiche Information. Angehörige können in diesem Fall eine Vermittlerrolle übernehmen und mit Videos, Fotos, Beschreibungen und mitgebrachten Gegenständen die Simulation realer machen.

2. **Festlegung des Anfangs- und Endpunktes der Betätigung:** Eine genaue Abgrenzung der Betätigung zu anderen Betätigungen ist sinnvoll, um den Fokus auf die zu beübende Sequenz beizubehalten. Dazu wird ein fester Anfangs- und Endpunkt festgelegt, die Klientin und Therapeut als passend einschätzen.
3. **Besprechung der identifizierten „Break-Down-Points"**: Bei der Betätigungsanalyse wurden vom Therapeuten Problempunkte, sog. „Break-Down-Points" identifiziert. Zweck des Trainings ist es, diese Punkte durch eine veränderte Durchführung zu korrigieren. Eine Besprechung der „Break-Down-Points" mit der Klientin ist also notwendig, damit sie sich dieser bewusst wird, weiß, wie sie sie verändern kann und den Sinn des Trainings versteht.
4. **Besprechung der genauen Schritte der Betätigung**: Vor dem Training wird die Betätigung genau definiert, um eine möglichst exakte Version der Tätigkeit zu üben. Für die Klientin nachvollziehbar ist dazu eine Aufteilung der Betätigung in Teilschritte. Dies wird ausführlich in Abschn. 14.1.4 (Aufteilung in Sequenzen) beschrieben.
5. **Besprechung der Durchführung unter Berücksichtigung vorbereiteter Aspekte**:
   - Evtl. Integration einzeln geübter Breakdown Points in Gesamtausführung (siehe Kap. 13),
   - evtl. Einsatz erlernter Strategien und Kompensationen (siehe Kap. 14, nach Symptomen sortiert),
   - evtl. Umsetzen der trainierten Körperfunktionen (siehe Kap. 14 nach Symptomen Sortiert),
   - evtl. Einsatz von Adaptationen (siehe Kap. 15).
6. **Durchführung des Trainings**: Nach der detaillierten Vorbereitung achtet der Therapeut nun auf die Umsetzung o. g. Punkte beim Training. Je eingehender die Beschäftigung mit der Betätigung **vor** der Durchführung ist, desto weniger muss der Therapeut während des Trainings intervenieren. Wann ein Einschreiten des Therapeuten notwendig ist und wann es besser ist, es „laufen zu lassen", muss der Therapeut mit Fingerspitzengefühl handhaben. Auf jeden Fall muss eine „falsche" oder fehlerhafte Ausführung der Betätigung vermieden werden. Eine Verhaltensänderung und somit erfolgreiche Therapie können nur erfolgen, wenn eine hohe Anzahl an „richtigen" Wiederholungen hintereinander gezeigt wird. Dies liegt an neuronalen Prozessen, die beim Lernen stattfinden. Neuronale Verknüpfungen und eine Festigung der Bahnen im Gehirn werden bei hoher Schnelligkeit, erhöhter Aufmerksamkeit, rhythmisiertem Training und einer großen Zahl an Repetitionen ausgelöst. Diese hohe Intensität und große Wiederholungszahl sind beim Training der kompletten Betätigung nicht so günstig umsetzbar wie beim Training einzelner Performance-Skills (siehe Kap. 13). Trotzdem sollten dem Therapeuten diese Trainingsfaktoren bekannt sein, um einer Verlangsamung im Training entgegenzuwirken.
7. **Zwischen-/Abschlussassessment**. Während des Trainings beobachtet der Therapeut konstant die Fortschritte der Klientin und spiegelt ihr diese. Zusätzlich ist es empfehlenswert, am Ende der Therapieeinheit jedes Mal eine Betätigungsanalyse (siehe Kap. 6) durchzuführen. Hierbei werden Anstrengung, Effizienz, Sicherheit und benötigte Hilfe festgehalten. Diese Messung der Verbesserung ist aus mehreren Gründen sinnvoll:
   1. Die Motivation der Klientin wird gesteigert, wenn der Fortschritt dokumentiert wird.
   2. Sie liefert konkrete Daten für Arztgespräche oder Berichte.
   3. Es wird aufzeigt, ob die Therapiemethode erfolgreich ist.

Die ausführliche Vorbereitung des Trainings und die konstanten Besprechungen mit der Klientin führen bei der Klientin zu einem tiefen Verständnis für den Inhalt der Therapie.

▶ Das stetige Miteinbeziehen der Klientin in die Therapieplanung und -durchführung ist wichtig, damit sie Eigenverantwortung übernimmt, aktiv an der Therapiegestaltung teilnimmt und das Ziel stets vor Augen hat.

Nicht selten kann bei einer solchen Arbeitsweise beobachtet werden, dass Klientinnen konkrete Vorschläge in die Therapie einbringen, sodass der Therapeut eher eine Berater- und Unterstützerrolle übernimmt. Die Kompetenz „Selbstmanagement" ist besonders bei einer chronischen Erkrankung wie M. Parkinson sehr wertvoll und stärkt die Klientin innerlich, damit sie sich auch in zukünftigen Therapiesituationen ganz selbstverständlich engagiert.

Kognitive Einschränkungen

Schon bei der Auswahl der Intervention hat sich der Therapeut gezielt Gedanken zur Effektivität des Trainings der kompletten Betätigung gemacht. Menschen mit (beginnender) Demenz werden meist eine geringere Umsetzung des veränderten Verhaltens zeigen, weswegen die Intervention in diesem Fall häufig im kompensatorischen oder adaptiven Bereich erfolgt. Entschließt sich der Therapeut dennoch dazu, trotz der kognitiven Einschränkungen der Klientin, die Betätigung mit der Klientin zu üben, sind einige Dinge zu beachten.

Der Ablauf der o. g. sieben Schritte wird ebenfalls durchlaufen. Gegebenenfalls werden sie leicht abgeändert.

Zu 1.: **Vorbereitung des Kontexts**: Die Nähe zum Alltag der Klientin während des Trainings ist bei kognitiven Einschränkungen besonders wichtig. Ein Übertrag von einer abstrakten Übungssituation in der Ergotherapie in den eigenen Kontext setzt eine kognitive Transferleistung voraus, die von Menschen mit kognitiven Schwierigkeiten nicht erwartet werden kann.

Zu 2.: **Festlegung des Anfangs- und Endpunkts**: Hier kann eine kurze Erinnerung vor Beginn des Trainings hilfreich sein.

Zu 3.: **Besprechung der identifizierten „Break-Down-Points"**: Wenn die Merkfähigkeit der Klientin eingeschränkt ist, ist eine Besprechung der Break-Down-Points wahrscheinlich nicht zielführend. Besser ist es, im genauen Moment der fehlerhaften Durchführung schnell einzugreifen und die Betätigung abzuändern; z. B. in dem Moment, wo die Klientin beginnt, das Gleichgewicht zu verlieren, die Klientin sichern und eine Anweisung einwerfen wie „Haltegriff!" oder „großer Schritt!". So kann eine Veränderung der Betätigung durch prozedurales Lernen erreicht werden.

Zu 4.: **Besprechung der genauen Schritte der Betätigung**: Anstatt nur zu besprechen, können Bilder mit den Betätigungsschritten als Visualisierung oder ein Video der Klientin bei der korrekten Durchführung als Erinnerungshilfe dienen. Dies kann dem Verständnis der Klientin sehr förderlich sein. Siehe Abb. 16.1, 16.2 und 16.3.

Und zu 5.: **Besprechung der Durchführung**: Die Besprechungen der Durchführung sollten kurzgehalten werden, um die Klientin nicht zu überfordern. Der Therapeut übernimmt mehr

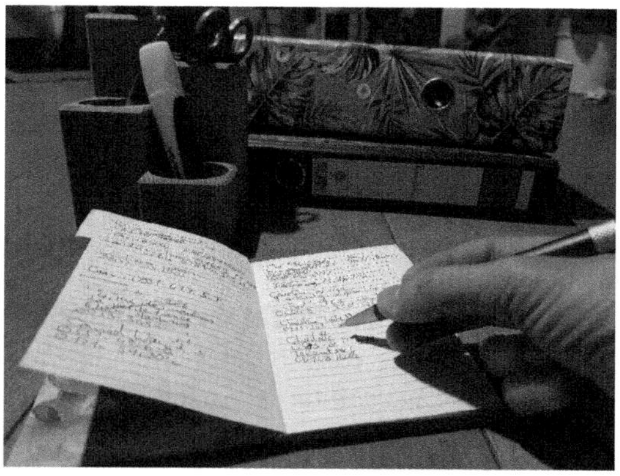

Abb. 16.1 Bei Klientinnen mit einer demenziellen Entwicklung ist, unterstützend zur Besprechung der Betätigungsschritte, die visuelle Veranschaulichung mit Fotos der Betätigung hilfreich. Hier z. B. Telefonnummer suchen …

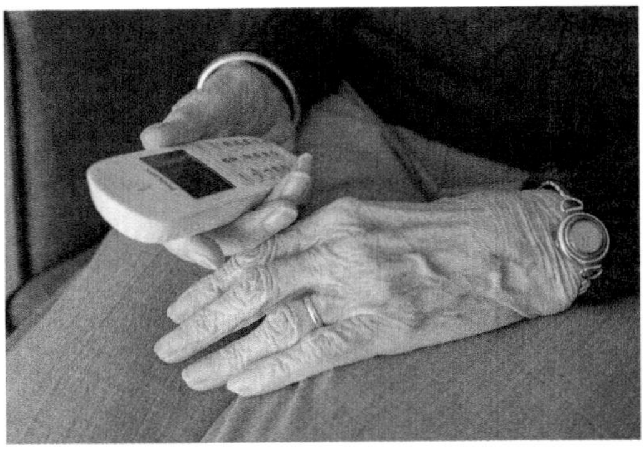

Abb. 16.2 … Telefonnummer eingeben…

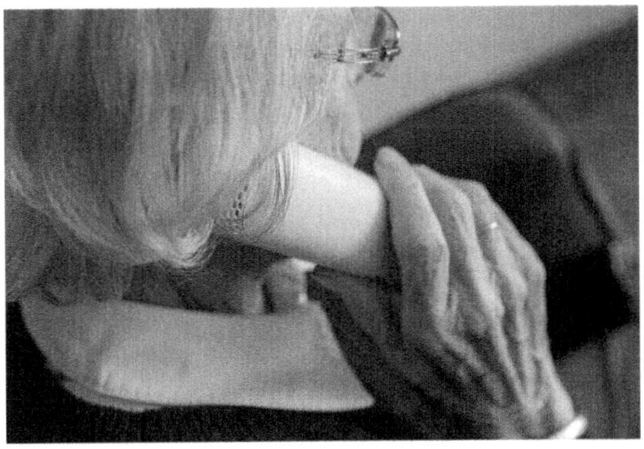

Abb. 16.3 … Klingeln lassen.

Verantwortung, bezieht die Klientin weniger in den Entscheidungsprozess ein.

Zu 6.: **Durchführung des Trainings**: Wenn die Merkfähigkeit der Klientin herabgesetzt ist, mag sie die korrekte Durchführung vergessen. Die Korrektur durch den Therapeuten sollte einfühlsam vermittelt werden. Die verbale Verbesserung wird von Klientinnen häufig als „belehrend" empfunden. Deswegen kann sie durch die o. g. Visualisierungen oder kurzes Führen der Bewegung abgelöst werden. Auch das Vormachen oder Paralleltrainieren von Therapeut und Klientin ist eine Möglichkeit.

Zu 7.: **Zwischen- und Abschlussassessment**: Die Betätigungsanalyse sollte auch bei kognitiv eingeschränkten Klientinnen am Ende jeder Therapieeinheit durchgeführt werden.

16.3 Begründung von betätigungsorientierter Therapie

Das Bild, das während dieser Art der Intervention „Betätigung trainieren" nach außen vermittelt wird, wirkt nicht immer professionell. Schließlich „steht der Therapeut nur daneben", während die Klientin etwas Alltägliches tut. So könnte es aus Sicht eines Außenstehenden, wie einer Ärztin, Physiotherapeutin oder Angehörigen scheinen. Natürlich ist es aus Sicht der Ergotherapeuten eine höchst professionelle und seriöse therapeutische Intervention. Denn schließlich…

- arbeitet der Therapeut nach einem Modell (z. B. OTIPM),
- hat die Intervention ein klientenzentriertes Betätigungsziel (z. B. Aufstehen aus dem Bett ohne Hilfe des Angehörigen),
- wurde die Interventionsart basierend auf wissenschaftlichen Erkenntnissen und praktischer Erfahrung sorgsam ausgewählt,
- wurden die Break-Down-Points der Betätigung vor der Durchführung mit der Klientin besprochen,
- hält er im Anschluss noch eine Angehörigenberatung zur Besprechung von Unterstützungsmöglichkeiten,
- wurde der Prozess und die Durchführung detailliert mit der Klientin besprochen und mit Fotos visualisiert.

Die Komponenten, die die Intervention sinnvoll machen, sind häufig nicht auf den ersten Blick sichtbar. Deswegen sind eine fachliche Ausdrucksweise und kompetente Kommunikation mit angrenzenden Berufsgruppen unabdingbar.

▶ Ergotherapeuten sollten bei jeder Möglichkeit ihre betätigungsorientierte Zielformulierung, ihr klientenzentriertes Denken und ihre evidenzbasierte Umsetzung fachlich mit Angehörigen und angrenzenden Berufsgruppen kommunizieren.

Der Therapeut sollte selbstbewusst die Gelegenheiten ergreifen (Visite, Bericht, Teambesprechungen) seine Professionalität darzulegen. Hierbei kann das Schreiben eines Therapieplans, z. B. mithilfe der o. g. sieben Schritte, zur Eigenstrukturierung hilfreich sein und der Selbstkontrolle dienen.

Beispiel

„So Herr N., für heute sind wir fast fertig. Sie haben einen großen Fortschritt gemacht. Sie haben Ihre Angst überwunden. Jetzt können Sie die Hände auf den Stuhl vor sich legen, ohne Angst zu haben. Jetzt möchte ich am Ende noch einmal, dass Sie Ihre Hose anziehen. Versuchen Sie es bitte so: Sie ziehen die Hose an. Vor Ihnen steht der Stuhl, auf dem Sie sich abstützen können, falls Sie Angst bekommen, und zusätzlich sichere ich Sie hier, von der Seite. Es kann also nichts passieren. Wir haben das Vorbeugen ja die ganze Stunde geübt, Sie können es gut. Gehen Sie Schritt für Schritt vor, Sie haben Zeit." ◀

Literatur und weiterführende Literatur

Fernandez L, Huys R, Issartel J, Azulay JP, Eusebio A (2018) Movement speed-accuracy trade-off in Parkinson's disease. Front Neurol 9:897. https://doi.org/10.3389/fneur.2018.00897. PMID: 30405521; PMCID: PMC6208126

Foster ER, Bedekar M, Tickle-Degnen L (2014) Systematic review of the effectiveness of occupational therapy-related interventions for people with Parkinson's disease. Am J Occup Ther 68(1):39–49. https://doi.org/10.5014/ajot.2014.008706. PMID: 24367954; PMCID: PMC4413458

Kakar C, Zia N, Sehgal S, Kushwaha S (2013) Effect of external and internal focus of attention on acquisition, retention, and transfer phase of motor learning in Parkinson's disease. Hong Kong Physiother J 31:88–94. https://doi.org/10.1016/j.hkpj.2013.02.001

Law M (2002) Participation in the occupations of everyday life. Am J Occup Ther 56(6):640–649. https://doi.org/10.5014/ajot.56.6.640

Law M, Baptiste S, Mills J (1995) Client-centred practice: what does it mean and does it make a difference? Can J Occup Ther 62(5):250–257. https://doi.org/10.1177/000841749506200504. PMID: 10152881

Law M, Steinwender S, Leclair L (1998) Occupation, health and well-being. Can J Occup Ther 65(2):81–91. https://doi.org/10.1177/000841749806500204

Mazzoni P, Hristova A, Krakauer J (2007) Why don't we move faster? Parkinson's disease, movement vigor, and implicit motivation. J Neurosci 27(27):7105–7116. https://doi.org/10.1523/JNEUROSCI.0264-07.2007. PMID: 17611263; PMCID: PMC6794577

Hubbard IJ, Parsons MW, Neilson C, Carey LM (2009) Task-specific training: evidence for and translation to clinical practice. Occup Ther Int 16(3–4):175–189. https://doi.org/10.1002/oti.275. PMID: 19504501

Radder DLM, Sturkenboom IH, van Nimwegen M, Keus SH, Bloem BR, de Vries NM (2017) Physical therapy and occupational therapy in Parkinson's disease. Int J Neurosci 127(10):930–943. https://doi.org/10.1080/00207454.2016.1275617

Sturkenboom I, Thijssen M, Gons-van Elsacker J, Jansen I, Maasdam A, Schulten M, Vijver-Visser D, Steultjens E, Bloem B, Munneke M (2008) Guidelines for occupational therapy in Parkinson's disease rehabilitation. ParkinsonNet/NPF, Nijmegen/Miami

17 Eigenübungen

Beispiel

Herr S. kracht mit dem Rollator gegen den Stuhl. Oh, den hat er nicht gesehen. In der Küche angekommen streckt er sich, um eine Tasse aus dem Schrank zu holen. Mit viel Mühe gelingt es ihm, bis zur Tasse zu greifen. Fast jede Tätigkeit im Alltag fällt Herrn S. wegen seiner vorgebeugten Haltung schwer. Außerdem tut ihm der Nacken ständig weh. Dabei übt er doch jede Woche in der Physiotherapie die Aufrichtung. ◀

17.1 Funktion von Eigenübungen

Eigenübungen sind ein elementarer Teil der ergotherapeutischen Intervention. Ohne Eigenübungen fehlt der Therapie die Wirksamkeit, ja die Vision. Folgende Funktionen werden hierbei erfüllt:

1. Klient übernimmt Eigenverantwortung
2. Repetitionszahlen werden erreicht
3. Übertrag in den Alltag kann stattfinden
4. Zwischenprüfung

1. **Klient übernimmt Eigenverantwortung**: Wie schon in Abschn. 10.1(Selbstmanagement) beschrieben, wird die Effektivität der Intervention wesentlich gesteigert, wenn der Klient „Herr der Lage" ist und seine eigenen Bedürfnisse, Ziele und Problemlösungsstrategien formuliert und anschließend aktiv wird. Dadurch empfindet sich der Klient als selbstwirksam und seine intrinsische Motivation wird gesteigert und der Antrieb wird größer. Das Gefühl des Klienten, dass die Krankheit ihn im Griff hat, nimmt ab, sobald er aktiv dagegenwirkt.
2. Repetition**szahlen werden erreicht**: Um eine neurophysiologische Veränderung zu erreichen und das Verhalten zu verändern, ist eine hohe Wiederholungszahl der zu trainierenden Betätigung oder Körperfunktion notwendig (siehe Abschn. 13.2). Diese sind innerhalb der Therapieeinheit selten erreichbar und müssen vom Klienten zu Hause bzw. auf dem Patientenzimmer (in der Klinik) selbständig geübt werden.
3. Übertrag in den Alltag: Die Kunst der Ergotherapie ist, das in der Therapieeinheit Trainierte in den Alltag zu übertragen, das sog. Carry-Over. Dies gelingt nur durch Übernahme von Eigenverantwortung in Form von Eigenübungen seitens des Klienten. Als Eigenübungen kann der Klient trainierte Inhalte zwischen den Therapieeinheiten regelmäßig in seinem Alltag ausprobieren und gegebenenfalls Schwierigkeiten an die Therapeutin zurückmelden.
4. **Kontrolle**: Die Eigenübungen dienen auch als eine Art Regulator. Macht der Klient seine Eigenübungen selbständig und regelmäßig, ist das ein Indikator für eine hohe Motivation des

A. Orellana, *Betätigungsorientierte Ergotherapie bei Morbus Parkinson*,
https://doi.org/10.1007/978-3-662-62583-5_17

Klienten. Ist dies nicht der Fall, müssen Therapeutin und Klient gemeinsam nach der Ursache suchen. Hilfreich hierfür ist das „Perfect fit" (siehe Abb. 4.4). Die nach oben führenden Pfeile auf der linken Seite stellen den Korrekturprozess dar.

17.2 Ziele von Eigenübungen

Eigenübungen richten sich meist nach dem Betätigungsziel; es kann aber auch sinnvoll sein, die Eigenübungen als eine Ergänzung der therapeutischen Intervention zu nutzen oder einen Teilaspekt der Betätigung als Eigenübung zu geben.

Beispiel Fr. F. möchte sich morgens wieder ohne Hilfe anziehen. Dies wird innerhalb der Therapieeinheit analysiert, besprochen, in Bewegungssequenzen eingeteilt und mithilfe von Selbstinstruktion geübt.

- **Eigenübung als Ergänzung**: Die positiven Einflussfaktoren, die in Kap. 10 ausführlich beschrieben sind, fördern die Effektivität der Therapie. Da sie meist nicht als Hauptziel genannt werden, kann es günstig sein, einen der positiven Einflussfaktoren durch Eigenübungen zu unterstützen, während in der Ergotherapie das Betätigungsziel im Vordergrund steht.

Beispiel Fr. F. hat aber auch beschrieben, dass sie immer weniger Lust und Energie hat, sich sportlich zu betätigen. Die Therapeutin erkennt, dass dies ein wichtiger positiver Einflussfaktor auf das ergotherapeutische Outcome ist (siehe Abschn. 10.3 „Allgemeines Kraft und Ausdauertraining") und erarbeitet mit Fr. F. einen Trainingsplan auf dem Hometrainer. Dazu trägt sie nach jeder durchgeführten Eigenübungssequenz einen Smiley auf einem Motivationsplan ein.

- **Teilaspekt als Eigenübung**: Eine andere Form der Ergänzung ist es, einen Teilaspekt als Eigenübung aufzugeben und den Rest innerhalb der Therapie umzusetzen.

  Beispiel: Da Fr. F. sich häufig gestresst fühlt, was ihre Symptome verstärkt, zeigt die Therapeutin Fr. F. eine Atemübung zur Entspannung. Diese kurze Übung spricht sie der Klientin auf das Smartphone, damit sie sie vor dem Anziehen und vor anderen für die Klientin schwierigen oder stressassoziierten Betätigungen, wie dem Einkaufen, selbständig durchführen kann.
- **Eigenübung, um Ziel zu unterstützen**: Je nachdem, welches Ziel Klient und Therapeutin formuliert haben, werden die Eigenübungen entsprechend geplant.

  Es ist förderlich, die in der Therapieeinheit besprochenen und geübten Inhalte im realen Kontext zu wiederholen. Wie im „Perfect fit" in Abb. 4.4 zu erkennen ist, gibt es vier mögliche Trainingsbereiche in der Ergotherapie. Anhand dieser Trainingsbereiche werden die Möglichkeiten zur Eigenübung aufgezeigt.

  1. **Betätigung trainieren**
     a) **Komplette Betätigung**
     Ganz gleich, welche Interventionsart gewählt wird, ein Carry-Over in den Alltag ist immer das übergeordnete Ziel. Deshalb ist die Umsetzung dessen, was in der Ergotherapie trainiert wurde, immer Bestandteil der Eigenübung. Die Therapeutin sollte dies auch so kommunizieren, z. B.: „Das Training in der Therapie reicht allein nicht, um Verbesserungen zu erzielen. Sie müssen zu Hause/auf dem Zimmer weiterüben und das Geübte anwenden. Dann erreichen Sie eine positive Veränderung."
     b) **Einzelne Performance-Skills**
     Beim Training der Betätigung ist die Repetition von essenzieller Bedeutung, um die neuronalen Strukturen zu verändern und die gelingende Betätigung zu festigen. Um auf die Zahl von mindestens 900 Wiederholungen in drei Wochen zu kommen, müssen 60 Wiederholungen pro Tag, 5 × pro Woche durchgeführt werden. Rechnet man dies auf einen Tag herunter, sind es 3 x 20 Wiederholungen pro Tag.

- Beim Training der kompletten Betätigung oder der einzelnen Performance-Skills sollte die Betätigung, wenn möglich, im originalen Kontext erfolgen. Das heißt, Ort, Zeitpunkt und Umgebungsfaktoren sollten in der Übungssituation so ähnlich sein wie im Alltag.

2. **Betätigung verändern/kompensieren**: (z. B. Cueing, Aufteilung in Bewegungssequenzen, Vermeidung von Dual-Tasks ...) Nachdem die veränderte Betätigung innerhalb der Therapieeinheit erarbeitet wurde, ist eine Anwendung des Gelernten im realen Kontext notwendig. Dies kann schrittweise oder als Ganzes erfolgen. Da eine korrekte Umsetzung der Veränderungen ohne Unterstützung der Therapeutin anfangs meist nicht möglich ist, kann ein späterer Beginn der Eigenübungen angebracht sein. So wird eine fehlerhafte Ausführung vermieden. Andernfalls kann evtl. eine Angehörige als Co-Therapeutin eingesetzt werden, die die Übungen mit dem Betroffenen gemeinsam durchführt.
3. **Körperfunktionen trainieren**: Auch beim Training von Körperfunktionen, z. B. Aufrichtung, Dehnung, Schmerzreduzierung, Gleichgewichtstraining, ist eine hohe Wiederholungszahl notwendig, um eine Veränderung zu erreichen. Aus diesem Grund ist der Aufenthalt in einer Rehabilitationsklinik oftmals sehr erfolgreich. Durch die intensive und repetitive Therapie werden strukturelle Veränderungen im Gehirn und im Körper erzielt. Eine höhere Repetitionszahl im Setting der ergotherapeutischen Praxis versucht man über Eigenübung zu erreichen.

Am Beispiel der **Dehnung der ventralen Muskelkette** werden mögliche Eigenübungen beschrieben, die in der therapeutischen Arbeit mit Klienten mit M. Parkinson Anwendung finden können. Diese Übungen wurden für zu Hause adaptiert (z. B. Durchführung im Bett statt auf Bank)

Beispiele, Dehnung der ventralen Muskelkette

Die zunehmende Immobilität führt zu einer häufigen Sitzposition, zusätzlich zeigt sich eine krankheitstypische kyphotische Körperhaltung. Infolgedessen ist bei vielen Menschen mit der Parkinson-Erkrankung eine Verkürzung der ventralen Muskelkette festzustellen. Dies wirkt sich wiederum negativ auf die Mobilität und die Körperaufrichtung aus.

Um den negativen Kreislauf zu durchbrechen, ist die Dehnung eine hilfreiche Methode.

Übung 1

Dazu kann der Klient angeleitet werden, sich täglich vor dem Aufstehen, im Bett oder auf einer Matte fünf Minuten auf den Bauch zu legen.

Es gibt drei Schwierigkeitsgrade:

1. **Flach auf dem Bauch liegen**:
   - Kopf in Verlängerung der Wirbelsäule, auf Stirn aufliegend (evtl. auf aufgerolltem Handtuch oder kleinem Kopfkissen)
   - Arme, wenn möglich, nach vorne neben dem Kopf ausgestreckt abgelegt oder unter der Stirn; sonst neben dem Körper
2. **Ausgangsstellung siehe Nr. 1**:
   - Kopf abgehoben, Blick geht nach vorne
   - Brustkorb wenige Zentimeter von Unterlage abheben
   - Tief ein- und ausatmen
3. **Ausgangsstellung siehe Nr. 1**
   - Kopf aufrecht, Blick schräg nach vorne, oben
   - Unterarme liegen auf Unterlage
   - Oberkörper in Dehnung nach oben gedrückt
   - Becken bleibt auf der Unterlage liegen, hebt nicht ab

Übung 2

Im Bett, in Ausgangslage auf dem Rücken am Rand des Bettes. Das Bein, welches an der Bettkante liegt, hängt locker nach unten, der Fuß berührt den Boden. Dadurch entsteht eine Dehnung der Hüftbeuger. Zur Verstärkung der Dehnung können die Arme in Verlängerung des Körpers gestreckt werden.

- ▶ Cave: Sturz aus Bett vorbeugen, z. B. durch Sicherung durch Angehörige.

1. **Kontextfaktoren verändern (Adaptation)** Wurden Kontextfaktoren verändert, z. B. Vermittlung von Hilfsmittel, Wohnraumanpassung, benötigt es unterschiedliche Übungsintensitäten zur konstanten Anwendung im Alltag.

   Es kann vorkommen, dass der Klient schon nach einmaliger Besprechung und/oder einmaligem Ausprobieren die Anwendung versteht und ohne weitere Anleitung im Alltag umsetzt. Oftmals benötigen Klienten mit M. Parkinson durch die Einschränkung der exekutiven Funktionen eine längere Gewöhnungsphase bis die Veränderung des Kontexts im Alltagsgeschehen angewandt wird. Bezugnehmend auf Kap. 15 (Kontextfaktoren verändern) werden hier beispielhaft Vorschläge gemacht, um veränderte Kontextfaktoren im Alltag des Klienten zu integrieren (Angehörigenberatung, Hilfsmittel, Wohnraumberatung)

Angehörigenberatung (Eigenübung)
Es empfiehlt sich, die mit Angehörigen besprochenen Themen oder geübten Handgriffe als Eigenübung mit nach Hause zu geben. So können Angehörige und Betroffene neue Verhaltensweisen ausprobieren und sie im Alltag festigen. Wird das im Therapiesetting Geübte auf den Alltagskontext übertragen? Müssen noch einzelne Aspekte adaptiert werden? Klappt die Zusammenarbeit auch gut, wenn die Therapeutin nicht anwesend ist? Entstehen Konflikte?

Hilfsmittel (Eigenübungen)
Bis Hilfsmittel absolut selbständig genutzt werden können, benötigt es meist eine wiederholte Verwendung. Auch dazu sollten Eigenübungen eingesetzt werden. Denkt der Klient selbst daran, das neue Hilfsmittel zu nutzen? Funktioniert der Gebrauch auch ohne die Hinweise und Sicherung der Therapeutin?

Wohnraumberatung (Eigenübungen)
Ähnlich wie der Gebrauch der Hilfsmittel muss auch die Nutzung eines optimierten Wohnraums implementiert werden. Findet sich der Klient in der veränderten Wohnumgebung zurecht? Kehrt er zu alten Mustern zurück? Fühlt er sich sicher und wohl mit der Erneuerung? Eine tägliche Dokumentation der Nutzung durch den Klienten oder Angehörigen ist empfehlenswert, um Schwierigkeiten oder Vergessen der Implementierung festzuhalten.

17.3 Ausführung von Eigenübungen

Die Umsetzung von Eigenübungen variiert von Fall zu Fall. Folgende Faktoren muss die Therapeutin bei der Planung von Eigenübungen berücksichtigen: Sicherheit, in On-Phase, Klientenfaktoren, Kontext, Ziel, Zeitfaktoren, Erinnerungs- und Motivationshilfen.

Sicherheit

▶ **Cave!** Die Sturzgefahr ist bei motorischen Eigenübungen stark erhöht, da die Therapeutin weder die Tagesverfassung des Klienten einschätzen noch als Sicherung danebenstehen kann.

Die Sicherheit ist der wichtigste Aspekt. Bei Sturzgefährdung, demenziellen Entwicklungen und plötzlich auftretenden Akinesen (Freezing) sind Eigenübungen im Stehen und Gehen risikoreich und müssen von der Therapeutin genau bedacht werden. Einem Sturz mit eventuellen Folgeschäden, wie Oberschenkelhalsbruch oder Platzwunde am Kopf, muss unbedingt vorgebeugt werden. Je nach Einschätzung der Therapeutin können Hilfsmittel oder -personen zur Sicherung nötig sein, um die Eigenübung realisierbar zu machen. Dazu zählen:

- Haltegriff
- Stuhl hinter Klient
- Bett hinter Klient

- feste Schuhe, nicht hinten offen!
- Sicherungsperson (Angehörige, Pflegeperson)

Viele Menschen mit M. Parkinson erleben große Tagesschwankungen. Dies kann mit Medikamentenfluktuation, Fatigue oder krankheits- oder medikamentenbedingten Stimmungsschwankungen zusammenhängen. Wenn solche Schwankungen, von Klient und Therapeutin unvorhersehbar, auftreten und ein Sturzrisiko zur Folge haben, ist die Therapeutin dazu verpflichtet, sehr vorsichtig vorzugehen. Entweder, es wird ein Training ohne Sturzgefahr erarbeitet, oder eine stabile Sicherungsperson muss in das Training miteinbezogen werden. Wenn beides nicht möglich ist, geht die Sicherheit vor und es wird kein motorisches Eigenübungsprogramm aufgegeben.

In On-Phase

Außerdem ist darauf zu achten, dass der Klient seine Übungen in der On-Phase durchführt, also wenn die Medikamente wirken. Dies beginnt meist 30 Minuten nach Medikamenteneinnahme und dauert, je nach Fluktuationskurve, unterschiedlich lang. In der Frühphase der Parkinson-Erkrankung kommt es kaum zu Fluktuationen, im Verlauf der Krankheit nehmen sie zu. In der Spätphase können die Medikamente auch schon nach 30 Minuten an Wirksamkeit verlieren. Es gibt zwei Gründe, weshalb in der On-Phase trainiert wird. Erstens ist die Effektivität durch die gute Versorgung des Gehirns mit Dopamin wesentlich größer, zweitens ist die Sicherheit in der Off-Phase nicht gewährleistet.

Klientenfaktoren

Folgende Klientenfaktoren beeinflussen die Wahl der Eigenübung:

- **Alter**: Natürlich werden ältere Klienten weniger gefordert als jüngere Klienten, da sie meist nicht derart belastbar, dafür gebrechlicher sind und evtl. unter mehr Komorbiditäten leiden.
- **Krankheitsstadium**: In den früheren Krankheitsstadien ist der Antrieb meist noch wenig gestört und die Symptome noch nicht stark ausgeprägt, sodass ein energischer Einstieg in die Eigenübungen wahrscheinlicher ist.
- **Demenzielle Entwicklung**: Bei einer beginnenden Demenz sind Eigenübungen mit Merkhilfen (Kalender, Mobiltelefon, Übungsplan) umsetzbar. Mit fortschreitender demenzieller Entwicklung können Angehörige als Co-Therapeutinnen in die Eigenübungen miteinbezogen werden. Bei einer stark ausgeprägten Demenz sind Eigenübungen kaum noch durchführbar und durch die stark herabgesetzte Lernfähigkeit auch selten sinnvoll. Hier gilt es, den Klienten durch Teilhabe an Aktivitäten im Familien- und Freundeskreis zu aktivieren.
- **Allgemeine Fitness**: Ein Klient, der schon vor der Diagnose einen aktiven Lebensstil hatte und sich evtl. sportlich betätigt hat, wird Eigenübungen wahrscheinlich konsequenter umsetzen als ein Klient, der eine passivere Lebensweise hatte und viel Zeit sitzend verbracht hat.
- **Erfahrung mit Training (Sportler)**: Menschen, die einen Beruf oder ein Hobby auf hohem Niveau haben oder hatten, welches regelmäßige Übungsdisziplin verlangt, kennen das intensive und selbständige Trainieren. So fällt es professionellen Sportlern oder Musikern leicht, sich diszipliniert auf einen Übungsplan einzulassen.
- **Intrinsische Motivation**: Je größer die intrinsische Motivation des Klienten ist, desto selbstverständlicher ist das Durchführen des selbständigen Trainings. Aus diesem Grund ist es sinnvoll, eine klientenzentrierte Intervention zu praktizierten. Je genauer das Ziel mit den Wünschen des Klienten übereinstimmt und je näher am Alltagskontext geübt wird, desto größer ist die intrinsische Motivation des Klienten und desto weniger muss die Therapeutin überzeugen und animieren.

Kontextfaktoren

Folgende mögliche Kontexte haben Einfluss auf die Wahl der Eigenübung:

- **Klinik (Patientenzimmer)**: Auf dem Patientenzimmer sind körpernahe Betätigungen wie Anziehen und Haare kämmen gut umsetzbar. Eine genaue Absprache mit der Pflege, dass dies ein therapeutisches Ziel darstellt, sollte

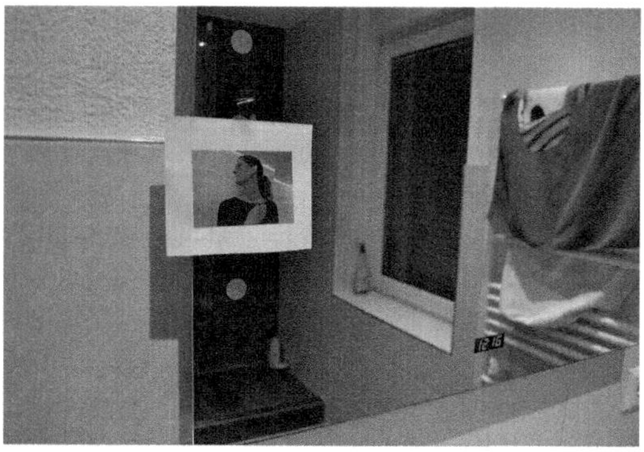

Abb. 17.1 Eine Erinnerungsnotiz hilft dem Klienten im Tagesablauf, an seine Eigenübungen zu denken, hier am Badspiegel

erfolgen, damit sie es nicht automatisch für den Klienten übernehmen.

Ein Zettel oder Bild am Spiegel kann als Erinnerungshilfe dienen (siehe Abb. 17.1).

- **Klinik (Übungsraum Ergotherapie)**: Eine gute Möglichkeit ist ein spezifischer Eigenübungsbereich in der Ergotherapie. Die genauen Rahmenbedingungen (Ort der Durchführung, Aufsicht, Klingel, Dokumentationspflicht, Art der Übungen) müssen mit dem Versicherer der Klinik besprochen werden, um sicherzugehen, dass eine Absicherung im Falle einer Verletzung besteht.
- **Gruppe „Eigenübungen"**: Sowohl in einer ergotherapeutischen Praxis als auch in einer Rehabilitationsklinik ist eine Gruppentherapie eine gute Möglichkeit, die Klienten an ihren eigenen Zielen arbeiten zu lassen. Dadurch entsteht eine positive Gruppendynamik, die motiviert. Die Therapeutin kann kleine Hilfestellungen und Tipps geben oder bei Bedarf sichernd danebenstehen.
- **Zu Hause**: Im Praxissetting sind Eigenübungen im häuslichen Umfeld die Regel. Dort sollte die Therapeutin mit dem Klienten genau besprechen, in welchem Raum, mit welchen Gegenständen und Sicherungen (z. B. bereitstehender Stuhl) trainiert werden sollte.
- **Außer Haus**: Hin und wieder kann eine Durchführung der Eigenübung außer Haus sinnvoll sein. Zum Beispiel zur Umsetzung von geübten Strategien beim Einkaufen, beim Ausdauertraining im Wald mit Walkingstöcken oder zur Übung der eigenständigen Nutzung von öffentlichen Verkehrsmitteln.

Zeitfaktoren

Die zeitliche Planung der Eigenübungen kann der ausschlaggebende Faktor sein, ob sie zu Hause durchgeführt werden oder nicht. Deshalb muss die Planung der Eigenübungen gut durchdacht werden. Folgende Faktoren sind zu bedenken.

- **Zeitpunkt**: Damit die Eigenübungen durchgeführt werden, ist eine wohlüberlegte Eingliederung in den Tagesablauf empfehlenswert. Es sollte ein Zeitpunkt gewählt werden, zu dem eine gute Beweglichkeit herrscht. Außerdem ist eine Regelmäßigkeit sinnvoll, damit die Übungen Teil der normalen Tagesroutine wird.
- **Verknüpfung**: Wird die Übung an eine Tätigkeit geknüpft, die schon fest in der Tagesroutine verankert ist, fällt es dem Klienten leichter, sich an die Übung zu erinnern, z. B. im Bett nach dem Mittagsschlaf, während die Partnerin das Essen zubereitet oder im Auto auf der Fahrt zum Stammtisch
- **Trainingshäufigkeit**: Beim intensiven Training eines Performance-Skills sollten fünf Mal pro Woche drei Mal pro Tag 20 Wiederholungen erfolgen (s. o.). Beim Training komplexerer Betätigungen oder Übungen wird diese Zahl der Wiederholung nicht möglich sein und richtet sich deswegen nach der Kapazität des Klienten. Grundsätzlich ist eine hohe Wiederholungszahl förderlich für eine Verbesserung. Setzt die Therapeutin die Häufigkeit zu hoch an, ist die Gefahr jedoch höher, dass der Klient die Übungen gar nicht durchführt. Eine kurze intensive Trainingseinheit mit anschließender Pause ist nachgewiesenermaßen effektiver als ein langes, aber langsames Training.

▶ Eine positive Formulierung der Trainingshäufigkeit ist förderlich, z. B.: „Machen Sie das Training fünf Mal die Woche 10 Minuten. Wenn Ihnen danach ist, ist länger natürlich super.".

- **Feste Gesamtzeit**: Für das Training sollte eine feste Gesamtzeit pro Woche festgelegt werden. Dieses genaue Ziel gibt eine klare Richtline vor und der Klient wird gestärkt, wenn er sein Wochenziel erreicht hat.

Erinnerungs- und Motivationshilfen
Eigenübungen sind selten aufregend und interessant. Die natürliche Trägheit, Übungen zu machen, wird von der Erkrankung durch Antriebsstörung und Fatigue noch verstärkt. Um dies zu überwinden und eine förderliche Disziplin aufrechtzuerhalten, können Erinnerungs- und Motivationshilfen eine gute Lösung sein.

- Einträge in Kalender des Klienten (mit fester Uhrzeit)
- Erinnerungsalarm auf Smartphone
- Apps, z. B. Therapio, mit Erinnerungsfunktion, Videoaufnahme-Möglichkeit, um Übungen nachzumachen
- Übungsplan: An sichtbarer Stelle einen Plan aufhängen, wenn durchgeführt abhaken oder Smiley eintragen
- Kleine Zettel an verschiedenen Orten im Haus anbringen, mit Mini-Übungen oder Erinnerungen. Z. B. an Badspiegel „Mimik-Übungen", im Büro „Entspannungsübung", in Flur „Arme schwingen", in Küche „5× Korb auf Regal"
- Auch Abbildungen der Übungen oder besser Fotos des Klienten bei der Durchführung der Übung dienen als Gedächtnisstütze
- Die Überprüfung des geleisteten Trainings durch die Ergotherapeutin ist wichtig, da die Motivation durch das Wissen gesteigert wird, dass es im Anschluss besprochen wird

Menschen mit einer chronischen Erkrankung, wie M. Parkinson, führen ihre Eigenübungen oftmals nicht oder nur zum Teil durch. Dies kann viele Gründe haben, wie Antriebsarmut, Depression, kognitive Einschränkung oder einfach eine Haltung von „Ich lebe das Leben, so gut es geht.". Für Therapeutinnen ist es oft schwer verständlich und auch nicht leicht zu akzeptieren, wenn Klienten ihre Eigenübungen nicht machen, schließlich hat die Therapeutin sich viele Gedanken gemacht und möchte dem Klienten wirklich helfen. Trotzdem sollte der von der Therapeutin angeschlagene Ton im Umgang mit Klienten, die ihre „Hausaufgaben" nicht machen, niemals urteilend oder belehrend sein. Der Klient hat seine Gründe. Die beste Umgangsweise ist, dass Therapeutin und Klient dies besprechen und gemeinsam versuchen zu ermitteln, ob die Änderung eines der o. g. Punkte zur vermehrten Eigenübung animieren würde.

Hilfsmittel für Eigenübungen
Da der Klient ohne die Kontrolle der Therapeutin trainiert, muss eine Selbstkontrolle erfolgen. Durch die Abnahme der Eigenwahrnehmung bei Parkinson-Klienten werden Bewegungen häufig nicht mit größtmöglicher Amplitude durchgeführt. Die innere Kontrolle im Gehirn ist defekt. Deshalb ist eine externe Kontrolle notwendig. Dazu sind folgende Hilfsmittel hilfreich:

- **Spiegel**: Ein Ganzkörperspiegel kann bei eingeschränkter Wahrnehmung die korrekte Durchführung sicherstellen, z. B. bei der Aufrichtung.
- **Videoaufnahme**: Zur anschließenden Selbstkontrolle, oder um der Therapeutin die genaue Ausführung der Eigenübung zu zeigen, ist eine Videoaufnahme mit dem Smartphone recht einfach möglich.
- **Referenzflächen** (s. Abb. 17.2): Wie in Abschn. 13.4 beschrieben, unterstützen Referenzflächen die externe Rückmeldung der ausgeführten Bewegung. Durch einen sensorischen Reiz (auditiv, visuell oder taktil/kinäs-

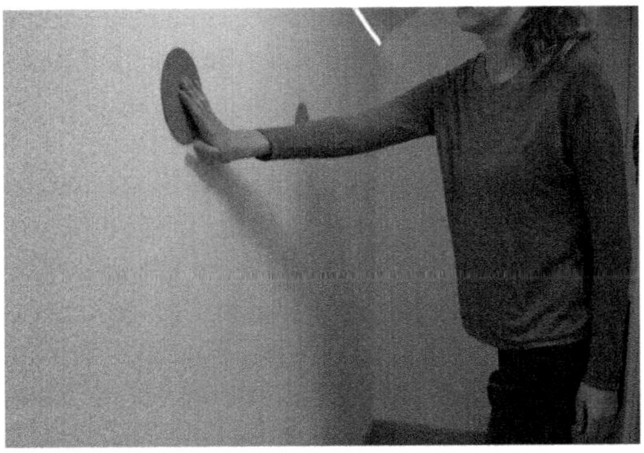

Abb. 17.2 Bei der Eigenübung helfen Referenzflächen dem Klienten dabei die größtmögliche Amplitude zu erreichen

thetisch) bekommt der Klient automatisch die Rückmeldung, dass er die Bewegung vollständig ausgeführt hat. Die Art der Referenzfläche wird innerhalb der Therapie besprochen und ausprobiert, sodass der Klient im Anschluss zu Hause allein damit zurechtkommt. Beispiele für Referenzflächen:
  - Auditiv: Stuhl, Wand, Tisch, Beine, festen Gegenstand mit Händen anklatschen
  - Visuell: Spiegel, Linie, farbiger Punkt, sichtbarer Gegenstand
  - Taktil/kinästhetisch: siehe „auditiv" und Berührung eines festen Gegenstandes mit Hand, Kopf, Fuß …
- **Angehörige als Co-Therapeuten**: Nach einer Einarbeitungszeit in der Therapieeinheit sind manche Angehörige fähig, eine Co-Therapeutenrolle zu übernehmen, um dem Klienten bei den Eigenübungen zu helfen. Sie fühlen sich wertgeschätzt und glücklich, dem Betroffenen Unterstützung bieten zu können. Erfahrungsgemäß ist die Beziehung zwischen Betroffenem und der Partnerin häufig durch das veränderte Verhältnis zueinander angespannt, sodass die Anleitung der Eigenübungen der Partnerin nicht immer reibungslos verläuft. Nimmt die Therapeutin eine negative Atmosphäre wahr, sollte die Zusammenarbeit vermieden werden und auf andere Methoden zurückgegriffen werden (s. o.).

Apps, Exergaming und Teletherapie

Seit einigen Jahren werden im Bereich der Entwicklung von Übungs-Apps und Exergaming-Geräten laufend Fortschritte gemacht. Erste Studien mit Parkinson-Betroffenen sind vielversprechend. Der spielerische Charakter erweist sich als stark motivationsfördernd, auch scheinen sie einen positiven Einfluss auf Lebensqualität, Motorik und Kognition zu haben. Vor allem in der Corona-Pandemie wurden die Vorteile der Teletherapie ersichtlich. Ergotherapeuten können mit Klienten in Kontakt bleiben, beratend unterstützen und Übungen anleiten, ohne Risikopatienten der Gefahr der Ansteckung auszusetzen. Die Akzeptanz von telemedizinischen und Exergaming-Angeboten ist bei Menschen mit M. Parkinson hoch. Besonders als Ergänzung zu konventionellen therapeutischen Methoden sind diese zukunftsgerichteten Angebote interessant.

Beispiel

Herr S. hat es jetzt verstanden. Nur wenn er auch im Alltag die Aufrichtung übt, wird es besser. Ein bis zwei Mal die Woche reichen nicht, um eine Veränderung zu erzielen. Gemeinsam mit der Ergotherapeutin hat er einen Übungsplan gemacht. Gleich morgens nach dem Aufstehen macht er Aufrichtungsübungen mit Musik. Morgengymnastik hat er schon immer gemacht, das macht ihn wach. Im Laufe des Tages haben sie zusammen überlegt, wo und wann sich kurze Bewegungsübungen gut integrieren lassen. Er hat sie an bestimmte Tätigkeiten geknüpft. Beim Zähneputzen vor dem Spiegel – Schultern zurück und im Spiegel Blickkontakt.

Vor dem Überqueren der Straße – aufrichten, bewusst nach links und rechts drehen, dann erst loslaufen. Vor jedem Loslaufen am Rollator – zwischen den Haltegriffen stehen, Schultern runter, Blick nach vorne (nicht nach unten). Abends hakt er stolz den Übungsplan ab. Fast alles geschafft, nur das Aufrichten beim Zähneputzen hat er vergessen. Aber daran arbeitet er noch. ◄

Literatur und weiterführende Literatur

van Beek J, van Wegen E, Bohlhalter S, Vanbellingen T (2019) Exergaming-based dexterity training in persons with Parkinson disease: a pilot feasibility study. J Neurol Phys Ther 43(3):168–174. https://doi.org/10.1097/NPT.0000000000000278. PMID: 31136450

Dias AE, Limongi JCP, Hsing WT, Barbosa ER (2016) Telerehabilitation in Parkinson's disease: influence of cognitive status. Dement Neuropsychol 10(4):327–332. https://doi.org/10.1590/s1980-5764-2016dn1004012

Foster ER, Bedekar M, Tickle-Degnen L (2014) Systematic review of the effectiveness of occupational therapy-related interventions for people with Parkinson's disease. Am J Occup Ther 68(1):39–49. https://doi.org/10.5014/ajot.2014.008706. PMID: 24367954; PMCID: PMC4413458

Garcia-Agundez A, Folkerts A, Konrad R, Caserman P, Tregel T, Goosses M, Goebel S, Kalbe E (2019) Recent advances in rehabilitation for Parkinson's disease with exergames: a systematic review. J Neuro Eng Rehabil. 16 LONDON: BMC. ISSN 1743-0003. https://doi.org/10.1186/s12984-019-0492-1

Hung KG, Fong KN (2019) Effects of telerehabilitation in occupational therapy practice: a systematic review. Hong Kong J Occup Ther 32(1):3–21. https://doi.org/10.1177/1569186119849119

van der Kolk NM, Overeem S, de Vries NM, Kessels RP, Donders R, Brouwer M, Berg D, Post B, Bloem BR (2015) Design of the Park-in-Shape study: a phase II double blind randomized controlled trial evaluating the effects of exercise on motor and non-motor symptoms in Parkinson's disease. BMC Neurol 15:56. https://doi.org/10.1186/s12883-015-0312-6. PMID: 25880966; PMCID: PMC4418070

Law M, Baptiste S, Mills J (1995) Client-centred practice: what does it mean and does it make a difference? Can J Occup Ther 62(5):250–257. https://doi.org/10.1177/000841749506200504. PMID: 10152881

Nieuwboer A, Weerdt W, Dom R, Truyen M, Janssens L, Kamsma Y (2001) The effect of a home physiotherapy program for persons with Parkinson's disease. J Rehab Med 33:266–272

Radder DLM, Sturkenboom IH, van Nimwegen M, Keus SH, Bloem BR, de Vries NM (2017) Physical therapy and occupational therapy in Parkinson's disease. Int J Neurosci 127(10):930–943. https://doi.org/10.1080/00207454.2016.1275617

Sturkenboom I, Thijssen M, Gons-van Elsacker J, Jansen I, Maasdam A, Schulten M, Vijver-Visser D, Steultjens E, Bloem B, Munneke M (2008) Guidelines for occupational therapy in Parkinson's disease rehabilitation. ParkinsonNet/NPF, Nijmegen/Miami

18 Gruppenangebote

Beispiel

Frau V. ist etwas nervös, heute wird das Thema in der Ergotherapiegruppe behandelt, das sie vorgeschlagen hat: „In der Öffentlichkeit mit dem Parkinson umgehen." Dieses Thema beschäftigt sie fast täglich und sie hat noch keinen guten Umgang damit gefunden. ◀

18.1 Integration in gemischte Gruppe

Vor allem in Kliniken sind Gruppenangebote ein wesentlicher Teil der ergotherapeutischen Behandlung. Inwieweit für Menschen mit M. Parkinson gemischte Gruppen, also mit Klientinnen mit unterschiedlichen Diagnosen, sinnvoll sind, ist fraglich. Im Folgenden sind ein paar Punkte aufgeführt, die helfen, damit Klientinnen mit M. Parkinson von einer Teilnahme an gemischten Gruppen profitieren.

Ablenkende Faktoren

Sobald Klientinnen mit Parkinson-Erkrankung abgelenkt sind, geraten sie oftmals in eine Freezing-Episode. Oder die Bewegungsfähigkeit bleibt zwar erhalten, ist jedoch weniger ausladend und flüssig. Auch die kognitive Verarbeitung von Anweisungen ist nur eingeschränkt möglich, wenn ablenkende Faktoren vorhanden sind. Aus diesem Grund ist es sinnvoll, wenn die Klientin mit M. Parkinson dem Therapeuten **gegenübersitzt**. So kann sie ihre Aufmerksamkeit durch visuelle Fixierung halten. Auch ein direktes Ansprechen mit Namen hat sich zur Fokussierung der Aufmerksamkeit bewährt.

Verlangsamung

Sowohl die Bewegung als auch Problemlösungsprozesse und Reaktion sind bei Menschen mit M. Parkinson verlangsamt. Dies kann zu einer Verzögerung der Ausführung führen und zu Missverständnissen bei der Kommunikation mit anderen Klientinnen. Eine direkte Kommunikation mit Blickkontakt und Namensnennung binden die Parkinson-Klientin in das Geschehen ein und signalisieren den anderen Klientinnen, dass auf die Antwort/Reaktion nun gewartet wird. Die Nutzung von auditiven Cues kann auch in einer gemischten Gruppensituation sinnvoll sein, z. B. klatschen beim Laufen oder ein „Und hoch!" beim Aufstehen.

Kommunikation

Die leise Sprache vieler Menschen mit M. Parkinson kann in der Gruppensituation die Kommunikation beeinträchtigen. Es hilft, wenn die Betroffene vom Therapeuten freundlich zum lauten Sprechen aufgefordert wird oder das Sprechen vor der ganzen Gruppe vermeidet, wenn dies mit Stress verbunden ist.

A. Orellana, *Betätigungsorientierte Ergotherapie bei Morbus Parkinson*,
https://doi.org/10.1007/978-3-662-62583-5_18

Sturzgefahr
Wenn durch Akinese oder posturale Instabilität Sturzgefahr besteht, sollte die Klientin direkt **neben** dem Therapeuten sitzen. Außerdem sollten Übungen, die Stürze provozieren können, immer im Sitzen durchgeführt werden können.

18.2 Parkinsongruppe

Sowohl in der Klinik als auch in der ergotherapeutischen Praxis können Parkinsongruppen eine Bereicherung sein, in der soziale Interaktionen mit Themen zu typischen Parkinson-Symptomen kombiniert werden. Es gibt eine Entwicklung im ergotherapeutischen Gruppenangebot, weg von funktionsfokussierten Gruppen, wie Feinmotorikgruppe oder Hirn-Leistungs-Trainingsgruppe, hin zu Betätigungsgruppen. Dieser Fortschritt ist auch für das Berufsbild der Ergotherapie prägend, da er den Paradigmenwechsel zu betätigungsorientiertem und klientenzentriertem Arbeiten repräsentiert.

▶ Der Ablauf einer betätigungsorientierten Gruppentherapie ist niemals gleich. Der Therapeut greift Themen auf, die den Klienten wichtig sind und setzt sie so um, dass alle Teilnehmerinnen sich einbringen können.

Im Folgenden werden Vorschläge zu Themen für Betätigungsgruppen gemacht. Dabei gibt es zwei Durchführungsarten. Einerseits kann ein Thema die Gruppe durchgehend begleiten, z. B. Schreiben, Fatigue. Andererseits kann aus einem Pool an Themen bei jedem Treffen der Gruppe ein für die Gruppe aktuelles oder interessantes Thema gewählt werden. Zum Beispiel:

- Schreibtraining
- Umgang mit Fatigue
- Parkinsonspezifische Hilfsmittel
- „Outing“: Wann sage ich es meinen Freunden?
- Partnerschaft
- Cueing im Alltag
- Krankheitsbewältigung
- Dual-Tasks vermeiden/Sequenzierung von Tätigkeiten
- Umgang mit Stress und Zeitdruck
- Negative Gedanken/Depressionen
- Praktische Merkstrategien
- Sport und Aktivität in den Alltag integrieren
- Balance von Aktivität und Ruhephasen im Tag
- Tagesstrukturierung
- Wohnraum
- Stürze vermeiden
- Was tun in der Off Phase?
- Effektive Kommunikation
- Nach Sturz wieder aufstehen
- Individuelle Eigenübungen
- …

Die Planung des Gruppenkonzepts, die Umsetzung in die Praxis und die Leitung einer Klientinnengruppe ist – genau wie die Einzeltherapieplanung, -umsetzung und -leitung – sehr individuell (je nach Klinik/Praxis und Persönlichkeit des Therapeuten). Damit wird der Therapeut der Einzigartigkeit der Klientinnen gerecht. Aus diesem Grund wird in dieser Veröffentlichung davon abgesehen, Gruppeneinheiten zu den einzelnen Themen auszuarbeiten. Es wird vielmehr dazu angeregt, aus den vorangegangenen Kapiteln zu den obigen Themen Informationen zusammenzustellen und speziell auf die Klientinnengruppe anzupassen. Beispielhaft wird eine mögliche Struktur für einen Gruppentherapieablauf dargestellt:

1. Die Teilnehmerinnen suchen sich einen Platz
2. Vorstellung der Klientinnen und Therapeuten (auch wenn schon bekannt, zur Auffrischung)
   - Reihum
   - Mit Ball zuwerfen
   - Namen auf Tafel schreiben
   - Namenskärtchen gemeinsam zuordnen
   - …
3. Austausch über Umsetzung des Themas der letzten Woche im Alltag der Klientinnen
4. Datum und Thema der heutigen Einheit an Tafel/Flipchart anschreiben
5. Informationen zum Thema geben

- Handout
- PowerPoint Präsentation
- Stichpunkte an Tafel/Flipchart
- Praktische Übungen
- …

6. Austausch zum Thema zwischen Teilnehmerinnen anregen
   - Arbeitsblätter
   - Fragen
   - Gedankenanregungen
   - Austausch/Rollenspiel in Zweier- oder Kleingruppen
   - Praktische Übungen
   - …
7. Zusammenfassung durch Therapeuten
8. Anregung, das Besprochene sofort im Alltag umzusetzen (Hausaufgaben)
9. Gemeinsame Auswahl eines Themas für nächste Gruppeneinheit
10. Abschlussritual
    - Gedicht
    - Zitat
    - Klatschspiel
    - …

Weitere Elemente

Es gibt eine große Auswahl an weiteren möglichen Elementen, die in eine Gruppentherapie einfließen können. Diese haben meist nicht direkt mit dem Thema zu tun, sondern unterstützen das Wohlbefinden und die Aufmerksamkeit, und verbessern die Zugänglichkeit der Klientinnen.

Übungen zur Auflockerung

Zur Auflockerung, wenn die Konzentration der Teilnehmerinnen nicht über die gesamte Einheit aufrechterhalten werden kann, oder wenn einzelne Klientinnen Apathie oder Tagesschläfrigkeit zeigen, sind Übungen zur Steigerung der Vigilanz und zur Aktivierung möglich, z. B.:

- Übungen zur Verbesserung der Aufrichtung
- Koordinationsübungen (z. B. mithilfe von Ball, Ballon, Tüchern)
- Konzentrationsübungen (z. B. Rhythmus nachklatschen, …)
- Steigerung der Vigilanz (z. B. Körper abklopfen, laute Sprechübungen, …)
- Bodypercussion vereint alle o. g. Punkte, zahlreiche Videos dazu findet man z. B. auf Youtube.de

Sozialer Austausch

Der soziale Austausch zwischen den Teilnehmerinnen ist ausschlaggebend dafür, dass sich die Teilnehmerinnen öffnen und sich als Teil der Gruppe gestärkt wahrnehmen können. Der Austausch untereinander über Tipps und Umgangsmöglichkeiten mit unterschiedlichen Hürden und Schwierigkeiten der Krankheit wird von Betroffenen meist als sehr wertvoll empfunden. Gelingt es dem Therapeuten, den Zusammenhalt der Gruppe zu fördern, kann ein offener Austausch über die aktuellen Themen zwischen den einzelnen Teilnehmerinnen erfolgen. Je nach Homogenität der Gruppe hinsichtlich Stadium und kognitiver Fähigkeiten, bedarf es für die erfolgreiche Kommunikation zwischen den Gruppenmitgliedern mehr oder weniger Hilfe vom Therapeuten. Die Vorstellungsrunde ist ein guter Start, um das Kennenlernen und Vertrauen untereinander zu fördern. Später können weitere niederschwellige Interaktionen dazukommen, z. B.:

- Igelballmassage am Rücken des Nachbarn
- Sammeln und Erraten von Interessen der Teilnehmer (z. B. Lieblingsblume, Hobbies, Lieblingsstadt …)
- Gegenseitiger Austausch in Zweiergruppen

Entspannung

Um den Teilnehmern Momente der Introspektion und Reflexion zu ermöglichen oder zur Fokussierung auf sich selbst und auf das zu besprechende Thema, sind Entspannungsübungen eine ideale Möglichkeit, z. B.:

- Achtsamkeitsübung
- Eigen-Handmassage
- Feldenkrais
- Für weitere Möglichkeiten siehe Abschn. 14.10.4

Übertrag in den Alltag

Das Ziel der Gruppentherapie ist der Übertrag des Besprochenen in den Alltag jeder Klientin. Dies stellt im Gruppensetting eine Herausforderung dar, da nicht auf jede Klientin einzeln eingegangen werden kann. Trotzdem ist es wichtig, mit den Teilnehmerinnen zu besprechen, wie ein Carry-Over gelingen kann.

Umstellung von Gruppentherapien in Kliniken

Anne Fischer und Abbey Marterella (2019) listen in ihrem Modell (OTIPM) die „Edukation" als eigenes Modell in der Interventionsphase. Sie heben hervor, dass diese Gruppeninterventionen, die in Form von Vorträgen oder Präsentationen stattfinden, streng betätigungsfokussiert sein müssen. Das Trainieren der Fertigkeiten sollte dagegen in einem anderen Setting stattfinden. Unserer Meinung nach muss hier nochmal genau differenziert werden. Der Fokus auf die Betätigung, auch im Gruppensetting, repräsentiert die moderne Ergotherapie und ist durchgängig zu beachten. Andererseits gibt es eine Reihe betätigungsorientierter Themen, die auch im Gruppensetting ideal praktisch umsetzbar sind (z. B. Aufstehen nach Sturz, effektive Kommunikation, Schreibtraining). Die Gruppenteilnehmer profitieren sogar vom Austausch untereinander mehr, als würden sie nur von einem Therapeuten angeleitet.

Gruppentherapien in Form von betätigungsfokussierten Vorträgen oder Präsentationen zu gestalten, wird in Deutschland bisher wenig praktiziert, kann jedoch eine bereichernde Ergänzung darstellen, wenn die Angehörigen dazu eingeladen werden. In Kliniken ist eine Umstellung von funktionellen Gruppen auf betätigungsorientierte Gruppen nicht immer ohne weiteres möglich. Schließlich wollen angrenzende Berufsgruppen wie Physiotherapeuten und Ärzte – die Gesamtorganisation im Blick – mitbestimmen: „Wer macht denn dann die Feinmotorikgruppe? Dafür war doch schon immer die Ergotherapie zuständig".

Dafür braucht es eine klare Positionierung der Ergotherapie, basierend auf aktuellen, betätigungsorientierten Modellen (z. B. OTIPM, CMOP-E). Außerdem müssen Ergotherapeuten Selbstbewusstsein zeigen, wenn sie repräsentativ auftreten: ob auf Bundesebene (Berufsverbände), in Institutionen (Leitung der Ergotherapie), bei Teamsitzungen auf Station oder während Interventionen mit Klientinnen. Je klarer sich die Ergotherapie Außenstehenden als betätigungsorientiert und klientenzentriert zeigt, desto leichter fällt folglich die Argumentation für die Umstellung von Gruppentherapien und die Abkehr von sonstigen funktionsorientierten Praktiken.

Beispiel

Frau V. ist überrascht, wie viele andere Patienten ähnliche Erfahrungen in der Öffentlichkeit gemacht haben wie sie: komische Blicke, ungeduldige Gesprächspartner, der Stress an der Supermarktkasse, … Gemeinsam haben sie eine lange Liste mit Ideen für Umgangsweisen auf einem Flipchart zusammengetragen: Menschen direkt ansprechen, zu ruhigen Zeiten einkaufen, Lebensmittel liefern lassen, … Die Kommunikation mit ungeduldigen Gesprächspartnern haben sie dann in Dreiergruppen geübt. Zwei stellen eine Situation nach, der Dritte gibt Rückmeldung über Formulierungen oder Alternativvorschläge. Frau V. geht nicht nur inspiriert aus der Stunde, sondern hat auch die anderen Betroffenen besser kennengelernt. Sie freut sich, dass sie sich getraut hat, dieses schwierige Thema auszusuchen. ◀

Literatur und weiterführende Literatur

Fischer A, Marterella A (2019) Powerful practice. CIOTS, Fort Collins, S 63–72, 207–211

Foster ER, Bedekar M, Tickle-Degnen L (2014) Systematic review of the effectiveness of occupational therapy-related interventions for people with Parkinson's disease. Am J Occup Ther 68(1):39–49. https://doi.org/10.5014/ajot.2014.008706. PMID: 24367954; PMCID: PMC4413458

Law M (2002) Participation in the occupations of everyday life. Am J Occup Ther 56(6):640–649. https://doi.org/10.5014/ajot.56.6.640

Law M, Baptiste S, Mills J (1995) Client-centred practice: what does it mean and does it make a diffe-

rence? Can J Occup Ther 62(5):250–257. https://doi.org/10.1177/000841749506200504. PMID: 10152881
Signer T, Weise A (2020) Betätigungsorientierte Patientenedukation und Kompensation im stationären Rehabilitations-Alltag: die „Energiemanagement-Schulung“ – ein Fallbeispiel. Schulz-Kirchner Verlag GmbH, Rheinsbreitbach, S 135–152
Sturkenboom I, Thijssen M, Gons-van Elsacker J, Jansen I, Maasdam A, Schulten M, Vijver-Visser D, Steultjens E, Bloem B, Munneke M (2008) Guidelines for occupational therapy in Parkinson’s disease rehabilitation. ParkinsonNet/NPF, Nijmegen/Miami

Teil V

Evaluationsphase

19 Evaluation

19.1 Zwischenevaluation

Im Laufe der therapeutischen Intervention sollte die Ergotherapeutin regelmäßig eine Evaluation über den Outcome der Therapie durchführen. Dies geschieht in einem kreisenden Muster, wie im „Perfect fit“ in Abb. 4.4 dargestellt. Nach jeder Interventionseinheit wird analysiert (siehe Kap. 6), wie der Klient nun die komplette Betätigung durchführt. Dadurch kann die Therapeutin konstant abgleichen, ob Fortschritte gemacht werden, ob die gewählte Intervention effektiv ist und ob dem Klienten ein Übertrag in den Alltag gelingt.

Zur Durchführung der Zwischenevaluation ist eine Betätigungsanalyse sinnvoll, bei der die Anstrengung, Effizienz, Sicherheit und benötigte Hilfe festgestellt wird. Dazu kann der Assessmentbogen (Betätigungsanalyse) im Anhang genutzt werden. Durch den Vergleich der Auswertungen der Betätigungsanalysen erkennt die Therapeutin unmittelbar, wenn die therapeutische Intervention nicht effektiv ist, und kann den Prozess anpassen, um das bestmögliche Ergebnis zu erreichen. Zusätzlich sollte der Klient befragt werden, wie zufrieden er mit der Durchführung der Betätigung ist und wo er noch Verbesserungsmöglichkeiten erkennt. Es ist wesentlich, den Klienten aktiv in das Interventionsgeschehen einzubeziehen. Dadurch wird gewährleistet, dass er ein Verständnis für den therapeutischen Prozess entwickelt und seinen eigenen Blickwinkel miteinbringen kann. So bleibt er interessiert und motiviert. Dazu kommt es nicht selten vor, dass der Klient während der Therapie feststellt, dass das von ihm gewählte Ziel nicht das wichtigste ist, sondern ein anderes Thema zurzeit im Vordergrund steht. In dem Fall hat die Ergotherapeutin die Möglichkeit, zeitnah umzuschwenken und den Fokus der Intervention zu verlegen. So vermeidet man langandauernde, ergebnislose Therapien.

Je nach angenommener Ursache für das Nicht-Gelingen der Therapie wird an unterschiedlicher Stelle weiter oben im therapeutischen Prozess angesetzt. Dies wird im „Perfect fit“ in Abb. 4.4 durch die nach oben führenden Pfeile auf der linken Seite veranschaulicht. Folgende veränderte Ansatzpunkte im Therapieprozess können zu einem erfolgreichen Outcome führen:

- Hat die Therapeutin eine wichtige Information nicht erhalten? Zum Beispiel, Pflegedienst kommt täglich zur Unterstützung beim Waschen → Ansatz beim ersten Punkt „Klientenzentrierte **Informationen** und Betätigungen sammeln“.
- Wurde das Ziel nicht klientenzentriert gewählt? Zum Beispiel, „Verbesserung der Aufrichtung“, da Therapeutin eine kyphotische Haltung erkannt hat. → Ansatz beim ersten Punkt „Klientenzentrierte Informationen und **Betätigungen** sammeln“.

A. Orellana, *Betätigungsorientierte Ergotherapie bei Morbus Parkinson*,
https://doi.org/10.1007/978-3-662-62583-5_19

- War die von der Therapeutin aufgestellte Hypothese nicht korrekt? Zum Beispiel, Tremor als Ursache für Unsicherheit beim Frühstück zubereiten. Auslöser ist jedoch der Zeitdruck beim Frühstück zubereiten. → Ansatz bei drittem Punkt „**Hypothese** über Ursache der problematischen Betätigung **bilden**".
- Wurde ein nicht idealer Therapieansatz gewählt? Zum Beispiel, wurde ein Training der Betätigung gewählt, durch eine beginnende Demenz ist diese jedoch nicht korrekt durchführbar; alternativ ist eine kompensatorische Methode sinnvoller. → Ansatz bei „Art der **Intervention festlegen**".
- Fehlt einer der **positiven Einflussfaktoren**? Zum Beispiel, durch mangelndes Selbstmanagement übernimmt der Klient wenig Verantwortung für seine therapeutischen Fortschritte. Das Üben erscheint ihm sinnlos → Ansatz bei „Selbstmanagement".

Diese Arbeitsweise ist evidenzbasiert. Die Therapeutin erweitert ihre Kenntnisse durch die regelmäßige systematische Überprüfung und Erfassung ihrer Interventionen. Ihr Wissen wächst sukzessive an.

19.2 Evaluation zu festgelegtem Zeitpunkt

Zu Beginn des therapeutischen Prozesses wurden Assessments durchgeführt. Dabei sollte die Therapeutin sofort ein Zeitpunkt für das Re-Assessment, die Evaluation, festgelegt haben.

Dieser Zeitpunkt kann sich nach dem natürlichen Ende der Therapie richten, z. B. bei einer Rehabilitation, oder nach dem Ende eines Rezepts. Die zweite Option ist die Wahl eines Zeitpunktes, zu dem die Therapeutin einschätzt, dass der Klient die Betätigung erfolgreich meistern kann. Es sollten dieselben Assessments wie zu Beginn der Assessmentphase durchgeführt werden, um einen direkten Vergleich zu haben und aussagekräftige Schlüsse ziehen zu können. Dabei gibt es zwei zu vergleichende Werte.

Objektive, von außen beobachtbare Veränderungen

Zum einen können objektive oder von außen beobachtbare Veränderungen von Körperfunktionen oder der Performanz festgestellt werden. Dazu dienen funktionelle Tests (z. B. PDQ39, Timed-up-and-go Test, MOCA-Test) und die Bewertung der Betätigungsperformanz durch die Therapeutin mithilfe einer Betätigungsanalyse (siehe Kap. 6). Diese Werte können angrenzenden Berufsgruppen kommuniziert werden, um erreichte Veränderungen aufzuzeigen.

Subjektive Einschätzung des Klienten

Zum anderen kann die Therapeutin eine subjektive Einschätzung des Klienten erfassen, ob sein Ziel oder eine ausreichende Verbesserung der Performanz der ihm wichtigen Betätigung erreicht wurde. Dazu dient das COPM (siehe Abschn. 5.4). Im COPM wird die Einschätzung des Klienten bezüglich der Performanz und der Zufriedenheit von 1–10 erfasst. Diese Zahlen können direkt mit den erfassten Zahlen bei der Aufnahme des Klienten verglichen werden, um festzustellen, ob eine Veränderung erzielt wurde und wie groß diese ist. Auch dieser Wert hilft der Therapeutin, stichhaltige Aussagen gegenüber Ärztinnen und anderen Berufsgruppen über den Therapieerfolg zu machen. Die Therapeutin gleicht die beiden erhaltenen Ergebnisse – die von der Therapeutin beobachtete und die durch den Klienten subjektiv wahrgenommene Veränderung – ab. Damit ermisst sie, ob das gesetzte Ziel erreicht wurde, ein Teilerfolg erzielt werden konnte, keine Verbesserung oder sogar eine Verschlechterung eingetreten ist.

Wenn das Ziel nicht erreicht wurde, setzt die Therapeutin den Behandlungsprozess wieder an der Stelle an, an dem sie Veränderungspotential sieht. Zum Beispiel kann eine Sammlung weiterer Informationen (z. B. Befragung von Angehörigen) neue Hinweise liefern oder es wird eine andere Interventionsmethode (z. B. Adaptation statt Körperfunktion trainieren) eingesetzt.

▶ Wenn das Ziel erreicht wurde und der Klient die Betätigung zu seiner Zufriedenheit meistert, sollte das gefeiert werden.

Das Feiern eines solchen Erfolgs ist in der Ergotherapie nicht immer üblich. Es wird ausdrücklich dazu geraten, am Ende der therapeutischen Intervention oder bei Erreichen eines Ziels die Leistung entsprechend zu würdigen. Besonders bei chronischen, degenerativen Erkrankungen sind Erfolge wertzuschätzen und wirken besonders motivierend für zukünftige Herausforderungen. Es sollte Zeit und Raum für einen offiziellen Abschluss geben. Wie der Abschluss gestaltet wird, liegt in der Hand der Therapeutin. Es folgen einige Anregungen:

- Mit Kaffee, Tee oder Saft auf den Erfolg anstoßen
- Ein Händedruck, Schulterklopfen
- Ein Zertifikat ausstellen: „Hiermit bestätigen wir offiziell das Erreichen des Ziels: …"
- Ein Gästebuch oder eine Wand mit den erreichten Zielen der Klienten
- Der verbale, persönliche Ausdruck der Anerkennung: „Ich bin stolz auf Sie." „Ich weiß, wie anstrengend das für Sie war." „Jetzt haben Sie es geschafft." „Hut ab!" „Glückwunsch."…

Literatur und weiterführende Literatur

Fischer A, Marterella A (2019) Powerful practice. CIOTS, Fort Collins, S 63–72, 207–211

Law M, Polatajko H, Carswell A, McColl MA, Pollock N, Baptiste S (1999) Das Kanadische Modell der Occupational Performance und das Canadian Occupational Performance Measure. In: Jerosch-Herold C, Marotzki U, Hack BM, Weber P (Hrsg) Konzeptionelle Modelle für die ergotherapeutische Praxis. Ergotherapie – Reflexion und Analyse. Springer, Berlin/Heidelberg. https://doi.org/10.1007/978-3-662-08173-0_7

Radder DLM, Sturkenboom IH, van Nimwegen M, Keus SH, Bloem BR, de Vries NM (2017) Physical therapy and occupational therapy in Parkinson's disease. International Journal of Neuroscience 127(10):930–943. https://doi.org/10.1080/00207454.2016.1275617

Sturkenboom I, Thijssen M, Gons-van Elsacker J, Jansen I, Maasdam A, Schulten M, Vijver-Visser D, Steultjens E, Bloem B, Munneke M (2008) Guidelines for occupational therapy in Parkinson's disease rehabilitation. ParkinsonNet/NPF, Nijmegen/Miami

Anhang

A. Orellana, *Betätigungsorientierte Ergotherapie bei Morbus Parkinson*,
https://doi.org/10.1007/978-3-662-62583-5

Betätigungsprofil

Name:______________________________ Datum__________________________

Ausgefüllt von: _________________________

Uhrzeit	Tätigkeit	Beschreibung der Ausführung	Wichtigkeit der Veränderung 1-10

Betätigungsanalyse

Datum________________________
Uhrzeit______________________
On/Off_______________________

Name:____________________
beobachtete Betätigung:____________________________
____

Performance Skills (Breakdown-points einkreisen!)	Durchführung	Hinderliche Kontextfatoren	Fördernde Faktoren

Qualitätsfaktoren der ganzen Performaz
Anstrengung:
Effizienz:
Sicherheit:
Selbständigkeit:
Soziale Effektivität:
Anschließende Gedanken:

Selbsteinschätzung der Klientin/des Klienten ____________________________
____
____

Hypothese des Therapeuten/der Therapeutin:____________________________
____
____

Selbstreflexion

Situation: ______________________________

Tragen Sie eine konkrete Situation ein, die Sie belastet.

Wünsche und Bedürfnisse	Eigene Ziele
Machen Sie ein Brainstorming zu Ihren eigenen persönlichen Wünschen und Bedürfnissen, zur obigen Situation.	Formulieren Sie Ziele, um Ihre Wünsche zu erfüllen • • • •

Informationssammlung

Tragen Sie hier ein, welche Quellen Sie nutzen um Informationen über das Thema (s.o) zu bekommen. (Websites, Broschüren, Therapeut)

Quellen	Gelesen

Selbstreflexion

Machen Sie sich Gedanken zur obigen Situation. Wann tritt die Situation ein? Wie fühlen Sie sich dabei? Was denken Sie dabei? Wie reagieren Sie darauf?

Gefühle	Gedanken	Reaktion

Problemlösungsstrategien/Alternative Umgangsweise

Welche Strategien können Sie anwenden, um die Situation zu verbessern.

Nach der Umsetzung der Problemlösungsstrategien, gehen Sie nochmals zur „Selbstreflexion" zurück und schreiben mit anderer Farbe ein, welche Gefühle, Gedanken und Reaktionen Sie jetzt haben und passen Sie die Problemlösungsstrategien gegebenenfalls an.

Wochenplan

	Montag	Dienstag	Mittwoch	Donnerstag	Freitag	Samstag	Sonntag
06:00							
07:00							
08:00							
09:00							
10:00							
11:00							
12:00							
13:00							
14:00							
15:00							
16:00							
17:00							
18:00							
19:00							
20:00							
21:00							
22:00							
23:00							

Mini Mental State Examination (MMSE)

Für jede der 5 zu bewertenden **Funktionen** gibt es eine dreispaltige Tabelle, die jeweils in Zeile 2 eine kurze Anleitung und in den folgenden Zeilen bis zu 10 Einzelfragen enthält. Die Spalte 3 enthält für jede links genannte Funktion die möglichen **Punkte**, die maximal erreichbare Punktzahl ist **30**.

Die beiden ersten Spalten benennen die Frage, die dritte Spalte gibt die mögliche Punktzahl an. Alle Fragen können mit 0 oder mit 1 Punkt bewertet werden, deshalb ist der Inhalt der Spalte immer gleich.

I. Orientierung		**Punkte**
Frage 1-5: Zuerst nach dem Datum fragen, dann gezielt nach den noch fehlenden Punkten (z. B. "Können Sie mir auch sagen, welche Jahreszeit jetzt ist?"). **Frage 6-10:** Zuerst nach dem Namen der Klinik fragen, dann nach Station/Stockwerk, Stadt/Stadtteil usw. fragen. In Großstädten sollte nicht nach Stadt und Landkreis, sondern nach Stadt und Stadtteil gefragt werden. Gefragt wird in jedem Fall nach dem aktuellen Aufenthaltsort und nicht nach dem Wohnort.		
1.	Datum	**1 / 0**
2.	Jahreszeit	**1 / 0**
3.	Jahr	**1 / 0**
4.	Wochentag	**1 / 0**
5.	Monat	**1 / 0**
6.	Bundesland	**1 / 0**
7.	Landkreis/Stadt	**1 / 0**
8.	Stadt/Stadtteil	**1 / 0**
9.	Krankenhaus	**1 / 0**
10.	Station/Stockwerk	**1 / 0**

Die beiden ersten Spalten benennen die Frage, die dritte Spalte gibt die mögliche Punktzahl an. Alle Fragen können mit 0 oder mit 1 Punkt bewertet werden, deshalb ist der Inhalt der Spalte immer gleich.

II. Merkfähigkeit		**Punkte**
Der Untersuchte muss zuerst gefragt werden, ob er mit einem kleinen Gedächtnistest einverstanden ist. Er wird darauf hingewiesen, dass er sich 3 Begriffe merken soll. Die Begriffe langsam und deutlich - im Abstand von jeweils circa 1 Sekunde - nennen. Direkt danach die 3 Begriffe wiederholen lassen, der erste Versuch bestimmt die Punktzahl. Gegebenenfalls wiederholen, bis der Untersuchte alle 3 Begriffe gelernt hat. Die Anzahl der notwendigen Versuche zählen und notieren (maximal 6 Versuche zulässig). Wenn nicht alle 3 Begriffe gelernt wurden, kann der Gedächtnistest nicht durchgeführt werden.		
11.	Apfel	**1 / 0**
12.	Pfennig	**1 / 0**
13.	Tisch	**1 / 0**

Die beiden ersten Spalten benennen die Frage, die dritte Spalte gibt die mögliche Punktzahl an. Alle Fragen bis auf 19 können mit 0 oder mit 1 Punkt bewertet werden, deshalb ist der Inhalt der Spalte immer gleich. Frage 19 ist alternativ zu den Fragen 14 bis 18 und kann mit 0 bis 5 Punkten bewertet werden.

III. Aufmerksamkeit und Rechenfertigkeit		**Punkte**
Beginnend bei 100 muss fünfmal jeweils 7 subtrahiert werden. Jeden einzelnen Rechenschritt unabhängig vom vorangehenden beurteilen, damit ein Fehler nicht mehrfach gewertet wird. Alternativ (z. B. wenn der Untersuchte nicht rechnen kann oder will) kann in Ausnahmefällen das Wort "STUHL" rückwärts buchstabiert werden. Das Wort sollte zunächst vorwärts buchstabiert und wenn nötig korrigiert werden. Die Punktzahl ergibt sich dann aus der Anzahl der Buchstaben, die in der richtigen Reihenfolge genannt werden (z. B. "LHTUS" = 3 Punkte).		
14.	< 93 >	**1 / 0**

15.	< 86 >	**1 / 0**
16.	< 79 >	**1 / 0**
17.	< 72 >	**1 / 0**
18.	< 65 >	**1 / 0**
19.	alternativ: "STUHL" rückwärts buchstabieren LHUTS	**5/4/3/2/1/0**

Die beiden ersten Spalten benennen die Frage, die dritte Spalte gibt die mögliche Punktzahl an. Alle Fragen können mit 0 oder mit 1 Punkt bewertet werden, weshalb der Inhalt der Spalte immer gleich ist.

IV. Erinnerungsfähigkeit		**Punkte**
Der Untersuchte muss die 3 Begriffe nennen, die er sich merken sollte.		
20.	Apfel	**1 / 0**
21.	Pfennig	**1 / 0**
22.	Tisch	**1 / 0**

Die beiden ersten Spalten benennen die Frage, die dritte Spalte gibt die mögliche Punktzahl an. Alle Fragen können mit 0 oder mit 1 Punkt bewertet werden, deshalb ist der Inhalt der Spalte immer gleich.

V. Sprache		**Punkte**
Eine Uhr und ein Stift werden gezeigt, der Untersuchte muss diese richtig benennen.		
23.	Armbanduhr benennen	**1 / 0**
24.	Bleistift benennen	**1 / 0**
25.	Nachsprechen des Satzes "Kein wenn und oder aber." (maximal 3 Wiederholungen) Der Satz muss unmittelbar nachgesprochen werden, nur 1 Versuch ist erlaubt. Es ist nicht zulässig, die Redewendung "Kein wenn und aber." zu benutzen.	**1 / 0**
26.	Kommandos befolgen: Der Untersuchte erhält ein Blatt Papier, der dreistufige Befehl wird nur einmal erteilt. 1 Punkt für jeden Teil, der korrekt befolgt wird.	
	- Nehmen Sie bitte das Papier in die Hand.	**1 / 0**
	- Falten Sie es in der Mitte.	**1 / 0**
	- Lassen Sie es auf den Boden fallen.	**1 / 0**
27.	Schriftliche Anweisungen befolgen "AUGEN ZU": Die Buchstaben ("AUGEN ZU") müssen so groß sein, dass sie auch bei eingeschränktem Visus noch lesbar sind. 1 Punkt wird nur dann gegeben, wenn die Augen wirklich geschlossen sind.	**1 / 0**
28.	Schreiben Sie bitte irgendeinen Satz: Es darf kein Satz diktiert werden, die Ausführung muss spontan erfolgen. Der Satz muss Subjekt und Prädikat enthalten und sinnvoll sein. Korrekte Grammatik und Interpunktion ist nicht gefordert. Das Schreiben von Namen und Anschrift ist nicht ausreichend.	**1 / 0**
29.	Fünfecke nachzeichnen: Auf einem Blatt Papier sind 2 sich überschneidende Fünfecke dargestellt, der Untersuchte soll diese so exakt wie möglich abzeichnen. Alle 10 Ecken müssen wiedergegeben sein und 2 davon sich überschneiden, nur dann wird 1 Punkt gegeben.	**1 / 0**

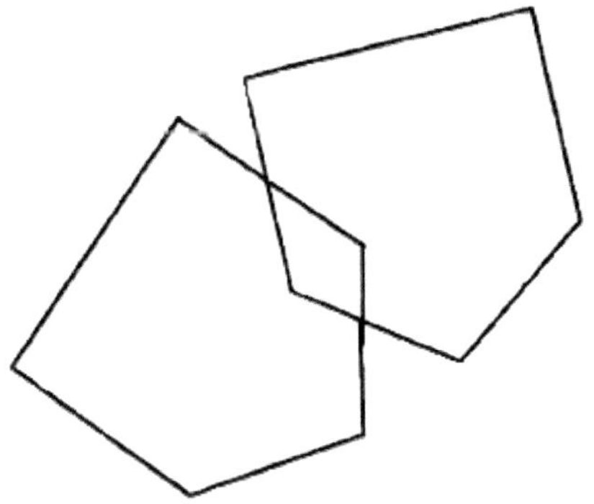

Uhrentest

Bitte zeichnen Sie eine Uhr. Die Zeiger stehen auf

11 Uhr 10 Minuten.

Parkinson-Tagebuch

	Mo.	Di.	Mi.	Do.	Fr.	Sa.	So.
07:00-8:00							
08:00-09:00							
09:00-10:00							
10:00-11:00							
11:00-12:00							
12:00-13:00							
13:00-14:00							
14:00-15:00							
15:00-16:00							
16:00-17:00							
17:00-18:00							
18:00-19:00							
19:00-20:00							
20:00-21:00							
21:00-22:00							
22:00-23:00							

Bitte Eintragen:

Name der eingenommenen Medikamente

U = Unterbeweglich
Ü = Überbeweglich
T = Tremor
St = Stimmung niedergeschlagen
Sch = Schmerzen
K = Konzentration, Gedächtnis eingeschränkt
= (sonstges Symptom)
= (sonstges Symptom)

WHO 5 – Fragebogen zum Wohlbefinden

In den letzten zwei Wochen…	Die ganze Zeit	Meistens	Etwas mehr als die Hälfte der Zeit	Etwas weniger als die Hälfte der Zeit	Ab und zu	Zu keinem Zeitpunkt
… war ich froh und guter Laune	5	4	3	2	1	0
… habe ich mich ruhig und entspannt gefühlt	5	4	3	2	1	0
…habe ich mich energisch und aktiv gefühlt	5	4	3	2	1	0
… habe ich mich beim Aufwachen frisch und ausgeruht gefühlt	5	4	3	2	1	0
… war mein Alltag voller Dinge, die mich interessieren	5	4	3	2	1	0

FSS-Fragebogen

Bitte geben Sie an, welchen Aussagen Sie mehr oder weniger zustimmen. Die Fragen beziehen sich auf die letzte Woche.

	Stimme nicht zu ⟷					Stimme zu
	1	2	3	4	5	6	7
1. Ich bin weniger motiviert, wenn ich müde bin.							
2. Körperliche Bewegung macht mich müde.							
3. Ich ermüde rasch.							
4. Meine Müdigkeit beeinträchtigt meine körperliche Leistungsfähigkeit.							
5. Meine Müdigkeit bereitet mir oft Probleme.							
6. Meine Müdigkeit verhindert länger dauernde körperliche Tätigkeiten.							
7. Meine Müdigkeit beeinträchtigt mich, gewisse Pflichten und Verantwortungen zu erfüllen.							
8. Meine Müdigkeit gehört zu den drei Beschwerden, die mich am meisten behindern.							
9. Meine Müdigkeit beeinträchtigt meine Arbeit, meine Familie oder mein soziales Leben							

FSS- Fatigue-Sevirity-Scale; Kleinman et al. 1989

Schreibtraining

Prinzipien des Schreibtrainings bei Parkinson

1. Größe trainieren, nicht Schnelligkeit
2. Nach jeder Übung–Pause
3. Keine Ablenkung
4. Täglich drei Mal Wiederholen (hohe Repetition)

1. Hand-Arm Transport

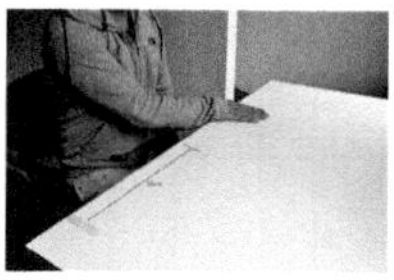

20 Mal

2. Handgelenk

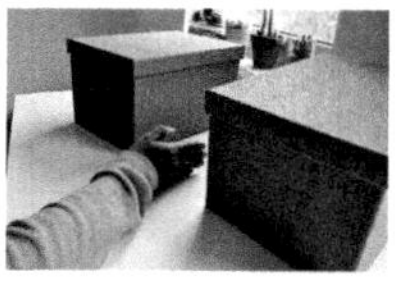

20 Mal

3. Finger vor-zurück

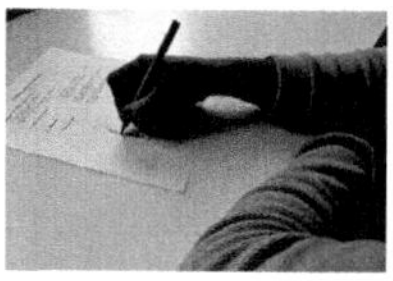

20 Mal

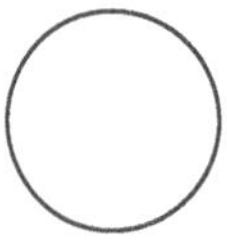

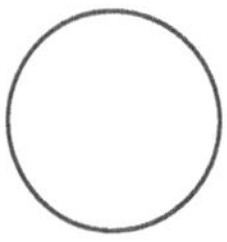

4. zwei Zeilen ℓℓℓ

Schreiben Sie mit Bleistift vier zusammenhängende ℓℓℓ, absetzen; wiederholen.

5. Satz Übung

Schreiben Sie mit einem Bleistift einen Satz, den Sie häufig verwenden (mit 4-8 Wörtern) z.B. „mit freundlichen Grüßen *Name*" Linien oben und unten berühren.

6. Satz Alltag

Schreiben Sie mit Ihrem Alltagsstift einen Satz, den Sie häufig verwenden (mit 4-8 Wörtern) z.B. „mit freundlichen Grüßen *Name*" Linien oben und unten berühren.

Stichwortverzeichnis

A. Orellana, *Betätigungsorientierte Ergotherapie bei Morbus Parkinson*,
https://doi.org/10.1007/978-3-662-62583-5

GPSR Compliance

The European Union's (EU) General Product Safety Regulation (GPSR) is a set of rules that requires consumer products to be safe and our obligations to ensure this.

If you have any concerns about our products, you can contact us on ProductSafety@springernature.com

In case Publisher is established outside the EU, the EU authorized representative is:

Springer Nature Customer Service Center GmbH
Europaplatz 3
69115 Heidelberg, Germany

Batch number: 10732823

Printed by Printforce, the Netherlands